AFB DIRECTORY OF SERVICES FOR BLIND AND VISUALLY IMPAIRED PERSONS IN THE UNITED STATES AND CANADA

AFB PRESS

New York

Directory of Services for Blind and Visually Impaired Persons in the United States and Canada, 25th edition is © 1997 by
American Foundation for the Blind
11 Penn Plaza, Suite 300, New York, NY 10001

Printed in the United States of America

ISBN 0-89128-301-3
ISSN 1067-5833

CD-ROM: ISBN 0-89128-243-2
CD-ROM with Print Edition: ISBN 0-89128-300-5

TABLE OF CONTENTS

Foreword *Carl R. Augusto* v

**How to Use This Directory
and Find Services**.........................A1

**A Brief Overview of Major
Federal Programs**.......................A5

Subject Index..............................B1

PART ONE—United States/State Listings

Alabama......................................3
Alaska 13
Arizona 16
Arkansas 25
California 31
Colorado 58
Connecticut 65
Delaware...................................70
District of Columbia 73
Florida......................................78
Georgia.....................................97
Guam......................................108
Hawaii.....................................109
Idaho.......................................113
Illinois.....................................117
Indiana....................................135
Iowa..144
Kansas.....................................148
Kentucky..................................155
Louisiana 161
Maine 167
Maryland.................................170

Massachusetts 178
Michigan..................................192
Minnesota................................206
Mississippi...............................213
Missouri...................................219
Montana...................................228
Nebraska..................................232
Nevada.....................................237
New Hampshire 240
New Jersey................................244
New Mexico.............................251
New York.................................255
North Carolina.........................286
North Dakota 294
Ohio...298
Oklahoma 313
Oregon 318
Pennsylvania............................325
Puerto Rico...............................351
Rhode Island 354
South Carolina 357
South Dakota 362
Tennessee.................................367
Texas 376
Utah...391
Vermont...................................396
Virginia 399
Virgin Islands...........................407
Washington 409
West Virginia............................417
Wisconsin.................................424
Wyoming 433

PART TWO—Canada/Provincial Listings

Alberta 437

British Columbia 439

Manitoba...442

New Brunswick 444

Newfoundland 446

Northwest Territories 447

Nova Scotia 448

Ontario..451

Prince Edward Island 456

Quebec 457

Saskatchewan.................................460

Yukon Territory..............................462

PART THREE—United States

Federal Agencies 465

National Organizations 472

National Consumer and Professional
Membership Organizations 487

PART FOUR—Canada

Federal Agencies 497

National Organizations. 499

National Consumer and Professional
Membership Organizations 501

PART FIVE—United States

Producers and Publishers of Braille
and Other Alternate Media...........507

Sources of Adapted Products
and Devices 519

PART SIX—Canada

Producers and Publishers of Braille
and Other Alternate Media...........539

Sources of Adapted Products
and Devices 543

Organization Index 545

FOREWORD

The American Foundation for the Blind (AFB) first published a directory of services in 1926. Since that time our *Directory of Services for Blind and Visually Impaired Persons in the United States and Canada* has become the most important reference and referral resource in the field of blindness and visual impairment. Although the contents and format of the *Directory* have changed over the years to reflect the nature and extent of the services available to blind and visually impaired persons at the time of publication, the purpose of the *Directory* has always been the same: to provide useful, comprehensive information that facilitates the delivery of services to persons who are blind or visually impaired.

This 25th edition of the *Directory* has the same purpose as previous editions and, in that sense, is no different from its predecessors. However, it differs dramatically from previous editions in that it is the first edition to appear in both print and electronic forms. Accompanying this printed book is a CD-ROM containing the same information, designed to be accessible with adaptive equipment, thus making the contents of the *Directory* available simultaneously to users who can read print and to users who cannot. In providing access to information to sighted and visually impaired readers alike, this *Directory* stands as a mark of AFB's continuing efforts to improve information and service delivery to blind and visually impaired persons and those who live and work with them.

Readers will find that the *Directory* continues to be organized for ease of use and still contains a remarkably wide range of services divided into clear categories that can be readily understood. Subject and organization indexes are also included as quick reference tools that help users find what they are looking for rapidly.

A reference work as comprehensive as this *Directory* requires the participation of many individuals and AFB staff in several departments. There are many to acknowledge and thank. AFB Press, the publishing arm of AFB, plays the central role in organizing and producing the *Directory of Services*. Barry Katzen, director, Natalie Hilzen, editor in chief, Stephanie Biagioli, marketing assistant, and Carol Wallace, executive secretary, deserve special credit, as do Irene DePonti, Beatrice Jacinto, John Lucas, and Albert Scé, who worked with the publications staff on gathering and checking the *Directory*'s data. Computer databases the AFB National Technology Center (NTC) maintains for other purposes were useful sources of information for the *Directory*, and Mark Uslan, manager of technical evaluation services, helped to make this information available. Other professional staff at AFB, including the staff of AFB's offices in Atlanta, Chicago, Dallas, San Francisco, and Washington, DC, play many roles in *Directory* development. They identify candidates for new listings, track down information that is difficult to obtain, and review listings for the states in their regions. Grace Daly, Frances Mary D'Andrea, Barbara Gallman, Sara Hayes, Elga Joffee, Gil Johnson, Linda Laubach, Barbara LeMoine, Alberta Orr, Frank Ryan, Paul Schroeder, Marlo Scoggins, Judy Scott, Mary Ann Siller, Susan Spungin, Karon Walker, and Penny Zibula provided help and valuable suggestions. Alan Dinsmore, AFB senior governmental relations representative, reviewed the United States federal listings and compiled the legislative overview.

A number of people outside AFB also provided important information on services. For this assistance, we thank Suzanne

Dalton, Yvonne Howze, Gale Malcolm, Linda Mamer, Ray Melhoff, Herb Miller, Linda Redmond, Carmen Tumac, and Todd Turansky.

Finally, we wish to thank all the organizations and individuals who supplied us with the information about programs included here. This book is based on the facts and descriptions they provide. Without them, there would be no *Directory*.

Carl R. Augusto
President
American Foundation for the Blind

HOW TO USE THIS DIRECTORY AND FIND SERVICES

The American Foundation for the Blind (AFB)'s *Directory of Services for Blind and Visually Impaired Persons in the United States and Canada* is a broad-based compilation of schools, agencies, organizations, and programs in the governmental and private, non-profit sectors that provide a wide variety of direct and indirect services, information, and other assistance to blind and visually impaired children and adults, their families, and professionals who work with them. Organized information on producers and distributors of alternate media, adapted devices, and other products useful to individuals who are blind or visually impaired are also included. A listing in the *Directory*, which is based on information supplied by the listee, does not imply endorsement or evaluation by AFB.

Evaluative information about an organization may sometimes be obtained by consulting local and state medical societies; health and welfare councils; Better Business Bureaus; the National Charities Information Bureau; university, school, medical, and rehabilitation accrediting bodies; or the National Accreditation Council for Agencies Serving the Blind and Visually Handicapped (NAC). A list of agencies and schools accredited by NAC at the time the *Directory* went to press appears at the end of this section.

Sections of the Directory

The *Directory* has separate sections for U.S. and Canadian services. Agencies and organizations have been listed according to whether they provide services to a local area, state, or province or on a national basis. The *Directory* has the following main sections:

1. "A Brief Overview of Major Federal Programs," a concise description of U.S. and Canadian legislative initiatives.

2. A comprehensive subject index that divides all entries into subject categories and lists them alphabetically within categories. One section of this index lists entries for the United States; another section lists entries for Canada.

3. Geographical listings arranged state by state (including U.S. territories) for the United States in one section, and province by province (including territories) for Canada in a separate section. Agencies in these listings generally provide services with-in their local area or state. In addition, state and provincial listings in this *Directory* contain cross-references to federal agencies and national organizations and the addresses and telephone numbers of local, state, and regional offices of national organizations.

4. Federal agency listings and listings of agencies and organizations that provide services and information nationally. Federal agencies, national organizations, and national consumer and professional membership organizations appear in one section for the United States and in a separate section for Canada.

5. Suppliers of braille, tape, large-print, and disk formats and manufacturers and distributors of adapted products and devices for people who are blind or visually impaired that provide services on a national basis. Listings for these organizations and companies appear in one section for the United States and in a separate section for Canada.

6. An alphabetical organization index containing all entries and separating them by alphabetical letter. One section of this index

lists entries for the United States; another section lists entries for Canada.

This *Directory* has been designed to help readers find information quickly and easily. It therefore contains two separate indexes and a number of sections separated into easy-to-locate categories. There are essentially three ways to locate an organization or service:

1. *By alphabetical order.* Consult the Organization Index at the back of the book. This index contains all entries listed alphabetically.

2. *By service category.* Consult the Subject Index at the front of the book. This index contains all entries divided into categories of services.

3. *By geographical location.* Consult the State or Provincial Listings for local, state, and regional services, or the sections listing national organizations for services delivered on a national basis. (However, when trying to locate services, keep in mind that some local agencies and organizations—for example, producers of braille and other media—may provide services beyond their local area.)

State and Provincial Listings

State and Provincial Listings are divided as follows (unless otherwise noted, all listings are in alphabetical order):

Educational Services: state or provincial services; programs for early intervention coordination; schools; infant and preschool programs; statewide outreach services; instructional materials centers; and university training programs.

Information Services: libraries; talking book machine distributors; media production services; radio reading; phone-in newspapers; and sources of information and referrals. Cross-references to national listings (that is, to agencies, organizations, or companies that are geographically located in a given state or province but that provide national services) appear at the end of Information Services. Many local, state, and regional offices of national organizations appear alphabetically in State or Provincial Listings under the category of Information and Referral.

Rehabilitation Services: state or provincial services (including cities, addresses, and telephone numbers of the local offices of state or provincial agencies); local private rehabilitation agencies; computer training centers; and dog guide schools.

Low Vision Services: state or provincial ophthalmological and optometric societies (appearing in that order); low vision clinics and centers.

Aging Services: For the United States, state units on aging; independent living programs funded by Title VII, Part C of the Rehabilitation Act of 1973.

Abbreviations

In the interests of space, a number of abbreviations are used in listings. Although some agencies have used abbreviations for services that are unique to their programs, many of the abbreviations are commonly known. The following abbreviations appear:

ADA (Americans with Disabilities Act)

ADL (activities of daily living)

AER (Association for Education and Rehabilitation of the Blind and Visually Impaired)

CMV (cytomegalovirus)

CCTV (closed-circuit television)

Est. (established)

HIV/AIDS (human immunodeficiency virus/acquired immune deficiency syndrome)

GED (general equivalency diploma)

IDEA (Individuals with Disabilities Education Act)

IEP (Individualized Education Program)

IFSP (Individualized Family Service Plan)

Inc. (incorporated)

K (kindergarten)

LEA (local education agency)

OCR (optical character recognition)

TDD (telecommunication device for deaf and hearing impaired persons)

TTY (teletype for deaf and hearing impaired persons)

URL (universal resource locator)

Y (yes)

No directory is ever completely up to date or perfect. As this book went to press, U.S. federal legislation was being reauthorized in Congress, and funding and service patterns in many sectors were undergoing change. In addition, many areas in the United States, such as California, were undergoing and will continue to experience extensive area code changes. Some of the information listed in this book will change as a result.

Readers should also keep in mind that many organizations such as state ophthalmological societies and membership organizations change their addresses and phone numbers annually, as their presidents or heads change. In such cases, attempts to find the service can be made through following forwarding at the previous listing; contacting the national organization, if any, affiliated with the local branch; or checking with local directory assistance.

Because of the constantly shifting nature of the data gathered for this *Directory*, AFB welcomes suggestions for corrections, deletions, and new listings. Such information should be sent in writing only to AFB Press, American Foundation for the Blind, 11 Penn Plaza, Suite 300, New York, NY 10001.

Members, National Accreditation Council for Agencies Serving the Blind and Visually Handicapped

The date accompanying each name for the organizations in the following listing represents the year through which accreditation has been awarded.

Alabama
Services for Blind and Visually Handicapped Children and Adults of the Alabama Institute for Deaf and Blind (1998)

Arizona
Foundation for Blind Children (1998)
Tucson Association for the Blind and Visually Impaired (1997)

Arkansas
Lions World Services for the Blind (1999)

California
Center for the Partially Sighted (1998)
Society for the Blind (1998)

Florida
Center for the Visually Impaired (1998)
Conklin Center for Multihandicapped Blind (1997)
Division of Blind Services (1999)
Florida Association of Workers for the Blind (Miami Lighthouse) (1998)
Florida School for the Deaf and Blind (1998)
Fort Lauderdale Lighthouse for the Blind (1999)
Independence for the Blind (2001)
Lighthouse for the Blind of Pasco and Hernando (2000)
Mana-Sota Lighthouse for the Blind (1997)
Pinellas Center for the Visually Impaired (1999)
Tampa Lighthouse for the Blind (1997)
Visually Impaired Persons of Southwest Florida (1998)

Georgia
Blind and Low Vision Services of North Georgia (2001)
Center for the Visually Impaired (1997)
Georgia Academy for the Blind (1998)
Savannah Association for the Blind (1999)

Hawaii
Ho'opono Services for the Blind Hawaii Department of Human Services (1997)

Illinois
Chicago Lighthouse for People Who Are Blind or Visually Impaired (2001)
Deicke Center for Visual Rehabilitation (2001)
Philip J. Rock Center and School (1999)

Indiana
Indiana School for the Blind (2000)

Iowa
Genesis Vision Rehabilitation Institute (2000)

Kansas
Wichita Industries and Services for the Blind (2000)

Maine
Maine Center for the Blind and Visually Impaired (1997)

Maryland
Maryland School for the Blind (1997)

Michigan
Association for the Blind and Visually Impaired (1999)
Upshaw Institute for the Blind (2001)
Visually Impaired Center (1998)

Minnesota
Duluth Lighthouse for the Blind (1998)

Missouri
Alphapointe Association for the Blind (1997)

New Hampshire
New Hampshire Association for the Blind (1999)

New York
Association for the Visually Impaired (2000)
Blind Association of Western New York (1997)
Catholic Guild for the Blind (1997)
Programs for the Visually Impaired/New York Institute for Special Education (1999)

North Dakota
North Dakota School for the Blind (1997)

Ohio
Cincinnati Association for the Blind (2000)
The Clovernook Center/Opportunities for the Blind (2001)

The Greater Akron Low Vision Clinic (1997)

The Toledo Society for the Blind (1998)

Vision Center of Central Ohio (1999)

Oklahoma

Parkview School (2001)

Visual Services Division (1998)

Pennsylvania

Greater Pittsburgh Guild for the Blind (1998) (now known as Pittsburgh Vision Services)

Pittsburgh Blind Association (1997) (now known as Pittsburgh Vision Services)

Susquehanna Association for the Blind and Vision Impaired (1997)

South Dakota

South Dakota School for the Visually Handicapped (1999)

Tennessee

Alliance for the Blind and Visually Impaired (1999)

Ed Lindsey Industries for the Blind (1997)

Lions Volunteer Blind Industries (1998)

Texas

Dallas Lighthouse for the Blind (1999)

Utah

Utah School for the Blind (2001)

Washington

Lighthouse for the Blind, Seattle (1997)

Canada

Centre for Sight Enhancement/University of Waterloo (1999)

A BRIEF OVERVIEW OF MAJOR FEDERAL PROGRAMS

Both the United States and Canada have undertaken important federal initiatives in regard to persons who are blind or visually impaired or who have other disabilities. On July 26, 1990, President George Bush signed the Americans with Disabilities Act (ADA), a landmark piece of legislation, into law in the United States. On September 6, 1991, Prime Minister Brian Mulroney announced the National Strategy for the Integration of Persons with Disabilities, a major five-year effort involving all levels of government and business, labor, community, and other groups in bringing persons with disabilities into the mainstream of society.

Key U.S. Legislation

The basic principles of disability policy in the United States are contained in the ADA (P.L. 101-336), the Rehabilitation Act of 1973, as amended, and the Individuals with Disabilities Education Act (IDEA) (P.L. 94-142, as amended). Policies and programs authorized by these laws do not provide a seamless transition through education, employment, health care, and civil rights for people with disabilities. However, each one of these laws

does provide important basic rights in each of those areas, and, when viewed in combination with the Social Security Act's disability insurance program, the Supplemental Security Income program, and Medicare and Medicaid programs, the laws provide the basis for integration of people who are blind or visually impaired into the mainstream of this country's social, political, and economic life.

The ADA is the most far-reaching civil rights legislation ever enacted in the history of disability policy in the United States. Prior to its enactment, federal nondiscrimination policy regarding persons with disabilities related only to programs receiving federal funds or employment by federal agencies. The ADA extends those policies to almost every segment of society. Discrimination against people with disabilities is prohibited in employment (Title I), state and local government services (Title II), transportation (Title II), public accommodations (Title III), and telecommunications services (Title IV). The ADA Accessibility Guidelines (ADAAG) were written by the Architectural and Transportation Barrier's Compliance Board (Access Board).

The ADA was intended to pro-

vide a clear national mandate for the elimination of discrimination against people with disabilities and to address the major areas of discrimination faced day to day by disabled individuals. What does it mean to people who are blind or visually impaired? It can mean that they have the same fair chance for consideration for employment that anyone else has, provided that they can perform the essential functions of the job, with or without a reasonable accommodation, and the employer is among those covered by the act. It also means that they should have the same fair chance to be considered for promotion and training by the employer once they are employed. It means that state and local government agencies cannot exclude them from participating in government services, programs, or other activities. And it means that the operator of a public transit system has the obligation to provide schedules and information in an accessible format for them. In a place of public accommodation like a motel, restaurant, movie theater, or doctor's office, policies must provide for a means of effective communication with the customer or recipient of services who is disabled.

The ADA provides a much more comprehensive list of circumstances and areas covered than those mentioned in this brief overview, and this *Directory* lists the governmental units that can provide additional information and are responsible for regulating and enforcing the ADA (see U.S. Federal Agencies listings and the table accompanying this discussion).

The authority for training and finding employment for people with mental, physical, and sensory disabilities is provided by the Rehabilitation Act of 1973. Training and employment services are provided through a federal-state partnership. Services for people who are blind or visually impaired are provided in many states through a separate state vocational rehabilitation agency for blind persons. In addition, the act, as amended in 1992, provides for independent living services for older blind persons, electronic equipment accessibility, employment with the federal government, and operation and funding of the Helen Keller National Center for Deaf-Blind Youths and Adults.

IDEA, a central piece of legislation relating to the education of persons with disabilities, was intended to ensure that all children with disabilities have available to them a free appropriate public education. The major components of IDEA are basic state formula grants to cover excess costs of special education and related services to children with disabilities; preschool state grants that are separate allotments to states to encourage services to preschool children with disabilities; and early intervention state grants to provide services for infants and toddlers and their families. IDEA provides for

discretionary grant programs like services to deaf-blind children and youths, technology development, personnel preparation, and descriptive video and captioning. It also provides authority for funding programs of financial assistance to state agencies for programs to meet the special education needs of children with disabilities in state-operated or state-supported schools in this country.

Other Legislation

A wide variety of additional legislation provides for significant rights and programs for persons who are blind or visually impaired.

The Fair Housing Act of 1988 prohibits discrimination in the sale or rental of private dwellings. The act does not cover discrimination in public housing. Title II of the ADA covers dwellings owned by state or local governments. The disability provisions of the Fair Housing Act do not supersede state laws or local ordinances that afford individuals with disabilities greater protection against housing discrimination. In addition to the Fair Housing Act, the Social Security Act contains provisions of great import to individuals with disabilities. As amended, the Act authorizes the Supplemental Security Income and the Social Security Disability Insurance programs.

Access to telecommunications equipment and services, an issue of increasing consequence in today's information age, is dealt with in the Telecommunications Act of 1996, which amends the Communications Act of 1934. The act provides that manufacturers of telecommunications equipment or customer premises equipment and telecommunications service

providers ensure that the equipment is accessible to and usable by people with disabilities, if readily achievable.

Library services, vital resources related to literacy, are covered by the Pratt-Smoot Act, which provides for books for children and adults who are blind or visually impaired. Services are provided through the National Library Service for the Blind and Physically Handicapped. P.L. 89-522 extended the availability of these services to individuals with disabilities who, because of their disability, are unable to handle standard printed material.

In the area of copyright, P.L. 104-97 allows authorized entities to reproduce or distribute copies or phono records of previously published nondramatic or literary works in specialized formats exclusively for use by blind or other persons with disabilities. Mailing privileges are another important right that has been extended, specifically through the Postal Reorganization Act of 1970, which provides for free mailing matter for blind and other disabled persons.

Transportation, a vital activity that is part of daily life, is covered in part by the Air Carrier Access Act (P.L. 99-435), which prohibits discrimination against any otherwise qualified disabled individual in the provision of air transportation. In addition, the Federal Transit Act establishes a formula assistance program that makes federal resources available to urban and rural areas. Urban area assistance may be for mass transit planning, capital, and operating assistance. The federal share may also be used for projects devoted to enhancing the accessibility and mobility of elderly individuals and people with disabilities.

The Vending Facility Program for Persons Who Are Blind was instituted by the Randolph-Sheppard Act (P.L. 74-732, as amended). This act provides persons who are blind with remunerative employment and self-support through the operation of vending facilities on federal and other property. Amendments to the act assured persons who are blind a "priority" in the operation of vending facilities.

Canadian Programs

The National Strategy for the Integration of Persons with Disabilities was announced in 1991. The goals of this five-year national initiative were equal access, economic integration, and effective participation intended to bring persons with disabilities into the social and economic mainstream of Canadian life. The strategy involved ten federal departments and agencies working together on a wide range of activities with disabled persons, other levels of government, and the private and nongovernmental sectors to resolve such issues as access to employment, training, housing, communications, transportation, public sensitivity, and community integration.

Other important initiatives in Canada were the enactment of the Canadian Human Rights Act, which prohibits discrimination, the inclusion of persons with a physical or mental disability in the wording of the Canadian Charter of Rights and Freedoms in 1982 to afford such persons the equal protection and benefit of the law, and the passage into law in 1992 of the Omnibus Bill to guarantee a large number of specific rights. Key legislation also includes the Employment Equity Act, passed in 1986, the Canada Assistance Plan of 1966, the Federal-Provincial Fiscal Arrangements and Established Programs Financing Act of 1977, and the National Training Act of 1982.

In addition to the federal agencies and programs in the Canadian Federal Agencies listings, the following information relates to federal structures in Canada.

Office for Disability Issues Human Resources Development Canada

The Office for Disability Issues is responsible for coordinating the government's overall strategy regarding persons with disabilities as well as carrying out activities specific to its mandate.
For further information: (819) 997-2412 (voice and TDD)

Canada Mortgage and Housing Corporation

The Canada Mortgage and Housing Corporation addresses the housing requirements of persons with disabilities.
For further information: (613) 748-2000

National Library of Canada

The National Library of Canada has developed and implemented technology and services that improve communications for persons with disabilities.
For further information: (613) 995-3904

Health Canada

Health Canada assists in the integration of persons with disabilities through its health programs, and with provinces and territories in their provision of health and social programs.
For further information: (613) 957-2991

Justice Canada

Justice Canada reviews federal legislation that affects persons with disabilities to identify existing legislative barriers to the full social and economic integration of disabled persons.
For further information: (613) 952-4222 or TDD (613) 992-4556

Transport Canada

Transport Canada improves access to transportation by providing financial incentives to industry to encourage the use of equipment and devices that would enhance accessibility.
For further information: (613) 991-6407

Canadian Transportation Agency

The Canadian Transportation Agency introduces regulations required to address the transportation needs of persons with disabilities.
For further information: (819) 953-2749

Treasury Board of Canada

The Treasury Board of Canada seeks to achieve equal employment and advancement opportunities for persons with disabilities.
For further information: (613) 952-2870

Canadian Human Rights Commission

The Canadian Human Rights Commission seeks to safeguard the rights of persons with disabilities and to monitor prohibitions against discrimination on the basis of disability.
For further information: (613) 995-1151 or TTY (613) 996-5211

Technical Assistance for Laws Affecting Individuals with Disabilities

Agency	Type of Assistance	Telephone	TDD
Americans with Disabilities Act: Title I Employment			
Equal Employment Opportunity Commission	ADA documents	(800) 669-3362	(800) 800- 3302
	ADA questions	(800) 669-4000	
National Institute on Disability and Rehabilitation Research	Disability and Business Technical Assistance Centers	(800) 949-4232	(800) 522-4369
President's Committee on Employment of People with Disabilities	Job Accommodation Network	(800) 526-7234	(800) 526-7234
	ADA Work Line	(800) 232-9675	
National Council on Disability	Technical Assistance	(202) 272-2004	(202) 272-2074
Americans with Disabilities Act: Title II State and Local Governments; Title III Public Accommodations			
Department of Justice	ADA documents; technical assistance	(800) 514-0301 (202) 514-0301	(800) 514-0383 (202) 514-0383
Department of Transportation	ADA documents; general questions	(202) 366-1656	
	Legal questions	(202) 366-1936	
	Complaints and enforcement	(202) 366-2285	(202) 366-0153
	Public transportation in general	(800) 527-8279	
National Institute on Disability and Rehabilitation Research	Disability and Business Technical Assistance Centers	(800) 949-4232	
National Council on Disability	Technical assistance	(202) 272-2004	(202) 272-2074
Americans with Disabilities Act: ADA Accessibility Guidelines (ADAAG)			
Architectural and Transportation Barriers Compliance Board	ADA documents and questions	(800) 872-2253 (202) 272-5434	(202) 272-5449
Americans with Disabilities Act: Title IV Telecommunications			
Federal Communications Commission	ADA documents; general questions	(202) 418-0200	(202) 418-2555
	Complaints and enforcement	(202) 632-7553	(202) 418-0484
Other Federal Laws			
Internal Revenue Tax Code: Internal Revenue Service	Information	(800) 829-1040	
	To order publication 907, *Tax Highlights for Persons with Disabilities*	(800) 829-3676 (202) 622-3110	(800) 829-4059
Fair Housing Act Amendments: Department of Housing and Urban Development	Technical assistance concerning accessibility standards that apply to privately owned residential facilities	(800) 795-7915	(800) 927-9275
Air Carrier Access Act: Department of Transportation	Technical assistance concerning air transportation accessibility standards	(202) 366-4859 (202) 366-9306	(202) 755-7687
	Complaints and enforcement	(202) 366-2220	(202) 755-7687
Hearing Aid Compatibility Act: Federal Communications Commission	Technical assistance concerning telephone accessibility standards	(202) 634-1808	(202) 632-0484
Telecommunications Act of 1996: Federal Communications Commission	Information	(202) 857-3800	
Free Matter for the Blind and Physically Handicapped Program: U.S. Postal Service Customer Response	Information	(202) 268-2284 (202) 268-6575	
Rehabilitation Act (Section 503): Department of Labor, Office of Federal Contract Compliance Programs	Information on antidiscrimination protection for qualified individuals with disabilities by federal contractors	(202) 219-9475	
Rehabilitation Act: National Association of Protection and Advocacy Systems	Information on the Client Assistance Program	(202) 408-9514	(202) 408-9521

SUBJECT
INDEX

UNITED STATES

◆ *Educational Services*

STATE SERVICES

Alabama State Department of Education (AL) 3

Alaska Department of Education (AK) 13

Arkansas Department of Education/Special Education
Department (AR) 25

Bureau of Instructional Support and Community
Services/Florida Department of Education (FL) 78

California Department of Education/Special Education
Division (CA) 31

Colorado Department of Education/Special Education
Services Unit (CO) 58

Connecticut State Board of Education and Services for
the Blind (CT) 65

Delaware Department of Public Instruction (DE) 70

District of Columbia Special Education Branch (DC) 73

Division for the Blind and Visually Impaired/Maine
Department of Human Services (ME) 167

Division of Special Education/Minnesota Department
of Children, Families and Learning (MN) 206

Exceptional Student Services/Arizona Department of
Education (AZ) 16

Georgia State Department of Education/Division of
Exceptional Students (GA) 97

Guam Department of Education (GU) 108

Hawaii Department of Education/Hawaii Center for
the Deaf and the Blind (HI) 109

Idaho State Department of Education (ID) 113

Illinois State Board of Education (IL) 117

Indiana Department of Education/Division of Special
Education (IN) 135

Iowa Department of Education (IA) 144

Kansas State Department of Education/Student
Support Services (KS) 148

Kentucky Department of Education/Division of
Exceptional Children Services (KY) 155

Louisiana Learning Resources System/Louisiana State
Department of Education (LA) 161

Maryland State Department of Education (MD) 170

Massachusetts Department of Education/Educational
Improvement Group (MA) 178

Michigan Department of Education/Special Education
Services (MI) 192

Mississippi Department of Education (MS) 213

Missouri Department of Elementary and Secondary
Education (MO) 219

Montana Department of Curriculum/Division of
Special Education (MT) 228

Nebraska Department of Education (NE) 232

Nevada Department of Education (NV) 237

New Hampshire Department of Education (NH) 240

New Mexico State Department of Education/Special
Education Office (NM) 251

New York State Education Department/Office for
Special Education Services (NY) 255

North Carolina Department of Public Instruction/
Exceptional Children Division (NC) 286

North Dakota Department of Public Instruction (ND) 294

Office of Programs for Exceptional Children/South
Carolina Department of Education (SC) 357

Office of Special Education/South Dakota Division of
Education and Resources (SD) 362

Office of Special Education Programs/New Jersey
Department of Education (NJ) 244

Ohio Department of Education/Division of Special
Education (OH) 298

Oklahoma State Department of Education/Special
Education Services (OK) 313

Oregon Department of Education (OR) 318

Pennsylvania Department of Education/Bureau of
Special Education (PA) 325

Puerto Rico Department of Education/Special
Education Program (PR) 351

Rhode Island Department of Education (RI) 354

Services for the Visually Impaired/Wyoming
Department of Education (WY) 433

Special Education Unit/Vermont Department of
Education (VT) 396

Tennessee Department of Education (TN) 367

Texas Education Agency (TX) 376

Utah State Office of Education/Special Education
Section (UT) 391

Virginia Department for the Visually Handicapped/
Program for Infants, Children, and Youth (VA) 399

Virgin Islands Department of Education/State Office of
Special Education (VI) 407

Washington Office of Superintendent of Public
Instruction/Special Education (WA) 409

West Virginia Department of Education (WV) 417

Wisconsin Department of Public Instruction/
Exceptional Education Team (WI) 424

EARLY INTERVENTION COORDINATION

Alabama's Early Intervention System/Alabama
Department of Rehabilitation Services (AL) 3

Baby Net/South Carolina Department of Health and
Environmental Control (SC) 357

Baltimore Infants and Toddlers Program (MD) 170

Birth to Three Early Intervention/Division of
Supportive Living/Wisconsin Department of Health
and Family Services (WI) 424

Birth to Three Early Intervention Program/
Washington Department of Social and Health
Services (WA) 409

Bureau of Developmental Disabilities/Idaho
Department of Health and Welfare (ID) 113

Bureau of Early Childhood Education and Social
Services/Connecticut Department of Education (CT) 65

Bureau of Special Education/Iowa State Department of
Education (IA) 144

California Early Intervention Technical Assistance
Network (CA) 31

Children's Medical Services (FL) 78

Developmental Disabilities Division/New Mexico
Department of Health (NM) 251

Developmental Disabilities Division/North Dakota
Department of Human Services (ND) 294

Developmental Disabilities Program/Department of
Public Health and Human Services (MT) 228

Developmental Disabilities Section/Division of Mental
Health, Mental Retardation and Substance Abuse
Services/North Carolina Department of Human
Services (NC) 286

Developmental Disabilities Services/Arkansas
Department of Human Services (AR) 25

Division of Community Program Development/Office
of Mental Retardation/Pennsylvania Department of
Public Welfare (PA) 325

Division of Developmental Disabilities/Wyoming
Department of Health (WY) 433

Division of Family Health/Rhode Island Department
of Health (RI) 354

Division of Health/Wisconsin Department of Health
and Family Services (WI) 424

Division of Management Services/Delaware Health
and Social Services Birth to Three (DE) 70

Division of Maternal and Child Health Care and
Crippled Children Services/Virgin Islands
Department of Health/Knud Hansen Complex (VI) 407

Early Childhood Division/Illinois State Board of
Education (IL) 117

Early Childhood Education/Michigan Department of
Education (MI) 192

Early Childhood Initiatives Unit/Colorado
Department of Education (CO) 58

Early Childhood Program/Texas Department of
Health (TX) 376

Early Childhood Services/Division of Child and
Family Services/Nevada Department of Human
Resources (NV) 237

Early Intervention and Early Childhood Special
Education Programs/Oregon Department of
Education (OR) 318

Early Intervention Program/Alaska Department of
Health and Social Services (AK) 13

Early Intervention Program/California Department of
Developmental Services (CA) 31

Early Intervention Program/District of Columbia
Department of Human Services (DC) 73

Early Intervention Program/Division of Family
Services/Utah Department of Health (UT) 391

Early Intervention Program/New York Department of
Health (NY) 255

Early Intervention Programs/Division of Public
Health/Georgia Department of Human
Resources (GA) 97

Early Intervention Services/Massachusetts
Department of Public Health (MA) 178

First Steps/Family and Social Services
Administration (IN) 135

Governor's Interagency Coordinating Council on
Infants and Toddlers/Arizona Department of
Economic Security (AZ) 16

Guam Department of Education/Division of Special
Education (GU) 108

Infant and Toddler Program/Mississippi Department
of Health (MS) 213

Infant and Toddler Program/Virginia Department of
Mental Health, Mental Retardation and Substance
Abuse Services (VA) 399

Infants and Toddlers with Handicaps/Puerto Rico
Department of Health (PR) 351

Infant-Toddler Program/Kentucky Department of
Mental Health and Mental Retardation Services (KY) ... 155

Interagency Coordinating Council for Early Childhood
Intervention/Oklahoma Commission on Children
and Youth (OK) 313

Interagency Early Intervention Planning Project/
Minnesota Department of Children, Families and
Learning (MN) 206

Interdepartmental Coordinating Council on Early
Intervention/Child Development Services (ME) 167

Kansas Department of Health and Environment (KS) 148

New Hampshire's Early Support and Services/
Division of Mental Health and Developmental
Services/New Hampshire Department of Health and
Human Services (NH) 240

Office for Special Education/Tennessee Department of
Education (TN) 367

Office of Early Intervention and School Readiness/
Florida Division of Public Schools/Department of
Education (FL) 78

Office of Maternal and Child Health/Children with
Special Health Care Needs Program/West Virginia
Department of Health and Human Resources (WV) 417

Office of Special Education/South Dakota Division of
Education and Resources (SD) 362

Office of Special Education Programs/New Jersey
Department of Education (NJ) 244

Office of Special Education Services (LA) 161

Ohio Department of Health/Bureau of Early
    Intervention Services (OH) 298

Oklahoma State Department of Education/Special
    Education Services/Sooner Start Program (OK) 313

Section of Special Education/Missouri Department of
    Elementary and Secondary Education (MO) 219

Special Education, Part H Program/Nebraska
    Department of Education (NE) 232

Special Education Unit/Vermont Department of
    Education (VT) 396

Zero to 3 Hawaii Project (HI) 109

SCHOOLS

Alabama School for the Blind/Alabama Institute for
    Deaf and Blind (AL) 3

Arizona State Schools for the Deaf and the Blind (AZ) 16

Arkansas School for the Blind (AR) 25

Blue Springs Special Services Center (MO) 219

Boston Center for Blind Children (MA) 178

California School for the Blind (CA) 31

Capital Area Intermediate Unit (PA) 325

Center for Blind and Visually Impaired Children (WI) 424

Children's Vision Center/Department of
    Ophthalmology/University of California, Davis
    Medical Center (CA) 32

Colorado School for the Deaf and the Blind (CO) 58

The Fernald Center (MA) 178

Florida School for the Deaf and Blind (FL) 78

Foundation for Blind Children (AZ) 17

Foundation for the Junior Blind (CA) 32

Georgia Academy for the Blind (GA) 97

Governor Morehead School (NC) 286

Hawaii Center for the Deaf and Blind (HI) 109

The Hope School (IL) 117

Idaho School for the Deaf and the Blind (ID) 113

Illinois School for the Visually Impaired (IL) 117

Indiana School for the Blind (IN) 135

Instituto Loaíza Cordero para Niños Ciegos (PR) 351

Iowa Braille and Sight Saving School (IA) 144

Kansas State School for the Blind (KS) 148

Kentucky School for the Blind (KY) 155

Lavelle School for the Blind (NY) 255

Louisiana School for the Visually Impaired (LA) 161

Maryland School for the Blind (MD) 170

Matheny School and Hospital (NJ) 244

Michigan School for the Deaf and Blind (MI) 192

Minnesota State Academy for the Blind (MN) 206

Mississippi School for the Blind (MS) 213

Missouri School for the Blind (MO) 219

Montana School for the Deaf and the Blind (MT) 228

Nebraska School for the Visually Handicapped (NE) 232

New Hampshire Educational Services for the Sensory
    Impaired (NH) 240

New Mexico School for the Visually
    Handicapped (NM) 251

New York Institute for Special Education (NY) 255

New York State School for the Blind (NY) 256

Northcentral Technical College (WI) 425

North Dakota Vision Services/School for the
    Blind (ND) 294

Northeast Vision Consultants (MA) 178

Oak Hill School/Connecticut Institute for the
    Blind (CT) 65

Ohio State School for the Blind (OH) 298

Oregon Office of Special Education/Services to
    Children and Youth with Deafblindness (OR) 318

Oregon School for the Blind (OR) 318

Overbrook School for the Blind (PA) 325

Parkview School (Oklahoma School for the Blind) (OK) .. 313

Perkins School for the Blind (MA) 179

Philip J. Rock Center and School (IL) 118

Program for Visually Impaired/Milwaukee Area
    Technical College (WI) 425

Rio Salado Community College (AZ) 17

Royer-Greaves School for Blind (PA) 326

St. Joseph's School for the Blind (NJ) 244

St. Lucy Day School for Children with Visual
    Impairments (PA) 326

Santa Barbara City Schools Program for Visually
    Impaired/Special Education Services (CA) 33

South Carolina School for the Deaf and the Blind (SC) 357

South Dakota School for the Visually
    Handicapped (SD) 362

Southwest Alabama Regional School for the Deaf and
    Blind (AL) 3

Special Education Services Agency (AK) 13

Tennessee School for the Blind (TN) 367

Texas School for the Blind and Visually Impaired (TX) 376

University of Kentucky Deafblind Project (KY) 155

Utah Schools for the Deaf and the Blind (UT) 391

Virginia School for the Deaf and Blind at
    Hampton (VA) 399

Virginia School for the Deaf and the Blind (VA) 399

Visually Impaired Program/Hillsborough County
    Schools (FL) 79

Washington State School for the Blind (WA) 409

Wausau School District (WI) 426

Western Pennsylvania School for Blind Children (PA) 327

West Virginia Schools for the Deaf and the Blind (WV) 417

Wisconsin School for the Visually Handicapped and
    Educational Services Center for the Visually
    Impaired (WI) 426

INFANT AND PRESCHOOL

Allegheny Intermediate Unit/Project Dart (PA) 327

Alpena-Montmorency-Alcona Intermediate
Schools (MI) 192

Anchor Center for Blind Children (CO) 59

Arizona State Schools for the Deaf and the Blind/
Visually Impaired Preschoolers Program (AZ) 17

Arkansas School for the Blind (AR) 26

BEGIN/(Babies Early Growth Intervention Network)/
Center for the Visually Impaired (GA) 98

Blind Babies Foundation (CA) 33

Blind Children's Center (CA) 33

Blind Children's Learning Center (CA) 34

Braille Institute of America, Inc./Youth Center (CA) 34

Center and Homebound Preschool Intervention
Program (UT) 391

Center for Blind and Visually Impaired Children (WI) 427

Cherry Creek School District (CO) 59

Chicago Lighthouse for People Who Are Blind or
Visually Impaired/Development Center (IL) 119

Child Development Center/The Lighthouse Inc. (NY) 256

Children's Center for the Visually
Impaired(CCVI) (MO) 220

Children's Rehabilitation Center/University of
Virginia Hospital (VA) 400

Cincinnati Association for the Blind (OH) 298

Cleveland Sight Center of the Cleveland Society for the
Blind (OH) 299

Connecticut State Board of Education and Services for
the Blind (CT) 66

Cooperative Preschool for Visually Handicapped (AZ) 18

Dallas Services for Visually Impaired Children (TX) 376

Debbie School/Mailman Center for Child
Development (FL) 79

Delaware Division for the Visually Impaired (DE) 70

Delta Gamma Center for Children with Visual
Impairments (MO) 220

Developmental Education Birth through Two (DEBT
Project) (TX) 377

Division of Blind Services/Florida Department of
Labor (FL) 79

DuPage/West Cook Regional Special Education
Association (IL) 119

Early Childhood Special Education Services/Omaha
Public Schools (NE) 232

Early Education Center/Training and Evaluation
Center of Hutchinson (KS) 148

Gary Community Public Schools Corporation (IN) 136

Helen Keller Services for the Blind (NY) 257

Hope Family Support Program (CA) 34

Idaho School for the Deaf and the Blind (ID) 113

Illinois School for the Visually Impaired (IL) 119

Infant and Child Development Program/Columbia
Lighthouse for the Blind (DC) 73

Infant-Family Program of the Foundation for the Junior
Blind (CA) 35

Jewish Guild for the Blind (The Guild) (NY) 257

J.I.S.D. #287 (MN) 206

Lavelle School for the Blind (NY) 258

LICA-NSSEO Infant Vision Program (IL) 120

The Lighthouse Inc./Hudson Valley (NY) 258

Little Light House, Inc. (OK) 314

Memphis City Schools (TN) 367

Merrick Educational Center (FL) 80

Metropolitan Nashville Public Schools/Visually
Impaired/Multihandicapped Program (TN) 368

Mississippi School for the Blind (MS) 213

Multi-Sensory Intervention Through Consultation and
Education (MICE) (NH) 240

Nebraska Department of Education (NE) 233

New Mexico School for the Visually Handicapped
Preschool (NM) 252

North Carolina Department of Human Resources/
Division of Services for the Blind (NC) 287

Oregon Department of Education (OR) 319

Oregon School for the Blind (OR) 319

Overbrook School for the Blind (PA) 327

Parkview School (Oklahoma School for the Blind) (OK) .. 314

Perkins School for the Blind (MA) 179

Services for the Blind/Tennessee Division of
Rehabilitation Services (TN) 368

South Carolina Commission for the Blind (SC) 358

Special Education Services Agency/Infant Learning
Program (AK) 13

Tennessee School for the Blind (TN) 368

Tri-Valley Developmental Services (KS) 149

Utah Schools for the Deaf and the Blind/Parent-Infant
Program (PIP) (UT) 392

Virginia Department for the Visually
Handicapped (VA) 400

Virginia School for the Deaf and Blind at
Hampton (VA) 401

Vision Rehabilitation Inc. (OH) 299

Vision Services/Early Childhood Learning Center/
Montgomery County Public Schools (MD) 171

Visually Impaired Preschool Services (VIPS) (KY) 156

West Virginia Schools for the Deaf and the Blind (WV) 418

Wisconsin School for the Visually Handicapped and
Educational Services Center for the Visually
Impaired (WI) 427

Wood County Office of Education (OH) 299

STATEWIDE OUTREACH SERVICES

Alabama Institute for Deaf and Blind (AL) 4

Arizona State Schools for the Deaf and the Blind (AZ).........18
California School for the Blind (CA) 35
Colorado School for the Deaf and the Blind (CO) 59
Educational Services for Visually Impaired / Arkansas
   School for the Blind (AR) 26
Georgia Academy for the Blind (GA) 98
Hawaii Center for the Deaf and Blind (HI) 109
Idaho School for the Deaf and the Blind (ID) 114
Illinois School for the Visually Impaired (IL)..............120
Indiana School for the Blind (IN)..................136
Instituto Loaíza Cordero para Niños Ciegos (PR) 351
Iowa Braille and Sight Saving School (IA) 144
Kansas State School for the Blind (KS) 149
Kentucky School for the Blind (KY) 156
Louisiana School for the Visually Impaired (LA)..................162
Maryland School for the Blind (MD) 171
Michigan School for the Deaf and Blind (MI) 193
Minnesota State Academy for the Blind (MN) 207
Missouri School for the Blind (MO) 221
Montana School for the Deaf and the Blind (MT) 229
Nebraska School for the Visually Handicapped (NE)........233
New Mexico School for the Visually
   Handicapped (NM).................252
Oak Hill School / Connecticut Institute for the
   Blind (CT) 66
Ohio State School for the Blind (OH) 299
Oregon School for the Blind (OR)................320
Outreach Services / Perkins School for the Blind (MA) 180
Parkview School (Oklahoma School for the Blind) (OK) .. 315
Resource Center for the Visually Impaired / New York
   State School for the Blind (NY).................259
South Carolina School for the Deaf and the Blind (SC) 358
South Dakota School for the Visually
   Handicapped (SD) 363
Tennessee School for the Blind (TN) 369
Texas School for the Blind and Visually Impaired (TX).....377
Utah Schools for the Deaf and the Blind (UT) 392
Virginia School for the Deaf and Blind at
   Hampton (VA) 401
Washington State School for the Blind (WA)...............410
West Virginia Schools for the Deaf and the Blind (WV) 418
Wisconsin School for the Visually Handicapped and
   Educational Services Center for the Visually
   Impaired (WI) 427

INSTRUCTIONAL MATERIALS CENTERS

Alabama Instructional Resource Center (AL)....................4
Arizona Instructional Resource Center (AZ)................18
Central Instructional Support Center (PA)...................328
Clearinghouse for Specialized Media and
   Technology / California Department of
   Education (CA)..................35

Colorado Instructional Materials Center for the
   Visually Handicapped (CO)...................59
Connecticut State Board of Education and Services for
   the Blind (CT)..................66
Delaware Division for the Visually Impaired (DE)................70
Educational Services for Visually Impaired / Arkansas
   School for the Blind (AR) 26
Florida Instructional Materials Center for the Visually
   Handicapped (FL) 80
George Meyer Instructional Resource Center (NJ)...............245
Idaho School for the Deaf and the Blind (ID) 114
Illinois Industrial Materials (IL)..................120
Independent Living Resources (OR) 320
Indiana Educational Resource Center / Indiana School
   for the Blind (IN)..................136
Instructional Materials Center for the Blind (ME) 167
Iowa Braille and Sight Saving School (IA) 145
Kansas Instructional Resource Center for the Blind and
   Visually Impaired (KS) 149
Kentucky Instructional Materials Resource Center (KY) .. 156
LEA Resource Center (GA) 98
Louisiana Learning Resources System / Louisiana State
   Department of Education (LA)..................162
Maryland School for the Blind (MD) 171
Minnesota Resource Center / Blind / Visually
   Impaired (MN) 207
Missouri School for the Blind (MO) 221
Montana School for the Deaf and the Blind (MT) 229
Nebraska School for the Visually Handicapped (NE)........233
New Hampshire Educational Services for the Sensory
   Impaired (NH) 241
New Mexico School for the Visually
   Handicapped (NM)..................252
North Dakota Vision Services / School for the
   Blind (ND) 294
ORCLISH (Ohio Resource Center for Low Incidence
   and Severely Handicapped) (OH) 300
Oregon Text and Media Center for the Visually
   Handicapped (OR) 320
PIA Media Center (MI)..................193
Resource Center for the Visually Impaired / New York
   State School for the Blind (NY)..................259
South Dakota State Library for the Handicapped (SD) 363
Southern Will County Cooperative (IL)..................120
Special Education Services Agency (AK)...................13
Tennessee Department of Education / Resource Center
   for the Visually Impaired (TN)..................369
Texas Instructional Materials Center for Students with
   Visual Handicaps / Texas Education Agency / Texas
   School for the Blind and Visually Impaired (TX)..............378
Utah Educational Resource Center (UT)..................392
Vermont Association for the Blind and Visually
   Impaired (VT)..................396

Virginia Department for the Visually Handicapped/
    Instructional Materials and Resource Center (VA)........... 401
Vision Resources Library (MA) 180
Washington Instructional Resource Center/
    Washington State School for the Blind (WA) 410
West Virginia Instructional Resource Center/West
    Virginia Schools for the Deaf and the Blind (WV)............. 418
Wisconsin Educational Services Center for the Visually
    Impaired (WI)... 427

UNIVERSITY TRAINING PROGRAMS

Boston College/Graduate School of Education (MA)........ 180
California State University at Sacramento (CA)...................... 35
California State University, Los Angeles (CA) 36
Dominican College (NY)... 259
D'Youville College/Division of Education (NY) 259
Eastern Michigan University (MI)... 193
Florida State University/Visual Impairments (FL) 80
Georgia State University (GA) 98
Hunter College, City University of New York/
    Department of Special Education (NY)................................ 259
Illinois State University (IL)... 120
Jackson State University/Department of Special
    Education and Rehabilitative Services (MS) 214
Kutztown University/Department of Special
    Education (PA)... 328
Mankato State University (MN)... 207
Michigan State University (MI)... 193
Mississippi State University/Rehabilitation Research
    and Training Center on Blindness and Low
    Vision (MS) 214
New York University/School of Education/
    Rehabilitation Counseling Program (NY) 259
Northeastern University (MA).. 180
Northern Illinois University (IL)... 120
Northern State College/Special Education
    Program (SD) 363
Ohio State University/School of Teaching and
    Learning (OH) 300
Peabody College of Vanderbilt University (TN).................... 369
Pennsylvania College of Optometry/Institute for the
    Visually Impaired (PA)... 328
Portland State University/Department of Special
    Education (OR) 320
Programs in Special Education (SC).. 358
San Francisco State University (CA) 36
Southern Illinois University (IL)... 121
Stephen F. Austin State University (TX) 378
Talladega College (AL)...4
Teachers College, Columbia University/Department
    of Health and Behavioral Studies (NY) 260
Texas Tech University/College of Education (TX) 378

University of Alabama at Birmingham (AL) 4
University of Arizona (AZ)... 19
University of Arkansas at Little Rock (AR) 27
University of Louisville/School of Education (KY)............. 156
University of Massachusetts at Boston (MA)........................... 180
University of Minnesota/Department of Educational
    Psychology (MN) 207
University of Nebraska (NE)... 233
University of North Dakota (ND) 295
University of Northern Colorado (CO)...................................... 60
University of Pittsburgh/School of Education/
    Department of Instruction and Learning (PA) 328
University of Puerto Rico (PR)... 352
University of Texas at Austin (TX)... 378
University of Toledo/Department of Special Education
    Services (OH).. 300
Wayne State University (MI)... 193
Western Michigan University/Department of Special
    Education (MI)... 193

◆ *Information Services*

LIBRARIES

Alabama Regional Library for the Blind and Physically
    Handicapped (AL).. 4
Alaska State Library/Talking Book Center (AK).................... 14
Albany Library for the Blind and Handicapped (GA) 99
Andrew Heiskell Library for the Blind and Physically
    Handicapped/New York Public Library (NY) 260
Arizona State Braille and Talking Book Library (AZ)........... 19
Bainbridge Subregional Library for the Blind and
    Physically Handicapped (GA)... 99
Bartholomew County Public Library (IN) 137
Blind and Physically Handicapped Services (IN) 137
Blue Water Library Foundation/Blind and Physically
    Handicapped Library (MI) 194
Braille Institute Library Services (CA) 36
Brevard County Library System Talking Books
    Library (FL).. 80
Broward County Talking Book Library (FL)............................ 80
Bureau of Braille and Talking Book Services (FL) 81
California State Library/Braille and Talking Book
    Services (CA) 36
Carnegie Library of Pittsburgh/Library for the Blind
    and Physically Handicapped (PA).. 328
Chicago Public Library/Illinois Regional Library for
    the Blind and Physically Handicapped (IL).................... 121
Chicago Public Library/Talking Book Center (IL)............... 121
Cleveland Public Library/Library for the Blind and
    Physically Handicapped (OH)... 300
Colorado Talking Book Library (CO).. 60

Connecticut State Library / Library for the Blind and Physically Handicapped (CT).................................. 66

Dade County Talking Book Library (FL).................................... 81

Department for the Blind and Physically Handicapped (AL).. 5

District of Columbia Library for the Blind and Physically Handicapped (DC)............................... 73

Downtown Detroit Subregional Library for the Blind and Physically Handicapped (MI)...................... 194

La Fayette Subregional Library for the Blind and Physically Handicapped (GA)........................... 99

Fort Smith Public Library for the Blind and Handicapped (AR).. 27

Fredericksburg Area Subregional Library (VA)................. 401

Free Library of Philadelphia / Library for the Blind and Physically Handicapped (PA)............ 329

Fresno County Free Library / Blind and Handicapped Services (CA)................................... 36

Georgia Regional Library for the Blind and Physically Handicapped (GA)........................... 99

Grand Traverse Area Library for the Blind and Physically Handicapped (MI)............................ 194

Guam Public Library for the Blind and Physically Handicapped (GU)................................ 108

Hampton Subregional Library for the Blind and Physically Handicapped (VA)............................ 401

Hawaii Library for the Blind and Physically Handicapped (HI).. 109

Heart of Illinois Talking Book Center (IL)..................... 121

Hillsborough County Talking Book Library (FL)................ 81

Huntsville Subregional Library for the Blind and Physically Handicapped (AL)............................. 5

Idaho State Library / Services for Blind and Physically Handicapped (ID)............................ 114

Indiana State Library / Special Services Division (IN)......... 137

Iowa Library for the Blind and Physically Handicapped / Iowa Department for the Blind (IA)......... 145

Kansas City, Kansas Public Library / Kansas Braille Library (KS)....................................... 149

Kansas Talking Book Service / Kansas State Library (KS)... 150

Kent County Library for the Blind and Physically Handicapped (MI)............................. 194

Kentucky Library for the Blind and Physically Handicapped (KY).................................. 157

Lee County Subregional Library for the Blind and Physically Handicapped (FL)........................ 81

Library and Resource Center / Virginia Department for the Visually Handicapped (VA)............ 401

Library and Resource Center for the Blind and Physically Handicapped (AL)......................... 5

Library for the Blind and Handicapped, Northwest (AR).................................... 27

Library for the Blind and Handicapped, Southwest (AR)................................... 27

Library for the Blind and Physically Handicapped (AL)......... 5

Library for the Blind and Physically Handicapped (AR)..... 27

Library for the Blind and Physically Handicapped (GA)..... 99

Library for the Blind and Physically Handicapped / Delaware Division of Libraries (DE)................ 70

Library for the Blind and Physically Handicapped / Newport News Public Library System (VA)............ 402

Library for the Blind and Print Handicapped (CA)............ 36

Library of Michigan / Services for the Blind and Physically Handicapped (MI)........................ 194

Louisiana State Library / Section for the Blind and Physically Handicapped (LA)..................... 162

Macomb Library for the Blind and Physically Handicapped (MI).................................. 194

Macon Subregional Library for the Blind and Physically Handicapped (GA)......................... 99

Maine State Library / Library Services for the Blind and Physically Handicapped (ME)................ 167

Manhattan Public Library (KS)......................... 150

Maryland State Library for the Blind and Physically Handicapped (MD)............................ 171

Massachusetts Braille and Talking Book Library (MA)...... 181

M.C. Migel Memorial Library / Information Center / American Foundation for the Blind (NY)............ 260

Mideastern Michigan Library Co-op / Library for the Blind and Physically Handicapped (MI)............ 195

Mid-Illinois Talking Book (IL)......................... 121

Minnesota Library for the Blind and Physically Handicapped (MN)............................. 207

Minnesota State Services for the Blind / Communication Center (MN)......................... 207

Mississippi Library Commission / Talking Book and Braille Services (MS)............................. 214

Montana Talking Books Library (MT).................... 229

Muskegon County Library for the Blind and Physically Handicapped (MI)......................... 195

Nevada State Library and Archives / Regional Library for the Blind / Talking Book Program (NV)............ 237

New Hampshire State Library / Library Services to the Handicapped Division (NH).................... 241

New Jersey Library for the Blind and Handicapped (NJ)................................. 245

New Mexico State Library for the Blind and Physically Handicapped (NM)......................... 252

New York Public Library Project ACCESS / Mid-Manhattan Library (NY)......................... 260

New York State Talking Book and Braille Library (NY).... 260

North Carolina Library for the Blind and Physically Handicapped (NC)............................. 287

North Dakota State Library Services for the Disabled (ND)...................................... 295

Northern Kentucky Talking Book Library (KY) 157

Northland Library Cooperative (MI) 195

Northwest Indiana Subregional Library for the Blind and Physically Handicapped (IN) 137

Northwest Kansas Library System / Talking Books (KS) ... 150

Oakland County Library for the Blind and Physically Handicapped (MI) 195

Oklahoma Library for the Blind and Physically Handicapped (OK) 315

Oregon State Library / Talking Book and Braille Services (OR) 320

Prescott Talking Book Library (AZ) 19

Public Library of Cincinnati and Hamilton County / Library for the Blind and Physically Handicapped (OH) 300

Puerto Rico Regional Library for the Blind and Physically Handicapped (PR) 352

Queens Borough Public Library / Special Services (NY) 261

Readers' Services Department (IN) 137

Rhode Island Regional Library for the Blind and Physically Handicapped (RI) 354

Roanoke City Public Library / Outreach Services (VA) 402

Rome Subregional Library for the Blind and Physically Handicapped (GA) 99

Ruth M. Shellens Library / The Lighthouse Inc. (NY) 261

Services for Blind and Physically Handicapped / Kanawha County Public Library (WV) 418

Services for the Blind and Physically Handicapped / Cabell County Public Library (WV) 418

Services for the Blind and Physically Handicapped / Ohio County Public Library (WV) 419

Services for the Blind and Physically Handicapped / Parkersburg and Wood County Public Library (WV) 419

South Carolina State Library / Department for the Blind and Physically Handicapped (SC) 358

South Central Kansas Library System / Talking Book Division (KS) 150

South Dakota State Library for the Handicapped (SD) 363

Southern Illinois Talking Book Center (IL) 121

Special Needs Center / Phoenix Public Library (AZ) 19

Special Needs Library (MD) 172

Special Services / Fairfax County Public Library (VA) 402

Special Services / Tulsa City-County Library System (OK) 315

Special Services Division / Virginia Beach Public Library (VA) 402

Stephanie Joyce Kahn Foundation (SJK) (NY) 261

Subregional Library for the Blind and Physically Handicapped (GA) 99

Subregional Library for the Blind and Physically Handicapped / Talking Book Center (GA) 100

Talking Book and Braille Service (NE) 233

Talking Book Center (GA) 100

Talking Book Center (MD) 172

Talking Book Center / Staunton Public Library (VA) 402

Talking Book Center of Northwest Illinois (IL) 121

Talking Book Library (KY) 157

Talking Book Library (MA) 181

Talking Book Library / Jacksonville Public Libraries (FL) 81

Talking Book Program / Las Vegas-Clark County Library / Subregional Library for the Blind and Handicapped (NV) 237

Talking Books (KS) 150

Talking Books / Nassau Library System (NY) 261

Talking Books / Palm Beach County Library Annex (FL) 81

Talking Books Department (KS) 150

Talking Book Service (FL) 81

Talking Book Service / Alexandria Library (VA) 402

Talking Book Service / Arlington County Department of Libraries (VA) 402

Talking Book Service / Library for the Blind and Physically Handicapped (KS) 150

Talking Book Services (IN) 137

Talking Books Plus / Outreach Services (NY) 261

Tennessee Library for the Blind and Physically Handicapped (TN) 369

Texas State Library / Talking Book Program (TX) 378

Tuscaloosa Subregional Library for the Blind and Physically Handicapped (AL) 5

Upper Peninsula Library for the Blind and Physically Handicapped (MI) 195

Utah State Library / Division for the Blind and Physically Handicapped (UT) 392

Vermont Department of Libraries / Special Services Unit (VT) 396

Virgin Islands Regional Library for the Visually and Physically Handicapped (VI) 407

Vision Resources Library / Massachusetts Department of Education (MA) 181

Washington Library for the Blind and Physically Handicapped (WA) 410

Washtenaw County Library for the Blind and Physically Handicapped (MI) 195

Wayne County Regional Library for the Blind and Physically Handicapped (MI) 195

West Florida Regional Library Subregional Talking Book Library (FL) 81

West Virginia Library Commission of Services for the Blind and Physically Handicapped (WV) 419

West Virginia Schools for the Deaf and the Blind (WV) 419

Wisconsin Regional Library for the Blind and Physically Handicapped (WI) 428

Wolfner Library for the Blind and Physically Handicapped (MO) 221

TALKING BOOK MACHINE DISTRIBUTORS

Indiana State Library/Special Services Division (IN) 137

Massachusetts Braille and Talking Book Library (MA) 181

North Dakota Vision Services/School for the
Blind (ND) 295

Services for the Visually Impaired/Wyoming
Department of Education (WY) 433

Special Library and Transcription Services/Minnesota
State Services for the Blind Communication
Center (MN) 208

Talking Book Program/State Library of Ohio (OH) 300

MEDIA PRODUCTION SERVICES

Aid to Visually Handicapped (OH) 301

Alabama Regional Library for the Blind and Physically
Handicapped (AL) 5

Allegheny Intermediate Unit Vision Program (PA) 329

American Red Cross/Braille Division (CA) 37

American Red Cross/Midway-Kansas Chapter (KS) 150

Arizona State Braille and Talking Book Library (AZ) 19

Arizona State Schools for the Deaf and the Blind (AZ) 19

Arkansas Department of Correction (AR) 27

Association of Pleasant Hills Community Church (PA) 329

ATLA Adaptive Materials Center (AK) 14

Atlanta Braille Volunteers (GA) 100

Barrett School (AL) 5

Beth Shalom Braille Committee (MO) 221

Blue Ridge Braillers (NC) 287

Boise Public Schools (ID) 114

Bower Hill Braille Foundation (PA) 329

Braille Association of Kansas (KS) 150

Braille Computer Center/Boulder Public Library (CO) 60

Braille Institute of America, Inc. (CA) 37

Braille Transcribers (CA) 37

Braille Transcribers Club of Illinois (IL) 121

Braille Transcribers of Central New York, Inc. (NY) 261

Braille Transcribers of Humboldt (CA) 37

Braille Transcription Project of Santa Clara County,
Inc. (CA) 37

Canton Program for the Visually Handicapped/
Canton City Schools (OH) 301

Capital Area Intermediate Unit (PA) 329

Castro Valley School District (CA) 37

Central Blind Rehabilitation Center (IL) 122

Central Instruction Support Center (PA) 329

Charleston County School District/Pupil Personnel
Services (SC) 359

Chicago Public Library/Illinois Regional Library for
the Blind and Physically Handicapped (IL) 122

Clark County School District (NV) 237

Clover Bottom Developmental Center (TN) 369

Colorado Talking Book Library (CO) 60

Columbia Lighthouse for the Blind (DC) 74

CompuBraille (CA) 37

Connecticut Braille Association (CT) 66, 67

Dallas Services for the Visually Impaired (TX) 379

Darien Community Association Program for the
Blind (CT) 67

Dayton Public Schools (OH) 301

DeKalb County School System (GA) 100

Delaware Association for the Blind (DE) 71

District of Columbia Library for the Blind and
Physically Handicapped (DC) 74

Educational Vision Services/New York City Public
Schools, District 75 (NY) 261

Escambia County School District (FL) 81

Exceptional Student Education (FL) 82

Father Palmer Memorial Braille Service/Lilac Blind
Foundation (WA) 411

Foundation for Blind Children (AZ) 20

Gary Public Schools, V.I.P. Resource Center (IN) 137

Georgia Division of Rehabilitation Services (GA) 100

Golden Gate Braille Transcribers, Inc. (CA) 37

Green Bay Public Schools (WI) 428

Guild for the Blind (IL) 122

Hawaii Library for the Blind and Physically
Handicapped (HI) 110

Helen Keller Services for the Blind/Braille
Library (NY) 262

Horizons for the Blind (IL) 122

Idaho State Library/Services for Blind and Physically
Handicapped (ID) 115

Illinois Instructional Materials Center (IL) 122

Illinois School for the Visually Impaired (IL) 122

Iowa Department for the Blind (IA) 145

Jefferson County Public Schools (KY) 157

Jewish Heritage for the Blind (NY) 262

Johanna Bureau for the Blind and Physically
Handicapped, Inc. (IL) 123

Kansas Rehabilitation Center for the Blind (KS) 150

Kings Tape Library for the Blind (CA) 38

Lehigh Valley Braille Guild (PA) 329

Library and Resource Center for the Blind and
Physically Handicapped (AL) 5

Library of Michigan/Services for the Blind and
Physically Handicapped (MI) 195

LICA-NSSEO Vision East (IL) 123

LICA-NSSEO Vision West (IL) 123

Lighthouse of Houston (TX) 379

Louisiana School for the Visually Impaired (LA) 162

Low Vision Library/Kansas City Association for the
Blind (MO) 221

Madison-Chatham Braille Association (NJ) 245

Maine Division for the Blind and Visually Impaired (ME) 167

Massachusetts Association for the Blind (MA) 181

Michigan Association of Transcribers for the Visually Impaired (MI) 195

Middle Tennessee Reception Center (TN) 369

Midwestern Braille Volunteers (MO) 222

Minnesota Library for the Blind and Physically Handicapped (MN) 208

Minnesota State Services for the Blind (MN) 208

Mississippi Library Commission/Talking Book and Braille Services (MS) 214

Mississippi School for the Blind (MS) 214

Montgomery County Public Schools Vision Services Center (MD) 172

Naperville Area Transcribing for the Blind (IL) 123

Nassau Community College Library (NY) 262

National Federation of the Blind of Utah (UT) 393

NEGA RESA (GA) 100

Nevada Bureau of Services to the Blind (NV) 237

Nevada State Library/Regional Library for the Blind (NV) 238

North Carolina Department of Human Resources/ Division of Services for the Blind (NC) 287

Northland Public Library (PA) 330

North Texas Taping and Radio for the Blind (TX) 379

Oakmont Visual Aids Workshop (CA) 38

Oklahoma Library for the Blind and Physically Handicapped (OK) 315

Onondaga Braillists (NY) 262

Oregon State Library/Talking Book and Braille Services (OR) 321

Owensboro Recording Unit (KY) 157

Palm Beach County Schools (FL) 82

Peoria Area Blind People's Center, Inc. (IL) 123

Petaluma Braille Transcribers, Inc. (CA) 38

Pinellas County Schools (FL) 82

Puerto Rico Department of Education/Special Education Program (PR) 352

Puerto Rico Regional Library for the Blind and Physically Handicapped (PR) 352

Quik-Scrybe (CA) 38

Recording for the Blind and Dyslexic (AZ) 20

Recording for the Blind and Dyslexic (CA) 38

Recording for the Blind and Dyslexic (CO) 60

Recording for the Blind and Dyslexic (GA) 100

Recording for the Blind and Dyslexic (IL) 123

Recording for the Blind and Dyslexic (KY) 157

Recording for the Blind and Dyslexic (MA) 181, 182

Recording for the Blind and Dyslexic (MI) 195

Recording for the Blind and Dyslexic (NJ) 245, 246

Recording for the Blind and Dyslexic (NY) 262

Recording for the Blind and Dyslexic (PA) 330

Recording for the Blind and Dyslexic (TN) 369

Recording for the Blind and Dyslexic (TX) 379

Recording for the Blind and Dyslexic (VA) 402

Recording for the Blind and Dyslexic/Connecticut Unit (CT) 67

Recording for the Blind and Dyslexic/Florida Unit (FL) 82

Recording for the Blind and Dyslexic of Metropolitan Washington (DC) 74

Recording Library for the Blind and Physically Handicapped (TX) 379

Region IV Education Service Center (TX) 379

Rodef Shalom Temple Sisterhood (PA) 330

Roosevelt Warm Springs Institute for Rehabilitation (GA) 101

San Gabriel Valley Braille Guild (CA) 38

Santa Barbara School District (CA) 38

Seattle Area Braillists, Inc. (WA) 411

Sequoia Transcribers (CA) 39

The Sight Center of the Toledo Society for the Blind (OH) 301

Sisterhood Braille Group of East Midwood Jewish Center (NY) 262

Sisterhood of Temple Beth Hillel (CA) 39

Sisterhood of Temple Sinai (NY) 262

Sisterhood Temple Israel of Jamaica (NY) 262

South Carolina Commission for the Blind (SC) 359

South Carolina School for the Deaf and the Blind (SC) 359

South Carolina State Library/Department for the Blind and Physically Handicapped (SC) 359

South Dakota Industries for the Blind (SD) 363

Southern Illinois University (IL) 123

Southwest Alabama Regional School for the Deaf and Blind (AL) 6

Special Education Media Center (NE) 234

Special School District, Saint Louis County (MO) 222

Spencerport Braille Association (NY) 262

Talking Book and Braille Service (NE) 234

Talking Book Center (GA) 101

Talking Book Program/Las Vegas–Clark County Library (NV) 238

Talking Tapes for the Blind (MO) 222

Temple Israel Sisterhood (TN) 369

Temple Sinai Sisterhood (PA) 330

Temple Sisterhood Braille Group (FL) 82

Temple Sisterhood Braille Group (OH) 301

Tennessee Library for the Blind and Physically Handicapped (TN) 370

Texas State Library/Talking Book Program (TX) 379

TFB Publications (NJ) 246

Theodore Lester Elementary School (SC) 359

Transcribers of Orange County (CA) 39

University of Illinois at Urbana-Champaign / Division of Rehabilitation Education Services (IL) 124

University of Washington (WA) 411

Utah Schools for the Deaf and the Blind (UT) 393

Ventura County Braille Transcribers Association (CA) 39

Vision Center of Central Ohio (OH) 301

Vision Resources Library / Massachusetts Department of Education (MA) 182

Visually Handicapped Materials Center / Cincinnati Public Schools (OH) 301

Volunteer Services for the Visually Handicapped (WI) 428

Volunteers for the Visually Handicapped (MD) 74, 172

Washington State Braille Access Center / Washington State School for the Blind (WA) 411

Wisconsin Educational Services Center for the Visually Impaired (WI) 428

Youngstown Braille Service (OH) 302

RADIO READING

A.I.R.R.E.S. Radio Reading Service (AK) 14

Alabama Radio Reading Service Network (AL) 6

APRIS (IL) 124

Arkansas Radio Reading Service (AR) 27

Audio Journal (MA) 182

Audio Reader of Cloud County (KS) 151

Audiovision / New Jersey Library for the Blind and Handicapped (NJ) 246

Audio Vision Radio Reading Service (CA) 39

Central Indiana Radio Reading, Inc. (IN) 138

Central Kentucky Radio Eye (KY) 157

Central Ohio Radio Reading Service (OH) 302

Central Piedmont Community College Radio Reading Service (NC) 287

Central Savannah River Area Radio Reading Service, Inc. (GA) 101

Chicagoland Radio Information Service, Inc. (IL) 124

Cleveland Radio Reading Service (OH) 302

Connecticut Radio Information System (CRIS) (CT) 67

Detroit Radio Information Service (MI) 196

Eastern Shore Radio Reading Service / WESM-FM (MD) .. 172

Education and Reading Service (EARS) (WI) 428

Electronic Information and Education Service (NJ) 246

El Paso Radio Reading Service (TX) 379

Evergreen Radio Reading Service (WA) 411

Georgia Radio Reading Service, Inc. (GA) 101

Golden Hours, Inc. (OR) 321

Hampton Roads Voice of the Print Handicapped (VA) 402

Harrisburg Area Radio Reading Service (PA) 330

Houston Taping for the Blind Radio (TX) 380

Idaho Radio Reading Service (ID) 115

Illinois Radio Reader (IL) 124

IN-SIGHT Radio—Division of IN-SIGHT (RI) 354

INSIGHT / WYMS (WI) 428

IN TOUCH Networks (NY) 263

Iowa Radio Reading Information Service (IRIS) (IA) 145

Kansas Audio-Reader Network (KS) 151

KBPS Seeing Sound (OR) 321

KCHO-FM Radio Reading Service (CA) 39

Keystone Radio Information Service / Blair County Association for the Blind and Visually Handicapped (PA) 330

KPBS-FM Radio Reading Service (CA) 39

KUT 90.5FM (TX) 380

LIFTT Radio Reading Service (MT) 229

Metropolitan Washington Ear, Inc. (MD) 74, 172

Neighborhood News for the Blind (NC) 288

Nevada Public Radio Corporation / KNPR (NV) 238

Niagara Frontier Radio Reading Service (NY) 263

North Central Sight Services (PA) 330

North Dakota State Library Services for the Disabled (ND) 295

North Eastern Indiana Radio Reading Service, Inc. (NEIRRS) (IN) 138

Northeast Radio Reading Service (NY) 263

Northern Illinois Radio Information Services / WNIJ (IL) 124

Northern Illinois Radio Information Services / WNIU-FM (IL) 124

North Texas Taping and Radio for the Blind (TX) 380

Ohio Educational Telecommunications Network Commission (OH) 302

Pennsylvania Association for the Blind and Handicapped (PA) 330

Radio Information Center for the Blind (RICB) (PA) 330

Radio Information Service (IL) 124

Radio Information Service for Blind and Print Handicapped (IL) 124

Radio Information Services (PA) 331

Radio Reading Network of Maryland (MD) 172

Radio Reading Service of Mississippi (MS) 215

Radio Reading Service of the Rockies (CO) 60

Radio Reading Service of Western New England (MA) 182

Radio Reading Services, Inc. (NC) 288

Radio Reading Services of Greater Cincinnati, Inc. (OH) 302

Radio Talking Book Network (MN) 208

Radio Talking Book Service (NE) 234

Radio Vision-Ramapo Catskill Library System (NY) 263

Reading Radio Service (KS) 151

Regional Audio Information Service Enterprise (RAISE) (NC) 288

RISE (NY) 263

Services to the Blind and Visually Impaired (SD) 363

Sight Center Audio Network (OH) 302
The Sight Seer (MI) 196
South Carolina Educational Radio for the Blind (SC) 359
Southeastern North Carolina Radio Reading
   Service (NC) 288
Southern Illinois Radio Information Service (IL) 125
Sun Sounds Radio Reading Service (AZ) 20
Talking Information Center (MA) 182
The Talking Library (TN) 370
Tri-Visual Services (CA) 39
University of Kansas Audio Reader Network (KS) ... 151
UPDATE (NY) 263
Utah State Radio Reading Service (UT) 393
Valley Voice Radio Reading Service (VA) 402
Virginia Tech Radio Reading Service (VA) 403
Virginia Voice for the Print Handicapped (VA) 403
Voice of the Peninsula (VA) 403
WCBU Radio Information Service (IL) 125
WCNY-READ-OUT Radio Reading Service (NY) 263
Western Montana Radio Reading Services (MT) 229
West Virginia Radio Reading Service (WV) 419
WGCU Radio Reading Service (FL) 82
Wichita Radio Reading Service (KS) 151
WIUM/WIUW Radio Information Service (IL) 125
WJGF Radio Station (WV) 419
WKAR Radio Talking Book (MI) 196
WLRH Radio (AL) 6
WLRN Radio Reading Service (FL) 82
WMFE Radio Reading Service (FL) 82
WNIN Radio Reading Service (IN) 138
WRBH-FM/Radio for the Blind (LA) 162
Written Communications Radio Service (WCRS) for
   the Print Handicapped (OH) 302
WRKC-Radio Home Visitor (PA) 331
WRRS/RADPRIN of Lehigh Valley (PA) 331
WTSU Radio Reading Service (AL) 6
WUAL Radio Reading Service (AL) 6
WUIS/WIPA Radio Information Service (IL) 125
WUSF Radio Reading Service (FL) 83
WXXI Reachout Radio (NY) 263
WYPL-FM (TN) 370
York County Blind Center Radio Reading Service (PA) 331
Youngstown Radio Reading Service (OH) 302

PHONE-IN NEWSPAPERS

Dialing-In/Metropolitan Washington Ear (MD) 172
Newsline for the Blind (NM) 252
Newspapers for the Blind (MI) 196

INFORMATION AND REFERRAL

Alabama Department of Rehabilitation/Volunteer
   Information Resource Center (AL) 6

American Foundation for the Blind (NY) 264
American Foundation for the Blind Midwest (IL) 125
American Foundation for the Blind Southeast (GA) 101
American Foundation for the Blind Southwest (TX) 380
American Foundation for the Blind West (CA) 39
American Optometric Association (VA) 403
Blind San Franciscans (CA) 40
Braille Institute of America, Inc. (CA) 40
Cattaraugus County Association for the Blind and
   Visually Handicapped, Inc. (NY) 264
The Foundation Fighting Blindness/Alaska
   Affiliate (AK) 14
The Foundation Fighting Blindness/Arizona
   Affiliate (AZ) 20
The Foundation Fighting Blindness/Arkansas
   Affiliate (AR) 27
The Foundation Fighting Blindness/Atlanta
   Affiliate (GA) 101
The Foundation Fighting Blindness/Bronx-
   Westchester-Rockland Affiliate (NY) 264
The Foundation Fighting Blindness/Brooklyn
   Affiliate (NY) 264
The Foundation Fighting Blindness/Central Florida
   Affiliate (FL) 83
The Foundation Fighting Blindness/Central Virginia
   Affiliate (VA) 403
The Foundation Fighting Blindness/Chicago
   Affiliate (IL) 125
The Foundation Fighting Blindness/Connecticut
   Affiliate (CT) 67
The Foundation Fighting Blindness/Dallas
   Affiliate (TX) 380
The Foundation Fighting Blindness/Delaware
   Affiliate (DE) 71
The Foundation Fighting Blindness/Eastern Kentucky
   Affiliate (KY) 157
The Foundation Fighting Blindness/Eastern Ohio
   Affiliate (OH) 303
The Foundation Fighting Blindness/Fresno
   Affiliate (CA) 40
The Foundation Fighting Blindness/Greater Kansas
   City Affiliate (MO) 222
The Foundation Fighting Blindness/Greater St. Louis
   Affiliate (MO) 222
The Foundation Fighting Blindness/Greater
   Washington, DC Chapter (DC) 74
The Foundation Fighting Blindness/Hawaii
   Affiliate (HI) 110
The Foundation Fighting Blindness/Iowa Affiliate (IA) ... 145
The Foundation Fighting Blindness/Long Island
   Affiliate (NY) 264
The Foundation Fighting Blindness/Maine
   Affiliate (ME) 167

The Foundation Fighting Blindness/Manhattan Affiliate (NY)...............264

The Foundation Fighting Blindness/Maryland Affiliate (MD)...............173

The Foundation Fighting Blindness/Massachusetts Affiliate (MA)...............182

The Foundation Fighting Blindness/Michigan Affiliate (MI)...............196

The Foundation Fighting Blindness/Minnesota Affiliate (MN)...............208

The Foundation Fighting Blindness/Nebraska/Iowa Affiliate (NE)...............234

The Foundation Fighting Blindness/New Jersey Affiliate (NJ)...............246

The Foundation Fighting Blindness/North Carolina Affiliate (NC)...............288

The Foundation Fighting Blindness/Northern California Affiliate (CA)...............40

The Foundation Fighting Blindness/Northern New Jersey Affiliate (NJ)...............246

The Foundation Fighting Blindness/North Florida Affiliate (FL)...............83

The Foundation Fighting Blindness/Ormond Beach Affiliate (FL)...............83

The Foundation Fighting Blindness/Philadelphia Affiliate (PA)...............331

The Foundation Fighting Blindness/Piedmont Affiliate (NC)...............288

The Foundation Fighting Blindness/Raleigh Affiliate (NC)...............288

The Foundation Fighting Blindness/Rhode Island Affiliate (RI)...............354

The Foundation Fighting Blindness/Rocky Mountain Affiliate (CO)...............60

The Foundation Fighting Blindness/San Diego Affiliate (CA)...............40

The Foundation Fighting Blindness/Seattle Affiliate (WA)...............411

The Foundation Fighting Blindness/Southern California Affiliate (CA)...............40

The Foundation Fighting Blindness/South Florida Affiliate (FL)...............83

The Foundation Fighting Blindness/Syracuse Affiliate (NY)...............264

The Foundation Fighting Blindness/Texas Panhandle Affiliate (TX)...............380

The Foundation Fighting Blindness/Toledo Affiliate (OH)...............303

The Foundation Fighting Blindness/Utah Chapter (UT)..393

The Foundation Fighting Blindness/Vermont Affiliate (VT)...............397

The Foundation Fighting Blindness (National Retinitis Pigmentosa Foundation, Inc.) (MD)...............173

Illinois Society for the Prevention of Blindness (IL)...............125

Institute for Families of Blind Children (CA)...............40

The Lighthouse Inc. (NY)...............264

Louisiana Council for the Blind (LA)...............162

Low Vision Information Center (MD)...............173

Maryland Society For Sight (MD)...............173

National Association for Visually Handicapped (CA)...............40

New Jersey College Resource Center for Adaptive Aids (NJ)...............246

Parent Advocates for Visually Impaired Children (PAVIC) (CO)...............61

Preserve Sight Colorado (CO)...............61

Preserve Sight Mississippi (MS)...............215

Prevent Blindness America (IL)...............125

Prevent Blindness Connecticut (CT)...............67

Prevent Blindness Florida (FL)...............83

Prevent Blindness Georgia (GA)...............101

Prevent Blindness Indiana (IN)...............138

Prevent Blindness Iowa (IA)...............145

Prevent Blindness Kentucky (KY)...............157

Prevent Blindness Massachusetts (MA)...............182

Prevent Blindness Nebraska (NE)...............234

Prevent Blindness New Jersey (NJ)...............246

Prevent Blindness New York (NY)...............264

Prevent Blindness North Carolina (NC)...............288

Prevent Blindness Northern California (CA)...............40

Prevent Blindness Ohio (OH)...............303

Prevent Blindness Oklahoma (OK)...............315

Prevent Blindness Southern California (CA)...............40

Prevent Blindness Tennessee (TN)...............370

Prevent Blindness Texas/Austin Branch (TX)...............380

Prevent Blindness Texas/Dallas Branch (TX)...............380

Prevent Blindness Texas/East Texas Branch (TX)...............380

Prevent Blindness Texas/El Paso Branch (TX)...............380

Prevent Blindness Texas/Fort Worth Branch (TX)...............381

Prevent Blindness Texas/Galveston/Gulf Coast Branch (TX)...............381

Prevent Blindness Texas/Lubbock Branch (TX)...............381

Prevent Blindness Texas/Midland Branch (TX)...............381

Prevent Blindness Texas/San Antonio Branch (TX)...............381

Prevent Blindness Texas/State Office (TX)...............381

Prevent Blindness Utah (UT)...............393

Prevent Blindness Virginia (VA)...............403

Prevent Blindness Wisconsin (WI)...............428

Prevention of Blindness Society of Metropolitan Washington (DC)...............74

Puerto Rico Deaf-Blind Parents Association/Projecto Ninos Sordos-Ciegos (PR)...............352

Saving Sight Rhode Island (RI)...............354

Sight and Hearing Association/Minnesota Society for the Prevention of Blindness and Preservation of Hearing (MN)...............208

♦ *Rehabilitation Services*

STATE SERVICES

Alabama Division of Rehabilitation Services (AL) 6

Alaska Division of Vocational Rehabilitation (AK) 14

Arkansas Division of Services for the Blind (AR) 28

Blind and Visually Impaired Services / Indiana Family and Social Services Administration (IN) 138

Bureau for Sensory Disabilities / Wisconsin Division of Supportive Living (WI) 429

Bureau of Blindness and Visual Services / Pennsylvania Department of Public Welfare (PA) 331

Commission for the Blind / Family Independence Agency (MI) 196

Connecticut State Board of Education and Services for the Blind (CT) 67

District of Columbia Rehabilitation Services Administration / Visual Impairment Section (DC) 75

Division for the Blind and Visually Impaired / Maine Department of Labor (ME) 168

Division for the Blind and Visually Impaired / Vermont Agency of Human Services (VT) 397

Division for the Visually Impaired / Delaware Department of Health and Social Services (DE) 71

Division of Blind Services / Florida Department of Labor (FL) 83

Division of Disabilities and Rehabilitation Services / Virgin Islands Department of Human Services (VI) 407

Division of Rehabilitation Services / West Virginia State Board of Rehabilitation (WV) 419

Division of Service to the Blind and Visually Impaired / South Dakota Department of Human Services (SD) 364

Division of Vocational Rehabilitation / Wyoming Department of Employment (WY) 433

Georgia Division of Rehabilitation Services (GA) 101

Guam Department of Vocational Rehabilitation (GU) 108

Ho'opono Services for the Blind / Hawaii Department of Human Services / Vocational Rehabilitation and Services for the Blind Division (HI) 110

Idaho Commission for the Blind and Visually Impaired (ID) 115

Illinois Department of Rehabilitation Services (IL) 126

Iowa Department for the Blind (IA) 145

Kansas Division of Services for the Blind (KS) 151

Kentucky Department for the Blind (KY) 158

Louisiana Rehabilitation Services (LA) 163

Maryland Division of Vocational Rehabilitation Services (MD) 174

Massachusetts State Commission for the Blind (MA) 183

Minnesota State Services for the Blind and Visually Handicapped (MN) 209

Missouri Rehabilitation Services for the Blind (MO) 222

Nebraska Division of Rehabilitation Services for the Visually Impaired (NE) 234

Nevada Bureau of Services to the Blind (NV) 238

New Jersey Commission for the Blind and Visually Impaired (NJ) 247

New Mexico Commission for the Blind (NM) 253

New York State Commission for the Blind and Visually Handicapped (NY) 265

North Carolina Department of Human Resources / Division of Services for the Blind (NC) 288

Office of Vocational Rehabilitation for the Blind / Mississippi Department of Rehabilitation Services (MS) 215

Ohio Rehabilitation Services Commission / Bureau of Services for the Visually Impaired (OH) 303

Oregon Commission for the Blind (OR) 321

Rehabilitation Services / Colorado Department of Human Services (CO) 61

Rehabilitation Services Administration / Arizona Department of Economic Security (AZ) 20

Services for the Blind / California Department of Rehabilitation (CA) 41

Services for the Blind and Visually Impaired (RI) 354

Services for the Blind and Visually Impaired / New Hampshire Division of Vocational Rehabilitation (NH) 241

Services for the Blind and Visually Impaired / Tennessee Division of Rehabilitation Services (TN) 370

South Carolina Commission for the Blind (SC) 360

Texas Commission for the Blind (TX) 381

Utah Division of Services for the Blind and Visually Impaired (UT) 393

Virginia Department for the Visually Handicapped (VA) 403

Visual Services Division / Oklahoma Department of Rehabilitation Services (OK) 315

Vocational Rehabilitation / North Dakota Department of Human Services (ND) 295

Vocational Rehabilitation / Blind and Low Vision Services / Montana Department of Public Health and Human Services (MT) 229

Vocational Rehabilitation Program / Puerto Rico Department of Social Services (PR) 352

Washington State Department of Services for the Blind (WA) 411

REHABILITATION

Addie McBryde Rehabilitation Center for the Blind (MS) 216

Akron Blind Center and Workshop (OH) 304

Alabama Industries for the Blind / Alabama Institute for Deaf and Blind (AL) 7

Alliance for the Blind and Visually Impaired (TN) 371
Alphapointe Association for the Blind (MO) 223
American Lake Blind Rehabilitation Clinic / U.S.
    Department of Veterans Affairs (WA) 412
Arizona Center for the Blind and Visually
    Impaired (AZ) 21
Arizona Industries for the Blind (AZ) 22
Arkansas Lighthouse for the Blind (AR) 28
Assistance League of Santa Clara County (CA) 42
Associated Blind (NY) 266
Associated Services for the Blind (PA) 332
Association for the Advancement of Blind and
    Retarded, Inc. (NY) 266
Association for the Blind (SC) 360
Association for the Blind and Visually Impaired /
    (formerly Vision Enrichment Services) (MI) 197
Association for the Blind and Visually Impaired of
    Greater Rochester, Inc. (NY) 266
Association for the Blind and Visually Impaired of
    Lehigh County / Pennsylvania Association for the
    Blind (PA) 332
Association for the Visually Impaired (NY) 267
Augusta Blind Rehabilitation Center / U. S. Department
    of Veterans Affairs (GA) 103
Aurora of Central New York (NY) 267
Badger Association for the Blind (WI) 429
Beacon Lighthouse for the Blind (TX) 382
Beaver County / Association for the Blind (PA) 333
Bedford Branch / Pennsylvania Association for the
    Blind (PA) 333
Berks County Association for the Blind / Pennsylvania
    Association for the Blind (PA) 333
BESB Industries (CT) 68
Bestwork Industries for the Blind (NJ) 247
Blair County Association for the Blind and Visually
    Handicapped (PA) 334
Blind and Low Vision Services of North Georgia (GA) 103
Blind and Visually Impaired Center of Monterey
    County (CA) 42
Blind Association of Western New York (NY) 268
Blind Enterprises of Oregon (OR) 322
Blind, Inc. (MN) 209
Blind Industries and Services of Maryland (MD) 174
Blind Industries and Services of Maryland / Eastern
    Shore Division (MD) 174
Blind Industries and Services of Maryland / Western
    Maryland Division (MD) 174
Blind Rehabilitation Center / U.S. Department of
    Veterans Affairs (TX) 382
Blind Relief Fund of Philadelphia (PA) 334
Blind Service Association (IL) 127
Blind Work Association (NY) 268
Bosma Industries for the Blind (IN) 139

Boston Aid to the Blind (MA) 183
Boston Center for Blind Children (MA) 184
Braille Institute of America, Inc. (CA) 42
Brooklyn Bureau of Community Service (NY) 268
Bucks County Association for the Blind / Pennsylvania
    Association for the Blind (PA) 334
Butler County Association for the Blind / Pennsylvania
    Association for the Blind (PA) 335
Cabell-Wayne Services for the Blind and Visually
    Impaired (WV) 420
Cambria County Association for the Blind and Visually
    Handicapped / Pennsylvania Association for the
    Blind (PA) 335
Camp Allen, Inc. (NH) 241
Carroll Center for the Blind (MA) 184
Catholic Charities / Office for Disabled Persons (NY) 269
Catholic Charities Services for Visually Impaired
    Persons (NY) 269
Catholic Community Services (NJ) 247
Catholic Guild for the Blind (NY) 269, 270
Center for Blind Adults (AK) 15
Center for Blindness and Low Vision / Rehabilitation
    Institute (MO) 223
Center for Independence (CO) 62
Center for Living Independence for Multi-
    Handicapped Blind (CLIMB) (CA) 43
Center for Sight and Hearing Impaired (IL) 127
Center for the Partially Sighted (CA) 43
Center for the Visually Impaired (GA) 103
Center for the Visually Impaired, Inc. (FL) 84
Central Alabama Easter Seal Rehabilitation
    Center (AL) 8
Central Association for the Blind and Visually
    Impaired (NY) 270
Central Blind Rehabilitation Center / U.S. Department
    of Veterans Affairs (IL) 128
Central Illinois Sight Center / TCRC Sight Center (IL) 128
Central Susquehanna Sight Services, Inc. (PA) 336
Chautauqua Blind Association, Inc. (NY) 271
Chester County Association for the Blind /
    Pennsylvania Association for the Blind (PA) 336
Chicago Lighthouse for People Who Are Blind or
    Visually Impaired (IL) 128
Cincinnati Association for the Blind (OH) 304
CITE (Center for Independence, Technology and
    Education) (FL) 85
Cleveland Sight Center of the Cleveland Society for the
    Blind (OH) 305
Cleveland Skilled Industries (OH) 305
The Clovernook Center / Opportunities for the
    Blind (OH) 306
Colorado Rehabilitation Center / Colorado Division of
    Vocational Rehabilitation (CO) 62

Columbia Lighthouse for the Blind (DC) 75

Community Blind Center (CA) 44

Community Services for the Blind and Partially
Sighted (WA) 412

Conklin Center for Multihandicapped Blind (FL) 86

Consolidated Industries of Greater Syracuse, Inc. (NY) 271

Dallas Lighthouse for the Blind, Inc. (TX) 382

Dallas Services for Visually Impaired Children (TX) 383

Delaware Association for the Blind (DE) 71

Delaware Industries for the Blind (DE) 71

Delco Blind/Sight Center (PA) 336

Desert Blind Association (CA) 44

Doran Resource Center for the Blind (CA) 44

East Bay Center for the Blind, Inc. (CA) 44

Eastern Blind Rehabilitation Center/U.S. Department
of Veterans Affairs (CT) 68

Easter Seals Occupational Rehabilitation Center (AL) 8

East Texas Lighthouse for the Blind (TX) 383

Edith R. Rudolphy Residence for the Blind (PA) 337

Ed Lindsey Industries for the Blind (TN) 372

E.H. Gentry Technical Facility/Alabama Institute for
Deaf and Blind (AL) 9

El Paso Lighthouse for the Blind (TX) 384

Emil Fries Piano Hospital and Training Center (WA) 412

Erie Center for the Blind and Visually Handicapped/
Pennsylvania Association for the Blind (PA) 337

Evansville Association for the Blind, Inc. (IN) 139

Fairfield Regional Vision Rehabilitation Center (OH) 306

Family and Social Service Federation (NJ) 248

Fayette County Association for the Blind/
Pennsylvania Association for the Blind (PA) 338

Ferguson Industries for the Blind (MA) 185

Florida Association of Workers for the Blind (Miami
Lighthouse) (FL) 86

Florida Center for the Blind Incorporated (FL) 87

Focus for Newly Blind and Family (WI) 429

Friendship Center for the Blind and Visually
Impaired (CA) 45

Georgia Industries for the Blind (GA) 104

Georgia Lions Lighthouse Foundation, Inc. (GA) 104

Glens Falls Association for the Blind (NY) 272

Goodwill Industries of Dayton (OH) 306

Goodwill Industries of Greater Detroit (MI) 198

Goodwill Industries of Mid-Michigan, Inc. (MI) 198

Goodwill Industries of the Coastal Empire, Inc. (GA) 104

Greater Pittsburgh Guild for the Blind (now known as
Pittsburgh Vision Services) (PA) 338

Greater Wilkes-Barre Association for the Blind (PA) 339

Guiding Light for the Blind (PA) 339

Hazleton Blind Association/Pennsylvania Association
for the Blind (PA) 339

Helen Keller National Center for Deaf-Blind Youths
and Adults/East Central Region Office (MD) 174

Helen Keller National Center for Deaf-Blind Youths
and Adults/Great Plains Region Office (KS) 152

Helen Keller National Center for Deaf-Blind Youths
and Adults/Mid-Atlantic Region Office (NY) 272

Helen Keller National Center for Deaf-Blind Youths
and Adults/New England Region Office (MA) 185

Helen Keller National Center for Deaf-Blind Youths
and Adults/North Central Region Office (IL) 129

Helen Keller National Center for Deaf-Blind Youths
and Adults/Northwest Region Office (WA) 413

Helen Keller National Center for Deaf-Blind Youths
and Adults/Rocky Mountain Region Office (CO) 63

Helen Keller National Center for Deaf-Blind Youths
and Adults/South Central Region Office (TX) 384

Helen Keller National Center for Deaf-Blind Youths
and Adults/Southeast Region Office (GA) 105

Helen Keller National Center for Deaf-Blind Youths
and Adults/Southwest Region Office (CA) 45

Helen Keller Services for the Blind (NY) 272

Ho'opono Workshop for the Blind (HI) 111

Independence for the Blind (FL) 88

Independent Living for Adult Blind (ILAB) (FL) 88

Independent Living Resources (OR) 322

Indiana County Blind Association (PA) 340

Industries for the Blind, Inc. (WI) 429

Industries for the Blind of New York State (NY) 273

Industries of the Blind (NC) 289

IN-SIGHT (Rhode Island Association for the Blind) (RI) .. 355

Intercommunity Blind Center (CA) 45

Jefferson County Association for the Blind (NY) 273

Jewish Guild for the Blind (The Guild) (NY) 273

Juniata Association for the Blind (PA) 340

Kagan Home for the Blind (IL) 129

Kansas Industries for the Blind (KS) 152

Kentucky Industries for the Blind (KY) 158

Keystone Blind Association (PA) 341

Lackawanna Branch/Pennsylvania Association for the
Blind (PA) 341

Lawrence County Branch/Pennsylvania Association
for the Blind (PA) 342

League for the Blind and Disabled, Inc. (IN) 140

Lighthouse for the Blind (MN) 209

Lighthouse for the Blind (MO) 224

The Lighthouse for the Blind, Inc. (WA) 413

Lighthouse for the Blind in New Orleans (LA) 164

Lighthouse for the Blind of Fort Worth (TX) 384

Lighthouse for the Blind of the Palm Beaches (FL) 89

Lighthouse for the Visually Impaired and Blind (FL) 89

The Lighthouse Inc. (NY) 274

Lighthouse of Broward County (FL) 90

Lighthouse of Houston (TX) 385

Lilac Blind Foundation (WA) 413

Lions Blind Center of Diablo Valley (CA)...................... 45

Lions Blind Center of the Santa Clara Valley (CA) 46

Lions Center for the Blind (CA).................................. 46

Lions Club Industries for the Blind, Inc. (NC)................ 289

Lions Industries for the Blind (NC)............................ 290

Lions Services (NC)... 290

Lions Volunteer Blind Industries (TN)......................... 372

Lions World Services for the Blind (AR)....................... 28

Living Skills Center for the Visually Impaired (CA)......... 46

Louisiana Association for the Blind (LA)...................... 164

Louisiana Center for the Blind (LA)........................... 164

Lowell Association for the Blind/Center for the Blind
and Visually Impaired (MA)................................... 185

Maine Center for the Blind and Visually Impaired (ME) .. 168

Mana-Sota Lighthouse for the Blind (FL)...................... 90

Mary Bryant Home for the Blind (IL).......................... 130

The Mary Culver Home (MO).................................... 224

Massachusetts Association for the Blind (MA)................ 185

Metrolina Association for the Blind (NC)...................... 290

Michigan Commission for the Blind Training
Center (MI).. 198

Midwest Enterprises for the Blind (MI)........................ 199

Mississippi Industries for the Blind (MS)..................... 216

Mobile Association for the Blind (AL)......................... 9

Mobility Services, Inc. (GA)................................... 105

Montgomery County Association for the Blind (PA) 342

Montgomery Home for the Blind/Wyoming Pioneer
Home (WY).. 434

Morgan Memorial Goodwill Industries, Inc. (MA)........... 186

New England Home for the Deaf (Aged, Blind or
Infirm) (MA).. 186

New Hampshire Association for the Blind (NH)............... 242

New Jersey Foundation for the Blind (NJ)..................... 248

New York City Industries for the Blind (NY)................. 275

North Carolina Lions Foundation (NC)........................ 290

North Central Sight Services/Pennsylvania
Association for the Blind (PA)............................... 342

North Country Association for the Visually
Impaired (NY).. 275

North Dakota Vision Services/School for the
Blind (ND).. 296

Northeastern Association of the Blind (NY)................... 276

Northern Indiana Independent Living Service/ADEC
Resources for Independence (IN)............................ 140

The Occupational Rehabilitation Group, Inc. (MA)........... 187

Ohio Valley Goodwill Industries/Rehabilitation
Center (OH)... 307

Oklahoma League for the Blind (OK).......................... 316

Outreach Services to Elders/Perkins School for the
Blind (MA).. 187

Peninsula Center for the Blind and Visually
Impaired (CA).. 47

Pennsylvania Association for the Blind (PA).................. 343

Pennsylvania Lions Beacon Lodge Camp (PA)................. 343

Penrickton Center for Blind Children (MI).................... 199

Peoria Area Blind People's Center, Inc. (IL)................. 130

Philomatheon Society of the Blind, Inc. (OH)................ 307

Pinellas Center for the Visually Impaired, Inc.
(PCVI) (FL)... 91

Pittsburgh Blind Association/Pennsylvania
Association for the Blind (now known as Pittsburgh
Vision Services) (PA).. 344

Pittsburgh Vision Services (PA)............................... 344

Program for Visually Impaired Adults/Family Service
Association (IN).. 141

Puerto Rico Blind Rehabilitation Center/U.S.
Department of Veterans Affairs (PR)........................ 353

Raleigh Lions Clinic for the Blind (NC)...................... 290

Rocky Mountain Development Council (MT)................... 230

Rose Resnick Lighthouse for the Blind and Visually
Impaired (CA).. 47

RP International (CA).. 48

St. John's Episcopal Home for the Aged and Blind (NY) .. 276

St. Joseph's Home for the Blind (NJ)......................... 248

St. Louis Society for the Blind and Visually
Impaired (MO).. 224

Samuel W. Bell Home for Sightless, Inc. (OH)............... 307

San Antonio Lighthouse (TX).................................. 385

San Bernardino Valley Lighthouse for the Blind,
Inc. (CA)... 48

San Diego Center for the Blind and Vision
Impaired (CA).. 48

Savannah Association for the Blind, Inc. (GA)............... 105

Seeing Hand Association (WV)................................. 421

Sensory Access Foundation (CA).............................. 49

Sensory Program/Rehabilitation Research and
Development Center (151 R)/U.S. Department of
Veterans Affairs (GA)... 106

Service Club for the Blind (MO).............................. 225

Services for Sensory Accommodations/University of
Illinois at Urbana-Champaign/Division of
Rehabilitation Education Services (IL)...................... 130

The Sight Center of the Toledo Society for the
Blind (OH).. 307

Sight Society of Ohio, Inc. (OH)............................. 308

Signature Works, Inc. (MS)................................... 216

Society for the Blind (CA).................................... 49

South Dakota Industries for the Blind (SD)................. 364

South Dakota Rehabilitation Center for the Blind (SD) ... 365

Southeastern Blind Rehabilitation Center/U.S.
Department of Veterans Affairs (AL)........................ 10

Southern Nevada Sightless (NV)............................... 239

Southern Tier Association for the Visually
Impaired (NY).. 276

South Texas Lighthouse for the Blind (TX).................. 386

Southwestern Blind Rehabilitation Center (AZ)........................ 22
Sunrise Care Center Inc. (WI) 430
Susquehanna Association for the Blind and Vision
  Impaired (PA) 344
Tampa Lighthouse for the Blind (FL) 91
Tennessee Rehabilitation Center/Visually Impaired
  Services (TN) 372
Texas Commission for the Blind/Criss Cole
  Rehabilitation Center (TX) 386
Therapeutic Living Centers for the Blind (CA) 50
Trade Winds Rehabilitation Center (IN) 141
Travis Association for the Blind (TX) 386
Tri-County Branch/Pennsylvania Association for the
  Blind (PA) 345
Tri-Visual Services (CA) 50
Tucson Association for the Blind and Visually
  Impaired (AZ) 22
Upshaw Institute for the Blind (MI) 199
Utah Industries for the Blind (UT) 394
Venango County Branch/Pennsylvania Association for
  the Blind (PA) 345
Vermont Association for the Blind and Visually
  Impaired (VT) 397
Vermont Association of Business, Industry, and
  Rehabilitation (VT) 398
Virginia Association of Workers for the Blind (VA) 405
Virginia Industries for the Blind/Virginia Department
  for the Visually Handicapped (VA) 405
Vision Center of Central Ohio (OH) 308
VISION Foundation (MA) 187
Vision Loss Resources (MN) 210
Vision Northwest (OR) 322
Vision Rehabilitation Inc. (OH) 309
VISIONS/Services for the Blind and Visually
  Impaired (NY) 277
Visual Impairment and Blindness Services of
  Northampton County, Inc. (VIABL) (PA) 346
Visually Handicapped Services/Detroit Receiving
  Hospital and University Health Center (MI) 200
Visually Impaired Center (MI) 200
Visually Impaired Persons of Southwest Florida (FL) 92
VITAL (Visually Impaired Training and Learning)
  Center (TN) 373
VITAL (Visually Impaired Training and Learning)
  Center of Nashville (TN) 373
Vocational Guidance Services (OH) 309
Volunteer Blind Industries (TN) 373
Volunteers for the Visually Handicapped (MD) 76, 174
Washington-Greene Blind Association (PA) 346
Welcome Home for the Blind (MI) 201
Westchester Independent Living Center, Inc. (NY) 277
Western Blind Rehabilitation Center/U.S. Department
  of Veterans Affairs (CA) 50

Westmoreland County Branch/Pennsylvania
  Association for the Blind (PA) 346
West Texas Lighthouse for the Blind (TX) 387
West Virginia Society for the Blind and Severely
  Disabled (WV) 421
Wichita Industries and Services for the Blind (KS) 152
Winston-Salem Industries for the Blind (NC) 291
Winston-Salem Industries for the Blind/Ashville
  Division (NC) 291
Wisconsin Council for the Blind (WI) 430
Wiscraft/Wisconsin Enterprises for the Blind (WI) 430
Workshops, Inc. (AL) 10
York County Blind Center (PA) 347
Yuma Center for the Visually Impaired (AZ) 23

COMPUTER TRAINING CENTERS

Addie McBryde Rehabilitation Center for the
  Blind (MS) 217
ADEC Resources for Independence (IN) 142
Affiliated Blind of Louisiana, Inc. (LA) 165
Arizona State Schools for the Deaf and the Blind (AZ) 23
Arkansas Division of Services for the Blind (AR) 29
Arkansas Technology Resource Center (AR) 29
Assistive Technology Center (RI) 355
Assistive Technology Clinics/The Childrens'
  Hospital (CO) 63
Assistive Technology Services/Kentucky Department
  for the Blind (KY) 159
Associated Services for the Blind (PA) 347
Association for the Blind and Visually Impaired
  (formerly Vision Enrichment Services) (MI) 201
Aurora of Central New York (NY) 278
Baruch College/Computer Center for Visually
  Impaired People (NY) 278
California School for the Blind (CA) 50
Center for Blind Adults (AK) 15
Center for Computer Assistance to the Disabled (TX) 387
Center for Independence (CO) 63
Center for the Blind and Visually Impaired (CA) 51
Central Blind Rehabilitation Center (IL) 131
Chicago Lighthouse for People Who Are Blind or
  Visually Impaired (IL) 131
Cincinnati Association for the Blind (OH) 309
CITE (Center for Independence, Technology and
  Education) (FL) 92
College of the Redwoods/High Tech Center (CA) 51
Colorado Easter Seal Society (CO) 63
Colorado Rehabilitation Center/Communications for
  the Visually Impaired (CO) 63
Colorado School for the Deaf and the Blind (CO) 63
Computer Access Laboratory/California State
  University, Students with Disabilities
  Resources (CA) 51

Computer Center for Citizens with Disabilities (UT).......... 394
Computers to Help People (WI).. 431
Connecticut State Board of Education and Services for
    the Blind (CT) 68
Crossroads Rehabilitation Center (IN) 142
Division for the Blind and Visually Impaired / Vermont
    Agency of Human Services (VT) 398
Division for the Visually Impaired / Delaware Health
    and Social Services (DE) 72
Division of Blind Services / Florida Department of
    Labor and Employment Security (FL) 92
Division of Rehabilitation Services / West Virginia
    Division of Rehabilitation Services (WV) 421
E.H. Gentry Technical Facility (AL)................................. 10
ENABLE (NY) 278
FACES Access Services (MN) 211
Finger Lakes Independent Center (NY)........................... 278
Florida Association of Workers for the Blind (FL) 92
Georgia Academy for the Blind (GA)............................. 106
Gillette Children's Hospital (MN) 211
Greater Pittsburgh Guild for the Blind (now known as
    Pittsburgh Vision Services) (PA)............................... 348
Helen Keller National Center for Deaf-Blind Youths
    and Adults (NY).. 278
Helen Keller Services for the Blind (NY) 278
Illinois Department of Rehabilitation Services / Bureau
    of Blind Services (IL) 131
Illinois School for the Visually Impaired (IL)................. 131
Independence for the Blind (FL) 93
Iowa Department for the Blind (IA)............................... 146
Kansas Rehabilitation Center for the Blind (KS)............ 153
Lavelle School for the Blind (NY) 278
League for the Blind and Disabled (IN).......................... 142
LIFT (NY).. 278
Lighthouse for the Blind of Fort Worth (TX).................. 387
Lighthouse for the Blind of the Palm Beaches (FL) 93
The Lighthouse Inc. (NY) 279
The Lighthouse Inc. / Hudson Valley (NY)...................... 279
Lighthouse of Houston (TX)... 387
Lions Center for the Blind (CA)....................................... 51
Low Vision Library / Kansas City Association for the
    Blind (MO).. 225
Maine Center for the Blind and Visually Impaired (ME) .. 169
Maryland Division of Vocational Rehabilitation
    Services (MD) 175
Maryland School for the Blind (MD) 175
Massachusetts State Commission for the Blind (MA)........ 188
Michigan Commission for the Blind Training
    Center (MI)... 201
Milwaukee Area Technical College (WI)......................... 431
Minnesota State Academy for the Blind (MN)................ 211
Mississippi School for the Blind (MS) 217

Missouri School for the Blind (MO)............................... 225
National Institute for Rehabilitation Engineering (NJ)...... 248
Nebraska Division of Rehabilitation Services for the
    Visually Impaired (NE) 235
Nebraska School for the Visually Handicapped (NE)........ 235
New Mexico School for the Visually
    Handicapped (NM).. 254
New York Institute for Special Education (NY) 279
North Carolina Rehabilitation Center for the
    Blind (NC) 291
Northcentral Technical College (WI) 431
Northeastern Association of the Blind (NY) 279
The Occupational Rehabilitation Group, Inc. (MA)......... 188
Ohio State School for the Blind (OH)............................. 309
Olympia Educational Service District 114 (WA) 414
Oregon Commission for the Blind (OR).......................... 322
Oregon School for the Blind (OR)................................... 322
Overbrook School for the Blind (PA).............................. 348
Palomar College (CA)... 51
Parents, Let's Unite for Kids (PLUK) (MT) 230
Parkview School (Oklahoma School for the Blind) (OK) .. 316
Project CABLE / Carroll Center for the Blind (MA) 188
Rhode Island Services for the Blind and Visually
    Impaired (RI) 356
Ruth Parker Eason School (MD) 175
Savannah Association for the Blind / Communications
    Department, Inc (GA)... 106
Services for the Blind and Visually Impaired / New
    Hampshire Division of Vocational
    Rehabilitation (NH)... 242
Service to the Visually Impaired / Business and
    Education Institute (SD)... 365
Sister Kenny Institute (MN)... 211
Southeastern Blind Rehabilitation Center (AL)................. 10
Special Education Technology Center (KS)...................... 153
Special Education Technology Center (WA)..................... 414
STORER Computer Access Center / Cleveland Sight
    Center of the Cleveland Society of the Blind (OH).......... 310
Tampa Lighthouse for the Blind (FL) 93
Technical Aids Center / New Jersey Commission for the
    Blind and Visually Impaired (NJ) 249
Technology Center / North Dakota School for the
    Blind (ND).. 296
Techspress / RCIL (NY) 279
Tennessee Rehabilitation Center (TN) 374
Tennessee School for the Blind (TN)............................... 374
Texas Commission for the Blind (TX)............................. 387
Texas School for the Blind and Visually Impaired (TX)..... 388
Tucson Association for the Blind and Visually
    Impaired (AZ).. 23
Virginia Rehabilitation Center for the Blind (VA)............ 405
Vision Center of Central Ohio (OH)............................... 310

Vision Loss Resources (MN) 211
Visually Handicapped Services/Detroit Receiving
    Hospital and University Health Center (MI)................. 201
Visually Impaired Center (MI) 202
Washington State School for the Blind/Technical
    Center for Blind and Visually Handicapped
    Students (WA).. 414
West Virginia Schools for the Deaf and the Blind (WV) 421
William Judson Center/San Antonio Lighthouse (TX)...... 388
Wisconsin School for the Visually Handicapped and
    Educational Services Center for the Visually
    Impaired (WI).. 431

DOG GUIDE SCHOOLS

Eye Dog Foundation for the Blind (CA)........................... 51
Eye of the Pacific Guide Dogs and Mobility Services,
    Inc. (HI).. 111
Fidelco Guide Dog Foundation (CT) 68
Guide Dog Foundation for the Blind, Inc. (NY) 279
Guide Dogs for the Blind (CA)....................................... 51
Guide Dogs for the Blind (OR)....................................... 323
Guide Dogs of America (CA).. 52
Guide Dogs of the Desert (CA)....................................... 52
Guiding Eyes for the Blind, Inc. (NY) 279
Kansas Specialty Dog Service (KS)................................ 153
Leader Dogs for the Blind (MI) 202
Pilot Dogs, Inc. (OH)... 310
Seeing Eye, Inc. (NJ)... 249
Southeastern Guide Dogs, Inc. (FL)............................... 93

♦ *Low Vision Services*

EYE CARE SOCIETIES

Alabama Academy of Ophthalmology (AL).................... 10
Alabama Optometric Association, Inc. (AL)................... 10
Alaska Optometric Association (AK).............................. 15
Alaska State Ophthalmological Society (AK)................. 15
Arizona Ophthalmological Society (AZ)........................ 23
Arizona Optometric Association (AZ)............................ 23
Arkansas Ophthalmological Society (AR)...................... 29
Arkansas Optometric Association (AR).......................... 29
California Association of Ophthalmology (CA).............. 52
California Optometric Association (CA)......................... 52
Colorado Ophthalmological Society (CO) 63
Colorado Optometric Association (CO)......................... 63
Connecticut Association of Optometrists (CT).............. 69
Connecticut Society of Eye Physicians (CT)................. 69
Delaware Academy of Ophthalmology/Delaware Eye
    Associates (DE) 72
Delaware Optometric Association, Inc. (DE)................. 72

Florida Optometric Association (FL)............................... 93
Florida Society of Ophthalmology (FL)........................... 93
Georgia Optometric Association (GA)............................. 106
Georgia Society of Ophthalmology (GA)........................ 106
Hawaii Ophthalmological Society (HI)............................ 111
Hawaii Optometric Association (HI)................................ 111
Idaho Optometric Association (ID)................................. 115
Idaho Society of Ophthalmology (ID) 115
Illinois Association of Ophthalmology (IL) 131
Illinois Optometric Association (IL)................................ 131
Indiana Academy of Ophthalmology (IN)....................... 142
Indiana Optometric Association (IN).............................. 142
Iowa Academy of Ophthalmology (IL)............................ 146
Iowa Optometric Association (IA)................................... 146
Kansas Optometric Association (KS)............................... 153
Kansas State Ophthalmological Society (KS)................... 153
Kentucky Academy of Eye Physicians and
    Surgeons (KY).. 159
Kentucky Optometric Association (KY).......................... 159
Louisiana Ophthalmological Association (LA) 165
Louisiana State Association of Optometrists (LA) 165
Maine Optometric Association, Inc. (ME)....................... 169
Maine Society of Eye Physicians and Surgeons (ME)........ 169
Maryland Optometric Association, Inc. (MD).................. 175
Maryland Society of Eye Physicians and
    Surgeons (MD)... 175
Massachusetts Society of Eye Physicians and
    Surgeons (MA)... 188
Massachusetts Society of Optometrists, Inc. (MA)........... 188
Michigan Ophthalmological Society (MI)........................ 202
Michigan Optometric Association (MI)............................ 202
Minnesota Academy of Ophthalmology (MN) 211
Minnesota Optometric Association (MN)......................... 211
Mississippi Eye, Ear, Nose, and Throat
    Association (MS).. 217
Mississippi Optometric Association, Inc. (MS)................ 217
Missouri Ophthalmological Society (IL).......................... 225
Missouri Optometric Association, Inc. (MO)................... 225
Montana Academy of Ophthalmology (MT) 230
Montana Optometric Association, Inc. (MT) 230
Nebraska Academy of Ophthalmology (NE) 235
Nebraska Optometric Association, Inc. (NE)................... 235
Nevada Ophthalmological Society (NV).......................... 239
Nevada Optometric Association, Inc. (NV)...................... 239
New Hampshire Optometric Association, Inc. (NH) 242
New Hampshire Society of Eye Physicians and
    Surgeons (NH)... 242
New Jersey Academy of Ophthalmology (NJ).................. 249
New Jersey Optometric Association (NJ)......................... 249
New Mexico Ophthalomological Society (NM)................ 254
New Mexico Optometric Association, Inc. (NM).............. 254
New York State Ophthalmological Society (NY)............... 280

New York State Optometric Association, Inc. (NY) 280
North Carolina Society of Eye Physicians and
    Surgeons (NC) 291
North Carolina State Optometric Society, Inc. (NC) 292
North Dakota Optometric Association, Inc. (ND) 296
North Dakota Society of Ophthalmology and
    Otolaryngology (ND) 296
Ohio Ophthalmological Society (OH) 310
Ohio Optometric Association, Inc. (OH) 310
Oklahoma Optometric Association (OK) 317
Oklahoma State Society of Eye Physicians and
    Surgeons (OK) 317
Optometric Society of the District of Columbia (MD) 76
Oregon Academy of Ophthalmology (OR) 323
Oregon Optometric Association (OR) 323
Pennsylvania Academy of Ophthalmology and
    Otolaryngology (PA) 348
Pennsylvania Optometric Association, Inc. (PA) 348
Puerto Rico Ophthalmological Society (PR) 353
Rhode Island Optometric Association (RI) 356
Rhode Island Society of Eye Physicians and
    Surgeons (RI) 356
South Carolina Optometric Association, Inc. (SC) 361
South Carolina Society of Ophthalmology (SC) 360
South Dakota Academy of Ophthalmology (MT) 365
South Dakota Optometric Society (SD) 365
Tennessee Academy of Ophthalmology (TN) 374
Tennessee Optometric Association, Inc. (TN) 374
Texas Ophthalmological Association (TX) 388
Texas Optometric Association, Inc. (TX) 388
Utah Ophthalmological Society (UT) 394
Utah Optometric Association (UT) 394
Vermont Ophthalmological Society (VT) 398
Vermont Optometric Association (VT) 398
Virginia Optometric Association (VA) 405
Virginia Society of Ophthalmology (VA) 405
Washington Academy of Eye Physicians and
    Surgeons (WA) 414
Washington Association of Optometric
    Physicians (WA) 414
Washington DC Ophthalmological Society (DC) 76
West Virginia Academy of Ophthalmology (WV) 421
West Virginia Optometric Association (WV) 422
Wisconsin Academy of Ophthalmology (IL) 431
Wisconsin Optometric Association, Inc. (WI) 431
Wyoming Ophthalmological Society (WY) 434
Wyoming Optometric Association (WY) 434

LOW VISION CENTERS

Asheville Lions Club Eye Clinic (NC) 292
Association for the Blind and Visually Impaired
    (formerly Vision Enrichment Services) (MI) 202

Association for the Blind and Visually Impaired of
    Greater Rochester, Inc. / Low Vision Clinic (NY) 280
Barnes Eye Clinic (MO) 225
Bascom Palmer Eye Institute / Anne Bates Leach Eye
    Hospital (FL) 93
Blind and Low Vision Services of North Georgia (GA) 106
Blind Association of Western New York (NY) 280
Boston Medical Center (MA) 188
Buffalo General Hospital / Wettlaufer Eye Clinic (NY) 280
Burns Clinic Medical Center / Low Vision Clinic (MI) 202
California Pacific Medical Center / Department of
    Ophthalmology / Low Vision Service (CA) 52
Camden Optometric Center (NJ) 249
Center for the Partially Sighted (CA) 53
Center for Vision Rehabilitation (PA) 348
Center for Visual Independence / Eye Foundation
    Hospital (AL) 10
Central Blind Rehabilitation Center (IL) 131
Chicago Lighthouse for People Who Are Blind or
    Visually Impaired (IL) 132
Children's Vision Rehabilitation Project / West Virginia
    University, Department of Ophthalmology (WV) 422
Cincinnati Association for the Blind (OH) 310
CITE (Center for Independence, Technology and
    Education) / Low Vision Screening and Education
    Clinic (FL) 94
Cleveland Sight Center of the Cleveland Society for the
    Blind (OH) 310
College of Optometry / Ferris State University (MI) 203
College of Optometry / Northeastern State
    University (OK) 317
Colorado Optometric Center / Low Vision Clinic (CO) 63
Columbia Lighthouse for the Blind / Ferd Nauheim
    Low Vision Clinic (DC) 76
Community Services for the Blind and Partially
    Sighted (WA) 414
Dallas Services for the Visually Impaired / Low Vision
    Clinic (TX) 388
Dean A. McGee Eye Institute (OK) 317
Deicke Center for Visual Rehabilitation (IL) 132
Detroit Institute of Ophthalmology / Low Vision
    Program / Friends of Vision (MI) 203
Devers Eye Institute (OR) 323
Duke University Eye Center / Duke University Medical
    Center (NC) 292
Eastern Blind Rehabilitation Center Eye Clinic (CT) 69
Eleanor E. Faye Low Vision Service / The Lighthouse
    Inc. (NY) 281
El Paso Lighthouse for the Blind / Low Vision
    Center (TX) 388
Erie County Medical Center (NY) 281
Erlanger Medical Center / Lions Low Vision
    Service (TN) 374

Eye and Ear Clinic (WA) 415

Eye Clinic/Grady Memorial Hospital (GA) 106

Eye Clinic, Children's Memorial Hospital (IL) 132

The Eye Institute/Pennsylvania College of
  Optometry/William Feinbloom Vision
  Rehabilitation Center (PA) 348

Eye Institute/St. Louis University (MO) 226

Eye Institute of New Jersey/University of Medicine
  and Dentistry (NJ) 249

Georgetown University Medical Center/Center for
  Sight (DC) 76

George Washington University Medical Center/
  Department of Ophthalmology (DC) 76

The Gerald E. Fonda, M.D., Low Vision Center of Saint
  Barnabas (NJ) 249

Greater Akron Low Vision Clinic (OH) 311

Greater Pittsburgh Guild for the Blind (PA) 349

Group Health Cooperative of Puget Sound (WA) 415

Halifax Hospital Medical Center Eye Clinic (FL) 94

Hope Haven Children's Clinic/Low Vision Clinic (FL) 94

Illinois Center for Rehabilitation and Education (IL) 133

Illinois Eye Institute/Illinois College of Optometry (IL) ... 133

Indianapolis Eye Care Center/Indiana University
  School of Optometry (IN) 142

IN-SIGHT (Rhode Island Association for the Blind) (RI) .. 356

Jewish Guild for the Blind/Home for Aged Blind/
  Kramer Vision Rehabilitation Center (NY) 281

Joslin Diabetes Center/William P. Beetham Eye
  Research and Treatment Unit (MA) 188

Jules Stein Eye Institute (CA) 53

Kansas City Veterans Affairs Medical Center/
  VICTORS Program (MO) 226

Kansas Eye Center/University of Kansas Medical
  Center/Low Vision Rehabilitation Service (KS) 153

Kentucky Clinic/University of Kentucky/Department
  of Ophthalmology (KY) 159

Kentucky Lions Eye Center, Low Vision Clinic/
  University of Louisville Department of
  Ophthalmology (KY) 159

King-Drew Medical Center (CA) 53

Kresge Eye Institute Low Vision Service (MI) 203

Lighthouse for the Blind of the Palm Beaches (FL) 94

Lighthouse of Houston/Low Vision Clinic (TX) 388

Lions Low Vision Clinic of the Inland Empire (WA) 415

Lions Vision Research and Rehabilitation Center/
  Wilmer Ophthalmological Institute (MD) 175

Lions World Services for the Blind (AR) 29

Liz Moore Low Vision Center (AL) 11

Long Island Jewish Medical Center/Eye Care
  Center (NY) 282

Louisiana State University Eye Center/Low Vision
  Clinic (LA) 165

Low Vision Center/Tampa Lighthouse for the
  Blind (FL) 95

Low Vision Clinic (LA) 165

Low Vision Clinic/Department of Ophthalmology,
  University of Iowa Hospitals and Clinics (IA) 146

Low Vision Clinic/Helen Keller Services for the Blind
  (HKSB) (NY) 282

Low Vision Clinic/Ho'opono Rehabilitation Center for
  the Blind and Visually Impaired (HI) 111

Low Vision Clinic/Nevada Bureau of Services to the
  Blind (NV) 239

Low Vision Clinic/University of California, San
  Francisco Eye Clinic (CA) 54

Low Vision Clinic/University of California School of
  Optometry (CA) 54

Low Vision Clinic/West Virginia University/
  Department of Ophthalmology (WV) 422

Low Vision Consultants (MI) 203

Low Vision/Contact Lens Service (IA) 146

Low Vision Facility of Boswell Eye Institute (AZ) 23

Low Vision Rehabilitation Center/Carroll Center for
  the Blind (MA) 189

Low Vision Rehabilitation Program/University of
  Missouri - Kansas City/Department of
  Ophthalmology (MO) 226

Low Vision Rehabilitation Service/University Station
  Clinics (WI) 431

Low Vision Service/The Lighthouse Inc. (NY) 282

Low Vision Service/Perkins School for the Blind (MA) 189

Low Vision Service/State University of New York/
  College of Optometry (NY) 283

Low Vision Service of Jessamine Optometric
  Association (KY) 159

Low Vision Services/The Lighthouse Inc. (NY) 283

Low Vision Services/Utah Division of Services for the
  Blind and Visually Impaired (UT) 394

Low Vision Services of Kentucky (KY) 160

Low Vision Unit/Hermann Eye Center (TX) 389

Loyola University Medical Center/Department of
  Ophthalmology (IL) 133

Marin Low Vision Clinic (CA) 54

Massachusetts Eye and Ear Infirmary/Vision
  Rehabilitation Services (MA) 189

Maxwell Low Vision Clinic/Center for the Visually
  Impaired (GA) 106

Mayo Clinic (MN) 211

Medical College of Georgia/Low Vision Clinic (GA) 107

Montana Low Vision Service, Inc. (MT) 230

Montefiore Hospital/Medical Center/Low Vision
  Service (NY) 283

Moore Eye Foundation (PA) 349

National Naval Medical Center/Ophthalmology
  Service (MD) 176

New England Eye Institute of the New England
  College of Optometry, Low Vision Clinic (MA) 190

New England Medical Center/New England Eye Center (MA) 190

New Hampshire Association for the Blind/Low Vision Program (NH) 242

New Mexico Commission for the Blind/Low Vision Clinic (NM) 254

New York Eye and Ear Infirmary (NY) 284

North Carolina Memorial Hospital/Low Vision Clinic (NC) 292

Northeastern Association of the Blind (NY) 284

Northeast Eye Institute (PA) 349

Northport Veterans Affairs Medical Center/Low Vision Clinic and VICTORS Program (NY) 284

North Shore University Hospital Low Vision Services (NY) 284

Northwestern Medical Faculty Foundation (IL) 133

Ohio State University College of Optometry/Low Vision Clinic (OH) 311

Ophthalmology Department/University of Nebraska Medical Center (NE) 235

Optometric Center of Los Angeles (CA) 54

Optometric Center of St. Louis (MO) 226

Oregon Health Sciences University/Department of Ophthalmology/Low Vision Aid Clinic (OR) 323

Pacific University/College of Optometry (OR) 323

Peninsula Center for the Blind and Visually Impaired (CA) 55

Porter Memorial Hospital/Porter Low Vision Service (CO) 64

Portland Family Vision Center (OR) 323

Programs for the Blind and Visually Impaired/ Wisconsin Division of Vocational Rehabilitation Low Vision Services (WI) 431

Raleigh Lions Clinic for the Blind/Evaluation Unit/ North Carolina Division of Services for the Blind (NC) 292

Rehabilitation Center Vision Rehabilitation Services (CT) 69

Richard E. Hoover Services for Low Vision and Blindness/Department of Ophthalmology/Greater Baltimore Medical Center (MD) 176

RP International/Low Vision (CA) 55

St. Joseph's Low Vision Services (AZ) 24

St. Louis Society for the Blind and Visually Impaired (MO) 227

St. Mary Low Vision Center (CA) 55

St. Paul-Ramsey Medical Center Low Vision Clinic (MN) 211

Santa Rosa Low Vision Clinic (TX) 389

Scheie Eye Institute Department of Ophthalmology/ University of Pennsylvania Health System/Low Vision Research and Rehabilitation Center (PA) 349

Schepens Retina Associates/Low Vision Rehabilitation Center (MA) 190

Scripps Memorial Hospital Mericos Eye Institute/ Partial Vision Center (CA) 55

Society for the Blind/Visual Services Center/Low Vision Clinic (CA) 56

South Carolina Commission for the Blind (SC) 361

South Carolina Commission for the Blind/Columbia Office (SC) 361

South Carolina Eye Institute/Department of Ophthalmology/University of South Carolina School of Medicine (SC) 361

South Dakota Low Vision Services/Service for the Blind and Visually Impaired (SD) 365

Southern California College of Optometry/Low Vision Clinic (CA) 56

Southern College of Optometry (TN) 374

Special Needs Vision Clinic (MI) 203

Stanford/Department of Ophthalmology, Low Vision Services (CA) 56

Temple University Hospital/Ophthalmology Department (PA) 350

Texas Tech University/School of Medicine/Health Sciences Center (TX) 389

Tulane Medical Center Hospital and Clinic (LA) 165

University Eye Institute/SUNY Health Science Center at Syracuse (NY) 285

University Medical Center/Department of Ophthalmology/John A. Moran Eye Center (UT) 395

University Medical Center, Department of Ophthalmology (MS) 217

University of Alabama at Birmingham/The Medical Center/School of Optometry/Low Vision Rehabilitation Clinic (AL) 11

University of Arkansas for Medical Sciences/ Department of Ophthalmology (AR) 30

University of California, Davis Department of Ophthalmology Low Vision Services (CA) 56

University of Florida/Eye Center, Low Vision Service (FL) 95

University of Maryland/Department of Ophthalmology/Low Vision Program (MD) 176

University of Minnesota/Department of Ophthalmology (MN) 212

University of Texas/Health Science Center at Dallas/ Department of Ophthalmology Low Vision Clinic (TX) 389

University of Texas, Health Science Center (TX) 390

Veterans Administration/West Side Medical Center/ VICTORS Program (IL) 134

Veterans Administration Center (WI) 432

Veterans Administration Hospital/Low Vision Service, Eye Clinic (FL) 95

Veterans Affairs Medical Center (CA) 56

Virginia Department for the Visually Handicapped (VA) 406

Virginia Optometric Center (VA) 406
Virginia Rehabilitation Center for the Blind (VA) 406
Vision Loss Resources (MN) 212
Vision Rehabilitation Center (KS) 154
Vision Rehabilitation Inc. (OH) 311
Vision Rehabilitation Institute / Genesis Medical
    Center (IA) 147
Vision Rehabilitation Institute, Sinai Hospital (MI) 204
Vision Rehabilitation Service / Wisconsin Council of the
    Blind (WI) 432
Visual Rehabilitation and Research Center of Southeast
    Michigan (MI) 204
Walter Reed Army Medical Center / Ophthalmology
    Service (DC) 76
Washington State School for the Blind (WA) 415
Washington University Eye Center / Department of
    Ophthalmology and Visual Sciences / Low Vision
    Service (MO) 227
Watts Health Foundation / United Health Plan (CA) 57
Western Blind Rehabilitation Center / U.S. Department
    of Veterans Affairs (CA) 57
Western Michigan University / Vision Rehabilitation
    Clinic (MI) 204
West Virginia Rehabilitation Center / Low Vision
    Clinic (WV) 422
White Station Lions Foundation (TN) 375
Wills Eye Hospital / Low Vision Service (PA) 350
W.K. Kellogg Eye Center / Low Vision Services /
    University of Michigan Medical Center (MI) 204

◆ *Aging Services*

STATE UNITS ON AGING

Aging and Adult Administration / Arizona Department
    of Economic Security (AZ) 24
Aging and Adult Services Administration / Washington
    State Department of Social and Health Services (WA) .. 415
Aging Services Division / North Dakota Department of
    Human Services (ND) 296
Aging Services Division / Oklahoma Department of
    Human Services (OK) 317
Board on Aging (MN) 212
Bureau of Aging / In-Home Services (IN) 143
Bureau of Aging / Wisconsin Division of Community
    Services (WI) 432
Bureau of Elder and Adult Services / Maine
    Department of Human Services (ME) 169
California Department of Aging (CA) 57
Commission on Aging (AL) 12
Commission on Aging (ID) 115
Commission on Aging (TN) 375
Connecticut Department of Social Services / Elderly
    Services Division (CT) 69

Council on Aging / Division of Aging and Adult
    Services (MS) 218
Department of Public Health and Human Services
    Office on Aging (MT) 231
Division for Aging Services / Nevada Department of
    Human Resources (NV) 239
Division of Aging (NC) 293
Division of Aging / Missouri Department of Social
    Services (MO) 227
Division of Aging and Adult Services / Arkansas
    Department of Human Services (AR) 30
Division of Aging and Adult Services / Colorado
    Department of Human Services (CO) 64
Division of Aging and Adult Services / Utah
    Department of Social Services (UT) 395
Division of Aging Services / Cabinet for Human
    Resources (KY) 160
Division of Elderly and Adult Services / New
    Hampshire Department of Health and Human
    Services (NH) 243
Division of Senior Citizens / Guam Department of
    Public Health and Social Services (GU) 108
Division of Senior Services / Alaska Department of
    Administration (AK) 15
Division of Services for Aging and Adults with
    Physical Disabilities / Delaware Department of
    Health and Social Services (DE) 72
Division on Aging (WY) 434
Division on Aging / New Jersey Department of
    Community Affairs (NJ) 250
Executive Office of Elder Affairs (MA) 190
Executive Office on Aging / Office of the Governor (HI) 112
Florida Department of Elder Affairs (FL) 95
Governor's Office for Elderly Affairs (PR) 353
Illinois Department on Aging (IL) 134
Iowa Department of Elder Affairs (IA) 147
Kansas Department on Aging (KS) 154
Nebraska Department on Aging (NE) 236
Office for the Aging (NY) 285
Office of Adult Services and Aging (SD) 365
Office of Aging (GA) 107
Office of Aging (WV) 422
Office of Elderly Affairs (LA) 166
Office of Services to the Aging (MI) 205
Office on Aging (DC) 77
Office on Aging (MD) 177
Ohio Department of Aging (OH) 311
Pennsylvania Department of Aging (PA) 350
Rhode Island Department of Elderly Affairs (RI) 356
Senior and Disabled Services Division (OR) 324
Senior Citizen Affairs / Virgin Islands Department of
    Human Services (VI) 408
South Carolina Commission on Aging (SC) 361

State Agency on Aging (NM)...................................... 254
Texas Department on Aging (TX)............................... 390
Vermont Department of Aging and Disabilities (VT) 398
Virginia Department for the Aging (VA)..................... 406

INDEPENDENT LIVING PROGRAMS

Bureau of Vocational Rehabilitation/New Hampshire
Department of Education (NH) 243
Commission for the Blind/Family Independence
Agency (MI).. 205
Connecticut Board of Education and Services for the
Blind (CT) 69
Department of Human Resources/Division of Services
for the Blind (NC)... 293
Department of Public Health and Human Services/
Blind and Low Vision Services (MT)........................ 231
Department of Rehabilitation Services (AL)................. 12
Department of Social Services/New York State
Commission for the Blind and Visually
Handicapped (NY).. 285
District of Columbia Department of Human
Services (DC) 77
Division for the Blind and Visually Impaired/Bureau
of Rehabilitation Services/Department of
Labor (ME).. 169
Division for the Blind and Visually Impaired/Vermont
Agency of Human Services (VT)............................... 398
Division for the Visually Impaired/Delaware
Department of Health and Social Services (DE)........ 72
Division of Services for the Blind/Arkansas
Department of Human Services (AR)......................... 30
Division of Service to the Blind and Visually
Impaired/South Dakota Department of Human
Services (SD) 366
Division of Supportive Living/Wisconsin Department
of Health and Family Services (WI).......................... 432
Division of Vocational Rehabilitation (AK).................. 15
Division of Vocational Rehabilitation/Hawaii
Department of Human Services (HI).......................... 112
Division of Vocational Rehabilitation/Wyoming
Department of Employment (WY)............................. 434
Family and Social Services Administration/Disability,
Aging and Rehabilitation Services (IN) 143
Florida Division of Blind Services (FL)........................ 96
Georgia Department of Human Resources/Division of
Rehabilitation Services (GA).................................... 107
Guam Department of Vocational Rehabilitation (GU) 108
Idaho Commission for the Blind and Visually
Impaired (ID)... 116
Illinois Department of Rehabilitation Services (IL)....... 134
Iowa Department for the Blind (IA)............................ 147
Kentucky Department for the Blind (KY).................... 160

Louisiana Rehabilitation Services/Department of
Social Services (LA) 166
Maryland Division of Vocational Rehabilitation
Services (MD) 177
Massachusetts Commission for the Blind (MA) 191
Minnesota Services for the Blind/Career and
Independent Living Services (MN)........................... 212
New Jersey Commission for the Blind and Visually
Impaired (NJ)... 250
New Mexico Commission for the Blind (NM) 254
North Dakota Department of Human Services (ND)......... 296
Office of Vocational Rehabilitation for the Blind/
Mississippi Department of Rehabilitation
Services (MS).. 218
Oregon Commission for the Blind (OR)...................... 324
Pennsylvania Department of Public Welfare (PA) 350
Rehabilitation Center for the Blind/Kansas
Department of Social Services (KS) 154
Rehabilitation Division/Nevada Department of
Human Resources (NV).. 239
Rehabilitation Services/Colorado Department of
Human Services (CO) 64
Rehabilitation Services Administration/Arizona
Department of Economic Security (AZ)...................... 24
Rehabilitation Services Commission/Bureau of
Services for the Visually Impaired (OH)................... 312
Rehabilitation Services for the Visually Impaired/
Nebraska Department of Public Institutions (NE).......... 236
Rhode Island Services for the Blind and Visually
Impaired/Rhode Island Department of Human
Services (RI)... 356
Services for the Blind/California Department of
Rehabilitation (CA).. 57
South Carolina Commission for the Blind (SC).......... 361
State Department of Rehabilitation/Visual Services
Division (OK) 317
Tennessee Department of Human Services/Division of
Rehabilitation Services (TN) 375
Texas Commission for the Blind (TX)......................... 390
Utah State Office of Rehabilitation (UT) 395
Virginia Department for the Visually Handicapped/
Services Division (VA).. 406
Virgin Islands Department of Human Services (VI) 408
Washington Department of Services for the Blind (WA) .. 416
West Virginia Division of Rehabilitation Services (WV) ... 422

♦ *Federal Agencies*

AMERICANS WITH DISABILITIES ACT AGENCIES

Architectural and Transportation Barriers Compliance
Board (DC).. 465

Equal Employment Opportunity Commission (DC) 465

Federal Transit Administration (DC) 465

National Institute on Disability and Rehabilitation
Research (DC) 465

U.S. DEPARTMENT OF EDUCATION

Assistant Secretary for Special Education and
Rehabilitative Services (DC) 466

Division of Blind and Visually Impaired (DC) 466

National Council on Disability (DC) 466

National Institute on Disability and Rehabilitation
Research (DC) 466

Office of Special Education Programs (DC) 466

Rehabilitation Services Administration (RSA) (DC) 466

U.S. Department of Education/Office of the
Secretary (DC) 465

U.S. DEPARTMENT OF HEALTH AND HUMAN SERVICES

Administration for Children and Families (DC) 467

Administration for Children, Youth, and Families (DC) ... 467

Administration on Aging (DC) 467

Health Care Financing Administration (DC) 467

Health Resources and Services Administration/Bureau
of Health Professions (MD) 467

Health Services Administration/Bureau for Maternal
and Child Health/Health Care Resources
Department (MD) 467

National Center for Health Statistics (MD) 468

National Institutes of Health/National Eye Institute
Information Center (MD) 468

National Institutes of Health/National Institute on
Aging (MD) 468

Social Security Administration (MD) 468

U.S. Department of Health and Human Services/Office
of the Secretary (DC) 467

U.S. DEPARTMENT OF LABOR

Employment Standards Administration/National
Office Program Administration (DC) 468

Office of Federal Contract Compliance Programs (DC) 468

U.S. Department of Labor/Office of the Secretary (DC) 468

U.S. Employment Service (DC) 468

U.S. DEPARTMENT OF TRANSPORTATION

Federal Transit Administration (DC) 468

U.S. Department of Transportation/Office of the
Secretary (DC) 468

U.S. DEPARTMENT OF VETERANS AFFAIRS

Blind Rehabilitation Service (DC) 469

U.S. Department of Veterans Affairs/Office of the
Secretary (DC) 469

Veterans Benefits Administration (VBA) (DC) 469

Veterans Health Administration (VHA) (DC) 469

OTHER AGENCIES

Architectural and Transportation Barriers Compliance
Board (DC) 470

Committee for Purchase from the Blind and Other
Severely Handicapped (VA) 470

Equal Employment Opportunity Commission (DC) 470

Library of Congress National Library Service for the
Blind and Physically Handicapped (DC) 470

President's Committee on Employment of People with
Disabilities (DC) 470

Small Business Administration (DC) 470

U.S. Department of Justice/Civil Rights Division/
Coordination and Review Section (DC) 471

U.S. Office of Personnel Management/Office of Human
Resources and Equal Employment (DC) 471

◆ *National Organizations*

American Diabetes Association/National Center (VA) 472

American Foundation for the Blind (NY) 472

American Society for Contemporary
Ophthalmology (IL) 473

AWARE (Associates for World Action in Rehabilitation
and Education) (NY) 473

Better Vision Institute/Vision Council of America (VA) .. 473

Blind Children's Fund (MI) 473

Blind Outdoor Leisure Development (CO) 473

Braille Authority of North America (BANA) (PA) 473

DB-LINK: The National Information Clearinghouse on
Children Who Are Deaf-Blind (OR) 474

Delta Gamma Foundation (OH) 474

Eye Bank Association of America (DC) 474

Eye Bank for Sight Restoration (NY) 474

Fight for Sight (NY) 474

The Foundation Fighting Blindness (National Retinitis
Pigmentosa Foundation Inc.) (MD) 475

4-Sights Network/Upshaw Institute for the Blind (MI) 472

The Glaucoma Foundation (NY) 475

Glaucoma Research Foundation (CA) 475

Governmental Relations Group/American Foundation
for the Blind (DC) 475

Hadley School for the Blind (IL) 475

Helen Keller International (NY) 476

Helen Keller National Center for Deaf-Blind Youths
and Adults (NY) 476

Hilton/Perkins Program/Perkins School for the
Blind (MA) 477

International Society on Metabolic Eye Disease (NY) 477

IN TOUCH Networks (NY) 478

Joint Commission on Allied Health Personnel in
Ophthalmology (MN) 478

Joslin Diabetes Center (MA) 478

Knights Templar Eye Foundation (IL) 478

The Lighthouse Inc. (NY) 478

Lions Clubs International (IL) 478

March of Dimes Birth Defects Foundation (NY) 479

Myasthenia Gravis Foundation (IL) 479

Myopia International Research Foundation (NY) 479

National Accreditation Council for Agencies Serving
the Blind and Visually Handicapped (NY) 479

National Association for Visually Handicapped (NY) 479

National Association of Area Agencies on Aging (DC) 480

National Association of Radio Reading Services (SC) 480

National Association of State Units on Aging (DC) 480

National Birth Defects Center (MA) 480

National Camps for Blind Children (NE) 481

National Council of Private Agencies for the
Blind (MA) 481

National Early Childhood Technical Assistance System
(NEC*TAS) (NC) 481

National Easter Seals Society (IL) 481

National Eye Care Project (NECP) (CA) 481

National Eye Research Foundation (Optometry) (IL) 482

National Glaucoma Research Program of the American
Health Assistance Foundation (MD) 482

National Industries for the Blind (VA) 482

National Information Center for Children and Youth
with Disabilities (DC) 482

National Multiple Sclerosis Society (NY) 483

National Self-Help Clearinghouse (NY) 483

New Eyes for the Needy (NJ) 483

NTAC (National Technical Assistance Consortium for
Children and Young Adults who are Deaf-Blind)/
Teaching Research Division (OR) 483

Orbis International (NY) 483

Overbrook International/Overbrook School for the
Blind (PA) 484

Prevent Blindness America (IL) 484

Research to Prevent Blindness (NY) 484

Schepens Eye Research Institute (MA) 485

Smith-Kettlewell Eye Research Institute/Rehabilitation
Engineering Center (CA) 485

Taping for the Blind (TX) 485

United Cerebral Palsy (DC) 485

United States Braille Chess Foundation (OH) 485

◆ Membership Organizations

Affiliated Leadership League of and for the Blind of
America (DC) 487

American Academy of Ophthalmology (CA) 487

American Association for Pediatric Ophthalmology
and Strabismus (CA) 487

American Association for the Deaf-Blind (MD) 487

American Association of Certified Orthoptists (FL) 487

American Association of Retired Persons/Disability
Initiative (DC) 487

American Blind Bowling Association (PA) 487

American Blind Lawyers Association (MS) 488

American Blind Skiing Foundation (IL) 488

American Council of the Blind (DC) 488

American Council on Rural Special Education
(ACRES) (UT) 488

American Optometric Association (MO) 488

American Society of Cataract and Refractive
Surgery (VA) 489

American Society of Ophthalmic Registered
Nurses (CA) 489

Association for Education and Rehabilitation of the
Blind and Visually Impaired (VA) 489

Association for Macular Diseases (NY) 489

The Association for Persons with Severe Handicaps
(TASH) (MD) 489

Association of Junior Leagues (NY) 489

Association of Visual Science Librarians (IN) 490

Association on Higher Education and Disability
(AHEAD) (OH) 490

Blinded Veterans Association (DC) 490

Contact Lens Association of Ophthalmologists (LA) 490

Council for Exceptional Children (VA) 491

Council of Citizens with Low Vision International (DC) .. 491

Council of Families with Visual Impairment (DC) 491

Council of Schools for the Blind (NJ) 491

Guide Dog Users (MD) 491

Independent Visually Impaired Enterprises (DC) 491

Laurence-Moon Bardet-Biedl Syndrome Self-Help
Support Network (MD) 491

National Association for Parents of the Visually
Impaired (MA) 492

National Association of Blind Teachers (DC) 492

National Association of State Directors of Special
Education (VA) 492

National Association of Vision Professionals (DC) 492

National Coalition on Deaf-Blindness (MA) 492

National Council of State Agencies for the Blind (DC) 492

National Federation of the Blind (MD) 493

National Marfan Foundation (NY)......................... 493

National Organization for Albinism and
  Hypopigmentation (NOAH) (PA) 493

Opticians Association of America (VA)................ 493

Randolph-Sheppard Vendors of America (LA)...... 494

RESNA (VA) 494

United States Association for Blind Athletes (CO)...... 494

United States Blind Golfers Association (FL)............ 494

◆ *Producers of Media*

MEDIA PRODUCERS AND PUBLISHERS

American Action Fund for Blind Children and
  Adults (CA) 507

American Bible Society (NY)................................. 507

American Foundation for the Blind (NY)............... 507

American Printing House for the Blind, Inc. (KY) 507

Associated Services for the Blind (PA).................. 507

Audio Studio for the Reading Impaired (KY)........... 508

Austin Junior Women's Federation (TX) 508

Bantam-Doubleday-Dell (NY)............................. 508

Beach Cities Braille Guild (CA)........................... 508

Bible Alliance (FL) 508

Blindskills, Inc. (OR) 508

Books Aloud (CA) 508

Braille Communication Services (MI).................... 509

Braille Inc. (MA).. 509

Braille International (FL) 509

Chivers North America (NH) 509

Choice Magazine Listening (NY)........................... 509

Christian Education for the Blind (TX) 509

Christian Mission for the Blind (IN) 509

Christian Record Services (NE) 510

Christian Science Publishing Society (MA)............ 510

Church of Jesus Christ of Latter-Day Saints/Special
  Curriculum (UT).. 510

Cleveland Sight Center of the Cleveland Society for the
  Blind (OH) 510

The Clovernook Center/Opportunities for the
  Blind (OH) 510

Contra Costa Braille Transcribers (CA) 510

Deaf-Blind Program/The National Academy,
  Gallaudet University (DC) 510

ELCA (Evangelical Lutheran Church in America)/
  Braille and Tape Service (MN) 511

G.K. Hall and Company/Simon and Schuster (NJ)..... 511

Gospel Association for the Blind (FL)..................... 511

Grey House Publishing Company (CT) 511

HarperCollins Publishers (NY)............................. 511

Helen Keller Services for the Blind/Braille
  Library (NY) 511

Herald House (MO)... 511

Howe Press of Perkins School for the Blind (MA) 511

Isis Large Print Books/Transaction Publishers (NJ) 511

Jewish Braille Institute of America (NY)............... 512

Jewish Guild for the Blind (The Guild) (NY)......... 512

John Milton Society for the Blind (NY) 512

Library Reproduction Service (CA) 512

Lutheran Braille Evangelism Association (MN) 512

Lutheran Braille Workers (CA) 512

Lutheran Library for the Blind (MO)..................... 513

Matilda Ziegler Magazine for the Blind (NY) 513

Metrolina Association for the Blind (NC) 513

Michigan Braille Transcribing Service (MI)............ 513

Monterey County Braille Transcribers (CA)........... 513

MSMT Braille Center (CA) 513

National Association for Visually Handicapped (NY)...... 513

National Association to Promote the Use of
  Braille (KY) 514

National Braille Association (NY).......................... 514

National Braille Press (MA) 514

Northern Nevada Braille Transcribers (NV) 514

Print Access Center/The Lighthouse Inc. (NY)....... 514

Prose & Cons Braille Unit (NE) 514

Random House Large Print (NY) 515

Recording for the Blind and Dyslexic (NJ)............. 515

Resources for Rehabilitation (MA)........................ 515

St. Martin's Press (NY) 515

Seedlings: Braille Books for Children (MI)............. 515

Services to the Blind/Reorganized Church of Jesus
  Christ of Latter-Day Saints (MO)....................... 515

Sight Line Productions (MA)................................ 515

Simon & Schuster Publishing (NJ)........................ 516

Theosophical Book Association for the Blind (CA)...... 516

Thorndike Press (MI).. 516

Ulverscroft Large Print Books Limited (NY)........... 516

Visual Aid Volunteers, Inc. (TX) 516

Volunteer Braille Services (MN)........................... 516

Volunteer Braillists and Tapists (WI) 516

Volunteers of Vacaville (CA)................................ 516

Volunteer Transcribing Services (CA).................... 517

Wheeler Publishing, Inc. (MA)............................. 517

Xavier Society for the Blind (NY) 517

Zondervan Publishing House (MI) 517

AUDIODESCRIPTION SERVICES

Audio Description/Metropolitan Washington
  Ear (MD) 517

Audio Optics, Inc. (NJ)....................................... 517

Audio Vision (CA) 517

Descriptive Video Service/WGBH-TV (MA) 517

Narrative Television Network (OK)........................ 517

National Academy of Audio Description/RP International (CA)..................518

◆ *Sources of Products*

MAIL ORDER, CATALOGS, AND DISTRIBUTORS

American Printing House for the Blind (KY) 519
Ann Morris Enterprises Inc. (NY)..................519
Automagic Corporation (CA)..................519
Carolyn's (FL)..................519
Enabling Technologies Company (FL)..................519
Enhanced Vision Systems, Inc. (CA) 519
Environmental Lighting, Inc (FL)..................519
Independent Living Aids, Inc. (NY)..................519
The Lighthouse Inc. (NY) 519
LS&S Group, Inc. (IL)..................519
Maddak, Inc. (NJ)..................519
Massachusetts Association for the Blind/The Store (MA)..................519
Maxi-Aids (NY)..................519
Mid-Michigan Center for the Blind (MI)..................519
National Federation of the Blind (MD)..................519
Rose Resnick Lighthouse for the Blind and Visually Impaired (CA)..................519
Science Products (PA)..................519
Visionics Corporation Inc. (MN)..................520

HOUSEHOLD, PERSONAL, AND INDEPENDENT LIVING PRODUCTS

Adaptive Living Institute (AZ)..................520
Ann Morris Enterprises Inc. (NY)..................520
Autofold, Inc. (MA)..................520
Braille Greeting Cards (OH)..................520
Fotofonics (GA)..................520
Gladys Loeb Foundation (MD)..................520
Howe Press of Perkins School for the Blind (MA)..................520
Innovative Rehabilitation Technology (CA) 520
Kentucky Industries for the Blind (KY)..................520
The Lighthouse Inc./Lighthouse Enterprises (NY)..................520
LS&S Group, Inc. (IL)..................520
Lucent/ACPC (MO)..................520
Maddak, Inc. (NJ)..................520
Massachusetts Association for the Blind/The Store (MA)..................520
Mattel Consumer Affairs/Mattel Toys (CA)..................520
Maxi-Aids (NY)..................520
Mid-Michigan Center for the Blind (MI)..................520
National Association for Visually Handicapped (NY)..................520
National Federation of the Blind (MD)..................520

Nurion Industries (PA)..................521
Phillip Barton Vision Systems (MD)..................521
Precision Grinding & Manufacturing (MD)..................521
Prophecy Designs (MA)..................521
Rainshine Company (WI)..................521
Rose Resnick Lighthouse for the Blind and Visually Impaired (CA)..................521
Rubbermaid Health Care Products (VA)..................521
Sears, Roebuck and Company/New Account Center (TN)..................521
Spectrum, The Lighthouse Store (NY)..................521
Technology for Independence (MA)..................521
Whirlpool Corporation/Appliance Information Services (MI)..................521
White Cane Institute for the Blind (MO)..................521
Wildlife Materials, Inc. (IL)..................521

LOW VISION

Audio Visual Marts (LA)..................521
Automagic Corporation (CA)..................521
Bausch & Lomb Company (NY)..................521
Bernell Corporation (IN)..................521
Big Eye Lamps, Inc. (NJ)..................521
Bossert Specialties, Inc./Magnification Center (AZ)..................521
Celexx Trading Company, Inc. (MI)..................521
Charles Nusinov and Sons, Inc. (MD)..................521
Coburn Optical Industries, Inc. (OK)..................522
Contact East, Inc. (MA)..................522
Dazor Manufacturing Corporation (MO)..................522
Deluxe Check Printers, Inc. (MN)..................522
Designs for Vision, Inc. (NY)..................522
Electronic Visual Aid Specialists (RI)..................522
Eschenbach Optik of America (CT)..................522
Exceptional Teaching Aids (CA)..................522
Fishburne Enterprises (CA)..................522
Florida New Concepts Marketing (FL)..................522
4X Products, Inc (NY) 521
Fred Sammons, Inc. (IL)..................522
General Electric (KY)..................522
Gladys Loeb Foundation (MD)..................522
Hexagon Products (IL)..................522
Honeywell Residential Controls (MN)..................522
HumanWare, Inc. (CA)..................522
Innoventions, Inc. (CO)..................522
Jesana Ltd. (NY)..................522
J P Trading, Inc. (CA)..................522
Keeler Instruments, Inc. (PA)..................522
The Lighthouse Inc./Lighthouse Enterprises (NY)..................523
LS&S Group, Inc. (IL)..................523
Luxo Corporation (NY) 523
Magnisight (CO)..................523

Maitland Vision Center (FL) 523

Massachusetts Association for the Blind/The
Store (MA) 523

Mattingly International, Inc. (CA) 523

Maxi-Aids (NY) 523

McLeod Optical, Inc. (RI) 523

Mons International (GA) 523

M-Tech Optics Corporation (MI) 523

National Association for Visually Handicapped (NY) 523

National Federation of the Blind (MD) 523

National Pen Corporation (TN) 523

New Concepts Marketing, Inc. (FL) 523

Ocutech, Inc. (NC) 523

Okay Vision-Aide Corporation (CA) 523

Overseer Electronic Visual Aids (MN) 523

Pencar Associates (NY) 523

Phillip Barton Vision Systems (MD) 523

Prodigy Products Company (OH) 523

PulseData International, Inc. (GA) 523

Reed EZ-Reader, Inc. (MD) 524

Reflection Technology (MA) 524

Replogle Globes, Inc. (IL) 524

Science Products (PA) 524

Sears, Roebuck and Company/New Account
Center (TN) 524

Seemore Vision Products (NY) 524

Sped Publications (CO) 524

Stocker and Yale, Inc. (NH) 524

Strieter Laboratories, Inc. (IL) 524

S. Walters, Inc. (CA) 524

Tagarno of America, Inc. (DE) 524

Talking and Visual Aids (MI) 524

Tekvision Products (CA) 524

TeleSensory Corporation (CA) 524

Typewriting Institute for the Handicapped (AZ) 524

Universal Low Vision Aids (OH) 524

Vision Technology, Inc. (MO) 524

Visual Methods, Inc. (NJ) 524

Winco Optical Inc. (PA) 524

Xerox Adaptive Products (MA) 524

COMPUTER HARDWARE

Acrontech International, Inc. (NY) 524

Adaptec Systems (TX) 525

AICOM Corporation (CA) 525

A.I. Kurzweil, Inc. (MA) 525

American Thermoform Corporation (CA) 525

Ann Morris Enterprises Inc. (NY) 525

Apple Computer, Inc. (CA) 525

Arkenstone, Inc. (CA) 525

Artic Technologies (MI) 525

Automated Functions, Inc. (VA) 525

Blazie Engineering (MD) 525

Braille Sterling/Christiansen Studios (NH) 525

Centigram Communications Corporation (CA) 525

ComputAbility Corporation (WI) 525

Cotrax Consumer Products Group (MI) 525

C TECH (NY) 525

Don Johnston Developmental Equipment (IL) 525

Dragon Systems, Inc. (MA) 525

Echo (CA) 525

Edmark (WA) 525

Electronic Learning Systems (FL) 525

Electronic Visual Aid Specialists (RI) 525

Enabling Technologies Company (FL) 525

First Byte Inc. (CA) 526

Health Science (NJ) 526

Henter-Joyce, Inc. (FL) 526

Hooleon Corporation (AZ) 526

HumanWare, Inc. (CA) 526

Hy-Tek Manufacturing CO. (IL) 526

IBM Special Needs Systems (TX) 526

Innovative Rehabilitation Technology (CA) 526

Institute on Applied Technology/Children's Hospital
of Boston (MA) 526

IntelliTools (CA) 526

Intex Micro Systems Corporation (MI) 526

Kinetic Designs, Inc. (WA) 526

Kurzweil Educational Systems (MA) 526

Maxi-Aids (NY) 526

OMS Development (IL) 526

Optelec (MA) 526

Personal Data Systems, Inc. (CA) 526

Personal Interface (CO) 526

Phillip Barton Vision Systems (MD) 526

Prodigy Products Company (OH) 526

R.C. Systems, Inc. (WA) 526

Reflection Technology (MA) 527

Royal Data Systems/Speech and Learning Center
Systems (NC) 527

Schamex Research (CA) 527

Science Products (PA) 527

Scientific Capital Corporation (FL) 527

Talking Computer Systems (MA) 527

Talktronics, Inc. (CA) 527

Technologies for the Visually Impaired, Inc. (NY) 527

TeleSensory Corporation (CA) 527

T.S. Microtech, Inc. (CA) 527

Western Center for Microcomputers (CA) 527

Words Plus, Inc. (CA) 527

Xerox Imaging Systems (MA) 527

Zygo Industries, Inc. (OR) 527

COMPUTER SOFTWARE

Access-Ability Systems (IL) 527
Adaptec Systems (TX) 527
Ai Squared (VT) 527
Alva Access (CA) 527
American Printing House for the Blind (KY) 527
Andromina, Inc. (VA) 527
Apple Computer, Inc. (CA) 527
Apple Talk (AR) 528
Aquarius Instructional (FL) 528
Aristo Computer, Inc. (OR) 528
Arkenstone, Inc. (CA) 528
Artic Technologies (MI) 528
Arts Computer Products, Inc. (MA) 528
Automagic Corporation (CA) 528
Automated Functions, Inc. (VA) 528
Blazie Engineering (MD) 528
Bobcat Computer Applications (KS) 528
Borland International (CA) 528
Boston Educational Computing, Inc. (MA) 528
Braille Sterling / Christiansen Studios (NH) 528
Castle Special Computer Services (NM) 528
Comp Tech Systems Design (MN) 528
ComputAbility Corporation (WI) 528
Cornucopia Software, Inc. (CA) 528
Cross Educational Software (LA) 528
Data Transforms (CO) 528
Digital Equipment Corporation (NH) 528
Don Johnston Developmental Equipment (IL) 528
Dunamis, Inc. (GA) 528
Duxbury Systems, Inc. (MA) 528
Electronic Learning Systems (FL) 529
Enabling Technologies Company (FL) 529
E.V.A.S. (RI) 529
Exceptional Teaching Aids (CA) 529
FDLRS (FL) 529
First Byte Inc. (CA) 529
Flexible Software / Laird Communications (MA) 529
GW Micro (IN) 529
Harbor Computing Services (WA) 529
Hartley Courseware, Inc. (CA) 529
Henter-Joyce, Inc. (FL) 529
Hexagon Products (IL) 529
HFK Software, Inc. (MA) 529
HumanWare, Inc. (CA) 529
IBM Special Needs Systems (TX) 529
Innovative Rehabilitation Technology (CA) 529
Intelligent Info Technologies Corporation (IL) 529
Interface Systems International (OR) 529
Kidsview Software, Inc. (NH) 529
Kinetic Designs, Inc. (WA) 529

Laureate Learning Systems, Inc. (VT) 529
Life Science Associates (NY) 529
Lorin Software (GA) 529
Marblesoft (MN) 530
Microsystems Software, Inc. (MA) 530
MicroTalk Software (TX) 530
Mirage Multimedia Systems, Inc. (CA) 530
Myna Corporation (MA) 530
National Institute for Rehabilitation Engineering (NJ) 530
Omnichron (CA) 530
OMS Development (IL) 530
One on One Computer Training (IL) 530
Optelec (MA) 530
PC-SIG (CA) 530
Peal Software, Inc. (CA) 530
Peripheral Technologies, Inc. (PA) 530
Personal Interface (CO) 530
Phillip Barton Vision Systems (MD) 530
Productivity Software International (NY) 530
The Productivity Works (NJ) 530
Raised Dot Computing, Inc. (WI) 530
R.C. Systems, Inc. (WA) 530
Replogle Globes, Inc. (IL) 530
Roundley Associates (MD) 530
Royal Data Systems / Speech and Learning Center
    Systems (NC) 530
Scholastic, Inc. (MO) 530
Seemore Vision Products (NY) 530
SkiSoft, Inc. (MA) 531
Soft Key International (MN) 531
Spies Laboratories (CA) 531
Stat Talk Computer Products (NJ) 531
Syn-Talk Systems and Services (CA) 531
Talking and Visual Aids (MI) 531
Talking Computer Products (KS) 531
Talking Computers, Inc. (VA) 531
Talking Computer Systems (MA) 531
Tandy / Radio Shack (TX) 531
Technologies for the Visually Impaired, Inc. (NY) 531
TeleSensory Corporation (CA) 531
Texas Instruments (TX) 531
T.F.I. Engineering, Inc. (MA) 531
Traxler Enterprises (WI) 531
Turbo Power (CO) 531
The Voice Connection (CA) 531
Worthington Data Solutions (CA) 531

BRAILLE AND OTHER LITERACY MATERIALS

Advanced Access Devices (CA) 531

American Printing House for the Blind (KY) 531
American Thermoform Corporation (CA) 531
Esselte Pendaflex Corporation (NY) 532
Fishburne Enterprises (CA) 532
General Electric (KY) 532
Howe Press of Perkins School for the Blind (MA) 532
HumanWare, Inc. (CA) 532
Learning Express (AR) 532
Mattel Consumer Affairs / Mattel Toys (CA) 532
Mid-Michigan Center for the Blind (MI) 532
National Federation of the Blind (MD) 532
Rose Resnick Lighthouse for the Blind and Visually
   Impaired (CA) 532
Sighted Electronics (NJ) 532

MEDICAL PRODUCTS

American Medical Alert Corporation (NY) 532
Andros Analyzers, Inc. (CA) 532
Becton-Dickinson (NJ) 532
Bentham International (FL) 532
Boehringer Mannheim Diagnostics (IN) 532
Conney Safety Products (WI) 532
Home Diagnostics, Inc. (FL) 532
Independent Living Aids, Inc. (NY) 532
LS&S Group, Inc. (IL) 532
Medical Monitoring System, Inc. (WI) 532
National Federation of the Blind (MD) 532
Palco Labs (CA) 532
Sears, Roebuck and Company / New Account
   Center (TN) 533
Tandy / Radio Shack (TX) 533

PRODUCTS FOR DEAF-BLIND/MULTIPLY DISABLED PERSONS

Beltone Hearing Aid Service (MA) 533
Canon, U.S.A., Inc. (NY) 533
Comp Tech Systems Design (MN) 533
Digital Equipment Corporation (NH) 533
Don Johnston Developmental Equipment (IL) 533
Dunamis, Inc. (GA) 533
Enable / Schneier Communication Unit (NY) 533
Fotofonics (GA) 533
Fred Sammons, Inc. (IL) 533
Haskill Hearing Aid Center (NJ) 533
Health Science (NJ) 533
Helen Keller National Center for Deaf-Blind Youths
   and Adults (NY) 533
Hitec Special Needs Center (IL) 533
Hy-Tek Manufacturing Company, Inc. (IL) 533
Independent Living Aids, Inc. (NY) 533

IntelliTools (CA) 533
Lucent / ACPC (MO) 533
Luminaud, Inc. (OH) 533
Maddak, Inc. (NJ) 533
National Catalog House of the Deaf (IL) 534
Royal Data Systems / Speech and Learning Center
   Systems (NC) 534
Science Applications International Corporation (MD) 534
Sonic Alert (MI) 534
Texas Instruments (TX) 534
Words Plus, Inc. (CA) 534
Zygo Industries, Inc. (OR) 534

AUDIBLE AND TACTILE SIGNS AND DETECTABLE WARNING SURFACES

Accessories Plus (IL) 534
AccuBraille (CA) 534
Advance Corporation (MN) 534
Advantage Metal Systems, Inc. (MA) 534
American Olean Tile Company (PA) 534
Balcon, Inc. (MD) 534
Best Manufacturing Company (CO) 534
Bomanite Corporation (CA) 534
Carsonite International (NV) 534
Castek, Inc. / Transpo Industries, Inc. (NY) 534
Crossville Ceramics (TN) 534
CT Concrete Company (PA) 534
Diversified Enterprises International (MI) 534
Emed Company, Inc. (NY) 534
Engineered Plastics, Inc. (NY) 535
G.A.L. Manufacturing Corporation (NY) 535
SCS (MN) 535
Stampcrete Decorative Concrete, Inc. (NY) 535
Summitville Tiles, Inc. (OH) 535
Suprarock Block Company (AL) 535
Traconex, Inc. (CA) 535
Truxes Company / Signage Division (IL) 535
Universal Engraving, Inc. (KS) 535

CANADA

◆ *Educational Services*

PROVINCIAL SERVICES

Atlantic Provinces Special Education Authority (APSEA)/Department of Education (NS)...................... 444, 446, 448, 456

Department of Education, Culture and Employment/ Early Childhood and School Services (NT) 447

Direction de l'Adaption Scolaire et des Services Complémentaires (PQ)..................... 457

Eastern School District Unit (PE) 456

Government of the Yukon/Special Programs/ Department of Education (YT) 462

Public Inquiries Unit/Communications Branch/ Ministry of Education and Training (ON)............ 451

Special Education Branch/Alberta Department of Education (AB)...................... 437

Special Education Unit/Saskatchewan Education (SK)..... 460

Special Materials Services/Manitoba Department of Education and Training (MWESM) (MB)................ 442

Special Programs Branch (BC)..................... 439

Student Services Branch (NB) 444

Student Services Division/Department of Education (NS)...................... 448

Student Support Services/Department of Education (NF) 446

SCHOOLS

Hollywood Public School (ON)..................... 451

Metro Special Program (Vision) (Itinerant Program- Public and Special Schools) (ON) 451

Montreal Association for the Blind (PQ)................. 457

Sir Frederick Fraser School/Atlantic Provinces Special Education Authority (NS)..................... 448

W. Ross Macdonald School (ON).................. 451

INFANT AND PRESCHOOL

High Park Forest School/Ontario Foundation for Visually Impaired Children Inc. (ON) 451

Montreal Association for the Blind (PQ)..................... 457

INSTRUCTIONAL MATERIALS CENTERS

Materials Resource Centre for the Visually Impaired/ Alberta Education (AEEM) (AB)..................... 437

Provincial Resource Centre for the Visually Impaired/ Ministry of Education and Ministry Responsible for Multiculturalism and Human Rights (BC).................. 439

Special Materials Services/Manitoba Department of Education and Training (MWESM) (MB)............... 442

W. Ross Macdonald School/Resource Services Library (ON)..................... 451

UNIVERSITY TRAINING PROGRAMS

Mohawk College of Applied Arts and Technology (ON).................. 452

University of British Columbia/Educational Psychology and Special Education (BC).................. 439

University of Sherbrooke/Faculty of Education (PQ)......... 457

◆ *Information Services*

LIBRARIES

British Columbia College and Institute Library Service for the Print Impaired (BC) 439

British Columbia Library Services to the Handicapped (BC)..................... 439

Crane Resource Centre/University of British Columbia (BC) 440

Direction des Bibliothèques Publiques/Ministère des Affaires Culturelles (PQ)..................... 458

Government of the Yukon/Libraries and Archives Branch/Department of Education (YT) 462

Library Services/Alberta Community Development (AB).................. 437

New Brunswick Library Service/Department of Municipalities, Culture and Housing (NB)............... 444

Newfoundland Provincial Public Libraries Board (NF)..... 446

Northwest Territories Library Services/Department of Education, Culture and Employment (NT) 447

Nova Scotia Provincial Library (NS)................ 449

Provincial Library (PE)..................... 456

Public Library InterLINK (BC)..................... 440

Saskatchewan Provincial Library (SK)............... 460

Stanley A. Milner Public Library (AB)................ 437

York Regional Library/Talking Book Service (NB)............ 444

MEDIA PRODUCTION SERVICES

Access 20/20 (ON)..................... 452

Audiobook Program/Province of British Columbia (BBLA) Library Services Branch (BC).................. 440

Computer Braille Facility/University of Western Ontario (ON)..................... 452

Ferguson Library for Print Handicapped Students (NS)... 449

Metropolitan Toronto Reference Library/Centre for People with Disabilities (ON) 452

Ontario Audio Library Service/Trent University (ON)..... 452

Resource Services/Atlantic Provinces Special Education Authority (NS)..................... 449

INFORMATION AND REFERRAL

Manitoba Blind Sport Association (MB)................................ 442
Organization for the Education of the Visually
　　Handicapped (OEVH) (ON) 452
Visually Impaired Persons' Action Council
　　(VIPAC) (SK) 460

◆ *Rehabilitation Services*

PROVINCIAL SERVICES

Community Living/Department of Social
　　Services (SK) 460
Community Support Services Division/Ministry of
　　Social Services (BC).. 440
Department of Family Services/Community Living
　　Division (MB).. 442
Department of Health and Social Services/
　　Government of the Yukon (YT) 462
Developmental Services Branch/Ministry of
　　Community and Social Services (ON)...................... 453
Family and Community Social Services/New
　　Brunswick Department of Health and Community
　　Services (NB) 444
Family and Rehabilitative Services/Department of
　　Social Services, Province of Newfoundland (NF) 446
Family and Social Services Department (AB)...................... 438
PEI Health and Community Services (PE)......................... 456
Policy and Planning/Family Services (MB)....................... 442
Service des Programmes aux Personnes Handicapées/
　　Ministère de la Santé et des Services Sociaux,
　　Gouvernement du Québec (PQ) 458
Stanton Regional House Board (NT)................................. 447
Strategic and Operational Planning and Policy
　　Development/Department of Community Services,
　　Province of Nova Scotia (NS) 449

REHABILITATION

Balance (ON) 453
Canadian National Institute for the Blind/Alberta–
　　Northwest Territories Division (AB)................... 438, 447
Canadian National Institute for the Blind/British
　　Columbia-Yukon Division (BC) 441, 462
Canadian National Institute for the Blind/Manitoba
　　Division (MB).. 442
Canadian National Institute for the Blind/New
　　Brunswick Division (NB) 444
Canadian National Institute for the Blind/
　　Newfoundland and Labrador Division (NF)............ 446
Canadian National Institute for the Blind/Nova
　　Scotia–Prince Edward Island Division (NS) 449, 456
Canadian National Institute for the Blind/Ontario
　　Division (ON) 453

Canadian National Institute for the Blind/Quebec
　　Division (PQ) 458
Canadian National Institute for the Blind/
　　Saskatchewan Division (SK)..................................... 460
Centre Louis-Hébert (PQ).. 458
Institut Nazareth et Louis-Braille (PQ)............................ 458
Montreal Association for the Blind (PQ)........................... 459

COMPUTER TRAINING CENTERS

Frontier Computing (ON)... 454

DOG GUIDE SCHOOLS

Canadian Guide Dogs for the Blind (ON)......................... 454
Canine Vision Canada/Lions Foundation of
　　Canada (ON)... 455
Foundation Mira (PQ).. 459

◆ *Low Vision Services*

EYE CARE SOCIETIES

Alberta Association of Optometrists (AB)......................... 438
Manitoba Association of Optometrists (MB)..................... 443

LOW VISION CENTERS

Centre for Sight Enhancement (ON) 455
Vision Institute (ON).. 455

◆ *Federal Agencies*

The Adaptive Computer Technology Centre (The ACT
　　Centre) (PQ)... 497
Canadian Human Rights Commission (ON)...................... 497
Canadian Transportation Agency/Accessible
　　Transportation Directorate (PQ) 497
Human Resources Development Canada/Office for
　　Disability Issues (PQ) 497
Human Resources Development Canada/Vocational
　　Rehabilitation of Disabled Persons Program (PQ)........... 497
National Library of Canada (ON)..................................... 497
The Public Works and Government Services Canada
　　(PWGSC)/Accessibility Office (PQ)......................... 497
Transport Canada/Accessible Transportation Policy
　　and Programs (ON) 497
Treasury Board of Canada (ON)....................................... 497
Veterans Affairs Canada/Health Care Division,
　　Veteran Services Branch (PE)................................... 498

◆ National Organizations

Alternate Media Canada / The National Broadcast
  Reading Service (ON) 499
Braille Authority of North America (DC) 499
Canadian Blind Sports Association (ON) 499
Canadian National Institute for the Blind / Department
  of Government Relations and International
  Services (ON) 499
Canadian National Institute for the Blind / National
  Office (ON) 499
Guide Dogs for the Blind (CA) 499
John Milton Society for the Blind in Canada (ON) ... 500
Leader Dogs for the Blind (MI) 500
National Camps for Blind Children (NE) 500
Operation Eyesight Universal (OEU) (AB) 500
Pilot Dogs, Inc. (OH) 500
Retinitis Pigmentosa Eye Research Foundation (ON) ... 500
The Seeing Eye, Inc. (NJ) 500
Ski for Light (Canada) Inc. (BC) 500

◆ Membership Organizations

Alberta Sports and Recreation Association for the
  Blind (AB) 501
American Optometric Association (MO) 501
Atlantic Provinces Special Education Authority (NS) ... 501
Canadian Association of Optometrists (ON) 501
Canadian Council for Exceptional Children / Division
  for the Visually Handicapped (ON) 501
Canadian Council of the Blind (ON) 501
Canadian National Society of the Deaf-Blind (ON) ... 501
Canadian Ophthalmological Society (ON) 501
CDBRA (Canadian Deaf Blind Research Association)
  National Office (ON) 502
Council for Exceptional Children (VA) 502
Council of Schools for the Blind (NJ) 502
Low Vision Association of Ontario (ON) 502
Regroupement des Aveugles et Amblyopes du
  Quebec (PQ) 502
VIEWS for the Visually Impaired (ON) 502

◆ Producers of Media

MEDIA PRODUCERS AND PUBLISHERS

Audio Studio for the Reading Impaired (KY) 539
Blindskills (OR) 539
Books Aloud (CA) 539

Braille International (FL) 539
Christian Blind Mission International (ON) 539
Christian Mission for the Blind (IN) 539
Christian Record Services (ON) 539
Church of Jesus Christ of Latter-Day Saints / Special
  Curriculum (UT) 539
Cleveland Sight Center of the Cleveland Society for the
  Blind (OH) 539
Crane Resource Centre / University of British
  Columbia (BC) 539
Eyes of Faith Ministries (TX) 540
Gospel Association for the Blind (FL) 540
I Can See Books (BC) 540
Institut Nazareth et Louis-Braille (PQ) 540
Library for the Blind / Canadian National Institute for
  the Blind (ON) 540
Lutheran Library for the Blind (MO) 540
Monterey County Braille Transcribers (CA) 540
Multi-Lingual Braille and Large Print Association (ON) .. 541
National Braille Association (NY) 541
National Braille Press (MA) 541
PAL Reading Services (ON) 541
People Helping People (ON) 541
Prose & Cons Braille Unit (NE) 541
Recording for the Blind and Dyslexic (NJ) 541
VoicePrint / The National Broadcast Reading Service,
  Inc. (ON) 541
Volunteers of Vacaville (CA) 541
Volunteer Transcribing Services (CA) 541
Xavier Society for the Blind (NY) 541

AUDIODESCRIPTION SERVICES

Audio Vision Canada / The National Broadcast
  Reading Service, Inc. (ON) 541

◆ Sources of Products

MAIL ORDER, CATALOGS, AND DISTRIBUTORS

Microcomputer Science Centre, Inc. (ON) 543

HOUSEHOLD, PERSONAL, AND INDEPENDENT LIVING PRODUCTS

AmbuTech / Melet Plastics, Inc. (ON) 543
Canadian National Institute for the Blind (ON) 543

LOW VISION

Acrontech (ON) 543

Microcomputer Science Centre, Inc. (ON) 543
Octopus Audio Visual (ON) 543

COMPUTER HARDWARE

Acrontech (ON) 543
Betacom Group/Montreal Betacom (PQ) 543
Betacom Group/Toronto Betacom (ON) 543
Canadian National Institute for the Blind (ON) 543
Frontier Computing (ON) 543
IBM/Special Needs Department (ON) 544
Microcomputer Science Centre, Inc. (ON) 544
Octopus Audio Visual (ON) 544
Syntha-Voice Computers, Inc. (ON) 544
Visualaide, Inc. (PQ) 544

COMPUTER SOFTWARE

Betacom Group/Montreal Betacom (PQ) 544
Betacom Group/Toronto Betacom (ON) 544
Frontier Computing (ON) 544
Microcomputer Science Centre, Inc. (ON) 544
Syntha-Voice Computers, Inc. (ON) 544

BRAILLE AND OTHER LITERACY MATERIALS

Inegra Products (BC) 544
Microcomputer Science Centre, Inc. (ON) 544

PRODUCTS FOR DEAF-BLIND/MULTIPLY DISABLED PERSONS

Canadian National Institute for the Blind (ON) 544
SuData Consulting (ON) 544

UNITED STATES
STATE LISTINGS

ALABAMA

♦ Educational Services

STATE SERVICES

Alabama State Department of Education
50 North Ripley Street
Montgomery, AL 36130
(334) 242-8114 or toll-free in
Alabama (800) 392-8020
FAX: (334) 242-9192
Dr. Ed Richardson, Superintendent
Bill East, Special Education
Services

Type of Agency: State.
Mission: Provides assistance for in-service teacher training through state workshops or technical assistance to individual programs.
Funded by: IDEA funds.
Hours of Operation: 7:30AM-5:00PM.
Area Served: Statewide.
Transportation: Y.
Age Requirements: 3-21 years.

Educational: Free appropriate public education for students 3-21 years who meet state eligibility requirements.

EARLY INTERVENTION COORDINATION

Alabama's Early Intervention System
Alabama Department of Rehabilitation Services
2129 East South Boulevard
Montgomery, AL 36111
(334) 281-8780, ext. 398
FAX: (334) 613-3494
Ouida G. Holder, Part H
Coordinator

Social work services; family training, counseling and home visits; assistive technology; evaluation and assessment; speech-language pathology; physical therapy; service coordination.

SCHOOLS

Alabama School for the Blind
Alabama Institute for Deaf and Blind
705 East South Street
P.O. Box 698
Talladega, AL 35161
(205) 761-3259
FAX: (205) 761-3362
E-mail: nstep@aidb.state.al.us
Dr. Joseph F. Busta, President,
Alabama Institute for Deaf and Blind
Noel E. Stephens, Principal

Type of Agency: State.
County/District Where Located:
Talladega County.
Mission: Services for totally blind, legally blind, visually impaired, mentally retarded, and orthopedically disabled persons.
Funded by: State appropriations.
Hours of Operation: 7:30AM-4:00PM.
Staff: 91 full time.
History/Date: Est. 1867.
Number of Clients Served: 1995-96: 128 on campus; 885 in Instructional Resource Center for the Blind.
Eligibility: Visually impaired (20/70 or less acuity).
Area Served: Alabama.
Transportation: Y.
Age Requirements: 3-21 years.

Health: Audiology, speech, physical therapy, general medical services. contracts for other health services.
Counseling/Social Work/Self-Help: Psychological testing and evaluation; individual, group, family/parent counseling; referral to community services. Provides consultation with other agencies as needed.
Educational: K-12 curriculum; general academic; vocational/skill development.
Professional Training: In-service.
Reading: Talking book record players and cassette players; braille books; large print books; braille magazines; recorded magazines.
Residential: Residential facilities available for students.
Rehabilitation: Personal management; braille; handwriting; listening skills; typing; computer keyboarding skills; home management; orientation/mobility; remedial education; sensory training.
Recreational: Extended day programs; swimming; track; wrestling. Summer camp for public school students.
Computer Training: Training on computer aids and devices.
Low Vision: Full-service clinic.
Low Vision Aids: Aids available for loan.
Low Vision Follow-up: Y.

Southwest Alabama Regional School for the Deaf and Blind
8901 Airport Boulevard
Mobile, AL 36608-9503
(334) 633-0241
FAX: (334) 633-9951
Mary Lou Casey, Director

Type of Agency: Public school.
County/District Where Located:
Mobile County.
Mission: Services for totally blind, legally blind, deaf-blind, and learning disabled persons.
Funded by: Mobile County public schools; state of Alabama.
Hours of Operation: 7:30 AM-3:30 PM.
Staff: 16 full time. Uses volunteers.

History/Date: Est. 1980.
Number of Clients Served: Students in 1992: 105.
Eligibility: Public school student; resident of Mobile, Baldwin, Clarke, Washington or Escambia County.
Area Served: Southwest Alabama with center in Mobile County.
Transportation: Y.
Age Requirements: 5-21 years.

Health: Audiology therapy; occupational therapy; speech therapy. Refers for other health services.
Counseling/Social Work/Self-Help: Social evaluation; psychological testing and evaluation; placement in school; training. Counselor on staff.
Educational: Grades K through 12. Accepts deaf-blind; emotionally disturbed; learning disabled. Programs for college prep; general academic; vocational/skill development.
Preschools: 0-5 as referred by state plan. Contact school directly—Mary Lou Casey.
Professional Training: Regular in-service training programs, open to enrollment from other agencies.
Reading: Talking book record player; cassette tape player; talking book records and tapes; braille and large print books; braille and recorded magazines. Information and referral.
Rehabilitation: Activities of daily living; braille; gesticulation; handwriting; typing; video magnifier; home management; orientation/mobility; remedial education; sensory training. Refers for other rehabilitation services.
Recreational: Refers for recreation services. Provides consultation to other agencies.
Employment: Prevocational evaluations; career and skill counseling. Contracts for other employment services. Provides consultation to other agencies.

STATEWIDE OUTREACH SERVICES

Alabama Institute for Deaf and Blind
205 East South Street
P.O. Box 698
Talladega, AL 35161
(205) 761-3206
FAX: (205) 761-3352
Terry Graham, Director, Office of Health, Evaluation, and Outreach
Lynn Hannez, Director of Institutional Relations

County/District Where Located: Talladega County.

Assessment: Multidisciplinary; comprehensive assessments as well as IEP activities.
Consultation to Public Schools: Available to schools and school systems.
Direct Service: Technical assistance and other services available to schools, school systems, and other agencies.
Parent Assistance: Counseling and instruction.
Materials Production: Instructional and other materials.

INSTRUCTIONAL MATERIALS CENTERS

Alabama Instructional Resource Center
P.O. Box 698
Talladega, AL 35161
(205) 761-3262
FAX: (205) 761-3337
E-mail: tlacy@aidb.al.state.us
Teresa Lacy, Director
Mike Jones, Assistant Director

Area Served: Alabama.
Groups Served: Newborns–adults.

Counseling/Social Work/Self-Help: Braille, large-print, and recorded textbooks.
Media Formats: Braille; large-print; tape.
Title Listings: None available.

UNIVERSITY TRAINING PROGRAMS

Talladega College
Rehabilitation and Special Education Department
Talladega, AL 35160
(205) 362-0206
FAX: (205) 761-6379
Dr. Elaine Sebera, Contact Person

County/District Where Located: Talladega County.

Programs Offered: Undergraduate program in blind rehabilitation.

University of Alabama at Birmingham
Department of Leadershiip, Special Education and Foundations
Education Building
Birmingham, AL 35294
(205) 934-4892
FAX: (205) 975-7581
Dr. Mary Jean Sanspree, Coordinator

County/District Where Located: Jefferson County.

Programs Offered: Graduate programs for teachers of the visually handicapped.

♦ Information Services

LIBRARIES

Alabama Regional Library for the Blind and Physically Handicapped
6030 Monticello Drive

Montgomery, AL 36130
(334) 213-3906 or toll-free in
Alabama (800) 392-5671 or TDD
(334) 213-3900
FAX: (334) 213-3993
E-mail: fzaleski@apls.state.al.
us
Fara Zaleski, Regional Librarian

Type of Agency: State library.
County/District Where Located:
Montgomery County.
Mission: To provide personalized
and efficient library services in
accessible format for persons with
qualifying disabilities.
Funded by: Federal and state
funds.
Budget: FY1996: $296,070.
Hours of Operation: Mon. - Fri.
8:00 AM - 5:00 PM.
Staff: 8.
History/Date: Est. 1965.
Number of Clients Served: 5,184.
Eligibility: Inability to use
standard print material due to
physical disability.
Area Served: Alabama.

Reading: Recreational reading and
basic reference.
Low Vision: Catalogs of products
for persons with low vision;
vertical files containing materials
of special interest to persons with
low vision.

Regional library of the Library of
Congress providing braille, talking
books and machines, tapes, and
tape cassette machines.

**Department for the Blind and
Physically Handicapped**
Houston-Love Memorial Library
P.O. Box 1369
Dothan, AL 36302
(334) 793-9767 or TDD (334) 793-
9767
FAX: (334) 793-6645
Linda Ruffner, Librarian

Subregional library.

**Huntsville Subregional Library
for the Blind and Physically
Handicapped**
P.O. Box 443
Huntsville, AL 35804
(205) 532-5980
FAX: (205) 532-5994
Joyce L. Smith, Librarian

Subregional library.

**Library and Resource Center for
the Blind and Physically
Handicapped**
Alabama Institute for Deaf and
Blind
705 East South Street
P.O. Box 698
Talladega, AL 35161
(205) 761-3287 or toll-free in
Alabama (205) 761-3288
FAX: (205) 761-3337
Teresa Lacy, Librarian

Subregional library.

**Library for the Blind and
Physically Handicapped**
Public Library of Anniston and
Calhoun County
P.O. Box 308
Anniston, AL 36202
(205) 237-8501
FAX: (205) 238-0474
Deenie M. Culver, Librarian

Subregional library.

**Tuscaloosa Subregional Library
for the Blind and Physically
Handicapped**
Tuscaloosa Public Library
1801 River Road
Tuscaloosa, AL 35401
(205) 345-3994 or TDD (205) 345-
3994
FAX: (205) 752-8300
Barbara B. Jordan, Librarian

Subregional library.

MEDIA PRODUCTION SERVICES

**Alabama Regional Library for
the Blind and Physically
Handicapped**
6030 Monticello Drive
Montgomery, AL 36130
(334) 213-3906
FAX: (334) 213-3993
E-mail: fzaleski@apls.state.al.
us
Fara Zaleski, Regional Librarian

County/District Where Located:
Montgomery County.
Area Served: Alabama.
Groups Served: Preschool–senior
citizens.

Types/Content: Recreational
reading and basic reference.
Media Formats: Braille books,
books on records or cassettes.
Title Listings: Subject listings
printed at no charge.

Barrett School
7605 Division Avenue
Birmingham, AL 35206
(205) 836-7173
Ann M. Connelly, Resource
Teacher for Visually Impaired
Students

County/District Where Located:
Jefferson County.
Area Served: Birmingham city
schools.
Groups Served: K-12.

Types/Content: Textbooks.
Media Formats: Braille/large-
print books.
Title Listings: No title listings
available.

**Library and Resource Center for
the Blind and Physically
Handicapped**
P.O. Box 698

Talladega, AL 35161
(205) 761-3287
FAX: (205) 761-3337
E-mail: tlacy@aidb.state.al.us
Teresa Lacy, Director
Martha Thompson, Reader
Advisor

Area Served: Talladega, St. Clair, and Coosa Counties.

Types/Content: Recreational; career/vocational; religious; leisure reading.
Media Formats: Braille books; talking books/cassettes.
Title Listings: No title listings available.

Southwest Alabama Regional School for the Deaf and Blind

8901 Airport Boulevard
Mobile, AL 36608
(334) 633-0241 or (334) 633-0323
FAX: (334) 633-9951
Mary Lou Casey, Director

County/District Where Located: Mobile County.
Area Served: Mobile County public schools. Resource: Baldwin, Clarke, Escambia, Washington Counties in southwest Alabama.
Groups Served: K-12.

Types/Content: Textbooks, career/vocational.
Media Formats: Braille books, talking books/cassettes, large print books.
Title Listings: No title listings available.

RADIO READING

Alabama Radio Reading Service Network

650 11th Street South
Birmingham, AL 35294
(205) 934-6576
FAX: (205) 975-6061
Charles Ewing, Director

County/District Where Located: Jefferson County.
Hours of Operation: Mon.-Fri. 7:00 AM-10:00 PM; Sat. 8:00 AM-12:00 noon; Sun. 12:00 noon-4:00 PM.
History/Date: Est. 1978 (WBHM-Birmingham).
Area Served: Three-quarters of Alabama.

WLRH Radio

4701 University Drive N.W.
Huntsville, AL 35899
(205) 895-9574
Scott Passmore, Volunteer Corp Reading Service
Cheryl Carlson, Director of Underwriting and Business Support

County/District Where Located: Madison County.
Hours of Operation: Mon.-Fri. 6:00 AM-4:00 PM.
History/Date: Est. 1980.
Area Served: 50-mile radius from Huntsville.

WTSU Radio Reading Service

207 Montgomery Street
Bell Building, Suite 1125
Montgomery, AL 36104
(334) 241-9574
John McVay, Station Manager

County/District Where Located: Montgomery County.
Hours of Operation: Mon.-Fri. 9:00 AM-5:00 PM; broadcast: 10AM-12noon; rebroadcast afternoon and evening hours.
Area Served: Coosa County to Tallapoosa County, Alabama; Columbus, Georgia; and northern panhandle of Florida.

WUAL Radio Reading Service

P.O. Box 870370
Tuscaloosa, AL 35487-0370
(205) 348-6644
Betty Jobe, Coordinator

County/District Where Located: Tuscaloosa County.
Funded by: Private donations; University of Alabama.
Hours of Operation: Broadcast 24 hrs per day; local broadcast 2:00PM-4:00PM weekdays.
Staff: Volunteers.
History/Date: Est. 1983.
Area Served: West Alabama.

INFORMATION AND REFERRAL

Alabama Department of Rehabilitation Volunteer Information Resource Center

P.O. Box 2388
Muscle Shoals, AL 35662
(205) 381-1110
Jill Murphy, Rehabilitation Teacher

Mission: To enable Alabama's adults and children with disabilities to achieve their maximum potential.
Age Requirements: None.

Counseling/Social Work/Self-Help: Career counseling.
Reading: Independent living skills.

♦ Rehabilitation Services

STATE SERVICES

Alabama Division of Rehabilitation Services

2129 East South Boulevard
P.O. Box 11586
Montgomery, AL 36111-0586
(334) 281-8780
Lamona Lucas, Director, Services to the Blind and Deaf
James G. Harris III, Supervisor, Services to the Blind and Deaf

Type of Agency: State.

County/District Where Located: Montgomery.

Mission: To enable Alabama children and adults with disabilities to achieve their maximum potential.

Funded by: State appropriation.

Hours of Operation: Mon.-Fri. 8:00 AM-5:30 PM.

Program Accessibility: Provides taped and brailled materials.

Staff: 63 full time.

History/Date: Est. 1926.

Number of Clients Served: 3,729.

Eligibility: Varies according to different programs. Vocational Rehabilitation Program–a mental or physical disability that creates a substantial barrier to employment and that will require vocational rehabitation services. OASIS program for older blind persons— an impairment that affects the performance of daily activities.

Area Served: State of Alabama.

Transportation: Y.

Age Requirements: Minimum age 16 years.

Health: Refers for all health services.

Counseling/Social Work/Self-Help: Individual, family/parent, couple counseling. Contracts and refers for other counseling/social work services.

Educational: Accepts deaf-blind, emotionally disturbed, learning disabled, mentally retarded, orthopedically disabled, and other multiply disabled persons. Programs for college prep; vocational skill development.

Preschools: Early intervention program serves children 0-2 years of age; serves all disabilities.

Professional Training: Internship/fieldwork placement in rehabilitation counseling. Regular in-service training programs. Short-term and summer training.

Residential: Contracts with Alabama Institute for Deaf and Blind for residential programming.

Recreational: Refers for recreation services.

Employment: Career and skill counseling; vocational placement; follow-up service. Contracts and refers for other employment-oriented services.

Computer Training: Access; training on computer aids and devices.

Low Vision: Exams.

Low Vision Aids: Purchased by program.

Low Vision Follow-up: Y.

Local Offices:

Andalusia: Division of Rehabilitation Services, 807 Eighth Avenue, Andalusia, AL 36420-2199, (334) 222-4114.

Anniston: Division of Rehabilitation Services, 1105 Woodstock Avenue, Anniston, AL 36201-4799, (205) 231-1025.

Auburn: Division of Rehabilitation Services, 1104 Haley Center, Auburn University, Auburn, AL 36849-3501, (334) 826-4475.

Bessemer: Division of Rehabilitation Services, P.O. Box 308, Bessemer, AL 35021-0308, (205) 426-1294.

Decatur: Division of Rehabilitation Services, P.O. Box 1686, Decatur, AL 35602-1686, (205) 353-2754.

Dothan: Division of Rehabilitation Services, P.O. Drawer 698, Dothan, AL 36302-0698, (334) 792-0022.

Gasden: Division of Rehabilitation Services, 1100 George Wallace Drive, Gasden, AL 35999-6501, (205) 547-6974.

Homewood: Division of Rehabilitation Services, 236 Goodwin Crest Drive, Homewood, AL 35219-0888, (205) 290-4400.

Huntsville: Division of Rehabilitation Services, 407 Governors Drive, S.W., Huntsville, AL 35804-0405, (205) 536-6621.

Mobile: Division of Rehabilitation Services, 2419 Gordon Smith Drive, Mobile, AL 36617-2395, (334) 479-8611.

Montgomery: Division of Rehabilitation Services, 2127 East South Boulevard, Montgomery, AL 36199-3801, (334) 288-0220.

Muscle Shoals: Division of Rehabilitation Services, P.O. Box 2388, Muscle Shoals, AL 35662-2388, (205) 381-1110.

Opelika: Division of Rehabilitation Services, 510 West Thomason Circle, Opelika, AL 36801-5499, (334) 749-1259.

Selma: Division of Rehabilitation Services, P.O. Box 1097, Selma, AL 36701-1097, (205) 872-8422.

Talladega: Division of Rehabilitation Services, #4 Medical Office Park, Talladega, AL 35160-2296, (205) 362-1300.

Troy: Division of Rehabilitation Services, 518 East Parklane Shopping Center, Troy, AL 36081, (334) 566-2491.

Tuscaloosa: Division of Rehabilitation Services, 922 Fifth Avenue, East, Tuscaloosa, AL 35401-2084, (205) 554-1300.

REHABILITATION

Alabama Industries for the Blind
Alabama Institute for Deaf and Blind

1241 McClellan Avenue
P.O. Box 698
Talladega, AL 35161
(205) 761-3510 or (205) 761-3513
FAX: (205) 761-3477
Billy Sparkman, General Manager

County/District Where Located: Talladega County.

Employment: Employs blind and deaf adults in a sheltered workshop and in one satellite operation.

Local Offices:

Birmingham: Industries for the Blind, Satellite Workshop, 220 34th Street South, Birmingham, AL 35212, (205) 252-3164, (205) 252-3957, FAX (205) 323-5897.

Central Alabama Easter Seal Rehabilitation Center

2125 East South Boulevard
Montgomery, AL 36116-2454
(344) 288-0240
FAX: (334) 288-7171
J. Larry Johnson, Administrator

Type of Agency: Private; non-profit.
County/District Where Located: Montgomery County.
Mission: To provide quality programs and services to enable people with disabilities to achieve their maximum potential.
Funded by: Fees and contributions.
Budget: $1,800,000.
Hours of Operation: Mon.-Fri. 8:00AM-4:30PM.
Staff: 60 full time/volunteers.
History/Date: Est. 1961.
Number of Clients Served: 1,700 annually.
Eligibility: Must have sponsorship.
Area Served: 11 counties: Montgomery, Elmore, Autauga, Macon , Lowndes, Crenshaw, Pike, Barbour, Conecuh, Coosa, Butler.
Transportation: Y.
Age Requirements: No age requirements.

Health: Audiology; occupational, physical and speech therapy.
Counseling/Social Work/Self-Help: Psychological testing and evaluation; counseling: individual, group. Placement in school and training. Referral to community services.
Educational: Tutor services for grades 1 through 12. Accepts deaf-blind; emotionally disturbed; learning disabled; mentally retarded; orthopedically handicapped; all other multiply handicapped. General academic programs; college preparatory; high school equivalency.
Professional Training: Internship/fieldwork placement in industrial arts; rehabilitation counseling; physical, speech and occupational therapy. In-service training programs.
Rehabilitation: Personal management; orientation/mobility; remedial education.
Low Vision Follow-up: Y.

Easter Seals Occupational Rehabilitation Center

1616 Sixth Avenue South
Birmingham, AL 35233
(205) 939-5800
FAX: (205) 939-5849
Richard Hinson, Administrator

Type of Agency: Private; non-profit.
County/District Where Located: Jefferson County.
Mission: To develop, deliver and manage vocational rehabilitation services to persons with disabilities to maximize their potential.
Funded by: Third party sponsorship; fee for service.
Budget: $ 1.4 million.
Hours of Operation: 8:00 AM - 4:30 PM.
Staff: 32 full time. Uses volunteers.
History/Date: Est. 1968.
Number of Clients Served: 60 average daily attendance.
Area Served: Jefferson, Shelby, Walker Counties. Other geographical areas upon request.

Age Requirements: Over 16 years.
Health: Clients in need of medical services are referred to appropriate agency.
Counseling/Social Work/Self-Help: Individual, group, couple counseling; training placement; referral to community services. Refers for other counseling/social work services.
Educational: K through 12th grade; adult basic education; general academic; vocational/skill development. Accepts persons who are deaf-blind, emotionally disturbed, learning disabled, mentally retarded, multiply disabled, physically disabled, or alcohol/drug abusers.
Professional Training: Internship/fieldwork placement in occupational therapy; rehabilitation counseling; special education. Affiliated with University of Alabama; University of Alabama in Birmingham; Auburn University; Talladega College. Regular in-service training programs.
Rehabilitation: CARF-accredited vocational evaluations, work adjustment training, job readiness training, job placement, and job skill clerical training.
Employment: Prevocational evaluation; career and skill counseling; job retention; vocational placement; follow-up services. Refers for other employment-oriented services.
Computer Training: CARF-accredited training.
Low Vision: Referral to low vision clinic.
Low Vision Aids: Voice synthesizer for computers; JAWS software; Kurzweil Voice for Windows.

E.H. Gentry Technical Facility Alabama Institute for Deaf and Blind

205 East South Street
P.O. Box 698
Talladega, AL 35161
(205) 761-3402
FAX: (205) 761-3450
Jim Hare, Dean

Type of Agency: State.
Mission: Provides services for totally blind, legally blind, visually impaired, deaf-blind, and deaf persons.
Funded by: State appropriation; fees; workshop sales; sub-contracts.
Budget: $3,600,000.
Hours of Operation: 8:00 AM-4:30 PM.
Staff: 92 full time. Uses volunteers.
History/Date: Est. 1968.
Number of Clients Served: 450 annually.
Eligibility: Must meet requirements of State Vocational Rehabilitation Service or U.S. Department of Veterans and be sponsored by State Vocational Rehabilitation Service.
Area Served: Unlimited.
Transportation: Y.
Age Requirements: At least 16 years old.

Health: Audiology therapy; general medical services; physical therapy; speech therapy. Contracts, refers for, and provides consultation to other agencies on other health services.
Counseling/Social Work/Self-Help: Social evaluation; individual, group, family/parent, couple counseling; placement in training; referral to community services.
Educational: Area secondary students; post-secondary and college preparatory; accepts deaf-blind, deaf, and blind. Programs for adult continuing education; college prep; general academic; vocational/skill development; technical training and evaluation.
Professional Training: Internship/fieldwork placement in industrial arts; low vision; orientation/mobility; rehabilitation counseling; special education; vocational rehabilitation. Has regular in-service training programs open to enrollment from other agencies.
Residential: Dormitories.
Recreational: Personal management; braille; handwriting; listening skills; typing; video magnifier; home management; orientation/mobility; home and community; remedial education; sensory training. Refers for other rehabilitation services.
Employment: Prevocational evaluation; career and skill counseling; occupational skill development; job retention; job retraining; sheltered workshops; vocational placement; vending stand training. Refers for and provides consultation to other agencies on other employment oriented services.
Computer Training: Access; training on computer aids and devices.
Low Vision Follow-up: Y.

Five campuses are located in Talladega, Alabama. Regional centers are located in Birmingham, Dotham, Huntsville, Auburn, Mobile, Muscle Shoals, Montgomery, Talladega, and Tuscaloosa.

Mobile Association for the Blind

2440 Gordon Smith Drive
Mobile, AL 36617
(334) 473-3585
FAX: (334) 470-8622
Mahlon P. McCracken, Executive Director

Type of Agency: Private; non-profit.
County/District Where Located: Mobile County.
Mission: Operates a sheltered workshop for visually impaired and deaf blind persons. Provides training in orientation and mobility, activities of daily living, recreation, and communication for visually impaired adults.
Funded by: Public funds, United Way, workshop sales, and sub-contracts.
Budget: $2.2 million.
Hours of Operation: 8:00 AM-4:30 PM.
Staff: 35.
History/Date: Est. 1926 and Inc. 1932.
Number of Clients Served: 1996: 450.
Eligibility: Determined by Adult Vocational Rehabilitation Service and/or Mobile Consortium–Private Industry Council (depending upon services client is seeking and agency applying through).
Area Served: Mobile, Baldwin, Choctow, Clarke, Escambia, Monroe, and Washington counties.
Transportation: Y.
Age Requirements: 16-65 years of age.

Counseling/Social Work/Self-Help: Offers individual counseling. Refers for group and family counseling and social work services.
Educational: Programs for skill development, job search.
Reading: Reading services provided through volunteers.
Rehabilitation: Work adjustment training; activities of daily living; mobility; communication skills for all disabilities; braille; typing.
Employment: Sheltered employment. Job coaches for on-the-job training.

Computer Training: Special software.
Low Vision: Limited staff assessments.
Low Vision Aids: Provided free of charge.
Low Vision Follow-up: Provided by rehabilitation teachers.
Professional Training: In-service training programs.

Local Offices:

Mobile: Better Employability Skills Training Plus Program, 521 Bayshore Avenue, Mobile, AL 36617, (334) 476-5881.

Southeastern Blind Rehabilitation Center
U.S. Department of Veterans Affairs
VA Medical Center
700 South 19th Street
Birmingham, AL 35233
(205) 933-8101
Y.C. Parris, Director

Type of Agency: Federal.
County/District Where Located: Jefferson County.
Mission: Provides residential rehabilitation services to eligible legally blind veterans.
History/Date: Est. 1982.

Referral applications by Visual Impairment Services Programs located at VA Medical Centers and Outpatient Clinics in the geographical area served by the Blind Rehabilitation Center or Clinic.

See U.S. Department of Veterans Affairs in U.S. Federal Agencies listings.

Workshops, Inc.
4244 Third Avenue, South
Birmingham, AL 35222
(205) 592-9683
FAX: (205) 592-9687
J. E Crim, Executive Director

County/District Where Located: Jefferson County.
Mission: Provides services to blind and visually impaired persons and all other persons with disabilities.
Funded by: Public funds, Community Chest, workshop sales.
History/Date: Est. 1955.
Area Served: Birmingham, Jefferson County, northern Alabama, and Shelby County.

Employment: Prevocational training; sheltered workshops.

COMPUTER TRAINING CENTERS

E.H. Gentry Technical Facility
P.O. Box 698
Talladega, AL 35161
(205) 761-3404
FAX: (205) 761-3450
Beauford Watson, Director, Vocational Training

Computer Training: Speech output systems; screen magnification systems; braille access systems; optical character recognition systems; closed-circuit television systems; word processing; database software; computer operating systems.

Technical assistance in modification and set-up.

Southeastern Blind Rehabilitation Center
VA Medical Center
700 South 19th Street
Birmingham, AL 35233
(205) 933-8101, ext. 6994
FAX: (205) 933-4484
B.C. Starkson, Supervisor

Computer Training: Braille and voice access systems; optical character recognition systems.

◆ Low Vision Services

EYE CARE SOCIETIES

Alabama Academy of Ophthalmology
500 Robert Jemison Road
Birmingham, AL 35209
(205) 942-7888
FAX: (205) 942-7882
Tonya Burnett, Executive Director

Alabama Optometric Association, Inc.
400 South Union Street
Suite 435
Montgomery, AL 36104
(334) 834-1057
FAX: (334) 834-1691
Virginia O. Campbell, CAE, Executive Director

LOW VISION CENTERS

Center for Visual Independence Eye Foundation Hospital
1201 11th Avenue South
Birmingham, AL 35205
(205) 933-2625 or (205) 930-4700
FAX: (205) 558-2553
Jessica Lambert, Low Vision Specialist/Director

County/District Where Located: Jefferson County.
Funded by: Client fees, Vocational Rehabilitation Service, and Alabama Sight (Lions Club funds).
Hours of Operation: Mon.- Fri. 8:00 AM - 5:00 PM.
Staff: Ophthalmologist, low vision director.
Area Served: United States, but primarily Alabama.

Educational: Referrals provided.
Preschools: Referrals provided.
Reading: Assistance provided.
Rehabilitation: Assistance provided.

Employment: Assistance provided.
Low Vision: Assistance provided.
Low Vision Aids: Provided for purchase; prescribed and fitted for variable charge. On-site training provided.
Low Vision Follow-up: Return appointment; phone interview; varies according to patient.

Local Offices:

Huntsville: Center for Visual Independence Eye Foundation Hospital, 204 Lowe, S.E., Suite 4, Huntsville, AL 35801, (205) 539-8851.
Montgomery: Center for Visual Independence Eye Foundation Hospital, 303 South Ripley, Suite 5900, Montgomery, AL 36104, (334) 263-0105.

Liz Moore Low Vision Center

50 Medical Park Drive, East Birmingham, AL 35235
(205) 838-3162
FAX: (205) 838-3515
E-mail: msanspree@icare.opt.uab.edu
Mary Jean Sanspree, Director

Type of Agency: Non-profit, community education, information and referral, and training center.
County/District Where Located: Jefferson County.
Mission: To provide support for persons with low visual acuity within Alabama and the southeastern United States.
Funded by: Eastern Health System, Inc., East End Memorial Foundation, private donors.
Budget: $200,000 (hospital support). Various private grants and foundation funds available.
Hours of Operation: 8:30 AM-5:00 PM.
Program Accessibility: Fully accessible.

Staff: 8 full time.
History/Date: Est. 1991.
Number of Clients Served: 2,000 per year.
Eligibility: Visual impairment, blindness and/or referral from physicians, social workers, or rehabilitation agencies.
Area Served: Alabama, Mississippi, and Georgia.
Transportation: Y.

Health: Referrals from physicians.
Counseling/Social Work/Self-Help: Referrals for counseling, social work. Assistance with classes and referrals for ADL. Monthly support group meetings.
Educational: Teacher training stipends, parent training, family education, community education. Summer "chill out" camp for children ages 2-14 years.
Preschools: Parent education, information and referral services.
Professional Training: Teacher training stipends in blindness and deaf-blindness. Video library available for check-out.
Reading: Resource room for use of closed circuit television, video education, and other educational opportunities. Weekly radio show "Low Vision and You" on statewide radio reading service for the blind.
Residential: none.
Rehabilitation: Through Outpatient Occupational Therapy Department and state rehabilition offices.
Recreational: Golf school, adapted art tours at Birmingham Museum of Art, Helen Keller Art show for Alabama and National shows.
Employment: Assistance with job accomodations.
Computer Training: Referrals to rehabilitation and employment training programs.
Low Vision: Training with ADLs and low vision devices.

Community and consumer education. Information and referral.
Low Vision Aids: Referral for prescriptions and evaluations.
Low Vision Follow-up: Training with low vision devices; support groups.

University of Alabama at Birmingham/The Medical Center School of Optometry
Low Vision Rehabilitation Clinic

1716 University Boulevard Birmingham, AL 35294-0010
(205) 934-2625 or (205) 934-3086
FAX: (205) 934-0911
Rodney W. Nowakowski, O.D., Ph.D., Director, Ocular Disease and Low Vision Service

Type of Agency: State University, Medical Center, School of Optometry.
County/District Where Located: Jefferson County.
Mission: Teaching and patient care.
Funded by: State and federal funds; registration fees and material fees.
Hours of Operation: By appointment, Mon., Tues., Thurs., Fri. 8:00 AM-12 noon, 1:00 PM-5:00 PM.
Program Accessibility: Wheelchair accessible.
Staff: Optometrists, ophthalmologist, optometric technicians.
Eligibility: No restrictions.
Area Served: No restrictions.
Age Requirements: None.

Low Vision: Comprehensive evaluation and treatment.
Low Vision Aids: Provided on loan for trial period; on-site training provided.
Low Vision Follow-up: By appointment within 3 weeks to 6 months.

Referrals made for other appropriate services.

♦ *Aging Services*

STATE UNITS ON AGING

Commission on Aging
770 Washington Avenue
Suite 470
Montgomery, AL 36130
(334) 242-5743 or Information &
Referral in state: (800) 243-5463
FAX: (334) 242-5594
Martha Murph Beck, Executive
Director

Provides referrals to Area Agencies on Aging and information on other local aging services.

INDEPENDENT LIVING PROGRAMS

Department of Rehabilitation Services
P.O. Box 11586
Montgomery, AL 36111-0586
(334) 281-8780 or (800) 441-7607
FAX: (334) 281-1973
Lamona Lucas, Commissioner
Rita Houston, Project Director

Provides independent living services for persons age 55 and over. For further information, contact the Project Director or general phone number listed.

ALASKA

♦ *Educational Services*

STATE SERVICES

Alaska Department of Education
801 West Tenth Street, #200
Goldbelt Building
Juneau, AK 99801-1894
(907) 465-2970
FAX: (907) 465-3396
Dr. Shirley Holloway,
Commissioner
Myra Howe, Director, Office of
Special Services

Mission: Administers special
educational programs through the
Division of Education Program
Support.
Funded by: Public funds.
Budget: $8 million.
Area Served: Alaska.

For further information, consult
the director of Education Program
Support or the administrator of the
Office for Exceptional Children.
For information about local
facilities, consult the
superintendent of schools in the
area.

EARLY INTERVENTION COORDINATION

**Early Intervention Program
Alaska Department of Health
and Social Services**
1231 Gambell Street
Anchorage, AK 99501
(907) 269-3400
FAX: (907) 269-3465
Jane Atuk, Part H Early Childhood
Coordinator

The State Infant Learning Program
funds an itinerant consulting
program for blind and visually
impaired children, birth-3 years,
and their families. Works with
local early intervention programs
to develop appropriate
Individualized Family Service
Plans (IFSPs).

SCHOOLS

**Special Education Services
Agency**
2217 East Tudor Road
Suite 1
Anchorage, AK 99507
(907) 562-7372
FAX: (907) 562-0545
E-mail: sesa@sesa.org
URL: http://www.sesa.org
Ron Jones, Program Administrator

Type of Agency: Private; non-
profit.
Mission: Services for totally blind
and legally blind persons.
Funded by: State funds.
Hours of Operation: Mon.-Fri.
8:00 AM-4:30 PM.
History/Date: Est. 1977.
Number of Clients Served: 80.
Eligibility: Visually impaired.
Students must be referred by
district Special Education Director.
Area Served: Statewide.
Age Requirements: 3-21 years.

Health: Refers for health services.
Educational: Ages 3-21. Accepts
deaf-blind, mentally retarded;
other multiply disabled students.
Special blind program. Programs
for college prep; general academic;
vocational/skills development;
parent-infant education. Itinerant
staff delivers on-site services
statewide to all local districts.
Rehabilitation: Activities of daily
living; braille; handwriting; typing;
video magnifier; Optacon;
electronic mobility aids; home
management; orientation/
mobility; rehabilitation teaching in
student's home and community;
sensory training.

Employment: Career and skill
counseling. Refers for other
employment services. Provides
consultation to other agencies.
Prevocational evaluation.
Computer Training: Training on
computer aids and devices.

Contact local school
superintendent for program
availability.

INFANT AND PRESCHOOL

**Special Education Services
Agency
Infant Learning Program**
2217 East Tudor Road
Suite 1
Anchorage, AK 99507
(907) 562-7372
FAX: (907) 562-0545
E-mail: sesa@sesa.org
URL: http://www.sesa.org
Julie Smith, Program Coordinator

Type of Agency: Private; non-
profit.
Funded by: State funds.
Hours of Operation: Mon.-Fri.
8:00AM-4:30PM.
Staff: 4 certified staff - full time.
History/Date: Est. 1977.
Number of Clients Served: 80.
Eligibility: Visually impaired,
with or without additional
disabilities.
Area Served: Alaska.
Age Requirements: 0-3 years.

Health: Refers for health services.
Educational: Provides instruction
in all developmental areas; parent
and teacher training. Consultant
services to other programs.

INSTRUCTIONAL MATERIALS CENTERS

**Special Education Services
Agency**
2217 East Tudor Road
Suite 1

Anchorage, AK 99507
(907) 562-7372
FAX: (907) 562-0545
E-mail: bmciver@sesa.org
William McIver, Specialist for
Blind and Visually Impaired

Area Served: Alaska.
Groups Served: Birth-21; college students; other adults.

Types/Content: Consultation in education of the visually impaired.
Title Listings: Provided at no charge.
Provides technical assistance, training, and consultation to school districts with students who are visually impaired.

◆ Information Services

LIBRARIES

Alaska State Library
Talking Book Center
344 West Third Avenue
Suite 125
Anchorage, AK 99501
(907) 269-6575
FAX: (907) 269-6580
Pat Meek, Library Assistant

Regional library for the blind and physically handicapped and distributor of talking book machines.

MEDIA PRODUCTION SERVICES

ATLA Adaptive Materials Center
2217 East Tudor #5
Anchorage, AK 99507
(907) 563-2599
FAX: (907) 563-0699
E-mail: atla@alaska.net
URL: http://www.alaska.net/
~atla
Cindy Davis, Director

Type of Agency: Non-profit.
Mission: To provide adaptive materials to people with special needs on a fee for service basis.
Funded by: State funds.
Budget: $96,000.
Hours of Operation: Mon-Fri. 9:30 AM-5:30 PM.
Staff: 2. Uses volunteers.
History/Date: Est. 1996.
Area Served: Statewide.
Age Requirements: None.

Educational: Provides adaptive materials to schools for students with special needs.

RADIO READING

A.I.R.R.E.S. Radio Reading Service
1102 West International Airport Road
Anchorage, AK 99518
(907) 563-2121
FAX: (907) 562-5951
Lynn Koral, Program Director

Hours of Operation: Mon.-Fri. 8:00 AM-5:00 PM.
History/Date: Est. 1986.
Area Served: Statewide.

INFORMATION AND REFERRAL

The Foundation Fighting Blindness
Alaska Affiliate
P.O. Box 22016
Juneau, AK 99802
(907) 586-2493
Norma Jean McCorcle, Contact Person

See The Foundation Fighting Blindness in U.S. national listings.

◆ Rehabilitation Services

STATE SERVICES

Alaska Division of Vocational Rehabilitation
1016 West Sixth
Suite 105
Anchorage, AK 99501
(907) 274-5630
FAX: (907) 274-5605
E-mail: dfrench@educ.state.ak.us
Duane French, Director

Type of Agency: State.
Funded by: Public funds.
Hours of Operation: Mon.-Fri. 8:00 AM-5:00 PM.
Area Served: Alaska.

Counseling/Social Work/Self-Help: Consultation services.
Employment: Prevocational evaluation; vocational training and placement; vending stand training.
Computer Training: Training in accessible technology.

Local Offices:

Anchorage: Counseling and Evaluation Center, 3600 South Bragaw, Anchorage, AK 99508, (907) 561-4466.
Bethel: P.O. Box 1507, Bethel, AK 99559-1507, (907) 543-4444.
Fairbanks: Office of Vocational Rehabilitation, 751 Old Richardson Highway, Suite 102, Fairbanks, AK 99701, (907) 451-6261.
Juneau: Office of Vocational Rehabilitation, 9085 Glacier Highway, Suite 102, Juneau, AK 99801-8033, (907) 465-8943.
Kenai: Office of Vocational Rehabilitation, 145 Main Street Loop, Suite 143, Kenai, AK 99611-7755, (907) 283-3133.

Ketchikan: Office of Vocational Rehabilitation, Tongass Commercial Center, Suite 220-A, Ketchikan, AK 99901, (907) 225-6655.
Kodiak: Office of Vocational Rehabilitation, 305 Center Street, Suite 5, Kodiak, AK 99615, (907) 486-5787.
Kotzebue: Office of Vocational Rehabilitation, P.O. Box 129, Kotzebue, AK 99752, (907) 442-3884.
Sitka: Office of Vocational Rehabilitation, 700 Katlian, Suite F, Sitka, AK 99835, (907) 747-4788.
Wasilla: Office of Vocational Rehabilitation, 867 West Commercial Drive, Wasilla, AK 99654-6937, (907) 352-2545.

REHABILITATION

Center for Blind Adults
3903 Taft Drive
Anchorage, AK 99517
(907) 248-7770
FAX: (907) 248-7517
Joe Pattison, Director

Type of Agency: Non-profit.
Mission: Services to help the adult student become independent and self-sufficient.
Funded by: State and federal rehabilitation funds and other contributions.
Hours of Operation: 8:00 AM - 5:00 PM.
Staff: 5.
Eligibility: Legally blind.
Area Served: Alaska.
Transportation: Y.
Age Requirements: 18 years and older.
Professional Training: Typing, computers.
Residential: Residential training facility for adults.
Rehabilitation: Independent travel; braille reading/writing; home economics; physical

education; computers; communications.
Recreational: Activities to aid in rehabilitation and reintegration of blind individuals to society.
Employment: Job placement assistance.
Computer Training: Training provided on talking computers and calculators.
Low Vision Aids: Screenings provided.

COMPUTER TRAINING CENTERS

Center for Blind Adults
3903 Taft Drive
Anchorage, AK 99517
(907) 248-7770
FAX: (907) 248-7517
James King, Rehabilitation Specialist

Computer Training: Speech output systems; screen magnification systems; braille access systems; optical character recognition systems; word processing; computer operating systems.

◆ Low Vision Services

EYE CARE SOCIETIES

Alaska Optometric Association
1345 West Ninth Avenue
Anchorage, AK 99501
(907) 272-2557
Maynard Falconer, Executive Director

Alaska State Ophthalmological Society
North 161 Binkley
Soldotna, AK 99669
(907) 262-4462 or (907) 262-1033
FAX: (907) 262-3914
Peter E. Cannava, M.D., President

◆ Aging Services

STATE UNITS ON AGING

Division of Senior Services Alaska Department of Administration
3601 C Street, #310
Anchorage, AK 99503
(907) 563-5654 or (800) 478-9996
FAX: (907) 562-3040
Connie Sipe, Director

Provides referrals to Area Agencies on Aging and information on other local aging services.

INDEPENDENT LIVING PROGRAMS

Division of Vocational Rehabilitation
801 West 10th Street
Suite 200
Juneau, AK 99801-1894
(907) 465-2814 or (800) 478-2815
FAX: (907) 465-2856
Duane M. French, Director
E. J. Reeder, Program Coordinator

Provides independent living services for persons age 55 and over. For further information, contact the Project Director or general phone number listed.

ARIZONA

◆ *Educational Services*

STATE SERVICES

Exceptional Student Services Arizona Department of Education
1535 West Jefferson Street
Phoenix, AZ 85007
(602) 542-3184
FAX: (602) 542-5404
E-mail: klund@mail.1.ade.state.az.us
URL: http://www.ade.state.az.us
Dr. Kathryn A. Lund, State Director of Exceptional Student Services
Dr. Lynn Busenbark, Preschool Project Specialist, (602) 542-3587
Dr. Julie Williams, Director of State and Federal Programs

Type of Agency: State.
Mission: Provides consultation on educational services for visually impaired students. Administers state funds available for blind children in public schools.
Funded by: Public funds.
Hours of Operation: 8:00AM-5:00PM.
History/Date: Est. 1961.
Area Served: Arizona.

Contact the Director of Exceptional Student Services for information about programs in local schools.

EARLY INTERVENTION COORDINATION

Governor's Interagency Coordinating Council on Infants and Toddlers Arizona Department of Economic Security
P.O. Box 6123, 801-A-6
Phoenix, AZ 85005
(602) 542-5577
FAX: (602) 542-5552
E-mail: azeip@aztec.asu.edu
Diane Renne, Ed.D., Executive Director

Coordination of multi-agency service system for infants and toddlers.

SCHOOLS

Arizona State Schools for the Deaf and the Blind
1200 West Speedway Boulevard
P.O. Box 87010
Tucson, AZ 85754
(520) 770-3738
FAX: (520) 770-3711
Dr. Lynne Albright, Principal, School for the Blind
Dr. Wilbur Lewis, Superintendent

Type of Agency: Public.
Mission: To provide quality, individualized programs for students who are blind or visually impaired.
Funded by: State appropriation with some Federal funds.
Hours of Operation: Office hours: Mon.-Fri. 7:30 AM - 4:00 PM.
Staff: Educational staff: 30; residential staff: 50; vocational/physical education staff: 12.
History/Date: Est. 1912.
Number of Clients Served: 1996-97: 110.
Eligibility: School age students with visual impairments whose needs cannot be met in a district program.
Area Served: State of Arizona. Out-of-state students accepted on tuition basis.
Transportation: Y.
Age Requirements: 0-21 years.

Health: Audiology; speech therapy; occupational and physical therapy.
Counseling/Social Work/Self-Help: Psychological testing and evaluation; individual, group counseling; refers for other counseling/social work services.
Educational: Grades K through 12; college prep; general academic; vocational skill development; activities of daily living; orientation/mobility; independent living program; parent outreach program.
Preschools: See listing under preschool.
Professional Training: Internship/fieldwork placement in orientation/mobility; rehabilitation counseling; special education. Regular in-service training programs, open to enrollment from other agencies.
Residential: Provides 24-hr. residential programming to students outside of day transportation area. All students within 125 miles travel home each weekend. All students return home during designated school break periods.
Rehabilitation: Students assigned rehabilitation counselor from State Blind Services as a part of Individual Transition Plan beginning at 14 years of age.
Recreational: Extracurricular activities: clubs, outdoor education program, swimming, and chorus. Athletics: football, volleyball, basketball, wrestling, track and field, Special Olympics, and other special sports.
Employment: Prevocational evaluation; career and skill counseling; occupational skill development. Refers and provides consultation to other agencies for other employment services.
Computer Training: Full array of computer education using technology which allows large-print, braille, and auditory output.

Low Vision: Evaluation, training and follow-up.
Low Vision Aids: Aids available for loan.
Low Vision Follow-up: Y.

Foundation for Blind Children

1235 E. Harmont Drive
Phoenix, AZ 85020
(602) 331-1470
FAX: (602) 678-5819
E-mail: tompkins@netzone.com
URL: http://www.the-fbc.org
Chris Tompkins, Executive Director

Type of Agency: Private; non-profit.
County/District Where Located: Maricopa County.
Mission: Services for blind and visually impaired; multiply disabled blind.
Funded by: United Way, government grants and contracts, fees for service, donations, and contributions.
Budget: $3 million.
Hours of Operation: Mon.-Fri. 8:00 AM - 5:00 PM.
Staff: 70. Uses volunteers.
History/Date: Est. 1952.
Number of Clients Served: 1996: 1,400.
Eligibility: Any child or adult with a vision loss; Arizona resident.
Area Served: Arizona.
Transportation: Y.
Age Requirements: Birth to 21 years.

Health: Contracts for audiology; physical, occupational and speech therapy for young children.
Counseling/Social Work/Self-Help: Counseling for young children and school age children, families, groups.
Educational: Grades preschool through 12 and nongraded. Serves blind and visually impaired,

multiply disabled blind persons. Operates cooperative preschool classes for blind and visually impaired and multiply disabled blind persons. Designated state depository for instructional materials for public and private schools.
Preschools: 10 month specialized preschool programs - 2 locations. 12 month, home-based infant program, and birth to 3 years.
Professional Training: Internships/fieldwork in special education/visually impaired. Regular in-service training programs.
Reading: Equipment available. Materials in braille, large print, supplemental media. Teaching tools and other materials available.
Rehabilitation: Orientation/mobility; rehabilitation teaching; communications. Conducts summer independent living program; prevocational counseling.
Recreational: Provides summer programs for blind and multiply disabled preschoolers; summer program for school age children.
Employment: Job development and job training.
Computer Training: Assistive technology training.

Local Offices:

Chandler: 191 West Oakland, Chandler, AZ 85224, (602) 963-9298.

Rio Salado Community College

2323 West Fourteenth Street
Tempe, AZ 85281
(602) 517-8000
FAX: (602) 517-8579
Erin Smith, Coordinator for Disabilities, Services and Resources
Linda Thor, President

County/District Where Located: Maricopa County.
Mission: Services for homebound individuals.
Eligibility: All are eligible.

Educational: Interactive classes via telephone on SUNDIAL teleconference system.
Computer Training: Internet classes; adaptive equipment available at campus lab sites.

INFANT AND PRESCHOOL

Arizona State Schools for the Deaf and the Blind
Visually Impaired Preschoolers Program

1200 West Speedway Boulevard
P.O. Box 87010
Tucson, AZ 85754
(520) 770-3002
FAX: (520) 770-3759
Susan Greer, Services Coordinator

Type of Agency: State; day preschool; infant outreach program.
Mission: Committed to looking at the whole child as a child first, who happens to have a visual impairment.
Funded by: Part H; private donations; state funds.
Hours of Operation: Mon.-Fri. 8:00 AM - 4:00 PM (center-based program). Flexible for outreach program.
Staff: 11.
History/Date: Est. 1975.
Number of Clients Served: Approximately 40-50 annually.
Eligibility: Visually impaired or multiply disabled.
Area Served: Statewide for infant outreach; Phoenix & Tucson for center based programs.
Transportation: Y.
Age Requirements: 0-5 years.

Health: Low vision and initial ophthalmological examinations.

Refers to other services for medical care.

Counseling/Social Work/Self-Help: Parent education and support groups. Also refers to other agencies.

Educational: All aspects of infant, toddler, and preschool activities with disability-specific emphasis.

Preschools: Classroom for visually impaired and multiply disabled.

Reading: Prebraille; braille; low vision materials.

Rehabilitation: Orientation/mobility; visual development; auditory/sensory training.

Low Vision: Functional vision assessments.

Local Offices:

Flagstaff: 2501 North 4th Street, Suite 20, Flagstaff, AZ 86004, (520) 774-0665.

Phoenix: Foundation for Blind Children, 1235 East Harmont Drive, Phoenix, AZ 85020, (602) 331-1470.

Cooperative Preschool for Visually Handicapped

1235 East Harmont Drive
Phoenix, AZ 85020
(602) 331-1470
FAX: (602) 678-5819
E-mail: tompkins@netzone.com
URL: http://www.the_fbc.org
Elaine Baldridge, Director

County/District Where Located: Maricopa County.
Mission: Services to visually impaired and multiply disabled persons.
Funded by: United Way, public and private contracts, Arizona State Schools for the Deaf and Blind, private donations.
Hours of Operation: Mon.-Thurs. 9:00 AM-2:30 PM (children); Fri. 9:00 AM-2:30 PM (infants).

Staff: 75. Includes administrator, teachers, paraprofessionals, family counselors (psychologist, attorney, pediatrician available on consultant basis). Orientation/mobility specialists, physical, occupational, and speech therapists, rehabilitation teachers, and librarian available to program. Uses volunteers.
Number of Clients Served: 200.
Eligibility: Any child with a visual loss, with or without multiple disabilities.
Area Served: Maricopa County.
Transportation: Y.
Age Requirements: Birth-6.

Health: Adaptive equipment; genetic counseling; low vision exams; immunizations; blood tests; other health services available on referral basis.
Counseling/Social Work/Self-Help: Parent and other counseling; financial assistance.
Educational: Provides instruction in all developmental areas. Home-based program with center component for infants; classrooms with home teaching component for infants and toddlers who are visually impaired, multiply disabled, or deaf-blind.
Preschools: Consultation to preschools when children are placed out of the center.
Professional Training: Workshops and in-service training for staff.

Outreach (satellite) programs set up with school districts as needed.

STATEWIDE OUTREACH SERVICES

Arizona State Schools for the Deaf and the Blind

1200 West Speedway Boulevard
P.O. Box 87010
Tucson, AZ 85754
(520) 770-3600
FAX: (520) 770-3759
Dennis Russell, Director

Funded by: State funds.
Located at: Tucson, Phoenix, and Flagstaff.
Age Requirements: Birth through 22 years.

Assessment: Developmental transdisciplinary assessments available.
Consultation to Public Schools: Consultation with preschool programs serving visually impaired children.
Direct Service: Through regional services program, and regional cooperative programs.
Parent Assistance: Parent education and counseling available.
Professional Training: Inservice training for teachers of the visually impaired.

INSTRUCTIONAL MATERIALS CENTERS

Arizona Instructional Resource Center

1235 East Harmont Drive
Phoenix, AZ 85020
(602) 678-5816
FAX: (602) 678-5819
E-mail: durre@enuxsa.esa.asu.edu
Ingrborg K. Durre, Contact Person

Area Served: Statewide.
Groups Served: K-12 (including age 21).

Types/Content: Textbooks; recreational reading material; literary material.
Media Formats: Braille and large print.

UNIVERSITY TRAINING PROGRAMS

University of Arizona

College of Education
Department of Special Education
Tucson, AZ 85721
(520) 621-0945
FAX: (520) 621-3821
E-mail: jerin@u.arizona.edu
Dr. Jane Erin, Visually
Handicapped
Dr. Irene Topor, Orientation and
Mobility
Dr. Stephanie MacFarland, Deaf-
Blindness

County/District Where Located:
Pima County.

Programs Offered: Graduate
(master's, educational specialist,
and doctoral) programs for
teachers of visually impaired,
multiply disabled, and deaf-blind
students and for orientation and
mobility specialists.
Distance Education: Y.

◆ *Information Services*

LIBRARIES

Arizona State Braille and Talking Book Library

1030 North 32nd Street
Phoenix, AZ 85008
(602) 255-5578 or toll-free in
Arizona (800) 255-5578
FAX: (602) 255-4312
E-mail: btbl@dlapr.lib.az.us
URL: http://www.dlapr.lib.az.us
Linda A. Montgomery, Librarian

Type of Agency: Regional library.
County/District Where Located:
Maricopa County.
Mission: To provide books,
magazines and other library
resources in alternate formats for
all Arizona residents whose visual
or physical disabilities prevent the
use of conventional print
materials.
Funded by: Foundation grants;
state funds.
Budget: $700,000.
Hours of Operation: Mon.-Fri.
8:00 AM-5:00 PM.
Program Accessibility:
Accessible.
Staff: 19.5.
History/Date: Est. 1969.
Number of Clients Served:
11,000.
Eligibility: Blind, visually
impaired, physically disabled, or
experiencing an organic learning
disability.
Area Served: Arizona.

Regional library providing disks,
braille, and cassettes. Distributes
talking books and tapes. Tapes
locally requested material on
cassettes.

Prescott Talking Book Library

215 East Goodwin Street
Prescott, AZ 86303
(520) 445-8110
FAX: (520) 445-1851
Jill North, Librarian

Subregional library.

Special Needs Center Phoenix Public Library

1221 North Central Avenue
Phoenix, AZ 85004
(602) 261-8690
FAX: (602) 534-4520
Cynthia Holt, Special Needs
Center Supervisor

Type of Agency: Municipal.
Mission: Information and library
services.
Funded by: City of Phoenix funds
for the Phoenix public library
system.
Staff: 5.1.
History/Date: Est. 1983.

Eligibility: Maricopa County
residents with disabilities.
Area Served: Maricopa County.
Age Requirements: None.

Educational: Library services;
readers advisory; reference
services.
Reading: Talking book records/
tapes; braille books/magazines;
transcriptions; large-print books;
video print enlarger; computers
with synthetic speech; screen
readers; Kurzweil personal reader.
Internet access on PC with
assistive technology. Internet and
Dial-IN access to the library's
catalog.
Computer Training: Training in
the use of the center's equipment.

MEDIA PRODUCTION SERVICES

Arizona State Braille and Talking Book Library

1030 North 32nd Street
Phoenix, AZ 85008
(602) 255-5578 or outside 602 area
code (800) 255-5578
FAX: (602) 255-4312
E-mail: btbl@dlapr.lib.az.us
URL: http://www.dlapr.lib.az.us
Linda A. Montgomery, Director

County/District Where Located:
Maricopa County.
Area Served: Arizona.
Groups Served: K-12, college
students, other adults.

Types/Content: Recreational,
informational.
Media Formats: Talking books/
cassettes; braille.
Title Listings: None specified.

Arizona State Schools for the Deaf and the Blind

Southeast Regional Cooperative
P.O. Box 87010

Tucson, AZ 85754
(520) 770-3757
FAX: (520) 770-3782
E-mail: sercoop@flash.net
Geri Nelson, Supervisor

Area Served: Southeastern Arizona.
Groups Served: K-12.

Types/Content: Textbooks; recreational; career/vocational; educational.
Media Formats: Braille books, talking books/cassettes, large-print books.
Title Listings: No title listings available.

Foundation for Blind Children
1235 E. Harmont Drive
Phoenix, AZ 85020
(602) 331-1470
FAX: (602) 678-5819
E-mail: tompkins@netzone.com
URL: http://www.the-fbc.org
Chris Tompkins, Executive Director

County/District Where Located: Maricopa County.
Area Served: Arizona.
Groups Served: Children and youths from birth through high school.

Types/Content: Education, counseling, technology, media, recreational, career/vocational, early intervention.
Media Formats: Braille/large-print books.
Title Listings: No title listings available.

Recording for the Blind and Dyslexic
9449 North 99th Avenue
Peoria, AZ 85345
(602) 977-6020
Robert J. Briscoe, Director

County/District Where Located: Maricopa County.

See Recording for the Blind and Dyslexic in U.S. national listings.

Recording for the Blind and Dyslexic
3627 East Indian School Road
Suite 108
Phoenix, AZ 85018
(602) 468-9144
FAX: (602) 553-0226
Marsha Mulcahy, Studio Director

See Recording for the Blind and Dyslexic in U.S. national listings.

RADIO READING

Sun Sounds Radio Reading Service
3124 East Roosevelt Street
Phoenix, AZ 85008
(602) 231-0500
FAX: (602) 220-9335
E-mail: pasco@rio.maricopa.edu
Bill Pasco, Director

County/District Where Located: Maricopa County.
Funded by: Grants, donations.
Hours of Operation: 24 hours per day.
Staff: 17.
History/Date: Est. 1979.
Area Served: State of Arizona.
Age Requirements: None.

Sun Sounds Radio Reading Service
7290 East Broadway
Suite K
Tucson, AZ 85710
(520) 296-2400
Mitzi Tharin, Station Manager

County/District Where Located: Pima County.
Hours of Operation: 24 hours.
History/Date: Est. 1979.
Area Served: Tucson.

INFORMATION AND REFERRAL

The Foundation Fighting Blindness
Arizona Affiliate
423 East Fairmont Drive
Tempe, AZ 85282-3720
(602) 894-0712
Jackie Olsen, Contact Person
Marvin Freeman, President

See The Foundation Fighting Blindness in U.S. national listings.

◆ Rehabilitation Services

STATE SERVICES

Rehabilitation Services Administration
Arizona Department of Economic Security
1789 West Jefferson Street (930A)
Phoenix, AZ 85007
(602) 542-6289 or toll-free in Arizona (800) 563-1221
FAX: (602) 542-3778
E-mail: azsbvi@cirs.org
Ed House, Section Manager

Type of Agency: State, a division of the Department of Economic Security.
Mission: To empower individuals with disabilities to achieve increased independence and/or gainful employment through the provision of quality services.
Funded by: Federal, state, and local funding.
Hours of Operation: Mon.-Fri. 8:00 AM-5:00 PM.
Program Accessibility: Accessible.
Staff: 91 full time. Uses volunteers.
History/Date: Est. 1966.
Number of Clients Served: 1996: 2,400.

Eligibility: Varies with individual program.
Area Served: Statewide.
Transportation: Y.
Age Requirements: Mostly adults.

Health: Sight conservation program, eye examinations, treatment, and eyeglasses for low-income persons. Contracts for other health services.
Counseling/Social Work/Self-Help: Psychological testing and evaluation; individual, group, family/parent, couple counseling. Contracts and/or refers for other counseling/social work services.
Educational: Transition rehabilitation program.
Professional Training: Internship/fieldwork placement in rehabilitation; counseling; teaching.
Reading: Lends talking book record players and cassette players and related equipment and accessories.
Rehabilitation: Personal management; communication skills, home management, orientation and mobility.
Recreational: By referral.
Employment: Vocational Rehabilitation Services, Business Enterprise Program, and Industries for the Blind program.
Computer Training: As part of vocational rehabilitation program.
Low Vision: Evaluation and referral.
Low Vision Aids: Aids and training available.

Local Offices:

Cottonwood: 1645 East Cottonwood Street, Cottonwood, AZ 86326, (520) 634-0063.

Flagstaff: RSA Region III (Coconino, Apache, LaPaz, Mohave, Navajo, and Yavapai Counties), 1510 South Riordan Ranch Street, Flagstaff, AZ 86001, (602) 779-4147.
Glendale: AZRSA, 4425 West Olive, Glendale, AZ 85302, (602) 842-1125.
Mesa: AZRSA, 225 East Main Street, Mesa, AZ 85210, (602) 962-7516.
Phoenix: RSA Region I (Maricopa, Gila, Pinal, and Yuma Counties), 1430 East Indian School Road, Suite 205, Phoenix, AZ 85014, (602) 255-5641.
Phoenix: Rehabilitation Instructional Services, 4620 North 16th Street, Phoenix, AZ 85016, (602) 266-9286.
Prescott: AZRSA, 1555 Ironsprings Road, Prescott, AZ 86302, (520) 445-6432.
Scottsdale: AZRSA, 10900 North Scottsdale Road, Scottsdale, AZ 85254, (602) 948-3819.
Tucson: Vocational Rehabilitation Office, 100 North Stone, Suite 500B, Tucson, AZ 85701, (520) 629-0225.
Tucson: RSA Region II (Pima, Cochise, Graham, Greenlee, and Santa Cruz Counties), 400 West Congress, Suite 420, Tucson, AZ 85701, (602) 628-6810.
Yuma: AZRSA, 1310 South Third Avenue, Yuma, AZ 85364, (520) 329-9462.

REHABILITATION

Arizona Center for the Blind and Visually Impaired
3100 East Roosevelt Street
Phoenix, AZ 85008
(602) 273-7411
FAX: (602) 273-7410
Jim La May, Executive Director

Type of Agency: Private; non-profit.

County/District Where Located: Maricopa County.
Mission: Services for persons who are visually impaired, 18 years of age and older.
Funded by: Contributions, fund raising, sub-contracts, United Way.
Budget: $800,000.
Hours of Operation: Mon.-Fri. 8:00 AM - 4:30 PM.
Staff: 19 full time. Uses volunteers.
History/Date: Est. 1947.
Number of Clients Served: 1,800.
Eligibility: Visually impaired; doctor's statement.
Area Served: Arizona.
Transportation: Y.
Age Requirements: 18 years of age or older.

Health: Refers for health services.
Counseling/Social Work/Self-Help: Social evaluation; individual, group, family/parent, couple counseling; referral to community services. Contracts and refers for other counseling/social work services.
Educational: Speakers' bureau.
Professional Training: Internships available.
Reading: Volunteer reading services.
Rehabilitation: Activities of daily living; home management; orientation/mobility; rehabilitation teaching in client's home and community; sensory training.
Recreational: Adult continuing education; arts and crafts; hobby groups; summer day camp; special programs for elderly; bowling; swimming; beep ball; skiing. Provides consultation to other agencies.
Employment: Refers for employment services.
Computer Training: Assistive technology program.

Low Vision: Functional assessments and clinical examinations; referrals.
Low Vision Aids: Training with variety of vision aids.
Low Vision Follow-up: Yes.

Local Offices:

Mesa: 247 North McDonald, Mesa, AZ 85201, (602) 273-7411.
Peoria: Arizona Center for the Blind & Visually Impaired, 9451 North 99th Avenue, Peoria, AZ 85345, (602) 273-7411.
Scottsdale: 7375 East 2nd Street, Scottsdale, AZ 85251, (602) 273-7411.

Arizona Industries for the Blind

3013 West Lincoln Street
Phoenix, AZ 85009
(602) 269-5131
FAX: (602) 269-9462
Donald H. Peterson, General Manager

Type of Agency: State.
County/District Where Located: Maricopa County.
Mission: To assist physically disabled adults (primarily those who are legally blind) to obtain their maximum level of vocational functioning and/or earned income by providing rehabilitation services and employment opportunities.
Funded by: Workshop sales, state appropriations, sub-contracts, fund raising, and State Vocational Rehabilitation.
Budget: $6 million.
Hours of Operation: Mon.-Fri. 8:00 AM - 5:00 PM.
Program Accessibility: Wheelchair accessible.
Staff: 45.
History/Date: Est. 1952.
Number of Clients Served: 300 annually.
Eligibility: Physically disabled adults (primarily legally blind).

Area Served: Maricopa County.
Age Requirements: Adults.

Health: Eye exams.
Rehabilitation: Work adjustment; job placement and development.
Employment: Vocational/prevocational evaluation and training; work adjustment/experience; job development/placement; follow-up; industrial workshop; work activities center.
Computer Training: Technology assessment.

Local Offices:

Phoenix: HANDILAB: 3122 West Indian School Road, Phoenix, AZ 85016, (602) 956-3451.
Phoenix: Lighting Distribution Center, 36 North 35th Avenue, Phoenix, AZ 85005, (602) 447-8272.
Phoenix: AIB, 1702 West Camelback Road, Suite 7, Phoenix, AZ 85015.

Southwestern Blind Rehabilitation Center

VA Medical Center
360 South Sixth Avenue
Tucson, AZ 85723
(520) 629-4643
Joseph J. Hennessey, Director

Referral applications by Visual Impairment Services programs located at VA Medical Centers and Outpatient Clinics in the geographical area served by the Blind Rehabilitation Center or Clinic. See U.S. Department of Veterans Affairs in U.S. Federal Agencies listings.

Tucson Association for the Blind and Visually Impaired

3767 East Grant Road
Tucson, AZ 85716
(520) 795-1331
FAX: (520) 795-1331
E-mail: tabvi@azstarnet.com
Gene Luini, Executive Director

Type of Agency: Private; non-profit.
County/District Where Located: Pima County.
Mission: TAB is committed to providing dynamic and progressive programs and services to meet the rehabilitation and social needs of individuals with vision loss; promoting individuals to become active participants in determining their success; and raising public awareness through community involvement and establishment of partnerships with others.
Funded by: Fees charged for services contracted by state of Arizona; contributions; bequests.
Budget: $ 800,000.
Hours of Operation: Mon.-Fri. 8:00 AM - 5:00 PM; special evening and weekend activities.
Program Accessibility: The facility and all programs are accessible to persons with disabilities.
Staff: 24 full-time, 7 part-time. Extensive use of volunteers.
History/Date: Inc. 1965.
Number of Clients Served: 900 annually.
Eligibility: Blind or visually impaired persons.
Area Served: Southern Arizona.
Age Requirements: 14 years or older.

Health: Refers for all health services.
Counseling/Social Work/Self-Help: Social evaluations; group and individual counseling; social work. Information and referral.
Educational: Scholarship program for visually impaired post-secondary students.
Reading: Lends talking book machines and provides referrals for adaptive reading resources: braille books; large-print books; braille magazines and books;

recorded magazines. Staffs a document conversion unit which provides transcription of braille; braille copying; reader service.
Residential: For Arizona residents in vocational rehabilitation programs. Short-term residential programs available.
Rehabilitation: Classes and training to promote emotional adjustment, consumer education and advocacy, and independent living skills. Group and individual training in home and personal management, to include braille, cooking, handwriting, adaptive aids, orientation and mobility; mentor program, counseling, outreach and referrals to community resources; rehabilitation, adjustment and employment services for developmentally disabled. Offers some social/recreational programs, job development, employment and technology services.
Recreational: Limited center-based programs and services directed toward participation in community activities.
Employment: Operates NIB switchboard contract at V.A. Medical Center, limited but individualized work adjustment services and extensive job development/job placement services.
Computer Training: Operates adaptive technology center offering individualized training in both screen reading and large-print programs.
Low Vision: Provides low vision education course prior to a clinical low vision evaluation.
Low Vision Aids: Referrals.

Private, non-profit independent living center.

Yuma Center for the Visually Impaired
2770 South Avenue B
Yuma, AZ 85364
(520) 726-1310
Cal Roberts, Executive Director

Type of Agency: Private; non-profit.
County/District Where Located: Yuma County.
Mission: Services for visually impaired and multihandicapped.
Funded by: Contracts, Community Chest, and fundraising.
History/Date: Est. 1972.
Eligibility: Visually impaired or multihandicapped.
Transportation: Y.

COMPUTER TRAINING CENTERS

Arizona State Schools for the Deaf and the Blind
1200 West Speedway Boulevard
P.O. Box 87010
Tucson, AZ 85754
(520) 770-3667
FAX: (520) 770-3752
E-mail: asdblrc@azstarnet.com
URL: http://www.azstarnet.com/~asdbhs
Carlton T. Wiens, Teacher

Computer Training: Speech output systems; screen magnification systems; braille access sytems; optical character recognition systems; computer operating systems.

Tucson Association for the Blind and Visually Impaired
3767 East Grant Road
Tucson, AZ 85716
(520) 795-1331
FAX: (520) 795-1331
Mimi Marsh, Director of Rehabilitation

County/District Where Located: Pima County.

Computer Training: Speech output systems; screen magnification systems; optical character recognition systems; word processing; computer operating systems.

Document conversion services: braille, large print, audio cassettes.

◆ Low Vision Services

EYE CARE SOCIETIES

Arizona Ophthalmological Society
810 West Bethany Home Road
Phoenix, AZ 85013
(602) 246-6053
FAX: (602) 242-6283
URL: http://www.armadoc.com
Patrice Hand, Executive Director

County/District Where Located: Maricopa County.

Arizona Optometric Association
3625 North 16th Street, Suite 125
Phoenix, AZ 85016
(602) 279-0055
FAX: (602) 264-6356
E-mail: azoa@aol.com
Alvin Levin, Executive Director

County/District Where Located: Maricopa County.

LOW VISION CENTERS

Low Vision Facility of Boswell Eye Institute
10541 West Thunderbird Boulevard
Sun City, AZ 85351
(602) 933-3402
FAX: (602) 972-5014
Albert L. Rhoades, M.D.

County/District Where Located: Maricopa County.

Mission: To assist visually impaired persons with optical and nonoptical aids; to help them cope with their visual impairment; to refer to local support agencies for assistance.

Funded by: Client fees and community grants.

Hours of Operation: Tue. 9:00 AM - 2:00 PM; Thurs. 9:00 PM - 1:00 PM; Fri. 10:00 AM - 2:00 PM.

Staff: Low vision assistant; ophthalmologist.

History/Date: Est. 1985.

Number of Clients Served: More than 200 annually.

Eligibility: Referral by ophthalmologist; current ophthalmological report.

Area Served: Unlimited.

Counseling/Social Work/Self-Help: Through local support groups.

Low Vision: On-site training provided.

Low Vision Aids: Prescribed; purchased at local optical shops.

Low Vision Follow-up: Return appointment; support group.

St. Joseph's Low Vision Services
350 North Wilmot
Tucson, AZ 85711
(520) 721-3862
FAX: (520) 750-5062
Tom Gagen, Senior Vice President/Administrator, St. Joseph's Hospital
Janet Dylla, Program Coordinator, Regional Eye Center/Low Vision Services

Type of Agency: Non-profit.
County/District Where Located: Pima County.
Funded by: Client fees.

Hours of Operation: Mon.-Fri. 7:30 AM-4:00 PM by appointment.

Staff: Vision specialist; psychologists; rehabilitation counselor; optician consultant.

Area Served: Southern Arizona, northern Sonora, Mexico.

Counseling/Social Work/Self-Help: Low vision support group.

Low Vision Aids: Sells and lends; on-site training provided.

Low Vision Follow-up: By return appointment.

◆ *Aging Services*

STATE UNITS ON AGING

Aging and Adult Administration Arizona Department of Economic Security
1789 West Jefferson Street
#950A
Phoenix, AZ 85007
(602) 542-4446 or Medigap Information and Referral
(800) 432-4040
FAX: (602) 542-6575
Art Olin, Director

Provides referrals to Area Agencies on Aging and information on other local aging services.

INDEPENDENT LIVING PROGRAMS

Rehabilitation Services Administration Arizona Department of Economic Security
1789 West Jefferson Street
930A
Phoenix, AZ 85007
(602) 542-6289 or (800) 563-1221
FAX: (602) 542-3778
Ed House, Administrator

Provides independent living services for persons age 55 and over. For further information, contact the Project Director or general phone number listed.

ARKANSAS

♦ Educational Services

STATE SERVICES

Arkansas Department of Education
Special Education Department
4 Capitol Mall
Education Building, Room 105-C
Little Rock, AR 72201
(501) 682-4221
FAX: (501) 682-4313
Dr. Diane Sydoriak, Associate
Director of Special Education
Bob Brasher, State Coordinator,
Educational Services for Visually
Impaired, Arkansas School for the
Blind, P.O. Box 668, Little Rock, AR
72203, phone (501) 296-1815, FAX
(501) 663-3536.

Type of Agency: State.
County/District Where Located:
Pulaski County.
Mission: Under the direct
supervision of Educational
Services for the Visually Impaired
of the Arkansas School for the
Blind, the Educational Materials
Center acts as a clearinghouse and
depository of large-print and
braille textbooks and adaptive
equipment for visually impaired
and blind students in Arkansas.
Regional vision consultants assist
local school districts by providing
technical assistance. Orientation
and mobility specialists provide
direct instruction. Preschool
consultants provide home
intervention.
Funded by: State and federal
funds.
Hours of Operation: 8:00 AM-
4:30 PM.
Staff: 16.
History/Date: Est. 1977.

Number of Clients Served: 120
families of preschoolers; 650
school-age students.
Eligibility: Visual impairment
that potentially affects education.
Area Served: Arkansas.
Age Requirements: Birth through
high-school age.

Educational: 5 vision consultants
provide technical assistance. 3
orientation and mobility specialists
provide instruction.
Preschools: 4 preschool
consultants provide home
intervention and center/day care
technical assistance.
Reading: Educational materials
center provides large-print/braille
textbooks statewide.
Recreational: 4-week summer
program for public school students
on Arkansas School for the Blind
campus.
Low Vision: Weekly low vision
clinic sees 150 preschool/public
school students annually plus all
residential students.

Education Services for the Visually
Impaired is the statewide program
of the Arkansas Department of
Education, Special Education. The
project is directly supervised by
the Arkansas School for the Blind.

EARLY INTERVENTION COORDINATION

Developmental Disabilities Services
Arkansas Department of Human Services
Donaghey Plaza North
Seventh and Main Streets
P.O. Box 1437
Slot 2520
Little Rock, AR 72203-1437
(501) 682-8676
FAX: (501) 682-8890
Sherry Cobb, Part H Early
Intervention Coordinator

County/District Where Located:
Pulaski County.

Evalutions, transportation, speech
therapy, occupational therapy,
physical therapy, early
intervention, targeted case
management, adaptive equipment,
family support, consultation.

SCHOOLS

Arkansas School for the Blind
2600 West Markham
P.O. Box 668
Little Rock, AR 72203
(501) 296-1810 or (501) 296-1815
(Educational Services for the
Visually Impaired-Preschool
Home Intervention Program)
FAX: (501) 663-3536
Dr. Ivan Terzieff, Superintendent
Bob Brasher, State Coordinator,
FSUI (Outreach)

Type of Agency: State.
County/District Where Located:
Pulaski.
Mission: Services for totally blind;
legally blind; deaf-blind; learning
disabled; mentally retarded;
orthopedically disabled.
Funded by: General State
Revenue; Department of
Education, PL94-142 funds.
Hours of Operation: 8:00AM-
5:00PM.
Staff: 109 full time. Uses
volunteers.
History/Date: Est. 1859. Home
Intervention/Technical Assistance
Program est. 1982.
Number of Clients Served: 110 on
campus, 760 off-site.
Eligibility: Legally blind,
Arkansas resident.
Age Requirements: 3-21 years.

Health: Diagnosis and evaluation
of eye health; treatment of eye
conditions; prescription of
spectacles or aids; has low vision
aids or devices; evaluation of eye
treatment or prescription; general

medical services; speech therapy. Refers for other health services.

Counseling/Social Work/Self-Help: Psychological testing and evaluation; individual counseling; placement in school.

Educational: Grades preschool through 12 and non-graded. Programs for general academic; vocational skill development.

Preschools: Programs for academic, concept, and skills development.

Professional Training: Internship/fieldwork placement in orientation/mobility. Regular in-service training programs.

Reading: Talking book machines, cassette players; talking book records and cassettes; braille books; large-print books; braille magazines; recorded magazines; Kurzweil reading machine.

Residential: Dormitories; on-site apartments for independent living.

Recreational: Afterschool programs; arts and crafts; hobby groups; summer day camp; swimming; track; wrestling. Refers for other recreation services.

Employment: Prevocational evaluation; career and skill counseling; occupational skill development; vocational placement; follow-up service; vending stand training. Refers for other employment-oriented services.

Computer Training: Training on computer aids and devices.

Low Vision: Evaluations and prescription of low vision aids.

Low Vision Aids: Available.

Low Vision Follow-up: Y.

INFANT AND PRESCHOOL

Arkansas School for the Blind
2600 West Markham
P.O. Box 668

Little Rock, AR 72203
(501) 296-1810
FAX: (501) 663-3536
Bob Brasher, State Coordinator

Type of Agency: State.

County/District Where Located: Pulaski County.

Mission: Provides instruction in all developmental areas; transportation; low vision exams.

Funded by: State funds, P.L. 94-142 incentive grants.

Hours of Operation: Mon.-Fri. 8:00 AM-5:00 PM.

Staff: 4 full time. Uses volunteers.

History/Date: Est. 1982.

Eligibility: Visual impairment, with or without other disabling conditions, 3-5 years old.

Area Served: Statewide.

Age Requirements: 5 years and under.

Health: Diagnosis and evaluation; referrals to other agencies.

Educational: Academic, concept and skills development programs.

Professional Training: Internships, technical assistance and inservice training programs.

Low Vision: Evaluations.

Low Vision Aids: Prescriptions and aids available.

Low Vision Follow-up: Y.

Outreach and consultant services also provided. For information, contact Bob Brasher, State Coordinator.

STATEWIDE OUTREACH SERVICES

Educational Services for Visually Impaired
Arkansas School for the Blind
2600 West Markham
P.O. Box 668
Little Rock, AR 72203
(501) 296-1815
FAX: (501) 663-3536
Bob Brasher, State Coordinator

Funded by: Arkansas Department of Education, Special Education (IDEA-6B) funds, and Arkansas School for the Blind.

Located at: Central Office: Arkansas School for the Blind, with four regional offices in Educational Service Coop locations.

History/Date: Est. 1978.

Age Requirements: Birth through high school age.

Professional Training: Local and statewide in-servicing annually.

Assessment: Provides weekly low vision clinic to public schools, preschool and residential students. (Other assessments by Arkansas School for the Blind on request).

Consultation to Public Schools: Five regional vision consultants provide technical assistance.

Direct Service: Three orientation and mobility specialists travel statewide.

Parent Assistance: Four preschool specialists provide home intervention and assistance to centers/day care programs.

Materials Production: Depository-style educational materials center provides all braille/large-print textbooks statewide and coordinates braille/large-print prison project.

INSTRUCTIONAL MATERIALS CENTERS

Educational Services for Visually Impaired
Arkansas School for the Blind
2600 West Markham
P.O. Box 668
Little Rock, AR 72203
(501) 296-1815
FAX: (501) 663-3536
Bob Brasher, State Coordinator

Area Served: Statewide (public, private and residential).

Groups Served: K-12.

Types/Content: Textbooks.
Media Formats: Braille and large-print textbooks.
Title Listings: No title listings.

UNIVERSITY TRAINING PROGRAMS

University of Arkansas at Little Rock

Department of Rehabilitation and Special Education
2801 South University Avenue
Little Rock, AR 72204
(501) 569-3169
FAX: (501) 569-8129
E-mail: pbsmith@ualr.edu
URL: http://www.ualr.edu/~rehdept/
Dr. Patricia Smith, Rehabilitation Teaching
Dr. William Jacobson, Orientation and Mobility
Dr. Cay Holbrook, Visually Handicapped, Teacher Education, (501) 569-3335

Programs Offered: Graduate (Master's) programs for teachers of visually impaired students, orientation/mobility specialists, and rehabilitation teachers of blind persons. Summer certification programs. Dual degree options. Certification in rehabilitation counseling.
Distance Education: Y.

◆ *Information Services*

LIBRARIES

Fort Smith Public Library for the Blind and Handicapped

61 South Eighth Street
Fort Smith, AR 72901
(501) 783-0229
FAX: (501) 782-8571
Larry Larson, Director

County/District Where Located: Sebastion County.

Subregional library.

Library for the Blind and Handicapped, Northwest

Ozarks Regional Library
217 East Dickson Street
Fayetteville, AR 72701
(501) 442-6253
Rachel Anne Ames, Librarian

County/District Where Located: Washington County.

Subregional library.

Library for the Blind and Handicapped, Southwest

CLOC Regional Library
P.O. Box 668
Magnolia, AR 71753
(501) 234-1991
FAX: (501) 234-5077
Christine McDonald, Librarian

Subregional library.

Library for the Blind and Physically Handicapped

One Capitol Mall
Little Rock, AR 72201-1081
(501) 682-1155
FAX: (501) 682-1529
John J.D. Hall, Regional Librarian

Funded by: Public funds.
Hours of Operation: Mon.-Fri. 8:00 AM - 5:00 PM.
Staff: 8.
History/Date: Est. 1969.
Number of Clients Served: 6,000.
Eligibility: Any visual or physical disability that makes it difficult to read regular printed material.
Area Served: Arkansas.

Regional library providing free loan of braille books and talking books, on record and cassette, and talking book machines.

MEDIA PRODUCTION SERVICES

Arkansas Department of Correction

P.O. Box 1000
Wrightsville, AR 72183
(501) 897-5806
FAX: (501) 897-5716
Clifford Terry, Warden

County/District Where Located: Pulaski County.
Groups Served: K-12.

Types/Content: Textbooks.
Media Formats: Braille books.
Title Listings: No title listings.

RADIO READING

Arkansas Radio Reading Service

2600 West Markham
P.O. Box 668
Little Rock, AR 72203
(501) 663-4540
FAX: (501) 663-4540
Randy Johnson, Executive Director

County/District Where Located: Pulaski County.
Hours of Operation: Office: Mon.-Fri. 8:00 AM-3:00 PM; on air 24 hours, 7 days.
History/Date: Est. 1981.
Area Served: 50-mile radius from Little Rock, covering central Arkansas.

INFORMATION AND REFERRAL

The Foundation Fighting Blindness
Arkansas Affiliate

Route 3
P.O. Box 337
Clinton, AR 72031
(501) 985-2202
Nancy Burgess

See The Foundation Fighting Blindness in U.S. national listings.

◆ Rehabilitation Services

Arkansas Division of Services for the Blind

522 Main Street, Suite 100
Little Rock, AR 72201
(501) 682-5463
FAX: (501) 682-0366
James C. Hudson, Director

Type of Agency: State rehabilitation.
County/District Where Located: Pulaski County.
Mission: To provide opportunities to individuals who are blind or visually impaired to achieve employment and/or independence.
Funded by: State funds; foundation grants.
Budget: 1993: $4.5 million.
Hours of Operation: 8:00AM-4:30PM.
Staff: 83 full time, 14 part time. Uses volunteers.
History/Date: Est. 1983.
Number of Clients Served: 1996: 3,645.
Eligibility: Legally blind or severely visually impaired persons.
Area Served: Statewide.
Health: Provides, purchases, or refers for the following health services: diagnosis and evaluation of eye health; treatment of eye conditions; prescription of spectacles or aids; low vision services; audiology therapy; occupational therapy; physical therapy; speech therapy.
Counseling/Social Work/Self-Help: Counseling and referral services.
Professional Training: Internships and supervised field placements in rehabilitation counseling, orientation/mobility, rehabilitation teaching and social work.
Rehabilitation: Provides or purchases the following services: personal management; communication skills; home management; orientation/mobility; rehabilitation teaching in client's home and community; remedial education; sensory training.
Employment: Provides or purchases the following services: prevocational evaluation; career and skill counseling; occupational skill development; vocational training; job retention and job retraining; sheltered workshops; vocational placement; follow-up service; vending stand training.
Computer Training: Training on computer aids and devices.

Local Offices:

Batesville: Division of Services for the Blind, 1652 White Drive, P.O. Box 3669, Batesville, AR 72503, (501) 793-4153, TDD (501) 793-4224.
El Dorado: Division of Services for the Blind, 123 West 18th, El Dorado, AR 71730, (501) 862-6631, TDD (501) 862-3729.
Fayetteville: Division of Services for the Blind, 4044 Frontage Road, Fayetteville, AR 72703, (501) 521-1270, TDD (501) 521-0103.
Fort Smith: Division of Services for the Blind, 616 Garrison Building, Garrison Avenue, Fort Smith, AR 72901, (501) 782-4555, TDD (501) 782-9873.
Harrison: Division of Services for the Blind, 2126 Copps Road, Harrison, AR 72601, (501) 741-6107.
Jonesboro: Division of Services for the Blind, 2920 McCellan Drive, Room 1106, Jonesboro, AR 77401, (501) 972-1732, TDD (501) 972-6013.
Pine Bluff: Division of Services for the Blind, Sixth and Mulberry, P.O. Box 5670, Pine Bluff, AR 71603, (501) 534-4200, TDD (501) 534-8976.
Texarkana: Division of Services for the Blind, 4425 Jefferson Avenue, #102, Texarkana, AR 71854, (501) 779-1141, TDD (501) 773-2807.

Arkansas Lighthouse for the Blind

69th and Murray Streets
P.O. Box 192666
Little Rock, AR 72219
(501) 562-2222
FAX: (501) 568-5275
James O. Avants, Executive Vice President

Type of Agency: Sheltered workshop.
County/District Where Located: Pulaski County.
Mission: Training and employment of blind individuals.
Funded by: Workshop sales.
Hours of Operation: 6:45 AM - 4:00 PM.
Program Accessibility: Fully accessible.
Staff: 8 full time.
History/Date: Est. and Inc. 1940.
Eligibility: Legally blind.
Area Served: Central Arkansas.
Age Requirements: 18 years and older.
Employment: Industrial evaluation; training.

Lions World Services for the Blind

2811 Fair Park Boulevard
P.O. Box 4055

Little Rock, AR 72204
(501) 664-7100
FAX: (501) 664-2743
E-mail: lwsb@mail.snider.net
URL: http://www.snider.net/
lions
Jim Cordell, Executive Director

Type of Agency: Private.
County/District Where Located:
Pulaski County.
Mission: To enable people who
are legally blind or visually
impaired to function
independently and live full,
productive lives with dignity &
self-respect.
Funded by: Tuition, contribution
and grants.
Budget: $2,500,000.
Hours of Operation: Mon.-Fri.
8:00 AM-4:30 PM.
Staff: 64 full time.
History/Date: Est. 1947.
Number of Clients Served: 300
annually.
Eligibility: Legally blind.
Area Served: Unlimited.
Transportation: Y.
Age Requirements: 16 years and
older.

Health: Provision, purchase or
referral for diagnosis and
evaluation of eye condition,
prescription of lenses and low
vision aids, audiological services,
occupational, physical or speech
therapy.
**Counseling/Social Work/Self-
Help:** Counseling and referral
services, psychological testing &
psychiatric evaluation.
Educational: Remedial services,
GED preparation.
Professional Training: Provides
internships and supervised field
placements for rehabilitation
counseling, orientation/mobility,
rehabilitation teaching & social
work students.
Reading: Remedial services.

Residential: Y.
Rehabilitation: Rehabilitation
teaching, communication skills,
orientation and mobility, low
vision evaluation and training.
Recreational: Leisure time
activities.
Employment: Provides vocational
evaluation, job readiness,
vocational training in 14 areas, job
development and placement and
follow-up services.
Computer Training: Operates
assistive technology laboratory
and provides training in computer
programming and computer
related areas.
Low Vision: Clinic and training.
Low Vision Aids: Y.
Low Vision Follow-up: Y.

COMPUTER TRAINING CENTERS

**Arkansas Division of Services
for the Blind**
522 Main Street, Suite 100
Little Rock, AR 72201
(501) 682-5463
FAX: (501) 682-0366
Larry Wayland, Sensory Aids
Specialist

County/District Where Located:
Pulaski County.

Computer Training: Speech
output systems; screen
magnification systems; braille
access systems; optical character
recognition systems; closed-circuit
television systems; word
processing; database software;
computer operating systems.

**Arkansas Technology Resource
Center**
3920 Woodland Heights Avenue
Little Rock, AR 72212
(501) 227-3602
FAX: (501) 227-3601
Joyce Arey, Director

County/District Where Located:
Pulaski County.

Computer Training: Speech
output systems; screen
magnification systems; braille
access systems; word processing;
database software; computer
operating systems; training for
instructors.

◆ Low Vision Services

EYE CARE SOCIETIES

**Arkansas Ophthalmological
Society**
305 North Monroe
Little Rock, AR 72205
(501) 663-5686
Stewart Bell, Executive Director

**Arkansas Optometric
Association**
100 South University Avenue
Suite 311
Little Rock, AR 72205
(501) 661-7675
FAX: (501) 661-1039
Betty Valachovic, CAE

County/District Where Located:
Pulaski County.

LOW VISION CENTERS

**Lions World Services for the
Blind**
2811 Fair Park Boulevard
P.O. Box 4055
Little Rock, AR 72204
(501) 664-7100 or (800) 248-0734
FAX: (501) 664-2743
E-mail: lwsb@mail.snider.net
URL: http://www.snider.net/
lions
Jim Cordell, Executive Director

Type of Agency: Private.
County/District Where Located:
Pulaski County.

Mission: To enable people who are blind or visually impaired to function independently and live full, productive lives with dignity and self-respect, as well as to promote a positive public awareness of blindness.

Funded by: Patient fees and contributions.

Hours of Operation: Mon.-Fri. 8:00 AM-4:30 PM.

Program Accessibility: Fully accessible.

Staff: Ophthalmologist; low vision assistant; psychologist / counselor; rehabilitation counselor; orientation / mobility instructor; rehabilitation teacher; special educator; licensed practical nurse; psychiatrist. Others available through referral.

History/Date: Est. 1947.

Number of Clients Served: 250 annually.

Eligibility: Legal blindness.

Area Served: Unlimited.

Age Requirements: 16 years and older.

Low Vision: Clinic and aids.

Low Vision Aids: Available for trial period, available for training, non-prescription low vision aids may be purchased at a discount through LWSB.

Low Vision Follow-up: Y.

University of Arkansas for Medical Sciences Department of Ophthalmology
4301 West Markham
Little Rock, AR 72205
(501) 686-5822
FAX: (501) 686-8560
Dr. John Shock, Department Chairman

County/District Where Located: Pulaski County.

Funded by: State government; fees.

Hours of Operation: Mon.-Fri. 8:00 AM-4:30 PM.

Staff: Ophthalmologist; low vision assistant; social worker.

Eligibility: Referrals from ophthalmologist prior to low vision examination.

Area Served: Unlimited.

Low Vision Aids: On-site training provided.

Low Vision Follow-up: By return appointment in one month.

◆ Aging Services

STATE UNITS ON AGING

**Division of Aging and Adult Services
Arkansas Department of Human Services**
Seventh and Main Streets
Little Rock, AR 72201
(501) 682-2441 or Information & Referral (501) 682-8150 or Adult Protective Services (800) 482-8049
FAX: (501) 682-8155
Herb Sanderson, Director

Provides referrals to Area Agencies on Aging and information on other local aging services.

INDEPENDENT LIVING PROGRAMS

**Division of Services for the Blind
Arkansas Department of Human Services**
522 Main Street
Suite 100
Little Rock, AR 72201
(800) 960-9270 or (501) 682-5463
FAX: (501) 682-0366
James C. Hudson, Director

Provides independent living services for persons age 55 and over. For further information, contact the Project Director or general phone number listed.

CALIFORNIA

♦ *Educational Services*

STATE SERVICES

California Department of Education
Special Education Division
515 L Street, Suite 270
Sacramento, CA 95814
(916) 445-4613
FAX: (916) 327-3516
Gabriel Cortina, Superintendent
Leo D. Sandoval, Director

Type of Agency: State; federal.
Mission: To provide assistance, information and coordination of services regarding the development and education of children with visual impairments, including those with multiple disabilities.
Funded by: State and federal funds.
Staff: 1 part time; variety of consultants available.
History/Date: Est. 1949.
Area Served: Statewide.
Transportation: Y.
Age Requirements: 0-21 years.

Health: Adaptive equipment; genetic and other counseling; low vision exams; immunizations; blood tests available on referral basis.
Counseling/Social Work/Self-Help: Parent counseling.
Educational: Provides instruction in all developmental areas. Home-based program for visually impaired children, with or without other handicaps; consultant services to other programs; referral; coordinates services between various agencies and programs.

EARLY INTERVENTION COORDINATION

California Early Intervention Technical Assistance Network
429 J Street
Plaza Level
Sacramento, CA 95814
(916) 492-9999
FAX: (916) 492-9995
Virginia Reynolds, Birth to Five Technical Assistant

County/District Where Located: Sacremento County.

Early Intervention Program
California Department of Developmental Services
1600 Ninth Street
Room 310
P.O. Box 944202
Sacramento, CA 95814
(916) 654-2777
FAX: (916) 654-3255
Ben Traverso, Manager
Beth Gould, Part H Coordinator, (916) 654-2773

County/District Where Located: Sacramento County.

Acts as lead agency for Part H of the Individuals with Disabilities Education Act (IDEA). Part H addresses the birth to 36 month population with developmental delays.

SCHOOLS

California School for the Blind
500 Walnut Avenue
Fremont, CA 94536
(510) 794-3800
FAX: (510) 794-3813
E-mail: swittens@supreme.cde.ca.gov
Dr. Stuart H. Wittenstein, Superintendent

Type of Agency: State.
County/District Where Located: Alameda County.

Mission: To provide educational services for blind children, including multiply disabled, deaf-blind.
Funded by: Public funds.
Budget: $7 million.
Hours of Operation: Sunday evening to Friday afternoon; some weekends.
Staff: 140 full time, 27 part time.
History/Date: Est. 1860.
Number of Clients Served: 130 on campus; more than 200 off campus.
Eligibility: Local school district unable to provide services, visual impairment is primary disability.
Area Served: California.
Transportation: Y.
Age Requirements: 3-22 years.

Health: On-campus infirmary. Provides comprehensive assessments to students with visual impairments throughout California.
Educational: Nongraded special classes and graded mainstream classes in local schools.
Preschools: One class.
Professional Training: Sponsors seminars with Northern California AER, San Francisco State University, and San Jose State University.
Reading: Braille and other literary media.
Residential: Dormitories for children and youths.
Rehabilitation: Orientation and mobility training, adapted physical education.
Recreational: Full range of activities.
Employment: Community-based transition-to-work program.
Computer Training: Y.

Extended school year offerred.

**Children's Vision Center
Department of Ophthalmology
University of California, Davis
Medical Center**
1603 Alhambra Boulevard
Sacramento, CA 95816
(916) 734-6959 or (800) 834-1007
Lois Harrell, Project Director

Type of Agency: Non-profit.
Mission: To help those who live
and work with a visually impaired
child to understand the unique
perspective of the child and how to
address related challenges.
Funded by: Grants and donations.
Budget: $100,000.
Hours of Operation: Mon.-Fri.
24-hour hotline (916) 734-6959.
Number of Clients Served: Over
200 families and children.
Eligibility: Any child under the
age of 18 years who will benefit by
diagnostically related (vision)
intervention.
Area Served: Northeastern
California.
Age Requirements: 0-18 years.

**Counseling/Social Work/Self-
Help:** Counseling for families
about their child's diagnosis and
needs.
Educational: Direct instruction in
adaptive techniques for children
and professionals working with
them.
Preschools: Visits and in-service
preschools with blind and low
vision children.
Professional Training: In-service
and a one-day monthly course.

Foundation for the Junior Blind
5300 Angeles Vista Boulevard
Los Angeles, CA 90043
(213) 295-4555
FAX: (213) 296-0424
Robert B. Ralls, M.S., President

Type of Agency: Private; non-
profit.

Mission: Services for blind,
visually impaired, and multiply
disabled blind children, birth to 21.
Services for blind and visually
impaired adults, 18 to 70.
Programs: Infant family program,
Children's Residential Center,
Summer camp program, Visions
Program, Special Education
School, and Davidson Program for
Independence.
Funded by: Fees for service
charged to public agencies; private
contributions.
Budget: $ 6,000,000.
Hours of Operation: Mon.-Fri.
8:00 AM-5:00 PM.
Program Accessibility: fully
accessible.
Staff: 120 full time. 500 volunteers.
History/Date: Est. 1953.
Number of Clients Served: 3,800.
Eligibility: Totally blind, legally
blind, partially sighted.
Area Served: California and other
western states.
Transportation: Y.
Age Requirements: 0-21 years
(children's program); 18-70 (adult
residential rehabilitation program).

Health: General medical and
nursing services; refers and
provides consultation to other
agencies for other health services.
**Counseling/Social Work/Self-
Help:** Social and vocational
evaluation; psychological testing
and evaluation; individual, group,
family/parent, couple counseling;
referral to community services;
placement. Refers and provides
consultation to other agencies on
other counseling/social work
services.
Educational: Nongraded. Accepts
emotionally disturbed, learning
disabled, mentally retarded,
orthopedically disabled, other
multiply disabled blind persons.
Programs for vocational/skill
development, adjustment training,

general academic. State-certified
nonpublic school and residential
living program for children and
youth.
Preschools: Non-center-based
preschool services.
Professional Training:
Internship/fieldwork placement;
in-service training programs.
Reading: Information and referral;
talking book records; braille books;
large print books; braille and
recorded magazines.
Residential: Seven-day-a-week
residential living for children and
six-day-a-week for adults.
Rehabilitation: Activities for daily
living; braille; typing; handwriting;
remedial education; home
management; orientation/
mobility; sensory communication
aid training; sensory training; low
vision training and electronic
travel aids; home repair; aids and
appliance store; sensory aids
center.
Recreational: Evening and
weekend programs; year-round
camp program; special interest
events; speakers and activities;
trips; bowling; swimming; arts and
crafts. Summer residential camp
program and day camp services
for children and youths. Refers for
and provides consultation to other
agencies on recreational/leisure
services.
Employment: Prevocational
evaluation and training;
occupational skill development;
job placement and retention
training; job retraining; follow-up
services. Refers for and provides
consultation to other agencies on
other employment-oriented
services.
Computer Training: Orientation
and training on computer aids and
devices.
Low Vision: Services provided on
campus; referrals to Center for the
Partially Sighted.

Low Vision Aids: Y.
Low Vision Follow-up: Y.

Home-based infant/family services for children birth to age 3, special education school and residential living program for multihandicapped blind children 5-21 years old; summer and year round residential camp for blind, visually impaired children and youths. Year-round recreational programs; adjustment training for adults in six-day-a-week residential living program; library and sensory aids, computer and technology training.

Santa Barbara City Schools Program for Visually Impaired Special Education Services

723 East Cota Street
Santa Barbara, CA 93103
(805) 966-7768
FAX: (805) 963-1992
Jan Ross, Program Chairperson

County/District Where Located: Santa Barbara County.
Mission: Services for visually impaired children, with or without additional handicaps.
Funded by: State funds.
Staff: 1 part-time administrator; 5 teachers (2 dual-certified, some early childhood); 2 aides.
Area Served: South Santa Barbara County.
Age Requirements: 0-22 years.

Educational: Provides instruction in all developmental areas; home teaching, itinerant teaching to other facilities and consultant services to other programs. Variety of support and related services available through other public school and community programs.
Preschools: Home teaching, infant and preschool.

INFANT AND PRESCHOOL

Blind Babies Foundation

1200 Gough Street
San Francisco, CA 94109
(415) 771-5464
FAX: (415) 771-9026
E-mail: 102052.303@compuserv. com
Dennak L. Murphy, Executive Director

Type of Agency: Private; non-profit.
Mission: Provides programs and services that enable families, professionals and the broader community to meet the unique needs of infants and preschool children who are blind or visually impaired.
Funded by: Fund raising, foundation grants, donations, bequests, and contract service fees.
Budget: $930,000 per year.
Hours of Operation: Mon.-Fri. 9:00 AM-5:00 PM.
Staff: 9 full time, 2 part time.
History/Date: Est. 1949.
Number of Clients Served: 400.
Eligibility: Visual impairment.
Area Served: Northern and central California.
Transportation: Y.
Age Requirements: 0-5 years.

Health: Home-based early intervention, functional vision and developmental assessment, information and referral and consultation.
Counseling/Social Work/Self-Help: Counseling for parents, siblings, extended family, and others involved with a preschool visually impaired child. Provides information to family, schools, medical professionals, and others regarding individual children. Refers to other appropriate services.
Educational: Provides instruction in developmental areas affected by

vision loss. Some direct teaching provided by staff, but emphasis is on teaching parents to become teachers. Home-based direct services and consultant services to other programs for visually impaired infants, and visually impaired children with or without other disabilities.
Professional Training: In-service training for health care professionals, special education teachers, and others.
Low Vision: Referrals to eye care professionals; home counselors provide training in visual functioning.
Low Vision Aids: Available on loan to clients.
Low Vision Follow-up: Home counselors follow progress of clients.

Blind Children's Center

4120 Marathon Street
Los Angeles, CA 90029
(213) 664-2153 or toll-free in California (800) 222-3567 or (800) 222-3566 out of state
FAX: (213) 665-3828
Midge Horton, Executive Director

Type of Agency: Private; non-profit.
Mission: Services to young children who are visually impaired.
Funded by: Private donations.
Staff: 25 full time; 15 part time.
History/Date: Est. 1938.
Eligibility: Visually impaired persons, with or without other disabilities.
Age Requirements: Birth to 5 years.

Counseling/Social Work/Self-Help: Family support services; parent support groups; advocacy training.
Educational: Infant stimulation program; educational preschool;

interdisciplinary assessment service; correspondence/toll-free phone line; publications.
Preschools: Center-based program.

Blind Children's Learning Center

18542-B Vanderlip Avenue
Santa Ana, CA 92705
(714) 573-8888
FAX: (714) 573-4944
Gabrielle Hass, Executive Director

Type of Agency: Private; non-profit.
County/District Where Located: Orange County.
Mission: To develop the full potential of visually impaired children and youth regardless of ability to pay.
Funded by: Grants, donations, and fees.
Budget: 1997: $1,300,000.
Hours of Operation: Mon.-Fri. 7:30 AM-5:30 PM.
Staff: 24 full time. Uses volunteers.
History/Date: Est. 1962.
Number of Clients Served: Over 100 annually.
Eligibility: Visually impaired; multiply disabled children.
Area Served: Greater Orange County community.
Transportation: Y.
Age Requirements: 0-6 years.

Counseling/Social Work/Self-Help: Social evaluation; psychological testing and evaluation; individual, group, family/parent, couple counseling. Consultation with other agencies in these areas. Information and referral systems.
Educational: Programs for preschoolers and infants on-site and in home. Consulting services to schools for K-12; itinerant teaching; orientation/mobility

counseling; teacher consultation and assessment.
Preschools: State accredited for childeren 6 months-6 years.
Professional Training: Internship/fieldwork placements in social work; special education; psychological testing; human services. Has regular in-service training program.
Low Vision: Work with Southern California College of Optometry to help children with low vision.

Braille Institute of America, Inc. Youth Center

3450 Cahuenga Boulevard West
Los Angeles, CA 90068
(213) 851-6122
FAX: (213) 851-6961
E-mail: communications @brailleinstitute.org
Mr. Leslie E. Stocker, President
Vicki Liske, Director of Child Development

Type of Agency: Private.
Mission: To promote a positive self-concept and increased independence by building on the child's strengths, overcoming delays in development and increasing the family's ability to respond to their child's strengths and special needs.
Funded by: Private donations.
Hours of Operation: Mon.-Fri. 8:30 AM - 5:00 PM.
Staff: 9 full time; 15 part time.
History/Date: Est. 1983.
Number of Clients Served: 250 families.
Eligibility: Visually impaired.
Area Served: Los Angeles, Orange, San Diego, Santa Barbara and parts of Riverside, San Bernardino counties.
Age Requirements: Birth - 6 years.

Counseling/Social Work/Self-Help: Parent counseling.

Educational: Provides instruction in all developmental areas.
Preschools: Option for mainstream experience in community preschools with assistance of on-site staff from Braille Institute.
Professional Training: In-services for professionals.

Local Offices:

Anaheim: Braille Institute, Orange County Center, 527 North Dale Avenue, Anaheim, CA 92801-4820, (714) 821-5000, Sheila Daily, Director.
Rancho Mirage: Braille Institute Desert Center, 70-251 Ramon Road, Rancho Mirage, CA 92270, (760) 321-1111, Jay Hatfield, Director.
Santa Barbara: Braille Institute, Santa Barbara Center, 2031 De La Vina, Santa Barbara, CA 93105-9990, (805) 682-6222, Joan Marcuse, Director.

Hope Family Support Program

c/o San Diego County Office of Education
6401 Linda Vista Road
San Diego, CA 92111-7399
(619) 292-3835
FAX: (619) 569-5394
Dr. Virginia McDonald, Director
Meryl Berk, Vision Specialist

Type of Agency: Public school.
Mission: Services to families with disabled and developmentally delayed infants, including visually impaired and multiply disabled infants, between birth and 3 years of age.
Hours of Operation: Mon.-Fri. 7:30 AM - 5:00 PM.
Staff: 80 instructional staff members.
History/Date: Est. 1975.
Eligibility: Infants showing delays in development or who are at risk for delay due to medical

conditions or diagnoses, including visual impairment, with or without other disabilities.
Area Served: San Diego County.
Age Requirements: 0-3 years.

Counseling/Social Work/Self-Help: Parent counseling.
Educational: Provides instruction in all developmental areas; home- or center-based consultation services in the following areas: nursing; speech and language; occupational therapy/physical therapy; social work/parent counseling; vision; deafness and hearing impairment; premature infant development; assistive technology and consultant services to other programs; occupational, speech, and music therapy; bilingual instruction available on consultant basis.

Infant-Family Program of the Foundation for the Junior Blind
5300 Angeles Vista Boulevard
Los Angeles, CA 90043
(213) 295-4555 or (800) 352-2290
FAX: (213) 296-0424
Mary Goldman, Intake Coordinator

Type of Agency: Private; non-profit.
County/District Where Located: Los Angeles County.
Mission: To help families understand the impact of visual impairment and multiple disabilities on their child's overall development.
Funded by: Private donations and state funds.
Hours of Operation: Mon.-Fri. 8:30 AM - 5:00 PM. Weekend camps and workshops.
Staff: 1 full-time administrator; 1 full time coordinator, 8 full time specialists. Members of other disciplines available as consultants. Has advisory board.

History/Date: Est. 1983.
Number of Clients Served: 225 a year.
Eligibility: Ages 0-3 years, visual impairment, and multiple disabilities.
Area Served: Los Angeles County area.
Age Requirements: 0-3 years.

Health: Adaptive equipment and toys on loan; free low vision exams.
Counseling/Social Work/Self-Help: Family support services and direct programming for families and infants in home-based program.
Educational: Provides instruction in all developmental areas.
Recreational: Family camps, picnics, and workshops on an on-going basis.
Low Vision: Free low vision exams provided by a developmental optometrist.

STATEWIDE OUTREACH SERVICES

California School for the Blind
500 Walnut Avenue
Fremont, CA 94536
(510) 794-3800
FAX: (510) 794-3813
E-mail: sgoodman@supreme.cde.ca.gov
Stephen A. Goodman, Contact Person

Funded by: California Department of Education, Special Education Division.
Age Requirements: 0-21 years.

Assessment: Comprehensive assessments in psychology, low vision, education, orientation and mobility, speech, and language.
Consultation to Public Schools: When requested, will provide technical assistance to local

agencies to develop and implement educational programs.
Parent Assistance: Week-long parent training provided during assessment of students.
Professional Training: Workshops are provided on assessment and programming of students with visual impairments. Other workshops and in-services offered when requested by local agencies.

INSTRUCTIONAL MATERIALS CENTERS

Clearinghouse for Specialized Media and Technology
California Department of Education
560 J Street
Room 390
Sacramento, CA 95814
(916) 445-5103 (voice/TDD)
FAX: (916) 323-9732
E-mail: rbrawley@cde.cq.gov
Rod Brawley, Director

Area Served: State of California.
Groups Served: California schools; students with print disabilities.

Types/Content: Textbooks, state adopted texts, recreational texts.
Media Formats: Braille, large print, books on tape.
Title Listings: Catalogs available.

UNIVERSITY TRAINING PROGRAMS

California State University at Sacramento
Department of Special Education, Rehabilitation, and School Psychology
6000 J Street
Sacramento, CA 95819
(916) 278-6622
FAX: (916) 278-5904
E-mail: fergi@csus.edu
Dr. Michael J. Lewis, Chairman

County/District Where Located: Sacramento County.

Programs Offered: Graduate (master's) programs for teachers of the learning handicapped and severely handicapped: school psychologist, special education, vocational rehabilitation. Call for course list.

California State University, Los Angeles

Division of Special Education
5151 State University Drive
Los Angeles, CA 90032
(213) 343-4411
FAX: (213) 343-5605
E-mail: dfazzi@calstatela.edu
URL: http://web.calstatela.edu/ academic/spec_ed/o_mobil/
Diane Fazzi, Orientation and Mobility, Teacher Education Programs in Visual Impairment
Dr. Martin Brodwin, Rehabilitation Counseling

County/District Where Located: Los Angeles County.

Programs Offered: Graduate (master's and credential) programs for teachers of the visually impaired and orientation and mobility specialists.
Undergraduate (bachelor's) program in rehabilitation counseling.
Distance Education: Y.

San Francisco State University

Department of Special Education
1600 Holloway Avenue
San Francisco, CA 94132
(415) 338-1245
FAX: (415) 338-0566
E-mail: srosen@sfsu.edu
Dr. Amanda Hall-Lueck, Visually Impaired
Dr. Sandra Rosen, Orientation and Mobility, Rehabilitation Teaching

Programs Offered: Graduate (master's, doctoral) programs for teachers of visually impaired students; orientation and mobility; rehabilitation teaching.
Distance Education: Y.

♦ Information Services

LIBRARIES

Braille Institute Library Services

741 North Vermont Avenue
Los Angeles, CA 90029
(213) 663-1111, ext. 358 or
(213) 660-3880 or toll-free in California (800) 808-2555
FAX: (213) 663-0867
E-mail: bils@brailib.org
Fekade Tadesse, Machine Lending Information
Henry C. Chang, Librarian

Type of Agency: Private, nonprofit. Regional library of the National Library Service.
Funded by: Contributions, bequests, and foundation grants.
Hours of Operation: Mon.-Fri. 8:30 AM - 5:00 PM.
History/Date: Est. 1919 and Inc. 1929.
Number of Clients Served: 21,000.
Area Served: Southern California.

Library provides braille, talking books and cassettes to blind and physically handicapped persons of southern California. Press produces *The Braille Mirror Magazine, Expectations,* an annual anthology for blind children, and other braille materials under contract for free distribution to blind persons who read braille in English. Recording and reading services primarily for students' textbooks and other educational material.

California State Library Braille and Talking Book Services

P.O. Box 942837
Sacramento, CA 94237-0001
(916) 654-0640 or toll-free in California (800) 952-5666
FAX: (916) 654-1119
E-mail: btbl@library.ca.gov
Donine Hedrick, Librarian

Type of Agency: State.
County/District Where Located: Sacramento County.
Mission: Library services for patrons unable to use print.
Funded by: State and federal funds, gifts.
Hours of Operation: Mon.-Fri. 9:30 AM - 4:00 PM.
Staff: 21.
History/Date: Est. 1904.
Number of Clients Served: 16,094.
Eligibility: Print impaired.
Area Served: Northern California.

Regional library for braille, talking books, and cassettes.

Fresno County Free Library Blind and Handicapped Services

Ted Williams Community Center
770 North Free Library
Fresno, CA 83728
(209) 488-3217 or toll-free in California (800) 742-1011
FAX: (209) 488-3209
Deborah Janzen, Librarian

Subregional library.

Library for the Blind and Print Handicapped

San Francisco Public Library
Civic Center
San Francisco, CA 94102
(415) 292-2022
FAX: (415) 557-4433
Martin Magid, Director

Subregional library.

MEDIA PRODUCTION SERVICES

American Red Cross Braille Division

10771 San Pablo
El Cerrito, CA 94530
(510) 526-7206

County/District Where Located:
Contra Costa County.
Groups Served: K-12, college students, other adults.

Types/Content: Miscellaneous.
Media Formats: Braille books.
Title Listings: No title listings available.

Braille Institute of America, Inc.

741 North Vermont Avenue
Los Angeles, CA 90029
(213) 663-1111
FAX: (213) 663-0867
E-mail: communications
@brailleinstitute.org
Carol Jimenez, Coordinator, Braille Transcription

Area Served: Primarily southern California.
Groups Served: K-12, college students, other adults.

Types/Content: Textbooks, recreational, career/vocational, religious, application instruction manuals.
Media Formats: Braille books, talking books/cassettes.
Title Listings: Print and braille lists available at no charge.

Braille Transcribers

4848 Cottage Way
Carmichael, CA 95608
(916) 971-7912
FAX: (916) 971-7410
Joanne Call, President

County/District Where Located:
Sacramento County.
Groups Served: K-12; college students; other adults.

Types/Content: Textbooks; recreational; career/vocational; religious; foreign language.
Media Formats: Braille books.
Title Listings: No title listings available.

Braille Transcribers of Humboldt

P.O. Box 6363
Eureka, CA 95502
(707) 442-4048
Pat Welsh, Chairperson

County/District Where Located:
Humbolt County.
Groups Served: K-12, college students, other adults.

Types/Content: Textbooks, recreational, career/vocational, religious.
Media Formats: Braille books.
Title Listings: No title listings available.

Braille Transcription Project of Santa Clara County, Inc.

101 North Bascom Avenue
San Jose, CA 95128
(408) 298-4468
Peggy Dodge, Executive Director

County/District Where Located:
Santa Clara County.
Area Served: Primarily Santa Clara county; also serves all of United States and Europe.
Groups Served: K-12, college students, other adults.

Types/Content: Textbooks, literature, recreational, career/vocational, any requests.
Media Formats: Braille books, tapes on request.
Title Listings: Listed with Library of Congress and American Printing House Central Catalog.

Maintains braille library.

Castro Valley School District

P.O. Box 2146
Castro Valley, CA 94546
(510) 537-3000
FAX: (510) 537-4754
E-mail: wagasa@aol.com
Jim Fitzpatrick, Assistant Superintentdent for Curriculum and Instruction

County/District Where Located:
Alameda County.
Area Served: San Leandro, Hayward, San Lorenzo, and Castro Valley school districts.
Groups Served: K-12.

Types/Content: Textbooks and other educational materials.
Media Formats: Braille, large print, audiotape.
Title Listings: None specified.

CompuBraille

2791 24th Street
Room 8
Sacramento, CA 95818
(916) 452-6189
Sandy Shubb, President

County/District Where Located:
Sacramento County.
Area Served: Primarily California; other states on request.
Groups Served: State schools, libraries, and individuals.

Types/Content: Embosses computer disks into braille.
Title Listings: No title listings available.

Golden Gate Braille Transcribers, Inc.

1466 44th Avenue
San Francisco, CA 94122
(415) 566-1641
Evelyn Daiss, President

Groups Served: K-12; adults.

Types/Content: Textbooks; recreational.
Media Formats: Braille books.
Title Listings: No title listings available.

Kings Tape Library for the Blind

202 West Grangeville Boulevard
Hanford, CA 93230
(209) 582-4843
E-mail: hmackey@aol.com
Caroline W. Mackey, Director

County/District Where Located:
Kings County.
Groups Served: Adults.

Types/Content: Recreational.
Media Formats: Talking books/
cassettes.
Title Listings: Printed and/or
cassette at no charge.

Oakmont Visual Aids Workshop

310 White Oak Drive
Santa Rosa, CA 95409-5942
(707) 539-0211
FAX: (707) 539-6537
Fern Harger, Co-chairperson
Betty Mann, Secretary, (707) 538-
0134

County/District Where Located:
Sonoma County.
Area Served: Worldwide.
Groups Served: Pre-K, K-12.

Types/Content: Tactile teaching
aids.
Media Formats: None specified.
Title Listings: Printed at no
charge.

Petaluma Braille Transcribers, Inc.

605 Reynolds Drive
Petaluma, CA 94592
(707) 763-6576
Eva Hoffman, Secretary

County/District Where Located:
Sonoma County.
Groups Served: None specified.

Types/Content: Textbooks;
recreational, career/vocational,
and religious materials.
Media Formats: Braille books,
talking books/cassettes, large-
print books.

Title Listings: Printed at no
charge.

Quik-Scrybe

14144 Burbank Boulevard, #4
Van Nuys, CA 91401
(818) 989-2137
FAX: (818) 989-5602
E-mail: sgstaley@netcom.com
Sue Staley, President

County/District Where Located:
Los Angeles County.

Types/Content: Textbooks,
computer manuals, and other text
materials other than music,
including computer-related
materials.
Media Formats: Braille
(Interpoint), large print.

Recording for the Blind and Dyslexic

5022 Hollywood Boulevard
Los Angeles, CA 90027
(213) 664-5525
FAX: (213) 664-1881
Carol Smith, Executive Director

County/District Where Located:
Los Angeles County.

See Recording for the Blind and
Dyslexic in U.S. national listings.

Recording for the Blind and Dyslexic

488 West Charleston Road
Palo Alto, CA 94306
(415) 493-3717 (as of 8/1/97 area
code 415 becomes 650)
FAX: (415) 493-5513
Howell Lovell, Jr., Contact Person

See Recording for the Blind and
Dyslexic in U.S. national listings.

Recording for the Blind and Dyslexic

3970 LaColina Road
Room 9

Santa Barbara, CA 93110
(805) 687-6393
Mary MacRae, Director

County/District Where Located:
Santa Barbara County.

See Recording for the Blind and
Dyslexic in U.S. national listings.

Recording for the Blind and Dyslexic

1844-C West 11th Street
Upland, CA 91786
(909) 949-4316
FAX: (909) 981-8457
E-mail: recblind@cyberg8t.com
URL: http://
www.cyberg8t.com/recblind/
Nancy Sjoholm, Studio Director

County/District Where Located:
San Bernardino County.

See Recording for the Blind and
Dyslexic in U.S. national listings.

San Gabriel Valley Braille Guild

3225 Charlinda
West Covina, CA 91791
(818) 331-2071
Susannah C. Mathews, President

County/District Where Located:
Los Angeles County.
Groups Served: K-12, college
students, other adults.

Types/Content: Career/
vocational, recreational.
Media Formats: Braille books.
Title Listings: No title listings
available.

Santa Barbara School District

723 East Cota Street
Santa Barbara, CA 93103
(805) 963-4331
FAX: (805) 963-1992
Janice W. Ross, Chairperson for
Visually Impaired

County/District Where Located:
Santa Barbara County.

Groups Served: K-12.

Types/Content: Textbooks, recreational, career/vocational.
Media Formats: Talking books/cassettes, large-print books.
Title Listings: Printed for a charge.

Sequoia Transcribers

2730 West Seeger Ave
Visalia, CA 93277
(209) 732-1912
Edith Pannell, Director

Groups Served: K-12; college students; other adults.

Types/Content: Textbooks; recreational.
Media Formats: Braille books.
Title Listings: Print and braille lists available at no charge.

Sisterhood of Temple Beth Hillel

12326 Riverside Drive
North Hollywood, CA 91607
(818) 763-9148
Julie Breitstein, Chairperson

Groups Served: College students, other adults.

Types/Content: Textbooks.
Media Formats: Talking books/cassettes.
Title Listings: None specified.

Transcribers of Orange County

10982 Paddock Lane
Santa Ana, CA 92705
(714) 731-5899
Alice Schultz, Assignment Chairperson

County/District Where Located: Orange County.
Groups Served: None specified.

Types/Content: None specified.
Media Formats: Braille books.
Title Listings: No title listings available.

Ventura County Braille Transcribers Association

P.O. Box 3353
Ventura, CA 93003
(805) 641-3963
John Calohan, President

Area Served: Ventura County.
Groups Served: K-12 and students at community college.

Types/Content: Textbooks; recreational; career/vocational.
Media Formats: Braille books; computer disk. Scanning and embossing available.
Title Listings: Available on request.

RADIO READING

Audio Vision Radio Reading Service

34475 Yucaipa
Suite 6
Yucaipa, CA 92399
(909) 797-4336
Tom Rash, Station Director/Executive Director

County/District Where Located: San Bernadino County.
Hours of Operation: Mon.-Sun. 5:00 AM - 12:00 midnight.
History/Date: Est. 1991.
Area Served: Riverside, Orange, Los Angeles and San Bernadino.

KCHO-FM Radio Reading Service

c/o California State University
Communications Department
Chico, CA 95929-0500
(916) 898-5896
FAX: (916) 898-4348
Joe Oleksiewicz, Director

County/District Where Located: Butte County.
Hours of Operation: 24 hours a day.
Area Served: Chico area, plus 75 miles to the north in Redding, 45 miles to the south in Maryville/Yuba City.

KPBS-FM Radio Reading Service

San Diego State University
San Diego, CA 92182
(619) 594-8170
FAX: (619) 594-2881
E-mail: keoni@kpbs.org
URL: http://www.kpbs.org
Mercedes Witherspoon, Director

County/District Where Located: San Diego County.
Hours of Operation: 24 hours.
Staff: Director and 1 staff member.
History/Date: Est. 1975.
Area Served: San Diego County.
Age Requirements: Over 18 years of age.

Tri-Visual Services

1713 J Street
Suite 211
Sacramento, CA 95814
(916) 447-7323
FAX: (916) 447-7324
Elena Negrete, Executive Director

County/District Where Located: Sacramento County.
Hours of Operation: Mon., Wed., Fri. 8:00-12:00 noon.

INFORMATION AND REFERRAL

American Foundation for the Blind West

111 Pine Street
Suite 725
San Francisco, CA 94111
(415) 392-4845
FAX: (415) 392-0383
E-mail: sanfran@afb.org
URL: http://www.afb.org

See American Foundation for the Blind in U.S. national listings.

Blind San Franciscans
1591 Jackson Street
Suite 8
San Francisco, CA 94109
(415) 931-8734
FAX: (415) 563-4896
Jewel McGinnis

Braille Institute of America, Inc.
741 North Vermont Avenue
Los Angeles, CA 90029
(213) 663-1111 or (800) 272-4453
Carlyle Rudkin, Director

Mission: To provide information, referrals and materials concerning services for the blind and visually impaired.
Hours of Operation: Mon.-Fri. 9:00AM-4:00PM.
Area Served: Nationwide.

**The Foundation Fighting Blindness
Fresno Affiliate**
1045 South Street
Fresno, CA 93721
(209) 439-7889
Jennifer Williamson, Director of Information Services

See The Foundation Fighting Blindness in U.S. national listings.

**The Foundation Fighting Blindness
Northern California Affiliate**
801 Goettel Court
Benicia, CA 94510
(707) 747-1008
FAX: (707) 747-1008
E-mail: vreikok@aol.com
Vicky Kennedy, President

County/District Where Located: Solano County.

See The Foundation Fighting Blindness in U.S. national listings.

**The Foundation Fighting Blindness
San Diego Affiliate**
2006 Chalcedony Street
San Diego, CA 92109-3411
(619) 595-3698
David Hopkins, President

See The Foundation Fighting Blindness in U.S. national listings.

**The Foundation Fighting Blindness
Southern California Affiliate**
10315 Missouri Avenue, Suite 400
Los Angeles, CA 90025-5059
(310) 274-5505
Cathy Barry, President
Evelyn Nidetz, Contact Person

See The Foundatiion Fighting Blindness in U.S. national listings.

Institute for Families of Blind Children
P.O. Box 54700
Mailstop#111
Los Angeles, CA 90054-0700
(213) 669-4649
FAX: (213) 666-6283
Nancy Chernus-Mansfield, Director
Marilyn Horn, Assistant Director

Type of Agency: Private; non-profit.
Mission: Provides consultation and therapy for parents, siblings and extended family members of children who are blind or visually impaired, refers parents and physicians to organizations specializing in meeting the needs of children with visual problems; writes and publishes journal articles, booklets and newsletters; and produces videotapes.
Funded by: Private donations.
Hours of Operation: Mon.-Fri. 9:00 AM-4:00 PM.
History/Date: Est. 1987.
Area Served: Unlimited.

Professional Training: In-service training for health care workers.

National Association for Visually Handicapped
3201 Balboa Street
San Francisco, CA 94121
(415) 221-3201
FAX: (415) 221-8754
E-mail: staffca@navh.org
Jeannine Louise

See National Association for Visually Handicapped in U.S. national listings.

Prevent Blindness Northern California
4200 California Street, #101
San Francisco, CA 94118-1395
(415) 387-0934 or (800) 338-3041
FAX: (415) 387-1689
E-mail: 104706.1110@compuserve.com
Peter Jamgochian, Executive Director

See Prevent Blindness America in U.S. national listings.

Prevent Blindness Southern California
3702 Ruffin Road
Suite 201
San Diego, CA 92123-1812
(619) 576-2122
FAX: (619) 576-2123
Linda R. Creel, President

County/District Where Located: San Diego County.

See Prevent Blindness America in U.S. national listings.

See also in national listings:

American Academy of Ophthalmology

American Action Fund for Blind Children and Adults

American Association for Pediatric Ophthalmology and Strabismus

American Society of Ophthalmic Registered Nurses

Audio Vision

Beach Cities Braille Guild

Books Aloud

Contra Costa Braille Transcribers

Glaucoma Research Foundation

Library Reproduction Service

Lutheran Braille Workers

Monterey County Braille Transcribers

MSMT Braille Center

National Academy of Audio Description
RP International

National Eye Care Project (NECP)

Smith-Kettlewell Eye Research Institute
Rehabilitation Engineering Center

Theosophical Book Association for the Blind

Volunteers of Vacaville

Volunteer Transcribing Services

♦ Rehabilitation Services

STATE SERVICES

Services for the Blind California Department of Rehabilitation
Central Office
830 K Street Mall
Room 208
Sacramento, CA 95814
(916) 323-2235 (voice/TDD)
FAX: (916) 327-6919
E-mail: doroa.rhblind@hw#1.cahwnet.gov
Brenda Premo, Director
Manuel S. Urena, Program Manager, Services for the Blind and Visually Impaired

Type of Agency: State.
County/District Where Located: Sacramento County.
Funded by: State and federal funds.
Budget: 1997-98: $358,819,000.
Hours of Operation: Mon.-Fri. 8:00 AM - 5:00 PM.
Staff: 70 rehabilitation counselors for the blind and counselor teachers.
History/Date: Est. 1963.
Number of Clients Served: 3,000.
Eligibility: The presence of a physical or mental disability that for the individual constitutes or results in a substantial handicap to employment; and a reasonable expectation that vocational rehabilitation services may benefit the individual in terms of employment.
Area Served: California.

Health: Diagnostic, medical and surgical treatment.
Counseling/Social Work/Self-Help: Consultation and referral service.
Reading: Reader services for clients and nonclients enrolled in community colleges, and private post secondary educational institutions.
Rehabilitation: Personal and home management; orientation/mobility; communications.
Employment: Evaluation, prevocational and vocational training; vocational placement; follow-up; vending stand training.

District Offices:

Anaheim: 2190 Towne Centre Place, Suite 200, Anaheim, CA 92806, (714) 935-2916.
Fresno: 2550 Mariposa Street, Room 2000, Fresno, CA 93721, (209) 445-6011.
Goleta: 5638 Hollister, Suite 200, Goleta, CA 92117, (805) 569-5586.
Long Beach: 4300 Long Beach Boulevard, Long Beach, CA 90807-2008, (310) 422-8325.
Los Angeles: 3251 West Sixth Street, Third Floor, Los Angeles, CA 90020-2591, (213) 736-3904.
Los Angeles: 11130 S. Western Avenue, Los Angeles, CA 90047-4896, (213) 241-1700.
Norwalk: 12440 E. Firestone Boulevard, Suite 215, Norwalk, CA 90650-4386, (310) 864-8521.
Oakland: 2229 Webster Street, Oakland, CA 94612, (510) 286-0511.
Pasadena: 150 South Los Robles Avenue, Suite 300, Pasadena, CA 91101-2497, (818) 304-8300.
Pleasant Hill: 2285 Morello Avenue, Pleasant Hill, CA 94523-1896, (510) 689-3010.
Riverside: 3130 Chicago Avenue, Riverside, CA 92507, (909) 782-6650.
Sacramento: 2225 19th Street, Sacramento, CA 95818-1690, (916) 322-8500.
San Bernardino: 303 W. Third Street, Room 300, San Bernardino, CA 92401-1885, (909) 383-4401.
San Diego: 5095 Murphy Canyon Road, Suite 330, San Diego, CA 92123, (619) 495-3600.
San Francisco: 185 Berry Street, Suite 180, San Francisco, CA 94107, (415) 904-7100.
San Jose: 100 Paseo de San Antonio, Room 324, San Jose, CA 95113-1479, (408) 277-1355.
Santa Rosa: 50 D Street, Suite 425, Santa Rosa, CA 95404-4764, (707) 576-2233.

Van Nuys: 5900 Sepulveda Boulevard, Suite 240, Van Nuys, CA 91411, (818) 901-5024.

Maintains the following center: Orientation Center for the Blind, 400 Adams Street, Albany, CA 94706, (510) 559-1208, Mike Cole, Administrator. Provides work adjustment and prevocational counseling; personal management; orientation/mobility; physical education; home management; industrial arts; braille; typing; business methods.

REHABILITATION

Assistance League of Santa Clara County

169 State Street
Los Altos, CA 94022
(415) 941-4625 (as of 8/1/97 area code 415 becomes 650)
Mary Kay McCarthy, Chairperson

County/District Where Located: Santa Clara County.

Educational: Piano lessons for the blind.

Blind and Visually Impaired Center of Monterey County

225 Laurel Avenue
Pacific Grove, CA 93950
(408) 649-3505
FAX: (408) 649-4057
Kathy Henson

Type of Agency: Non-profit.
Mission: To help blind and visually impaired adults become independent, contributing members of society.
Funded by: Private donations.
Budget: $209,000.
Program Accessibility: Wheelchair accessible.
Staff: Orientation and mobility specialists; low vision specialist.
History/Date: Est. 1971.
Number of Clients Served: Approximately 500.

Eligibility: Blind or visually impaired adults.
Area Served: Monterey County.
Age Requirements: 18 years or older.

Educational: Braille instruction.
Rehabilitation: Home-based instruction in daily living skills.
Recreational: Exercise program, lunch, and ceramics class on Tuesdays.
Low Vision: Clinic open four days a month; full-time low vision specialist available.
Low Vision Aids: Y.
Low Vision Follow-up: Y.

Braille Institute of America, Inc.

741 North Vermont Avenue
Los Angeles, CA 90029
(213) 663-1111
FAX: (213) 663-0867
E-mail: communications @brailleinstitute.org
Leslie E. Stocker, President

Type of Agency: Private; non-profit.
Mission: Free services for adults, youths, and preschool children who are legally blind.
Funded by: Contributions, bequests, grants.
Budget: 1995-96 (including capital expenditures): $18 million.
Hours of Operation: Mon.-Fri. 8:30 AM - 5:00 PM.
Staff: 363 full-time equivalents; 5,170 volunteers.
History/Date: Est. 1919; inc. 1929.
Number of Clients Served: 1996: 41,779.
Eligibility: Visual impairment.
Area Served: Southern California.
Age Requirements: Varies with program.

Health: Refers to other agencies for health services.

Counseling/Social Work/Self-Help: Psychological counseling and referral.
Educational: Programs for adults, youth, and preschool children in a broad curriculum with over 200 courses and 282,000 hours of instruction.
Preschools: Integrated with community.
Professional Training: Internship and fieldwork; in-service training programs and seminars for professionals in allied fields.
Reading: Talking book records and cassettes; braille books, large print materials; information and referral; volunteer reading and tape recording services. Southern California Regional Library of the National Library Service.
Rehabilitation: Independent living skills; orientation/mobility on site and at home.
Recreational: Adult and youth programs; summer youth camp experiences; swimming, sports, arts and crafts, physical education, woodshop, and music activities.
Employment: Prevocational evaluation; career and skill development; refers and provides consultation to other agencies.
Computer Training: Training varies depending upon individual needs (usually between 12 weeks and 1 year). Access/training on computer aids and devices, microcomputer classes. Subsidy program for equipment needed in employment (southern California only). Contact: Director, Admitting Services (213) 663-1111.
Low Vision: Visual aids, consultations and demonstrations.

Local Offices:

Anaheim: Orange County Center, 527 North Dale Avenue, Anaheim, CA 92801-4820, (714) 821-5000.

Los Angeles: Sight Center, 741 North Vermont Avenue, Los Angeles, CA 90029, (213) 663-1111.
Los Angeles: Youth Center, 3450 Cahuenga Boulevard West, Los Angeles, CA 90068, (213) 851-6122.
Rancho Mirage: Desert Center, 70-251 Ramon Road, Rancho Mirage, CA 92270, (760) 321-1111.
San Diego: San Diego Center, 4510 Executive Drive, Suite 100, San Diego, CA 92121, (619) 452-1111.
Santa Barbara: Santa Barbara Center, 2031 De La Vina, Santa Barbara, CA 93105, (805) 682-6222.

Community outreach programs are conducted in more than 40 locations throughout Southern California.

Center for Living Independence for Multi-Handicapped Blind (CLIMB)

161 West Sierra Madre Boulevard
Sierra Madre, CA 91024
(818) 355-1447
FAX: (818) 289-5378
William Young, Executive Director
Chris Onye, Director of Operations

Type of Agency: Private; non-profit.
County/District Where Located: Los Angeles County.
Mission: Residential and community services for multiply handicapped blind adults.
Funded by: Client fees and workshop sales.
Hours of Operation: 24 hours, 7 days a week.
Staff: 75.
History/Date: Est. 1977.
Number of Clients Served: 130.
Eligibility: Visually impaired, multiply handicapped. Referral by state regional center.
Area Served: Statewide.
Transportation: Y.

Age Requirements: Over 18 years of age.

Health: Refers for diagnosis, evaluation, treatment, and prescriptions for eye health.
Counseling/Social Work/Self-Help: Provides social evaluation, psychological evaluation/testing, and individual counseling.
Educational: Social/vocational/skill development.
Professional Training: Internships in orientation/mobility.
Reading: Talking book records/tapes; braille/large print books; braille/recorded magazines; book selection service; Optacon and other equipment.
Residential: Dormitories for multiply handicapped adults.
Rehabilitation: Daily living/communication skills; orientation/mobility; sensory training.
Recreational: Continuing education; arts/crafts; hobbies; bowling; swimming; track.
Employment: Vocational training/evaluations; career/skill counseling; occupational skill development; sheltered workshops; placement.
Computer Training: Voice synthesizer training.
Low Vision: Refers for prescriptions and fittings for aids.

Center for the Partially Sighted

720 Wilshire Boulevard
Suite 200
Santa Monica, CA 90401-1713
(310) 458-3501
FAX: (310) 458-8179
E-mail: lovision@ix.netcom.com
LaDonna Ringering, Ph.D., Executive Director

Type of Agency: Private; non-profit.

County/District Where Located: Los Angeles County.
Mission: Rehabilitation services for partially sighted/legally blind persons.
Funded by: Government grants; private donations; fees.
Budget: 1996: $1,450.00.
Hours of Operation: Mon.-Fri. 8:00 AM - 5:00 PM.
Program Accessibility: Fully accessible.
Staff: 16 full time, 13 part time. Uses volunteers.
History/Date: Est. 1978.
Number of Clients Served: 1,800 annually.
Eligibility: Visually impaired (visual acuity in the better eye not exceeding 20/70, but better than light perception; or visual field not greater than 30 degrees).
Area Served: Unlimited.
Transportation: Y.
Age Requirements: None.

Health: Evaluation of functional vision; prescription and training in the use of spectacles/aids; sells or lends low vision aids or devices; diabetic support group; follow-up evaluation. Refers for, or provides consultation to other agencies for other health services.
Counseling/Social Work/Self-Help: Psychological evaluation; individual, family, and group counseling; peer phone counseling; referral to community services. Refers for other counseling/social work services. Provides consultation to other agencies.
Professional Training: Residency internship/fieldwork placement in rehabilition training, orientation and mobility, low vision, optometry. Open to enrollment from other agencies.
Reading: Information and referral for large-print and recorded materials; closed-circuit televisions

and computers for demonstration and limited use.

Rehabilitation: Orientation/ mobility and independent living skills instruction. Refers for other rehabilitation services.

Recreational: Limited recreational program for clients. Refers for recreational/leisure services.

Employment: Refers for employment-oriented services.

Computer Training: Demonstrations and training in access technology.

Low Vision: Evaluations and prescriptions of low vision devices by licensed optometrists.

Low Vision Aids: Provided on loan for trial purposes; individualized prescriptions; sale of optical/nonoptical devices.

Low Vision Follow-up: Recheck appointments; scheduled phone follow-ups.

Community Blind Center

130 West Flora Street
P.O. Box 467
Stockton, CA 95202
(209) 466-3836
FAX: (209) 466-5692
Patrick Moore, Executive Director

Type of Agency: Private; non-profit.

County/District Where Located: San Joaquin County.

Mission: Services for totally blind, legally blind, and visually impaired persons.

Budget: $260,000.

Hours of Operation: Mon.- Fri, 8:30 A.M.- 5:00 P.M.

Staff: 4 full time, 6 part time. Uses volunteers.

History/Date: Est. 1949.

Eligibility: Vision impairment.

Area Served: San Joaquin County and surrounding areas.

Counseling/Social Work/Self-Help: Outreach; social evaluation;

individual, family and couple counseling; information and referral services.

Rehabilitation: Orientation/ mobility; daily living skills; braille; English as a second language.

Recreational: Adult education; afterschool youth program; arts and crafts; bowling; swimming; summer session for youth.

Employment: Training in job-seeking skills.

Computer Training: Skill testing for employment.

Low Vision: Low vision aids and appliances.

Low Vision Follow-up: Y.

Desert Blind Association

800 Vella Road
P.O. Box 66
Palm Springs, CA 92263
(619) 323-4414
D. Elaine Clark, Director

Type of Agency: Private; non-profit.

County/District Where Located: Riverside County.

Mission: Services for visually impaired, physically disabled and elderly.

Funded by: United Way and contributions.

Hours of Operation: Mon.-Fri. 8:00 AM-5:00 PM.

Staff: 3 full time, 2 part time. Uses volunteers.

History/Date: Est. 1972.

Number of Clients Served: 480 annually.

Eligibility: Sixty years of age and over.

Area Served: Coachella Valley.

Transportation: Y.

Age Requirements: 60 years or older.

Health: Outreach.

Rehabilitation: Through outreach.

Doran Resource Center for the Blind

413 Laurel Street
Santa Cruz, CA 95060
(408) 458-9766
Sheila Vaughn, Executive Director

Type of Agency: Resource center providing programs and services for blind and visually impaired persons.

Mission: To provide resources, programs, and services that encourage independence for blind and visually impaired persons.

Funded by: Private contributions.

Hours of Operation: Mon.-Fri. 9:00 AM-5:00 PM.

Program Accessibility: Fully accessible.

Staff: 2 full time, 2 part time.

History/Date: Est. 1980.

Number of Clients Served: Approximately 150 per month.

Eligibility: Any level of visual impairment.

Area Served: Santa Cruz County.

Transportation: Y.

Counseling/Social Work/Self-Help: Available.

Educational: Independent living skills and orientation and mobility training.

Reading: Braille books, large print, library of books on tape.

Rehabilitation: Daily living skills.

Recreational: Crafts, exercises, outings.

Low Vision: Clinic staffed by professionals.

Low Vision Aids: Prescribed through clinic; non-optical aids available for sale.

Low Vision Follow-up: Home visit to assist in use of low-vision aids.

East Bay Center for the Blind, Inc.

2928 Adeline Street

Berkeley, CA 94703-2503
(510) 843-6935
Grant Metcalf, Executive Director

County/District Where Located:
Alameda County.
Hours of Operation: Mon.-Fri.
9:00 AM-4:00 PM.

**Friendship Center for the Blind
and Visually Impaired**
2032 Kern Mall
Fresno, CA 93721
(209) 266-9496
FAX: (209) 266-6879
Phillip Kimble, Director

Type of Agency: Private; non-
profit.
Funded by: Donations; city and
county contracts.
Budget: $ 180,000.
Hours of Operation: Mon.-Fri.
8:00 AM - 4:30 PM.
Program Accessibility:
Wheelchair accessible.
Staff: 4 full time; 2 part time. Uses
volunteers.
History/Date: Est. 1973.
Number of Clients Served: 1996:
444.
Eligibility: Totally blind; legally
blind; severely visually impaired.
Area Served: Fresno County.
Transportation: Y.

**Counseling/Social Work/Self-
Help:** Social evaluation; peer
support groups; individual, group,
family/parent counseling. Referral
to community services, refers and
provides consultation to other
agencies for other counseling/
social work services.
Professional Training: Placement
in training; regular in-service
training programs; open to
enrollment from other agencies.
Rehabilitation: Activities of daily
living; gesticulation; video
magnifier; home management.
Recreational: Arts and crafts;
therapeutic recreation activities;

special programs for elderly;
bowling; swimming; fishing.
Employment: Refers for
employment services.
Low Vision: Low vision service
and referrals.
Low Vision Aids: Low vision aids
and devices.

**Helen Keller National Center for
Deaf-Blind Youths and Adults
Southwest Region Office**
18345 Ventura Boulevard
Suite 505
Tarzana, CA 91356
(818) 757-8921 or TDD (818) 757-
8922
FAX: (818) 757-8965
E-mail: hkncsw@aol.com
Rustie Rothstein, Regional
Representative

See Helen Keller National Center
for Deaf-Blind Youths and Adults
in U.S. national listings.

Intercommunity Blind Center
7702 South Washington Avenue
Whittier, CA 90602
(562) 945-8771
FAX: (562) 945-0051
Gerald R. Konsler, Executive
Director

Type of Agency: Non-profit
human services agency.
County/District Where Located:
Los Angeles County.
Mission: To integrate blind and
visually impaired persons into all
aspects of the sighted world and
thus to improve their overall
quality of life.
Funded by: Private donations;
foundations; city grants; United
Way; fundraisers, corporations and
service clubs.
Budget: $100,000.
Hours of Operation: Mon.-Fri.
9:00 AM-5:00 PM.
Program Accessibility: Fully
accessible.

Staff: 1 full time, 4 part time.
History/Date: Est. 1967.
Number of Clients Served: Over
350.
Eligibility: Visual impairment
that cannot be corrected with
normal eye wear.
Area Served: Unlimited, but,
primarily southeastern Los
Angeles County area.
Age Requirements: 6 years and
older.
**Counseling/Social Work/Self-
Help:** Support group.
Educational: Braille instruction.
Reading: Talking books library.
Rehabilitation: Independent
living skills education and training
(cooking, homemaking, house
management).
Recreational: Youth group (6-19
years); adult recreational outings
(44 years and older); arts and crafts
instruction.
Computer Training: Assistive
technology training.

**Lions Blind Center of Diablo
Valley**
175 Alvarado Avenue
Pittsburg, CA 94565
(510) 432-3013 or (800) 750-3937
(750-EYES)
FAX: (510) 432-7014
Helen Breeding, Office Manager
Denise Cintron-Perales, Executive
Director

Type of Agency: Private; non-
profit.
County/District Where Located:
Contra Costa County.
Mission: Services for totally blind;
legally blind adults.
Funded by: Grants, income from
fund-raising events, Lions Clubs.
Hours of Operation: Mon.-Fri.
9:00 AM-5:00 PM.
Staff: 3 full time, 4 part time. Uses
volunteers.

History/Date: Est. 1954.
Eligibility: Legally blind or severely visually impaired adults.
Area Served: Contra Costa County.
Transportation: Y.
Age Requirements: 21 years and older.

Health: Low vision aids and devices. Refers for other health services.
Counseling/Social Work/Self-Help: Social evaluation; individual and group counseling; referral to community services. Refers for other counseling/social work services.
Educational: Program for adult continuing education; cooking; crafts; talking book discussion group.
Professional Training: In-service training for staff and community.
Reading: Talking book record player; cassette player; talking book records and tapes; braille and large-print books; braille and recorded magazines. Information and referral.
Rehabilitation: Activities of daily living; braille; handwriting; video magnifier; electronic mobility aids; home management; orientation/mobility; rehabilitation teaching in client's home and community; sensory training.
Recreational: Adult continuing education; arts and crafts; bowling; fishing; field trips.
Employment: Refers for employment services.
Computer Training: Classes available.
Low Vision: Refers for some low vision screening.
Low Vision Aids: For loan and sale.

Lions Blind Center of the Santa Clara Valley

101 North Bascom Avenue

San Jose, CA 95128
(408) 295-4016
FAX: (408) 295-1398
E-mail: lbcscv@aol.com
Ed Thomas, Director

Type of Agency: A recreational, social and theraputic center for the blind and visually impaired.
County/District Where Located: Santa Clara County.
Mission: Living skills, counseling, braille instruction, recreation and social activities, information and referral.
Funded by: Lions Clubs, city of San Jose, and community donations.
Budget: $150,000.
Hours of Operation: Mon.-Fri. 9:00 AM - 4:00 PM.
Staff: 2 full time, 4 part time.
History/Date: Est. 1952.
Number of Clients Served: 100 monthly.
Eligibility: Legally blind.
Area Served: Santa Clara Valley.
Transportation: Y.

Counseling/Social Work/Self-Help: Support groups at local senior residences.
Educational: Cooking, Spanish, sewing, English as a second language, braille, computer training.
Reading: Volunteers on site to read mail, low vision reading machines.
Recreational: Monthly field trips, dance classes, self-defense, bingo.
Employment: Referrals.
Computer Training: Word processing, basic database programs.

Lions Center for the Blind

3834 Opal Street
Oakland, CA 94609
(510) 450-1580
FAX: (510) 654-3603
Charles Boyer, Executive Director

Type of Agency: Private; non-profit.
County/District Where Located: Alameda County.
Mission: Services for blind, visually impaired, deaf-blind, and developmentally disabled persons.
Budget: 1997: $538,000.
Hours of Operation: Mon.-Fri. 7:30 AM-4:30 PM.
Staff: 14 full time. Uses volunteers.
History/Date: Est. 1942.
Number of Clients Served: 250 annually.
Eligibility: Blind, visually impaired or deaf-blind.
Area Served: Alameda and Contra Costa counties.
Age Requirements: 18 and over.

Counseling/Social Work/Self-Help: Counseling/social work services.
Educational: Adult continuing education; vocational skill development.
Professional Training: Internship/supervised field work placement in orientation/mobility; social work; special education. Regular in-service training programs.
Reading: Volunteers.
Rehabilitation: Living skills; orientation and mobility.
Recreational: Life enrichment programs; exercise; field trips; arts and crafts; hobby groups; programs for the elderly; bowling.
Employment: Job development and placement.
Computer Training: Speech output software.
Low Vision: Referrals.

Living Skills Center for the Visually Impaired

13830 San Pablo Avenue
Suite B

San Pablo, CA 94806-3704
(510) 234-4984
FAX: (510) 234-4986
Patricia Williams, Executive
Director

Type of Agency: Private, non-profit agency administered by the Research and Service Foundation for the Handicapped.
Mission: Services for totally blind, legally blind, multiply disabled, and deaf-blind persons.
Funded by: California Department of Rehabilitation.
Staff: 6 full time, 1 part time.
History/Date: Est. 1972.
Eligibility: Legally blind; eligible for California Department of Rehabilitation services.
Area Served: California.
Age Requirements: Over 18 years.

Health: Refers for medical services; assists in obtaining low vision evaluations and service; fosters medical awareness through evaluations.
Counseling/Social Work/Self-Help: Assertiveness training; referral to community services. Refers for other counseling/social work services.
Educational: Independent living skills. Transition skills for college success. Accepts deaf-blind; additional disabilities considered on individual basis.
Professional Training: In-service training of others working with visually impaired people.
Residential: Clients share apartments in the community; instruction occurs in clients' apartments and in local area.
Rehabilitation: Personal management; signature writing; home management; orientation/mobility; rehabilitation teaching in client's home and community; listening and vision skills; financial skills training; broad evaluations and training in areas of cooking,

cleaning, care of clothing, social skills, personal hygiene.
Recreational: Recreational outings, i.e. camping, skiing, sea kayaking, shopping, hiking; regular informal exercise program; jogging; swimming.
Employment: Prevocational evaluation and training; career/skill counseling; follow-up service. Refers for other employment-oriented services.

Staff activities also include extensive information and referral service via telephone and participation in outreach programs; involvement in community affairs, including task force participation on public transportation, city planning, housing, and technical assistance in areas affecting visually impaired persons.

Peninsula Center for the Blind and Visually Impaired

2470 El Camino Real
Suite 107
Palo Alto, CA 94306-1701
(415) 858-0202 (as of 8/1/97 area code 415 becomes 650)
FAX: (415) 858-0857
Pam Brandin, Executive Director

Type of Agency: Private; non-profit.
Mission: Home-based services for blind and visually impaired persons of all ages.
Funded by: United Way; fees; contributions; fundraisers.
Budget: $ 890,000.
Hours of Operation: Mon.-Fri. 9:00 AM - 5:30 PM.
Staff: 10 full time, 6 part time; low vision optometrists on contract part time.
History/Date: Est. 1936 and Inc. 1945.
Number of Clients Served: 820/year.

Eligibility: Resident of Santa Clara or San Mateo County; visually impaired.
Area Served: San Mateo and Santa Clara Counties.
Transportation: Y.

Health: Low vision clinic.
Counseling/Social Work/Self-Help: Psycho-social evaluation; individual and group counseling; family counseling; support groups; referral to community services. Consultation to other agencies.
Educational: Contracts with school districts and youth group.
Professional Training: Internship/fieldwork placement.
Reading: Information and referral. Kurzweil reader available to clients.
Rehabilitation: Personal management; medical management; home management; orientation/mobility; communication skills, including braille.
Recreational: Enrichment program.
Low Vision: Low vision evaluation, prescriptions, aids, and appliances.
Low Vision Aids: Y.
Low Vision Follow-up: Y.

Rose Resnick Lighthouse for the Blind and Visually Impaired

214 Van Ness Avenue
San Francisco, CA 94102-4508
(415) 431-1481
FAX: (415) 863-7568
Anita Shafer Baldwin, Executive Director

Type of Agency: Private; non-profit.
County/District Where Located: San Francisco County.
Mission: Services for blind and visually disabled children and adults.

Funded by: Private donations.
Hours of Operation: Mon.-Fri.
8:30 AM-5:00 PM; resource center,
Mon.-Fri. 10:00 AM-4:00 PM and
first Sat. of each month 10:00 AM-
2:00 PM.
Staff: 25 (plus counselors during
the summer). Fully trained
volunteers available for reading,
in-home personal assistance.
History/Date: Est. 1902.
Number of Clients Served: 1,500.
Transportation: Y.
Age Requirements: Program
specific.

**Counseling/Social Work/Self-
Help:** Information and referral;
intake evaluation; crisis
intervention; workshops and
seminars for professionals and
families.
Educational: Adult continuing
education classes taught through
the San Francisco Community
College, specializing in braille,
arts/crafts, ceramics, and
introductory typing.
Reading: Braille library.
Volunteers available for reading
services.
Rehabilitation: Braille instruction;
orientation and mobility
instruction; daily living skills.
Recreational: Recreational and
social programs for seniors and
adults including dances, field trips,
and hot lunch on two weekdays;
Enchanted Hills Camp, residential
summer camp for children and
adults.
Employment: Job training;
employment search assistance;
resume preparation.
Low Vision: Low vision center.
Low Vision Aids: Visual and
adaptive aids available for
purchase in person and by mail.
Low Vision Follow-up: As
needed.

Local Offices:

Napa: Enchanted Hills Camp,
3410 Mt. Veeder Road, Napa, CA
94558, Phone main office:
(415) 431-1481.

RP International
P.O. Box 900
Woodland Hills, CA 91365
(818) 992-0500 or (800) FIGHT RP
FAX: (818) 992-3265
Helen Harris, President

Type of Agency: Non-profit.
Mission: To find a cure or
treatment for retinal degenerative
eye disease, disseminate
information and provide human
services.
Funded by: Donations and grants.
Budget: $300,000.
Hours of Operation: 9:00 AM-
6:00 PM daily; 24-hour crisis line.
Program Accessibility: Van
transport; bus access.
Staff: 4 full time. Uses volunteers.
History/Date: Est. 1975.
Area Served: Southern California.
Support group formed nationally.

**Counseling/Social Work/Self-
Help:** Provided at center and
through 24-hour crisis line.
Educational: Classes in mobility,
braille, arts and crafts, life
adjustment.
Reading: At vision clinic.
Recreational: Bowling team and
other school functions.
Low Vision: Clinic one morning a
week.
Low Vision Aids: Available.

San Bernardino Valley Lighthouse for the Blind, Inc.
762 North Sierra Way
San Bernardino, CA 92410
(909) 884-3121
FAX: (909) 884-2964
Robert G. McBay, Executive
Director

Type of Agency: Private; non-
profit.
Funded by: Thrift store,
donations.
Budget: $500,000.
Hours of Operation: Mon.-Fri
8:00 AM-5:00 PM.
Program Accessibility: Fully
accessible.
Staff: 17.
History/Date: Est. 1938.
Number of Clients Served:
Average 90 per day.
Eligibility: Legally blind.
Area Served: Inland Empire area.
Transportation: Y.
Age Requirements: Over 13 years.

**Counseling/Social Work/Self-
Help:** Counseling available on
adjusting to visual impairment.
Reading: Braille Institute sublending library.
Rehabilitation: Orientation/
mobility; home economics.
Recreational: Woodwork; sewing;
macrame; ceramics; braille; arts
and crafts.
Low Vision: Vision consultant
visits once a month.

San Diego Center for the Blind and Vision Impaired
5922 El Cajon Boulevard
San Diego, CA 92115
(619) 583-1542
FAX: (619) 583-2335
Kim Gibbens, Executive Director

Type of Agency: Non-profit.
Mission: To rehabilitate blind and
visually impaired individuals so
they might reach their highest
potential of independence and
self-reliance.
Funded by: Private donations,
bequests, grants, foundations, state
and local governments.
Budget: $740,000.
Hours of Operation: Mon.-Fri.
8:30 AM-4:30 PM.

Program Accessibility: Accessible to persons with disabilities. The building has received national recognition regarding the accessibility design features.
Staff: 31. 134 volunteers.
History/Date: Est. 1972.
Number of Clients Served: 1995-1996: Approximately 1,000.
Eligibility: Vision loss.
Area Served: San Diego County.
Transportation: Y.
Age Requirements: Primary age group served is adults 18 years of age or older.

Counseling/Social Work/Self-Help: Individual, group, family, and outreach counseling.
Professional Training: Undergraduate and graduate internship training.
Reading: Volunteer reading services; braille instruction.
Rehabilitation: Activities of daily living, orientation/mobility, braille, typing, handwriting, resource information, sensory awareness, clothing construction, kitchen skills, transition.
Low Vision: Provides low vision screening.
Low Vision Aids: Sells aids.
Low Vision Follow-up: Follow-up and training provided.

Local Offices:

Vista: 1385 Bonair Road, Vista, CA 92084, (619) 758-5956, FAX (619) 758-6296.

Sensory Access Foundation
385 Sherman Avenue
Suite 2
Palo Alto, CA 94306-1840
(415) 329-0430 (as of 8/1/97 area code 415 becomes 650)
FAX: (415) 323-1062
E-mail: saf@gbx.org
Diana L. Drews, Executive Director

Type of Agency: Private; non-profit.
County/District Where Located: Santa Clara County.
Mission: Services for totally blind and legally blind persons.
Funded by: Government grants, donations, fee-for-service programs and services.
Budget: $718,000.
Hours of Operation: Mon.-Fri. 8:00 AM-12:00 Noon; 1:00 PM-5:00 PM.
Staff: 12 full-time, 3 part-time. Uses volunteers.
History/Date: Est. 1973.
Number of Clients Served: Direct services 188/year; information and referral 800/year.
Eligibility: Referral by State Department of Rehabilitation, counselor or employer. Self-referral for information and referral program.
Area Served: Direct services, California; information and referral, unlimited.
Age Requirements: Working age primarily.

Employment: Employment services include: job preparation and placement; access technology evaluations, both on-site and in our Computer Education, Training and Evaluation Center (CETEC); employer/employee education; ADA consultation; on-the-job equipment loan; individualized access technology training; installation and configuration of systems; and the Work Incentive Program.

Society for the Blind
2750 24th Street
Sacramento, CA 95818
(916) 452-8271
FAX: (916) 452-2622
Thomas Ryan, Executive Director

Type of Agency: Non-profit.
Mission: Services for totally blind, legally blind, and visually impaired persons.
Funded by: Contributions; fees; bequests; fundraising.
Budget: $743,404.
Hours of Operation: Mon.-Fri. 8:00 AM - 4:30 PM.
Program Accessibility: All programs totally accessible.
Staff: 12 full-time, 2 part-time. Uses volunteers.
History/Date: Est. 1954.
Number of Clients Served: 1996: 2,241.
Eligibility: Visually impaired and blind persons able to benefit from our services.
Area Served: Sacramento area except for low vision clinic, which serves 26 counties of northern California. Products for Independence Store will do mail order.

Health: Low vision clinic.
Counseling/Social Work/Self-Help: Social services, family, and group counseling; peer support group.
Professional Training: Internships in mobility/orientation and rehabilitation teaching.
Residential: In-home volunteer service, reading mail, shopping, paying bills.
Rehabilitation: Orientation/mobility; activities of daily living; braille; support groups.
Recreational: Adult education, arts, crafts, special programs for elderly persons.
Employment: Refers for employment services.
Computer Training: Computer literacy and typing; training on computer aids and devices.
Low Vision: Y.
Low Vision Aids: Y.
Low Vision Follow-up: Y.

Operates Products for Independence, a retail store that sells products that blind and visually impaired people use to enhance independence.

Therapeutic Living Centers for the Blind

7955 Lindley Avenue
Reseda, CA 91335
(818) 708-1740
FAX: (818) 708-7899
Lynn Robinson, Executive Director

Type of Agency: Private; non-profit.
County/District Where Located: Los Angeles County.
Mission: Services for blind and developmentally disabled persons.
Funded by: Private, federal, and state funds.
Budget: $2,500,000.
Program Accessibility: Program sites accessible to wheelchairs.
Staff: 100.
History/Date: Est. 1975.
Number of Clients Served: Day program: 55; residential: 60.
Eligibility: Developmentally disabled and visually impaired may have additional disabilities, such as hearing loss, epilepsy, cerebral palsy, and/or behavioral deficits.
Age Requirements: 18-65 years.

Health: Monitoring and assistance with management of health issues.
Counseling/Social Work/Self-Help: Training and assistance.
Educational: Tutorial services available to persons unable to attend day program on site.
Residential: Various residential programs to serve clients with behavioral/self-help deficits, as well as medical problems.
Recreational: Comprehensive programming available.
Employment: Pre-employment training available.

Low Vision: On-site training provided.

Tri-Visual Services

1713 J Street, Suite 211
Sacramento, CA 95814
(916) 447-7323
FAX: (916) 447-7323
Elena Negrete, Executive Director

Type of Agency: Non-profit.
County/District Where Located: Sacramento County.
Mission: Strengthen services to visually impaired and blind people of Northern California.
Funded by: Grants; fund raising; private donations.
Hours of Operation: Mon.-Fri. 8:30 AM-3:00 PM.
History/Date: Est. 1981.
Area Served: Northern California.

Rehabilitation: Independent living program; daily living skills.
Recreational: Travel club has several field trips for youths and adults; bowling; beep baseball.
Computer Training: Computer literacy workshop; BCUG, quarterly meetings; resource computer guide.

Western Blind Rehabilitation Center
U.S. Department of Veterans Affairs

VA Medical Center
3801 Miranda Avenue
Palo Alto, CA 94304
(415) 493-5000, ext. 4358 (as of 8/1/97 area code 415 becomes 650) or (415) 858-3921
FAX: (415) 852-8472
William Ekstrom, Director

Type of Agency: Federal.
Mission: Provides residential rehabilitation services to eligible legally blind veterans.
Funded by: Federal government.

Hours of Operation: Mon.-Fri. 7:30 AM-4:00 PM.
Staff: Optometrist; optometry students and residents; low vision specialist; social worker; orientation/mobility instructor; rehabilitation teachers; psychologist/counselor; manual skills instructor; ophthalmologist; ophthalmology residents; occupational therapist; rehabilitation counselors; audiologist; recreational therapist; computer access training instructors.
History/Date: Est. 1967.
Eligibility: Legally blind veterans; opthalmology report.
Area Served: California, Montana, Utah, Wyoming, Nevada, Hawaii.

Low Vision Aids: Provided when prescribed.

Referral applications by Visual Impairment Services programs located at VA Medical Centers and Outpatient Clinics in the geographical area served by the Blind Rehabilitation Center or Clinic.

See U.S. Department of Veterans Affairs in U.S. Federal Agencies listings.

COMPUTER TRAINING CENTERS

California School for the Blind

500 Walnut Avenue
Fremont, CA 94536
(510) 794-3800, ext. 237
FAX: (510) 794-3813
Jim Carreon, Technology Coordinator

Computer Training: Speech output systems; screen magnification systems; braille access systems; closed-circuit television systems; word processing.

Center for the Blind and Visually Impaired

1124 Baker Street
Bakersfield, CA 93305
(805) 322-5234
FAX: (805) 322-7754
Sandra Quigley, Executive Director

County/District Where Located:
Kern County.

Computer Training: Available free of charge to the visually impaired; classes are scheduled on an as needed basis.

College of the Redwoods High Tech Center

7351 Tompkins Hill Road
Eureka, CA 95501
(707) 445-6825
FAX: (707) 445-6990
Julie Wells, Technical Specialist

County/District Where Located:
Humboldt County.

Computer Training: Speech output systems; screen magnification systems; optical character recognition systems; word processing; computer operating systems; training for instructors.

Computer Access Laboratory California State University, Students with Disabilities Resources

18111 Nordhoff Street
Northridge, CA 91330-8264
(818) 677-2684
FAX: (818) 677-4932
E-mail: mark.sakata@csun.edu
URL: http://www.csun.edu/cod/
Mark Sakata, Assistant Technical Specialist, Rehabilitation Counselor

County/District Where Located:
Los Angeles County.

Computer Training: Speech output systems; screen magnification systems; braille access systems; optical character recognition systems; closed-circuit television systems; word processing, speech recognition and readback; gui internet access; screen readers.

Lions Center for the Blind

3834 Opal Street
Oakland, CA 94609
(510) 450-1580
FAX: (510) 654-3603
Charles Boyer, Executive Director
Gerry Newell, Coordinator

County/District Where Located:
Alameda County.

Computer Training: Screen magnification systems; braille access systems; closed-circuit television systems; word processing; database software; computer operating systems.

Palomar College

1140 Mission Road
San Marcos, CA 92069
(619) 744-1150
Sherry Goldsmith, Computer Specialist

Computer Training: Speech output systems; screen magnification systems; optical character recognition systems; word processing.

DOG GUIDE SCHOOLS

Eye Dog Foundation for the Blind

211 South Montclair Street, Suite A
Bakersfield, CA 93309-3165
(805) 831-1333
FAX: (805) 831-0681
Lequita J. McKay, Executive Director
David A. Hagemann, Director of Training

Type of Agency: Non-profit.
County/District Where Located:
Kern County.

Mission: Trains dog guides and blind individuals with the dog guides. Dog guides are given to blind persons at no cost.
Funded by: Public donations, trusts, wills, and endowments.
History/Date: Est. 1952.
Area Served: Unlimited.

Local Offices:

Phoenix: Eye Dog Foundation for the Blind, Training Center, 8252 South 15th Avenue, Phoenix, AZ 85041, (602) 276-0051.

Guide Dogs for the Blind

P.O. Box 151200
San Rafael, CA 94915
(415) 499-4000 or (800) 295-4050
FAX: (415) 499-4035
Richard A. Bobb, President and CEO
Sue Sullivan, Admissions

Type of Agency: Private; non-profit.
County/District Where Located:
Marin County.
Mission: Trains and supplies dog guides to blind persons at no cost. Provides follow-up services for clients and an annual stipend for veterinary services.
Funded by: Contributions and endowment.
Budget: $16 million.
Hours of Operation:
Administrative offices: Mon.-Fri. 8:00 AM-5:00 PM.
Staff: 220.
History/Date: Est. and Inc. 1942.
Number of Clients Served: More than 350 annually.
Eligibility: At least 16 years of age, legally blind and physically and emotionally capable of undergoing required four-week in-residence training program.
Area Served: United States and Canada.
Transportation: Y.

Age Requirements: Minimum age: 16 years.

Health: Able to walk at fairly brisk pace to allow dog to work safely.
Counseling/Social Work/Self-Help: Counselor on staff.
Professional Training: Trains own instructors and breeds own dogs.
Residential: Dormitories for 24 trainees.

Local Offices:

Topanga: Field Office, 1776 Old Topanga Canyon Road, Topanga, CA 90290, (310) 455-1095.

Guide Dogs of America
13445 Glenoaks Boulevard
Sylmar, CA 91342
(818) 362-5834
FAX: (818) 362-6870
Andi Krusoe, Admissions and Graduate Services Manager

County/District Where Located: Los Angeles County.
Mission: Trains and supplies dog guides to blind persons free of charge. Provides consultation and referral and follow-up services for clients.
Funded by: Contributions.
Budget: $1.5 million.
Hours of Operation: Mon.-Fri. 8:00 AM-5:00 PM.
Staff: 27.
History/Date: Inc. 1948.
Number of Clients Served: More than 250 active.
Eligibility: Individually evaluated for acceptance to program.
Area Served: United States and Canada.
Transportation: Y.
Age Requirements: 16 years or older.
Educational: Tours, speakers bureau.
Residential: 28 day, in-residence training course.

Rehabilitation: Guide dog mobility training.

Guide Dogs of the Desert
P.O. Box 1692
Palm Springs, CA 92263
(619) 329-6257
FAX: (619) 329-2127
James O. Hyatt, CEO.

Type of Agency: Non-profit.
County/District Where Located: Riverside County.
Mission: To provide independent mobility to blind persons through the companionship and assistance of a guide dog.
Funded by: Donations.
Budget: $500,000.
Hours of Operation: Mon.-Fri. 8:00 AM-5:00 PM, Sat. 8:00 AM-12:00 PM.
Staff: 15.
History/Date: Est. 1972.
Number of Clients Served: 30 new graduates each year. Approximately 140 provided with postgraduate assistance.
Eligibility: Legally blind.
Area Served: United States, Canada and Mexico.
Age Requirements: At least 16 years.

Residential: 28 days, free boarding.

♦ Low Vision Services

EYE CARE SOCIETIES

California Association of Ophthalmology
605 Market Street
Suite 1109

San Francisco, CA 94105-3213
(415) 777-3937
FAX: (415) 777-1082
E-mail: starrs 2020@aol.com
Starr E. Shulman, Executive Director
Martin L. Fishman, M.D., M.P.A., President

County/District Where Located: San Francisco County.

California Optometric Association
P.O. Box 2591
Sacramento, CA 95812
(916) 441-3990
FAX: (916) 448-1423
URL: http://www.coavision.org
Claudia Foutz, Executive Director

County/District Where Located: Sacramento County.

LOW VISION CENTERS

California Pacific Medical Center Department of Ophthalmology Low Vision Service
2340 Clay Street
Fifth Floor
San Francisco, CA 94115
(415) 923-3933
FAX: (415) 923-3945
August Colenbrander, M.D., Director
Anna E. Ortiz-Harder, M.A., Coordinator

Type of Agency: Non-profit; full-service eye department.
Mission: Low vision rehabilitation, education, and research.
Funded by: Patient fees.
Hours of Operation: Mon.-Fri. 8:30 AM-5:30 PM.
Staff: Ophthalmologist, low vision specialist, full-service eye department.
History/Date: Est. 1960.
Eligibility: Ophthalmology report.

Area Served: Unlimited.
Transportation: Y.

Professional Training: Internship site for San Francisco State University residency training program.
Rehabilitation: Rehabilitation services by referral.
Low Vision Aids: Provided on loan for trial purposes; no rental fee; on-site training provided.
Low Vision Follow-up: As needed. Long-term follow-up by questionnaire.

Center for the Partially Sighted
720 Wilshire Boulevard
Suite 200
Santa Monica, CA 90401-1713
(310) 458-3501
FAX: (310) 458-8179
E-mail: lovision@ix.netcom.com
LaDonna Ringering, Ph.D., Executive Director
Phyllis Amaral, Ph.D., Director of Clinical Services

Type of Agency: Private; non-profit.
County/District Where Located: Los Angeles County.
Mission: Rehabilitation services for partially sighted/legally blind persons.
Funded by: California Department of Rehabilitation; private donations; client fees (sliding scale); third-party payers; city of Santa Monica; and County of Los Angeles.
Budget: $1,450,000.
Hours of Operation: Mon.-Fri. 8:00 AM-5:00 PM.
Program Accessibility: Fully accessible.
Staff: Optometrists; optometric interns; optometric technicians; psychologists; peer counselors; orientation/mobility instructors; independent living skills

instructors; social service and follow-up counselors.
History/Date: Est. 1978.
Number of Clients Served: 1,800 annually.
Eligibility: Low vision.
Area Served: Unlimited.
Transportation: Y.
Age Requirements: None.

Health: Off-site evaluations for physically frail.
Counseling/Social Work/Self-Help: Psychological evaluations and therapy by licensed clinical psychologists; peer counseling; diabetes support group.
Educational: In-service training and workshops on low vision.
Professional Training: Optometric residence and internship; psychology, gerontology and orientation and mobility field placement.
Rehabilitation: Independent living skills classes; orientation and mobility.
Computer Training: Access technology demonstrations.
Low Vision: Evaluations and prescriptions of low vision devices by licensed optometrists.
Low Vision Aids: Provided on loan for trial purposes; no rental fees; on-site and off-site training provided.
Low Vision Follow-up: Phone interview after 1 week; second appointment 2 weeks after initial visit; periodic phone calls and home/school/work site follow-up visits as needed; 6 month and 1 year recall.

Local Offices:

Torrance: 3537 Torrance Boulevard, Suite 18, Torrance, CA 90503 . Call for appointment, (310) 458-3501.

Jules Stein Eye Institute
University of California at Los Angeles
100 Stein Plaza
Los Angeles, CA 90095-7000
(310) 825-5053
Bartly J. Mondino, M.D., Director and Chairman, Department of Ophthalmology

County/District Where Located: Los Angeles County.
Funded by: Client fees; state funds; contributions.
Hours of Operation: Mon.-Fri. by appointment, or emergency clinic at all times.
History/Date: Est. 1966.
Area Served: Unlimited.
Age Requirements: None.

Professional Training: Residency and Fellowship program.
Reading: When available, on case by case basis.
Low Vision: Evaluation by appointment.
Low Vision Aids: On-site training provided.
Low Vision Follow-up: By return appointment in 6 months.

King-Drew Medical Center
12021 South Wilmington Avenue
Los Angeles, CA 90059
(310) 668-4531
FAX: (310) 537-9446
Dr. Richard Casey, Chief of Ophthalmology
Candace Chandler, Administrator

Type of Agency: Non-profit.
County/District Where Located: Los Angeles County.
Hours of Operation: Mon.-Fri. 8:00 AM-4:30 PM.
Staff: Ophthalmologist; ophthalmology residents; optometrist; social worker; orientation/mobility instructor; rehabilitation teacher; special educator; occupational therapist; psychologist/counselor;

rehabilitation counselor; audiologist; genetic counselor.
Area Served: County of Los Angeles.

Low Vision Aids: On-site training provided.
Low Vision Follow-up: After 3 months by return appointment.

Low Vision Clinic
University of California, San Francisco Eye Clinic
400 Parnassus Avenue
Seventh Floor
P.O. Box 0344
San Francisco, CA 94143
(415) 476-5022
FAX: (415) 502-6334
Dr. Roland Jung, Coordinator

Type of Agency: University medical center.
Mission: To provide evaluations for low vision devices, nonoptical assistive devices, counseling, and referrals as necessary.
Funded by: University of California, San Francisco.
Hours of Operation: Mon., Thurs., Fri. 8:00 AM-11:30 AM.
Staff: Optometrist, ophthalmic technician, ophthalmologist, ophthalmology residents.
History/Date: Est. 1984.
Number of Clients Served: Approximately 125 patients per year.
Eligibility: Referral by ophthalmologist, optometrist, State Department of Rehabilitation, or other physicians.
Area Served: San Francisco Bay area, northern and central California.
Transportation: Y.
Age Requirements: 5 years and older.

Health: Full scale ophthalmology clinic; accessibility to campus medical facilities.

Counseling/Social Work/Self-Help: Social work services available through university hospitals and clinics and local non-profit agencies.
Low Vision: Evaluations; training and prescription of devices; low vision devices available on loan.
Low Vision Follow-up: Y.

Low Vision Clinic
University of California School of Optometry
Berkeley, CA 94720-2020
(510) 642-5726
FAX: (510) 643-5109
Ian L. Bailey, O.D., Director

Mission: Provide clinical low vision care and training for optometrists.
Funded by: State funds; client fees.
Hours of Operation: Mon.-Fri. 9:00 AM-5:00 PM.
Staff: Optometrists; optometry residents; special educators; low vision mobility specialists.
History/Date: Est. 1960.
Eligibility: None.
Area Served: Unlimited.

Counseling/Social Work/Self-Help: Peer support group for adults.
Educational: Educational assessments within special vision assessment clinic for disabled children.
Professional Training: Training for undergraduate and graduate students in optometry.
Rehabilitation: Information and referral services; mobility assessments.
Low Vision: Comprehensive assessments of visual capabilities for all ages.
Low Vision Aids: May be purchased by client or provided on loan for trial period; on-site training provided.

Low Vision Follow-up: After 1 month with additional services as needed.

Marin Low Vision Clinic
930 Tamalpais Avenue
San Rafael, CA 94901
(415) 457-8890
Dr. Howard A. Levenson, O.D., Clinic Administrator

Type of Agency: Public.
County/District Where Located: Marin County.
Mission: Provide therapy and low vision aids for patients to maintain independence.
Funded by: Lions Club, various foundations, donations.
Budget: $30,000.
Hours of Operation: Mon. 10:00 AM-4:00 PM.
Program Accessibility: Referral from ophthalmologist or optometrist only.
Staff: 2 optometrists and support staff.
History/Date: Est. 1991.
Number of Clients Served: 150 annually.
Area Served: Marin and Sonoma Counties.
Transportation: Y.
Age Requirements: None.

Counseling/Social Work/Self-Help: Y.
Low Vision: Comprehensive services, including follow-up and dispensing of aids.
Low Vision Aids: Extensive inventory.
Low Vision Follow-up: Yes.

Optometric Center of Los Angeles
Southern California College of Optometry
3916 South Broadway

Los Angeles, CA 90037
(213) 234-9137
FAX: (213) 235-6203
Tony Carnevali O.D., Director
Robert L. Gordon O.D.,
Coordinator, Low Vision Services

Type of Agency: Non-profit.
County/District Where Located:
Los Angeles County.
Funded by: Client fees.
Hours of Operation: Mon.-Fri.
8:00 AM - 5:00 PM, Sat. 8:00 AM-
3:00 PM.
Area Served: Unlimited.

Low Vision: Complete low vision
services.
Low Vision Aids: Provided on
loan for trial purposes through
Lions Loaner Library; on-site
training provided.
Low Vision Follow-up: Complete
follow-up services provided.

Peninsula Center for the Blind and Visually Impaired

2470 El Camino Real
Suite 107
Palo Alto, CA 94306-1701
(415) 858-0202 (as of 8/1/97 area
code 415 becomes 650)
FAX: (415) 858-0857
Pam Brandin, Executive Director
Selma Chin, O.D., Low Vision
Director

Type of Agency: Private; non-
profit.
Mission: To provide low vision
evaluations, low vision aids and
technology, and training in their
use.
Funded by: Client fees and
donations.
Budget: $110,000 (low vision clinic
only).
Hours of Operation: Tues., Thurs.
and Fri. 9:00 AM - 4:30 PM.
Staff: Optometrist; social worker;
orientation/mobility instructor;
rehabilitation teacher.

Number of Clients Served: 375/
year.
Area Served: San Mateo and Santa
Clara Counties.

**Counseling/Social Work/Self-
Help:** Information and referral,
counseling, and support groups.
Rehabilitation: Y.
Low Vision Aids: Provided on
loan for trial purposes; available
for purchase; on-site training
provided; prescriptions ordered.
Demonstrations of adaptive
technology for low vision.
Low Vision Follow-up: By return
appointment as needed.

RP International Low Vision

23241 Ventura Boulevard
Suite 117
Woodland Hills, CA 91365
(818) 992-0500 or (800) FIGHT RP
Helen Harris, President

Staff: Optometrist, mobility
instructor.

Low Vision: Low vision exams,
prescriptions for devices free of
charge.
Low Vision Aids: Available for
sale.
Low Vision Follow-up: As
needed.

St. Mary Low Vision Center

1050 Linden
Long Beach, CA 90813
(310) 491-9275
FAX: (310) 491-9934
Bonnie Steinberg Solberg,
Coordinator
Florence Traub, RN, Assistant
Coordinator

Type of Agency: Private; non-
profit.
County/District Where Located:
Los Angeles County.
Funded by: Foundation grants;
donations.

Hours of Operation: Mon.-Fri. by
appointment only.
Eligibility: Written referral from
ophthalmologist.
Area Served: Unlimited.
Age Requirements: 5 years and
up. Special programs geared
toward older adults.

Rehabilitation: Independent
living classes instructed on an on-
going basis. Orientation and
mobility training on a limited
basis. Braille instruction provided
on request.
Low Vision Aids: Provided on
loan for trial purpose at no charge.
On-site training provided.
Low Vision Follow-up: By return
appointment.

Scripps Memorial Hospital Mericos Eye Institute Partial Vision Center

P.O. Box 28
La Jolla, CA 92038-0028
(619) 626-6571
FAX: (619) 626-6560
Linda Van der Plaats, Contact
Person

Type of Agency: Private; non-
profit.
Mission: To serve as a resource
center for visually impaired
persons.
Funded by: Donations.
Hours of Operation: Mon.-Fri.
9:00 AM-4:00 PM.
Staff: Staff and volunteers
demonstrate low vision
equipment, magnifiers, and
illumination.
Eligibility: Unlimited.
Area Served: Unlimited.
Transportation: Y.

Educational: Free brochures
provided on request.
Rehabilitation: On-site training
and referral services.

Low Vision: Evaluation by a specialist available with a referral from an ophthalmologist.
Low Vision Aids: Prescriptive devices provided on loan for trial purposes.
Low Vision Follow-up: Y.

Society for the Blind
Visual Services Center
Low Vision Clinic

2750 Twenty-Fourth Street
Sacramento, CA 95818
(916) 452-8271
FAX: (916) 452-2622
Stephen J. Ingman, O.D., Director
Jean Autrey, Clinic Manager

Type of Agency: Rehabilitation and low vision clinic.
County/District Where Located: Sacramento County.
Funded by: Client fees.
Hours of Operation: Mon.-Fri. 8:00 AM-4:30 PM.
Staff: Optometrist; low vision assistant; social worker; orientation/mobility instructor; rehabilitation teacher; resource specialist.
Number of Clients Served: Over 1,000 patients annually.
Eligibility: Visual impairments.
Area Served: Unlimited.

Professional Training: On-site training provided.
Low Vision: Low vision assessments.
Low Vision Aids: Provided on loan for trial purposes; no rental fee. Nonoptical products.
Low Vision Follow-up: By return appointment in 1 month; by visit to place of employment or school at that time, if necessary.

Southern California College of Optometry
Low Vision Clinic

2575 Yorba Linda Boulevard

Fullerton, CA 92831
(714) 449-7415
FAX: (714) 992-7811
Dr. Pamela Thomas, Chief

Type of Agency: Private; non-profit.
County/District Where Located: Orange County.
Mission: To provide comprehensive low vision examinations.
Funded by: Medicare; sliding fee scale for medical examinations available.
Hours of Operation: Tues. 8:00 AM-5:00 PM; Wed. 11:30 AM-3:30 PM; Thurs. 11:30 AM-3:30 PM.
Staff: Optometrist; optometry student/residents; service coordinator.
Area Served: Unlimited.

Low Vision: Evaluations provided.
Low Vision Aids: Provided on loan for trial purposes; rental fee charged; on-site training.
Low Vision Follow-up: By recall system within 6 months.

Stanford
Department of Ophthalmology, Low Vision Services

300 Pasteur Drive
Palo Alto, CA 94305-5308
(415) 723-6995 (as of 8/1/97 area code 415 becomes 650)
FAX: (415) 725-6619
Dr. Peter D'Alena, Low Vision Specialist

Type of Agency: Non-profit.
County/District Where Located: Santa Clara County.
Hours of Operation: 1st and 3rd Friday of every month.
Eligibility: Doctor's referral.
Area Served: California.

Low Vision: Prescription of aids; follow-up available.

University of California, Davis
Department of Ophthalmology
Low Vision Services

1611 Alhambra Boulevard
Sacramento, CA 95816
(916) 734-6602
FAX: (916) 734-6992
Janis Lightman, O.D., Director

Type of Agency: University.
County/District Where Located: Sacramento County.
Funded by: Client fees; county and state funds.
Hours of Operation: Mon.-Fri. 9:00 AM - 11:30 AM; Tues. and Fri. 8:30 AM - 3:30 PM.
Staff: Ophthalmology resident; ophthalmologist; optometrist.
Number of Clients Served: 4-10 per week.
Eligibility: Self-referral and OD/MD referral welcome.
Area Served: Unlimited.
Age Requirements: None.

Health: Associated with University Medical Center.
Counseling/Social Work/Self-Help: Referrals.
Low Vision Aids: Prescribed and fitted for variable charge.
Low Vision Follow-up: By return appointment.

Veterans Affairs Medical Center

11301 Wilshire Boulevard
Los Angeles, CA 90073
(310) 268-3396
FAX: (310) 268-4806
Gary N. Holland, M.D., Chief, Ophthalmology Clinic
Martin Maharis, Secretary, Ophthalmology Clinic
Dr. David Bright, Optometry Department

County/District Where Located: Los Angeles County.
Funded by: Federal government.
Hours of Operation: Mon.-Fri. 8:00 AM-4:30 PM.

Staff: Ophthalmologist; ophthalmology residents; optometrist; ophthalmic assistant/technician, ophthalmic photographer.
Eligibility: Visually impaired veterans.
Area Served: United States.

Counseling/Social Work/Self-Help: Services available.
Professional Training: On-site training available.
Rehabilitation: Services available.
Low Vision: Provided for eligible veterans.
Low Vision Aids: Provided on loan for trial purposes; no rental fee.
Low Vision Follow-up: Provided to all veterans.

Watts Health Foundation United Health Plan
10300 Compton Avenue
Los Angeles, CA 90002
(213) 564-4331
Leonida Johnson, Chief, Optometry Department

County/District Where Located: Los Angeles County.
Funded by: Grants; patient fees; Medicare; Medicaid.
Hours of Operation: Mon.-Fri. 8:00 AM-5:00 PM.
Area Served: South central Los Angeles and additional local areas.

Low Vision Follow-up: By return appointment after 1 month.

Western Blind Rehabilitation Center
U.S. Department of Veterans Affairs
VA Medical Center
3801 Miranda Avenue

Palo Alto, CA 94304
(415) 858-3921 (as of 8/1/97 area code 415 becomes 650)
FAX: (415) 852-3472
William Ekstrom, Director

Mission: Provides residential rehabilitation services to eligible legally blinded veterans.
Funded by: Federal government.
Hours of Operation: Mon.-Fri. 7:30 AM-4:00 PM.
Staff: Optometrist; optometry students and residents; low vision specialist; social worker; orientation/mobility instructor; rehabilitation teachers; psychologist/counselor; manual skills instructor; ophthalmologist; ophthalmology residents; occupational therapist; rehabilitation counselors; audiologist; recreational therapist; computer access training instructors.
History/Date: Est. 1967.
Eligibility: Legally blind veterans only; ophthalmology report.
Area Served: California, Montana, Utah, Wyoming, Nevada, Hawaii.

Low Vision Aids: Provided when prescribed.

Referral applications by Visual Impairment Services programs located at medical centers and outpatient clinics in the geographic area served by the Blind Rehabilitation Center or Clinic.

See U. S. Department of Veterans Affairs in U.S. Federal Agencies listings.

◆ *Aging Services*

STATE UNITS ON AGING

California Department of Aging
1600 K Street

Sacramento, CA 95814
(916) 322-5290 or in-state only
(800) 510-2020
FAX: (916) 324-1903
Arlene Davidson, Interim Director

Provides referrals to Area Agencies on Aging and information on other local aging services.

INDEPENDENT LIVING PROGRAMS

Services for the Blind California Department of Rehabilitation
P.O. Box 944222
Sacramento, CA 94244
(916) 445-9040
Manuel Urena, Program Director

Provides independent living services for persons age 55 and over. For further information, contact the Project Director or general phone number listed.

COLORADO

♦ *Educational Services*

STATE SERVICES

Colorado Department of Education
Special Education Services Unit
201 East Colfax Avenue
Denver, CO 80203
(303) 866-6694
FAX: (303) 866-6811
Tanni Anthony, Deaf-Blind
Consultant Unit

Type of Agency: State.
County/District Where Located:
Denver County.
Mission: Provides consultation in educational services for visually impaired children.
Funded by: Public funds.
Area Served: Colorado.

For information about local facilities, consult the superintendent of schools in the area.

EARLY INTERVENTION COORDINATION

Early Childhood Initiatives Unit
Colorado Department of Education
201 East Colfax Avenue
Room 305
Denver, CO 80203
(303) 866-6710
FAX: (303) 866-6662
Diane Turner, Part H Early Childhood Coordinator

County/District Where Located:
Denver County.

SCHOOLS

Colorado School for the Deaf and the Blind
33 North Institute Street
Colorado Springs, CO 80903-3599
(719) 578-2100 or (719) 578-2201
FAX: (719) 578-2239
Marilyn Jaitly, Superintendent
Dave Farrell, Principal, School for the Blind
Mike McCarthy, Outreach Coordinator
Debra Pike-Thomas, Parent/Child Advocate

Type of Agency: State.
Mission: Services for totally blind, visually impaired, learning disabled, moderately mentally retarded, and orthopedically disabled persons.
Funded by: State funds.
Hours of Operation: Offices: 8:00 AM - 2:55 PM. Residential: Sun. evening - Fri. afternoon.
Program Accessibility: Wheelchair accessible.
Staff: 68 full time. Uses volunteers.
History/Date: Est. 1874.
Number of Clients Served: 210.
Eligibility: School has enrollment criteria. Educable.
Area Served: Statewide.
Transportation: Y.
Age Requirements: 0-21 years.

Health: Audiology therapy; general medical services; speech therapy. Contracts and refers for other health services.
Counseling/Social Work/Self-Help: Social evaluations; psychological testing and evaluation; individual, group counseling; placement in school, training. Refers and provides consultation to other agencies for other counseling/social work services.
Educational: Grade range: K through 12 and nongraded.

Programs for infants, preschool; college prep; general academic; remedial education.
Preschools: Includes opportunities for integration with non-disabled peers.
Professional Training: Internship/fieldwork placement in orientation/mobility; special education; vocational rehabilitation.
Reading: Talking book record players and cassette players; talking book records and cassettes; braille books; large-print books; braille magazines; recorded magazines.
Residential: Dormitories.
Rehabilitation: Personal management; braille; gesticulation; handwriting; low vision training; listening skills; Optacon; typing; video magnifier; electronic mobility aids; home management; orientation/mobility; sensory training. Provides consultation to other agencies for rehabilitation teaching in client's home and community.
Recreational: Afterschool programs; arts and crafts; hobby groups; bowling; swimming; track; wrestling. Refers for other recreational services. Music (handbells, choir, band).
Employment: Prevocational evaluation; career and skill counseling; occupational skill development; job retention. Refers and provides consultation to other agencies for other employment services.
Computer Training: Access; training on computer aids and devices.
Low Vision: Evaluations on functional vision. Large-print texts.
Low Vision Aids: Closed-circuit television, magnifers, and reading stands.

Regular in-service training programs, open to enrollment from other agencies.

Contact Superintendent for program availability.

INFANT AND PRESCHOOL

Anchor Center for Blind Children
3801 Martin Luther King Boulevard
Denver, CO 80205
(303) 377-9732
FAX: (303) 377-9744
Alice Applebaum, Director
Patty Garfield, Office Manager

Type of Agency: Private.
Mission: To foster the unique potential of children who are visually impaired, deaf-blind or blind/multi-challanged, from birth through age five, by providing exemplary education, therapy, and family support services.
Funded by: Private donations and foundation grants.
Budget: $350,000.
Hours of Operation: Mon.-Fri. 8:00 AM - 4:00 PM.
Staff: 2 full time, 10 part time.
History/Date: Est. 1982.
Number of Clients Served: 50-100 children and their families.
Eligibility: Birth to 5 years old with visual impairment.
Area Served: All of Colorado.
Transportation: Y.
Age Requirements: Birth through age 5.

Health: Functional vision exams and play based assessment for all children are provided. Hearing exams or genetic counseling is referred out.
Counseling/Social Work/Self-Help: Parent counseling is available.
Educational: Provides instruction in all developmental areas.

Home-based and classroom program for visually impaired infants, 0-3 years. Classroom for 3-5 year olds, plus consultant services to other programs. Parent group component.

Cherry Creek School District
4700 South Yosemite
Englewood, CO 80111
(303) 486-4234
FAX: (303) 486-4272
Dr. Edward Steinberg, Associate Director of Student Achievement Services

Type of Agency: Public school itinerant vision program.
County/District Where Located: Arapahoe County.
Funded by: State and federal funds.
Staff: 3 full-time, dually certified teacher. Has advisory board for overall program.
History/Date: Est. 1973.
Area Served: Cherry Creek School district.
Age Requirements: 3-5 years.

Health: Genetic counseling and low vision exams available on referral basis.
Counseling/Social Work/Self-Help: Parent counseling. Variety of support and related services available.
Educational: Provides instruction in developmental areas related to vision. Home-teaching, multihandicapped classes, consultant services to other programs for visually handicapped children, with or without other handicaps.

Generic program (CHEER) also offered to children, 0-5 years, with itinerant vision support. Includes home teaching, parent-child groups, family workshops, preschool classes.

STATEWIDE OUTREACH SERVICES

Colorado School for the Deaf and the Blind
33 North Institute Street
Colorado Springs, CO 80903-3599
(719) 578-2100
FAX: (719) 578-2239
E-mail: irishfolk@aol.com
Mike McCarthy, Contact Person

Funded by: State funds; foundation grants.
History/Date: Est. 1875.
Age Requirements: 0-21 years.

Assessment: On request, on site or in home/school.
Consultation to Public Schools: On request.
Direct Service: Adaptive technology for the blind in conjunction with standard application; computer assisted instruction.
Parent Assistance: Family learning seminars/workshops.
Materials Production: Braille, large-print.
Professional Training: In-service training.

INSTRUCTIONAL MATERIALS CENTERS

Colorado Instructional Materials Center for the Visually Handicapped
1015 High Street
Colorado Springs, CO 80903
(719) 578-2195
FAX: (719) 578-2207
E-mail: cimc@pcisys.net
Lucia Hasty, Consultant

Area Served: State of Colorado.
Groups Served: 0-21 years, students with visual impairment in public schools.

Types/Content: Textbooks; equipment; professional resources.
Media Formats: Braille; large-print.

Title Listings: No title listings available.

UNIVERSITY TRAINING PROGRAMS

University of Northern Colorado

Division of Special Education
McKee Hall, Room 318
Greeley, CO 80639
(970) 351-2691
FAX: (970) 351-1061
David L. Kappan, Orientation & Mobility, (970) 351-1666
Kay Ferrell, Visually Handicapped, (970) 351-1653

County/District Where Located: Weld County.

Programs Offered: Master's programs for dual competency teachers of visually impaired students. Orientation and mobility specialists with emphases available in early childhood, deaf-blindness, and multiple disabilities. Graduate (master's, doctoral) level programs in education of visually impaired students, orientation & mobility.
Distance Education: Y.

◆ Information Services

LIBRARIES

Colorado Talking Book Library

180 Sheridan Boulevard
Denver, CO 80226
(303) 727-9277 or toll-free in Colorado (800) 685-2136
FAX: (303) 727-9281
Barbara J. Goral, Supervisor
Charmayne Wood, Machine Lending Information

Type of Agency: Library.
County/District Where Located: Denver County.

Funded by: Public funds; private donations.
Budget: $449,518.
Hours of Operation: Mon.-Fri. 8:00 AM-5:00 PM.
Program Accessibility: Fully accessible.
Staff: 10.5 full-time equivalents.
History/Date: Est. 1931.
Number of Clients Served: 10,500.
Eligibility: Blind, visually impaired, physically and reading disabled persons.
Area Served: Colorado.

Low Vision Aids: CCTV available.

Regional library providing braille, disks, cassettes, and large-type books and magazines. Recording and transcription services.

MEDIA PRODUCTION SERVICES

Braille Computer Center Boulder Public Library

P.O. Drawer H
Boulder, CO 80306
(303) 441-3098
FAX: (303) 442-1808
E-mail: gartenmannd@boulder.lib.co.us
Donna Gartenmann, Contact Person

Area Served: Primarily Colorado but other states as well.

Types/Content: Text materials other than mathematics or music, including computer-related materials.
Media Formats: Braille.

Colorado Talking Book Library

180 Sheridan Boulevard
Denver, CO 80226
(303) 727-9277
FAX: (303) 727-9281
Barbara J. Goral, Supervisor

Area Served: Colorado.
Groups Served: K-12; college students; other adults.

Types/Content: Recreational.
Media Formats: Talking books/cassettes.
Title Listings: Provided at no charge.

Recording for the Blind and Dyslexic

2696 South Colorado Boulevard
Suite 330
Denver, CO 80222
(303) 757-0787
Nireen King, Executive Director
Maureen Hart, Studio Director
Bob Rubin, Board Chairman

See Recording for the Blind and Dyslexic in U.S. national listings.

RADIO READING

Radio Reading Service of the Rockies

5290 Arapahoe Avenue, Unit G
Boulder, CO 80303
(303) 786-7777
David Dawson, Director

County/District Where Located: Boulder County.
Hours of Operation: Mon. - Sun. 24 hours a day.
History/Date: Est. 1900.
Area Served: Colorado and Wyoming.

INFORMATION AND REFERRAL

The Foundation Fighting Blindness
Rocky Mountain Affiliate

5026 E. Weaver Avenue
Littleton, CO 80121-3519
(303) 841-4202
Robert E. Lee II, President
Kathy Young, Contact Person

See The Foundation Fighting Blindness in U.S. national listings.

Parent Advocates for Visually Impaired Children (PAVIC)
17011 East Berry Avenue
Aurora, CO 80015
(303) 693-0959
Gayle Scheihing, President

Type of Agency: Private; non-profit.
County/District Where Located: Arapahoe County.
Mission: Maintains parent support group, advocacy regarding care and education of visually impaired children.
History/Date: Est. 1981.
Eligibility: Visually impaired and blind.
Age Requirements: 0-21 years.

Counseling/Social Work/Self-Help: Referrals.
Reading: Information and referral services available.

Preserve Sight Colorado
3500 East 12th Avenue
Denver, CO 80206
(303) 399-8090
FAX: (303) 399-9434
Clem Spainhower, Executive Director

Mission: To preserve sight and prevent blindness.
Funded by: Private and public contributions only.
Budget: $200,000.
Hours of Operation: Mon.-Fri. 8:30 AM-4:30 PM.
Staff: 3. Uses volunteers.
History/Date: Est. 1951; Inc. 1964.
Area Served: Statewide.
Age Requirements: None.

Health: Glaucoma screening for adults.
Educational: Eye safety programs in schools and for industry.
Preschools: Preschool vision screening.
Low Vision: Evaluations and referrals.

Low Vision Aids: Referrals.

See Prevent Blindness America in U.S. national listings.

See also in national listings:

Blind Outdoor Leisure Development

United States Association for Blind Athletes

♦ Rehabilitation Services

STATE SERVICES

Rehabilitation Services Colorado Department of Human Services
110 16th Street
Denver, CO 80203
(303) 620-2152
FAX: (303) 620-4189
Kenneth Schmidt, Ph.D., Administrator of Field Services
Diana Huerta, Director

Type of Agency: State.
Mission: To assist individuals with physical and/or mental disabilities to attain a level of functioning that will enable them to enter, reenter, or maintain employment and enhance skills necessary for living independently.
Funded by: Federal, state funds.
Hours of Operation: Mon.-Fri. 8:00 AM - 5:00 PM.
Program Accessibility: Fully accessible.
Staff: 200. Uses volunteers.
Eligibility: Visual impairment that interferes with employment or independent living.
Area Served: Statewide.

Health: Low vision aids or devices. Contracts and refers for other health services.

Counseling/Social Work/Self-Help: Vocational evaluation; individual counseling. Contracts and refers for other services.
Professional Training: Internship/fieldwork placement; orientation/mobility; rehabilitation counseling and teaching; in-service programs.
Rehabilitation: Personal management; braille; handwriting; listening skills; typing; video magnifier; home management; orientation/mobility; rehabilitation teaching in client's home and community. Contracts and refers for other rehabilitation services.
Recreational: Special programs for elderly, deaf-blind, blind and deaf persons.
Employment: Prevocational evaluations; occupational skill development; vocational training; placement; follow-up service; vending stand training. Contracts for other services.
Computer Training: Access.

Local Offices:

Alamosa: Division of Rehabilitation, 422 Fourth Street, P.O. Box 990, Alamosa, CO 81101, (303) 589-5158.
Boulder: 207 Canyon Boulevard, Suite 202, Boulder, CO 80302, (303) 444-2816.
Colorado Springs: Division of Rehabilitation, 1322 North Academy Boulevard, Colorado Springs, CO 80909-3316, (719) 574-2200.
Denver: Two Denver Highlands Bldg., 10065 E. Harvard, Suite 809, Denver, CO 80231, (303) 745-8112.
Denver: Rehabilitation Center, 2211 West Evans Avenue, Denver, CO 80223, (303) 937-1226.
Denver: Services for Individuals Who Are Blind or Deaf, 600 Grant Street, Suite 302, Denver, CO 80203, (303) 894-2515.

Durango: 425 West Building, 835 Second Avenue, Durango, CO 81301, (970) 247-3161.

Fort Collins: Division of Rehabilitation, 2850 McClelland Drive, Fort Collins, CO 80525, (970) 223-9823.

Fort Morgan: 625 W. Platte Avenue, P.O. Box 429, Fort Morgan, CO 80701, (970) 867-3068.

Glenwood Springs: Executive Plaza, 1512 Grand Avenue, Glenwood Springs, CO 81601, (970) 945-9174.

Golden: Human Service Building, Suite 290, 900 Jefferson County Parkway, Golden, CO 80401, (303) 271-4888.

Grand Junction: Divison of Rehabilitation, 222 South Sixth Street, Room 215, Grand Junction, CO 81501, (970) 248-7103.

Greeley: Division of Rehabilitation, 822 7th Street, Suite 4, Greeley, CO 80631, (970) 352-5180.

Lamar: Cedar Main Building, 1006 South Main Street, Lamar, CO 81052, (719) 336-7712.

Limon: PO Box 910, 820 Second Street, Limon, CO 80828, (719) 775-2342, ext. 7.

Littleton: 609 West Littleton Boulevard, Suite 100, Littleton, CO 80120, (303) 795-7954.

Longmont: 1707 North Main Street, Suite 302, Longmont, CO 80501, (303) 772-2612.

Montrose: 1010 South Cascade Avenue, Montrose, CO 81401, (970) 249-4468.

Northglenn: 11990 Grant Street, Suite 201, Northglenn, CO 80233, (303) 452-5875.

Pueblo: Services for Individuals Who Are Blind or Deaf, 720 North Main Street, Suite 320, Pueblo, CO 81003, (719) 544-1406.

Rocky Ford: 409 South Main, Rocky Ford, CO 81067, (719) 254-3358.

Sterling: 220 South Third Street, P.O. Box 592, Sterling, CO 80751, (970) 522-3737.

Trinidad: 134 West Main, Suite 2-4, Trinidad, CO 81082, (719) 846-4431.

REHABILITATION

Center for Independence
1600 Ute Avenue
Suite 100
Grand Junction, CO 81501
(970) 241-0315 (voice/TDD)
FAX: (970) 245-3341
E-mail: nconklin@csn.org
Mary Lynn McNutt, Executive Director

Type of Agency: Private; non-profit.
Mission: Provides services to people with disabilities, encouraging control, direction, and independence in their lives.
Funded by: Grants, donations.
Hours of Operation: Mon.-Thurs. 7:00 AM-5:00 PM.
Staff: 6 full time, 3 part time. Volunteers for reading.
History/Date: Est. 1984.
Number of Clients Served: 1,200/year.
Eligibility: Physical disability.
Area Served: 13 counties on western slope of Colorado.
Transportation: Y.

Counseling/Social Work/Self-Help: Individual and group counseling; support groups; also refers for community services.
Educational: Vocational and skill development for deaf, blind, and multiply disabled persons.
Reading: Information and referral services; braille instruction; reading aids.
Rehabilitation: Daily living, communication skills; orientation/mobility; off-site training.
Recreational: Arts and crafts.
Employment: Occupational skill development, job retraining.
Computer Training: Available for training.
Low Vision Aids: Aids and magnifiers.
Low Vision Follow-up: Home visits, outreach.

Colorado Rehabilitation Center
Colorado Division of Vocational Rehabilitation
2211 West Evans Avenue
Denver, CO 80223
(303) 937-1226
Ron Landwehr, Manager

Type of Agency: Non-profit.
Mission: To assist individuals whose disabilities result in barriers to employment.
Funded by: State and federal funds.
Staff: 8 full time rehabilitation teachers, 2 vocational development counselors, 1 vocational evaluator, 4 business enterprise consultants.
Eligibility: Blind and visually impaired persons who have a disability that has a significant impact on employment or independent living.
Area Served: Colorado.

Rehabilitation: Comprehensive training in braille, typing, home and personal management, orientation/mobility and related training for personal and/or vocational use, either at home or in the rehabilitation center. Referrals for other services.
Recreational: Recreation and social activities.
Employment: Vocational assessment and consultation; job seeking and job skills services; job training and business and employment opportunities under the Randolph Shepherd Act.

Computer Training: Keyboarding and computer access.

For further information on local offices, see listing under State Services.

Helen Keller National Center for Deaf-Blind Youths and Adults Rocky Mountain Region Office

1880 South Pierce Street
Suite 5
Lakewood, CO 80232-7143
(303) 934-9037 (voice/TDD)
FAX: (303) 934-2939
Maureen McGowan, Regional Representative

County/District Where Located: Jefferson County.
Mission: To provide comprehensive rehabilitation training and advocacy for deaf-blind persons.
Funded by: Federal funds.
Hours of Operation: Mon.-Fri. 9:00AM - 5:00PM.
Staff: 2.
Age Requirements: Fourteen years and older.

See Helen Keller National Center for Deaf-Blind Youths and Adults in U.S. national listings.

COMPUTER TRAINING CENTERS

Assistive Technology Clinics The Childrens' Hospital

1056 East 19th Avenue
P.O. Box 410
Denver, CO 80218
(303) 861-6250
FAX: (303) 764-8214
E-mail: lange.michelle@tchden.org
Michelle L. Lange, OTR

Computer Training: Speech output systems; screen magnification software; word processing; database software.

Center for Independence

1600 Ute Avenue
Suite 100
Grand Junction, CO 81501
(970) 241-0315
FAX: (970) 245-3341
E-mail: nconklin@csn.org
Mary Lynn McNutt, Executive Director

Computer Training: Speech output systems; screen magnification systems; braille access systems; word processing; database software; computer operating systems; closed-circuit television systems; mpu; training for instructors; optical character recognition systems.

Colorado Easter Seal Society

5755 West Alameda Avenue
Lakewood, CO 80226
(303) 233-1666
Barbara Janes, Director of Rehabilitation Services
Christine Newell, Camp Specialist

County/District Where Located: Jefferson County.

Computer Training: Broad spectrum of assistive technology.

Colorado Rehabilitation Center Communications for the Visually Impaired

2211 West Evans Avenue
Denver, CO 80223
(303) 937-1226
Candiss Leathers, Services Coordinator

Computer Training: Speech output systems; screen magnification systems; braille access systems; optical character recognition systems; closed-circuit television systems; word processing; database software; computer operating systems.

Colorado School for the Deaf and the Blind

33 North Institute Street
Colorado Springs, CO 80903
(719) 578-2100
FAX: (719) 578-2239
E-mail: bonnielee@kktv.com
Bonnie Snyder, Educational Technologist

Computer Training: Speech output systems; screen magnification systems; braille access systems; closed-circuit television systems; word processing; database software; telecommunication systems; training for instructors.

◆ Low Vision Services

EYE CARE SOCIETIES

Colorado Ophthalmological Society

1945 West 102 Avenue
Denver, CO 80221-6346
(303) 741-3937
FAX: (303) 438-9062
E-mail: eyesociety@aol.com
David R. Scott, Executive Director

County/District Where Located: Denver County.

Colorado Optometric Association

1600 Broadway
Denver, CO 80202
(303) 863-9778
FAX: (303) 863-9775
Gwenne Hume, Executive Director

LOW VISION CENTERS

Colorado Optometric Center Low Vision Clinic

2736 Welton Street
Suite 200

Denver, CO 80205
(303) 295-2402
FAX: (303) 295-1067
Peggy Futch, Executive Director
Julia Lampo, O.D., Clinical
Director
Dr. Alpa Patel O.D., Director, Low
Vision Service

Type of Agency: Non-profit.
County/District Where Located:
Denver County.
Mission: To diagnose and prevent
eye disease and disability through
comprehensive vision care,
including low vision services.
Funded by: Client fees; United
Way; corporate and foundation
support.
Budget: $500,000.
Hours of Operation: Tues.-Thurs.
7:30 AM - 6:30 PM; Sat. 9:00 AM -
2:00 PM.
Program Accessibility:
Wheelchair-accessible. Some
services delivered at home or job
site.
Staff: Optometrist; optometry
intern; low vision therapist;
orientation/mobility instructor;
opthalmologist; special educator,
by referral.
History/Date: Est. 1961.
Eligibility: None.
Area Served: Unlimited.

Low Vision Aids: Provided on a
trial basis; rental fee; on-site
training provided.
Low Vision Follow-up: Return
appointment in one month.

Porter Memorial Hospital
Porter Low Vision Service
2525 South Downing Street
Denver, CO 80210
(303) 778-5707
Barbara Meyer, Low Vision
Consultant

Type of Agency: Public.
Mission: To assist the visually
impaired with optical aids, non-

optical aids, daily living skills
training, education and counseling.
Funded by: Client fees;
foundation grants.
Hours of Operation: Mon.-Thurs.
9:00 AM-5:00 PM.
History/Date: Est. 1985.
Area Served: Unlimited.

**Counseling/Social Work/Self-
Help:** Counseling available.
Educational: Educate patients on
optics, the eye, community
resources and available assistive
devices.
Rehabilitation: Functional
training.
Employment: Training for specific
job needs.
Low Vision Aids: Provided on
loan for trial purpose at no charge.
Low Vision Follow-up: Return
appointment; phone interviews
when necessary.

◆ Aging Services

STATE UNITS ON AGING

**Division of Aging and Adult
Services
Colorado Department of Human
Services**
110 16th Street
Suite 200
Denver, CO 80202-5202
(303) 620-4147 or Adult Protection
and Elder Rights (800) 773-1366
FAX: (303) 620-4189
Rita Barreras, Manager

Provides referrals to Area Agencies
on Aging and information on other
local aging services.

INDEPENDENT LIVING PROGRAMS

**Rehabilitation Services
Colorado Department of Human
Services**
110 16th Street
Suite 200
Denver, CO 80202
(303) 620-4152 or (303) 620-4181
Sharon Mikrut, Administrator
Ken Schmidt, Field Services
Director

Provides independent living
services for persons age 55 and
over. For further information,
contact the Project Director or
general phone number listed.

CON- NECTICUT

♦ *Educational Services*

STATE SERVICES

Connecticut State Board of Education and Services for the Blind
170 Ridge Road
Wethersfield, CT 06109
(860) 249-8525
FAX: (860) 278-6920
Kenneth R. Tripp, Executive Director

Type of Agency: State.
County/District Where Located: Hartford County.
Mission: To provide the most appropriate individualized education programs in the least restrictive settings possible for every eligible blind or visually impaired student.
Funded by: Public funds.
Budget: $8.7 million.
Hours of Operation: Mon.-Fri. 8:30 AM-4:00 PM.
Program Accessibility: Fully accessible.
History/Date: Est. 1966.
Number of Clients Served: 950.
Eligibility: Statutory blindness or impaired vision.
Area Served: Statewide.
Age Requirements: 5-21.

Counseling/Social Work/Self-Help: Full range of counseling programs available.
Educational: Instruction in specialized curriculum related to blindness. Provides adapted books, supplies, and assistive technology.
Recreational: Summer camp opportunities.

Employment: Transition school-to-work programs.
Computer Training: Assistive technology training.
Low Vision: Evaluations and referrals.
Low Vision Aids: Available on case basis.
Low Vision Follow-up: Y.
Professional Training: Development programs for regular and special education teachers.

For information about local facilities, contact the superintendent of schools in the area.

EARLY INTERVENTION COORDINATION

Bureau of Early Childhood Education and Social Services Connecticut Department of Education
25 Industrial Park Road
Middletown, CT 06457
(860) 638-4208
FAX: (860) 638-4218
George Coleman, Part H Coordinator

SCHOOLS

Oak Hill School Connecticut Institute for the Blind
120 Holcomb Street
Hartford, CT 06112
(860) 242-2274
FAX: (860) 242-3103
Lars Guldager, Ph.D., Executive Director

Type of Agency: Private; non-profit.
County/District Where Located: Hartford County.
Mission: To set the standard for the quality of life of, and to advance the inherent dignity of people with blindness, visual impairment and other physical and mental disabilities through safe, cost-effective training, education, vocational and residential programs.
Funded by: Public funds, federal grants, contributions, and endowment.
Budget: $40 million.
Hours of Operation: 24 hours/day.
Program Accessibility: Fully accessible.
Staff: Almost 1,000 (full and part time).
History/Date: Est. and inc. 1893.
Number of Clients Served: 375.
Eligibility: Children and adults with multiple disabilities.
Area Served: Unlimited.
Transportation: Y.
Age Requirements: Over 2 years, 8 months.

Health: Occupational, physical, speech therapies; medical; dental; 24-hour nursing services; numerous consultants.
Counseling/Social Work/Self-Help: Social casework; social and rehabilitation guidance.
Educational: Individualized Education Programs (IEPs) for each student; overall plans of service (OPs) for each adult.
Professional Training: Coordinated by full-time staff development specialist. Initial and on-going training for all direct care staff, professionals and paraprofessionals.
Reading: Large-print books and cassettes.
Residential: 75 group homes in 41 towns serving students and adults.
Rehabilitation: Emphasis on daily living skills; personal management; behavior management; orientation/mobility; leisure time activities.
Recreational: Age-appropriate activities utilizing community facilities; summer camp on shores

of Long Island Sound; greenhouse program for elderly people.
Employment: Supported employment in community.
Computer Training: Available for people with visual impairments.
Low Vision: Text to Braille translation available.
Low Vision Aids: Adaptive computer equipment such as speech synthesizers and enlarged screens.

INFANT AND PRESCHOOL

Connecticut State Board of Education and Services for the Blind
170 Ridge Road
Wethersfield, CT 06109
(860) 249-8525
FAX: (860) 278-6920
Kenneth R. Tripp, Executive Director

Type of Agency: State.
County/District Where Located: Hartford County.
Mission: To provide the most appropriate, individualized education services and programs for each eligible blind or visually impaired child in his or her natural environment.
Funded by: State funds.
Budget: $960,000.
Hours of Operation: Mon.-Fri. 8:30 AM-4:00 PM.
Program Accessibility: Fully accessible.
Staff: 7 full time (teachers of visually impaired children).
History/Date: Est. 1974.
Number of Clients Served: 250.
Eligibility: Statutory blindness or impaired vision.
Area Served: Statewide.
Transportation: Y.
Age Requirements: 0-5 years.

Health: Adaptive equipment; low vision exams. Home-based and

itinerant vision services to public schools and private agencies for preschool visually handicapped children, with or without other handicaps.
Counseling/Social Work/Self-Help: Parent counseling. Variety of support and related services available by consultation.
Educational: Provides instruction in all developmental areas. Home-based and consultant services to other programs for visually handicapped infants, toddlers and preschoolers.
Preschools: Instruction in all developmental areas.
Computer Training: Pre-braille computer training.
Low Vision: Evaluations.
Low Vision Follow-up: Y.
Professional Training: In-service training for teachers and aides. Consultation available for schools and private agencies.

STATEWIDE OUTREACH SERVICES

Oak Hill School
Connecticut Institute for the Blind
120 Holcomb Street
Hartford, CT 06112
(860) 242-2274
FAX: (860) 769-3807
Anna Eddy, Director

Funded by: Local school districts.
Located at: Group homes and classrooms in various community settings.
Age Requirements: Ages 6-22.

Assessment: Multi-handicap with mental retardation.

Operates satellite programs throughout the state.

INSTRUCTIONAL MATERIALS CENTERS

Connecticut State Board of Education and Services for the Blind
170 Ridge Road
Wethersfield, CT 06109
(860) 566-5800, ext. 211
FAX: (860) 278-6920
William Dessin, Contact Person

Groups Served: PreK-12.

◆ Information Services

LIBRARIES

Connecticut State Library
Library for the Blind and Physically Handicapped
198 West Street
Rocky Hill, CT 06067
(860) 566-2151 or toll-free in Connecticut (800) 842-4516
FAX: (860) 566-6669
URL: http://www.cslnet.ctstate.edu/lbph.htm
Carol A. Taylor, Library Director
Gordon Reddick, Circulation Librarian

Hours of Operation: Mon.- Fri., 10:00 A.M.- 3:00 P.M.

Regional library supplying recorded and braille books and magazines and necessary playback equipment to eligible state residents unable to read conventional print because of a visual or physical disability.

MEDIA PRODUCTION SERVICES

Connecticut Braille Association
664 Oakwood Avenue

West Hartford, CT 06110
(860) 953-9692
FAX: (860) 953-9692
Yolanda M. Rossi, Executive
Secretary, Large Type Division

Area Served: Primarily
Connecticut but will copy our
master for any out-of-state source.
Groups Served: K-12, college
students, other adults.

Types/Content: Textbooks.
Media Formats: Large-print
books.
Title Listings: None specified.
Listings available from American
Printing House for the Blind,
Louisville, Kentucky.

Connecticut Braille Association
44 Imperial Avenue
Westport, CT 06880
(203) 227-5243
Eileen Akers, President
Marguerite Smith, Vice President

Area Served: Nationwide.
Groups Served: None specified.

Types/Content: None specified.
Media Formats: Braille/large-
print books. Computer braille.
Title Listings: None specified.

**Darien Community Association
Program for the Blind**
274 Middlesex Road
Darien, CT 06820
(203) 655-8554
Siv Safwat, Chairperson

Area Served: Connecticut.
Groups Served: K-12; college
students; other adults.

Types/Content: Textbooks;
recreational.
Media Formats: Talking books/
cassettes.
Title Listings: None specified.

**Recording for the Blind and
Dyslexic
Connecticut Unit**
209 Orange Street
New Haven, CT 06510
(203) 624-4334
FAX: (203) 865-0203
E-mail: connecticut@rfbd.org
Ann Fortunato, Studio Director
Peter DiLeo, Executive Director

County/District Where Located:
New Haven County.

See Recording for the Blind and
Dyslexic in U.S. national listings.

RADIO READING

**Connecticut Radio Information
System (CRIS)**
589 Jordan Lane
Wethersfield, CT 06109
(860) 956-3579
FAX: (860) 956-2658
E-mail: crisrad@courant.infi-net
Mary Clare Quirk, Executive
Director

Funded by: Public contributions
and grants.
Hours of Operation: 24 hours a
day.
Staff: 2 full-time, 3 part-time. 350
volunteers.
History/Date: Est. 1979.
Area Served: Statewide.
Age Requirements: None.

INFORMATION AND REFERRAL

**The Foundation Fighting
Blindness
Connecticut Affiliate**
P.O. Box 5162
Hartford, CT 06518
(203) 268-4538
Leonard Roberto, President

See The Foundation Fighting
Blindness in U.S. national listings.

Prevent Blindness Connecticut
1275 Washington Street
Middletown, CT 06457
(860) 347-2020 or toll-free in
Connecticut (800) 850-2020
FAX: (860) 347-0613
E-mail: 104706.1100
@compuserve.com
Paul L. Blawie, President and CEO

See Prevent Blindness America in
U.S. national listings.

See also in national listings:

Grey House Publishing Company

◆ Rehabilitation Services

STATE SERVICES

**Connecticut State Board of
Education and Services for the
Blind**
170 Ridge Road
Wethersfield, CT 06109
(860) 566-5800
FAX: (860) 278-6920
Brian Sigman, Vocational
Rehabilitation Director

Type of Agency: State.
Mission: Administers the federal-
state vocational rehabilitation
program.
Funded by: Public funds.
Staff: 130 full time.
History/Date: Est. 1893.
Eligibility: Severe visual
impairment.
Area Served: Connecticut.

Health: Low vision service; aids
and appliances. Diagnosis and
evaluation of eye health;
evaluation of eye treatment or
prescription.
**Counseling/Social Work/Self-
Help:** Consultation and referral

service; psychological testing and evaluation.

Educational: Preschool; elementary; secondary; college.

Rehabilitation: Optacon; personal management; orientation/mobility training.

Recreational: Refers for summer camp program.

Employment: Evaluation and prevocational and vocational training; vocational placement; follow-up service; sheltered workshop; vending facility training; home employment programs.

Computer Training: Access; training on computer aids and devices.

REHABILITATION

BESB Industries
114 Shield Street
West Hartford, CT 06110
(860) 566-1331 or (860) 566-8144
FAX: (860) 953-4519
N. J. (Chip) Gorra, Director, Division of Industries

Type of Agency: State.
Mission: Provides business enterprise programs, vocational rehabilitation, adult services, and children's services to visually impaired and blind children and adults.
Funded by: State of Connecticut.
Budget: $6 million.
Hours of Operation: 8:00 AM-4:00 PM.
Program Accessibility: Fully accessible.
Staff: 30.
Number of Clients Served: 242.
Eligibility: Legally blind (adults); visually impaired (children).
Area Served: Connecticut.

Counseling/Social Work/Self-Help: On an individual basis.
Professional Training: Workshops on site; training in

collaboration with local colleges and universities; in-service training for staff.
Reading: Instruction in using braille and adaptive reading devices.
Recreational: On individual basis in homes and schools.
Employment: Job development; job placement.
Computer Training: Individual training. Voice output, large-print output, braille output, CCTVs.
Low Vision Aids: Works in conjunction with Lions Vision Center for prescription devices; non-prescription devices available on site.
Low Vision Follow-up: Refers.

Local Offices:

West Haven: 281 Dogburn Street, West Haven, CT 06516, (203) 795-1390.

Eastern Blind Rehabilitation Center
U.S. Department of Veterans Affairs
VA Medical Center
950 Campbell Avenue
West Haven, CT 06516
(203) 932-5711
Mark Hieftje, Director

Type of Agency: Federal.
Mission: Provides residential rehabilitation services to eligible legally blind veterans.
History/Date: Est. 1969.

Referral applications by Visual Impairment Services programs located at VA Medical Centers and Outpatient Clinics in the geographical area served by the Blind Rehabilitation Center or Clinic.

See U.S. Department of Veterans Affairs in U.S. Federal Agencies listings.

COMPUTER TRAINING CENTERS

Connecticut State Board of Education and Services for the Blind
170 Ridge Road
Wethersfield, CT 06109
(860) 249-8525
FAX: (860) 278-6920
Brian Sigman, Vocational Rehabilitation Director

Computer Training: Speech output systems; screen magnification systems; braille access systems; optical character recognition systems; closed-circuit television systems; word processing; database software; computer operating systems.

DOG GUIDE SCHOOLS

Fidelco Guide Dog Foundation
P.O. Box 142
Bloomfield, CT 06002
(860) 243-5200
FAX: (860) 243-7215
Charles Kaman, President

Type of Agency: Private, non-profit.
Mission: Mobility training with dog guides.
Funded by: Income from capital funds; voluntary donations.
Hours of Operation: Mon.-Fri. 8:00 AM - 4:30 PM.
Staff: 17.
History/Date: Breeding program est. 1962; training program est. 1981.
Eligibility: Serious visual impairment; good physical/mental health, and character.
Area Served: New England; New York.
Age Requirements: At least 16 years.

Professional Training: Orientation/mobility.

◆ Low Vision Services

EYE CARE SOCIETIES

Connecticut Society of Eye Physicians
782 Bantam Road
Bantam, CT 06750
(860) 567-3787
Debbie Osborn, Executive Director

Connecticut Association of Optometrists
638 Prospect Avenue
Hartford, CT 06105-4298
(203) 586-7508 or (800) 677-7714
Sharon S. Bruce, Executive Director

LOW VISION CENTERS

Eastern Blind Rehabilition Center Eye Clinic
VA Medical Center
950 Campbell Avenue
West Haven, CT 06516
(203) 932-5711
Charles Haskes, Optometrist

Funded by: Federal government.
Hours of Operation: Mon.-Fri. 8:00 AM - 4:30 PM.
Eligibility: Legally blind veterans only; referral by local Veterans Administration coordinator or social worker.
Area Served: East Coast from Maine to Virginia.

Low Vision Aids: On-site training provided.
Low Vision Follow-up: By telephone and questionnaire.

Rehabilitation Center Vision Rehabilitation Services
95 Hamilton Street
New Haven, CT 06511
(203) 777-2000, ext. 270
William V. Padula, O.D., Director

Funded by: Client fees; state funds.
Hours of Operation: Mon., Tues., Wed., Fri., 8:00 AM-4:00 PM.
Staff: Low vision assistant; occupational therapist; counselors; optometrist; speech therapists; physical therapist.
Eligibility: Vision impairment, neurological impairment, or physical disability.

Low Vision: On-site/in-home/place of employment training available.
Low Vision Aids: Provided on loan or purchase.
Low Vision Follow-up: Return appointment.

◆ Aging Services

STATE UNITS ON AGING

Connecticut Department of Social Services Elderly Services Division
25 Sigourney Street
10th floor
Hartford, CT 06106-5033
Information & Referral in state
(800) 443-9946
FAX: (860) 424-4966
Christine Lewis, Director of Community Services

Provides referrals to Area Agencies on Aging and information on other local aging services.

INDEPENDENT LIVING PROGRAMS

Connecticut Board of Education and Services for the Blind
170 Ridge Road
Wethersfield, CT 06109
(860) 249-8525 or (800) 842-4510
Tom Grossi, Director

Provides independent living services for persons age 55 and over. For further information, contact the Project Director or general phone number listed.

DELAWARE

♦ Educational Services

STATE SERVICES

Delaware Department of Public Instruction
John G. Townsend Building
P.O. Box 1402
Dover, DE 19903
(302) 739-4601
FAX: (302) 739-4654
Michael C. Ferguson,
Superintendent
Martha Brooks, Director for
Exceptional Children

Type of Agency: State.
County/District Where Located:
Kent County.
Mission: To ensure a free,
appropriate public education for
children and youth with
disabilities.
Funded by: Public funds.
Hours of Operation: Mon.-Fri.
8:00 AM - 4:30 PM.
Program Accessibility: Fully
accessible.
Area Served: Delaware.

For information about local
facilities, consult the
superintendent of schools in the
area.

EARLY INTERVENTION COORDINATION

**Division of Management
Services
Delaware Health and Social
Services Birth to Three**
2nd Floor, Main Bldg.
1901 North DuPont Highway

Newcastle, DE 19720
(302) 577-4647
FAX: (302) 577-4083
Rosanne Griff-Cabelli, Part H
Coordinator

INFANT AND PRESCHOOL

**Delaware Division for the
Visually Impaired**
305 West Eighth Street
Wilmington, DE 19801
(302) 577-3333
FAX: (302) 577-6100
E-mail: lyoung@state.de.us
Lynne Young, Principal

Type of Agency: State.
Mission: Services for all visually
handicapped persons from birth,
with or without other handicaps.
Funded by: Federal funds, private
donations, state funds.
Hours of Operation: 8:00 AM-
4:30 PM.
Staff: 13 full time (includes
teachers of visually handicapped
children and of orientation/
mobility). Has advisory committee
with parent member.
History/Date: Est. 1971.
Number of Clients Served: 175.
Area Served: Statewide.
Transportation: Y.

Health: Adaptive equipment.
Genetic counseling and other
health services available by
referral.
**Counseling/Social Work/Self-
Help:** Child and parent
counseling.
Educational: Full itinerant
teaching services.
Preschools: Day care program.
Instruction in all developmental
areas.
Recreational: Beach house
weekend for children; summer
camp through the Association for
the Blind; state chapter of
Association of Blind Athletes.

Low Vision: Low vision exams;
eye exams if not covered by
insurance.
Low Vision Follow-up: Yes.

INSTRUCTIONAL MATERIALS CENTERS

**Delaware Division for the
Visually Impaired**
305 West Eighth Street
Wilmington, DE 19801
(302) 577-6200, ext. 13
FAX: (302) 577-6100
Ann Hitchcock, Director, Materials
Center

Area Served: State of Delaware.
Groups Served: Ages 0-21 and
adults.

Types/Content: Textbooks.
Media Formats: Braille books,
large-print books.
Title Listings: No title listings
available.

♦ Information Services

LIBRARIES

**Library for the Blind and
Physically Handicapped
Delaware Division of Libraries**
43 South DuPont Highway
Dover, DE 19901
(302) 739-4748 or TDD (302) 739-
4739 or toll-free in Delaware
(800) 282-8676
FAX: (302) 739-6787
E-mail: norman@lib.de.us
URL: http://www.lib.de.us
Anne E. Norman, Librarian

Type of Agency: Library for the
blind and physically handicapped.
Funded by: Public funds.
Hours of Operation: Mon.-Fri.
8:00 AM - 4:30 PM.
Staff: 4 full time.

History/Date: Est. 1971.
Number of Clients Served: 1,400.
Eligibility: Unable to read standard print; national library service requirements.
Area Served: Delaware.

Regional library that is a division of the Department of State Services. Supplies talking books and playback equipment.

MEDIA PRODUCTION SERVICES

Delaware Association for the Blind

2915 Newport Gap Pike
Wilmington, DE 19808
(302) 994-9478
Linda S. Lauria, Executive Director
Robert Emrick, Coordinator

County/District Where Located: New Castle County.
Groups Served: College students, other adults.

Types/Content: Recreational, career/vocational, religious, personal needs and local publications.
Media Formats: Talking books/cassettes.
Title Listings: As requested.

INFORMATION AND REFERRAL

The Foundation Fighting Blindness
Delaware Affiliate

Ten South Market Street Plaza
Smyrna, DE 19977
(302) 653-9200
Marsha Ross Berman, O.D.,
Contact Person

See The Foundation Blindness in U.S. national listings.

◆ Rehabilitation Services

STATE SERVICES

Division for the Visually Impaired
Delaware Department of Health and Social Services

Herman Holloway Campus
1901 North DuPont Highway
Biggs Building
New Castle, DE 19720
(302) 577-4731
Debra A. Wallace, Acting Director
Beverly Eustis, Training Center Supervisor
Dianne Grambau, Independent Living Services Supervisor

Type of Agency: State.
County/District Where Located: New Castle County.
Mission: Services to all visually handicapped persons from birth, with or without other handicaps.
Funded by: Public funds, state and federal funds.
History/Date: Est. 1909.
Transportation: Y.

Counseling/Social Work/Self-Help: Consultation services.
Educational: Preschool and supportive services.
Employment: Prevocational evaluation; vocational training; vocational placement; vending facility training; sheltered workshops. Business enterprise services; sheltered workshop service.
Computer Training: Access; training on computer aids and devices.
Low Vision: Exams.

REHABILITATION

Delaware Association for the Blind

800 West Street

Wilmington, DE 19801
(302) 655-2111 or (888) 777-3925
Linda S. Lauria, Executive Director

Type of Agency: Private; non-profit.
Staff: 5 full time, 7 part time, 12 seasonal. Uses volunteers.
History/Date: Est. 1948.
Eligibility: Legally blind or severe visual impariment; Delaware resident.
Area Served: Statewide.

Counseling/Social Work/Self-Help: Referral to community services; peer counseling.
Residential: 22-bed camp dormitory for adults.
Recreational: Trips; arts and crafts; residential summer camps for adult blind; summer children's day camp; swimming; transportation.

Delaware Industries for the Blind

1901 North DuPont Highway
Biggs Building, Health and Social Services Campus
New Castle, DE 19720
(302) 577-4760
FAX: (302) 577-4763
Alan B. Wingrove, General Manager, (302) 577-4751

Type of Agency: Affiliated with National Industries for the Blind.
Mission: Providing employment for blind and visually impaired individuals.
Funded by: State funds; sale of products.
Budget: $1 million.
Hours of Operation: 8:00 AM-4:30 PM.
Staff: 10.
History/Date: Est. 1909.
Number of Clients Served: 40.
Area Served: Statewide.

COMPUTER TRAINING CENTERS

Division for the Visually Impaired
Delaware Department of Health and Social Services
13 S.W. Front Street, MSSCA, Suite 105
Milford, DE 19963
(302) 422-1570
FAX: (302) 422-1419
E-mail: beustis@state.de.us
Beverly Eustis, Sr. Rehabilitation Instructor

County/District Where Located:
Sussex County.

Computer Training: Speech output systems; screen magnification systems; braille access systems; optical character recognition systems; closed-circuit television systems; word processing; database software; computer operating systems; training for instructors.

♦ Low Vision Services

EYE CARE SOCIETIES

Delaware Academy of Ophthalmology
Delaware Eye Associates
2006-B Foulk Road
Wilmington, DE 19810
(302) 475-2500
Dorothy M. Moore, M.D., President

Delaware Optometric Association, Inc.
11 Par Haven, Building L
Dover, DE 19904
(302) 734-3511
Zannis Bousses, Executive Director

♦ Aging Services

STATE UNITS ON AGING

Division of Services for Aging and Adults with Physical Disabilities
Delaware Department of Health and Social Services
1909 North DuPont Highway
Administration Building, Annex
Second Floor
New Castle, DE 19720
(302) 577-4791 or Information & Referral in state, University Plaza Office (800) 223-9074 or Milford office (800) 292-1515
FAX: (302) 577-4793
Eleanor Cain, Director

Provides referrals to Area Agencies on Aging and information on other local aging services.

INDEPENDENT LIVING PROGRAMS

Division for the Visually Impaired
Delaware Department of Health and Social Services
Health and Social Services Campus
1901 North DuPont Highway
Biggs Building
New Castle, DE 19720
(302) 577-3333
FAX: (302) 577-4758
Deborah Wallace, Acting Director
Charles Gebhart, Director

Provides independent living services for persons age 55 and over. For further information, contact the Project Director or general phone number listed.

DISTRICT OF COLUMBIA

♦ *Educational Services*

STATE SERVICES

District of Columbia Special Education Branch
Goding School
920 Tenth Street N.E.
Washington, DC 20002
(202) 724-4800 or (202) 724-7833
FAX: (202) 724-5116
Jeff Myers, Acting Director

Type of Agency: State.
Mission: Administers supplemental funds for visually handicapped students in local schools. Maintains special teachers or sight conservation and braille programs on both the elementary and secondary levels.
Funded by: Public funds.

EARLY INTERVENTION COORDINATION

Early Intervention Program District of Columbia Department of Human Services
609 H Street, N.E.
Fifth Floor
Washington, DC 20002
(202) 727-5930
FAX: (202) 727-1687
Joan Christopher, Program Manager

INFANT AND PRESCHOOL

Infant and Child Development Program
Columbia Lighthouse for the Blind
1421 P Street, N.W.

Washington, DC 20005
(202) 462-2900
FAX: (202) 667-8095
Dale Otto, President and CEO
Peishi Wang, Director, Children's Program

Type of Agency: Private; non-profit.
Mission: To provide blind and visually impaired people with programs, services and information that advances their ability to lead independent and fulfilling lives.
Funded by: Private donations and foundation grants.
Budget: $2.5 million.
Hours of Operation: Mon.-Fri. 8:00 AM-4:00 PM. Special children's events on some Saturdays.
Staff: 31 full time; 12 part time; uses volunteers. Has board of trustees for overall program.
History/Date: Est. 1900.
Number of Clients Served: 5,400 annually.
Area Served: Metropolitan Washington, DC.
Transportation: Y.
Age Requirements: None.

Health: Adaptive equipment; low vision exams.
Counseling/Social Work/Self-Help: Parent and family support groups. Other related and support services available on referral.
Educational: Provides direct instruction in developmental areas. Home-based and consultant services to other programs for visually impaired infants, with or without other disabilities. Education series offered for schools, churches, civic groups and corporations.
Professional Training: Career services available.
Rehabilitation: Adaptive skills; orientation and mobility training.

Recreational: Tours and activities with sighted guides.
Computer Training: Assistive technology; speech synthesizers; braille printers; large print software programs.

♦ *Information Services*

LIBRARIES

District of Columbia Library for the Blind and Physically Handicapped
901 G Street, N.W., Room 215
Washington, DC 20001
(202) 727-2142 or TDD (202) 727-2255
Grace J. Lyons, Librarian

Mission: Perform all duties involved with Library of Congress services to blind and physically disabled persons.
Funded by: Public funds.
Budget: $275,000.
Hours of Operation: Mon.-Fri. 8:45 AM-5:30 PM.
Staff: 11.
History/Date: Est. 1974.
Number of Clients Served: 2,000.
Eligibility: All those who meet criteria set by the National Library Service of Congress.
Area Served: District of Columbia.

Reading: Taping service, some in-person reading.

Regional library supplying talking books, braille, tape and large-type books. Kurzweil Reading Machine and closed-circuit television. Provides training on computer aids and devices.

MEDIA PRODUCTION SERVICES

Columbia Lighthouse for the Blind

1421 P Street, N.W.
Washington, DC 20005
(202) 462-2900
FAX: (202) 667-8095
Dale Otto, President and CEO

Area Served: Washington
metropolitan area: District of
Columbia, Maryland, and Virginia.
Groups Served: Adults.

Types/Content: Short items.
Media Formats: Braille and
cassette tape and large print.
Title Listings: Prices supplied on
request.

District of Columbia Library for the Blind and Physically Handicapped

901 G Street, N.W., Room 215
Washington, DC 20001
(202) 727-2142
Grace J. Lyons, Librarian

Groups Served: K-12, college
students, other adults.

Types/Content: Textbooks,
recreational, career/vocational.
Media Formats: Talking books/
cassettes.
Title Listings: Provided at no
charge.

Recording for the Blind and Dyslexic of Metropolitan Washington

5225 Wisconsin Avenue, N.W.
Washington, DC 20015
(202) 244-8990
FAX: (202) 244-1346
Kay Marshall, Deputy Director

Area Served: Maryland and
Virginia.
Groups Served: Visually
handicapped and reading disabled.

Types/Content: Educational
reading matter.
Media Formats: Audio tapes and
computer disk.

See Recording for the Blind and
Dyslexic in U.S. national listings.

Volunteers for the Visually Handicapped

8720 Georgia Avenue
Suite 210
Silver Spring, MD 20910
(301) 589-0894
FAX: (301) 589-7281

See Volunteers for the Visually
Handicapped in Maryland state
listings.

RADIO READING

Metropolitan Washington Ear, Inc.

35 University Boulevard East
Silver Spring, MD 20901
(301) 681-6636
FAX: (301) 681-5227
E-mail: washear@his.com
URL: http://www.his.com/
~washear/
Nancy Knauss, Administrative
Director

Hours of Operation: Mon.-Fri.
8:30AM-5:00PM.
History/Date: Est.1974.
Area Served: Maryland and
Virginia.

See Metropolitan Washington Ear,
Inc. in Maryland state listings.

INFORMATION AND REFERRAL

The Foundation Fighting Blindness Greater Washington, DC Chapter

P.O. Box 255
Washington, DC 20038
(202) 362-3277
Bonnie Seaton, President

See The Foundation Fighting
Blindness in U.S. national listings.

Prevention of Blindness Society of Metropolitan Washington

1775 Church Street, N.W.
Washington, DC 20036
(202) 234-1010
FAX: (202) 234-1020
E-mail: prvblind@pop.erols.com
Arnold Simonse, Executive
Director

Type of Agency: Non-profit.
Mission: Prevents blindness by
public/professional education
screening programs, provision of
care.
Funded by: United Way.
Budget: $900,000.
Hours of Operation: Mon.-Fri.
9:00 AM - 4:00 PM.
History/Date: Est. 1936.
Number of Clients Served:
35,000.
Area Served: Washington, DC
metropolitan area.

**Counseling/Social Work/Self-
Help:** Y.
Educational: Videos and
pamphlets on eye health and
safety.
Professional Training: Nurses
and allied health personnel.
Low Vision: Resource
information.
Publications: Newsletter.

See also in national listings:

**Affiliated Leadership League of
and for the Blind of America**

**American Association of Retired
Persons
Disability Initiative**

American Council of the Blind

Blinded Veterans Association

**Council of Citizens with Low
Vision International**

Council of Families with Visual Impairment

Deaf-Blind Program
The National Academy, Gallaudet University

Eye Bank Association of America

Governmental Relations Group
American Foundation for the Blind

Independent Visually Impaired Enterprises

National Association of Area Agencies on Aging

National Association of Blind Teachers

National Association of State Units on Aging

National Association of Vision Professionals

National Council of State Agencies for the Blind

National Information Center for Children and Youth with Disabilities

United Cerebral Palsy

♦ Rehabilitation Services

STATE SERVICES

District of Columbia Rehabilitation Services Administration Visual Impairment Section
800 Ninth Street, S.W.
4th Floor
Washington, DC 20024
(202) 645-5807
FAX: (202) 645-3857
Carolyn Wells, Supervisor

Type of Agency: State.
Staff: 6 full time. Uses volunteers.
Eligibility: Resident of D.C.; disability imposes vocational handicap; potential for benefit from vocational rehabilitation; of an age still able to work.

Health: Contracts for most health services.
Counseling/Social Work/Self-Help: Social evaluation; individual counseling; referral to community services. Contracts for other counseling/social work services.
Educational: College programs; vocational/skill development.
Professional Training: Internship/fieldwork placement in vocational rehabilitation. Regular in-service training programs. Short-term or summer training.
Rehabilitation: Contracts or refers for all rehabilitation services.
Employment: Career and skill counseling; vocational placement; follow-up service; vending facility training. Contracts for other employment services.
Low Vision Follow-up: Y.

REHABILITATION

Columbia Lighthouse for the Blind
1421 P Street, N.W.
Washington, DC 20005
(202) 462-2900
FAX: (202) 667-8095
Dale Otto, President and CEO

Type of Agency: Private; non-profit.
Mission: To provide blind and visually impaired people with programs and services that advances their opportunity to lead independent and fulfilling lives.
Funded by: District of Columbia government contract, contributions, product sales, investments, wills, and bequests.
Budget: $2.5 million.
Hours of Operation: Mon.-Fri. 8:00 AM-4:30 PM.

Program Accessibility: Fully accessible.
Staff: 32 full time, 13 part time.
History/Date: Est. 1900.
Eligibility: Anyone with a vision impairment that is not correctible with conventional lenses or medical treatment.
Area Served: Metropolitan Washington DC.
Transportation: Y.
Age Requirements: None.

Health: Refers for all health services.
Counseling/Social Work/Self-Help: Individual, group, family/parent, couple counseling; placement in training; referral to community services.
Educational: Infant and early intervention program for children with visual impairments, including multiple disabilities.
Professional Training: Internship/student teaching in orientation/mobility; rehabilitation and counseling.
Reading: Talking book record players and cassette players; talking book records and cassettes; braille books; large-print books; braille magazines; recorded magazines; information and referral special collection; transcription to braille.
Rehabilitation: Personal management; braille; handwriting; listening skills; typing; electronic mobility aids; home management; orientation/mobility; remedial education; sensory training.
Recreational: Adult program of recreational and social activities. Provides consultation to other agencies on special programs for visually impaired persons. Summer camp.
Employment: Prevocational evaluation; occupational skill development; vocational training; job retention; job retraining;

sheltered workshops; vocational placement. Refers for other employment services. Provides consultation to other agencies in vending facility training.
Computer Training: Basic word processing, training using assistive technology.
Low Vision: Evaluation and referral.
Low Vision Aids: Training in use of devices. Aids available for loan or purchase.
Low Vision Follow-up: Y.

Volunteers for the Visually Handicapped
8720 Georgia Avenue
Suite 210
Silver Spring, MD 20910
(301) 589-0894
FAX: (301) 589-7281

See Volunteers for the Visually Handicapped in Maryland state listings.

◆ Low Vision Services

EYE CARE SOCIETIES

Washington DC Ophthalmological Society
1145 19th Street, N.W.
Suite 500
Washington, DC 20036
(202) 833-1328
Mary Henegan, Executive Director

Optometric Society of the District of Columbia
7705 Cayuga Avenue
Bethesda, MD 20817
(301) 229-4990
Virginia Martin, Director

LOW VISION CENTERS

Columbia Lighthouse for the Blind
Ferd Nauheim Low Vision Clinic
1421 P Street, N.W.
Washington, DC 20005
(202) 462-2900
FAX: (202) 667-8095
Stephen J. Feinberg, O.D., Director

Type of Agency: Private; non-profit.
Hours of Operation: Tues. and Wed. afternoons; Fri.
Staff: Low vision assistant; orientation/mobility instructor; ophthalmology resident; ophthalmologist; rehabilitation counselor. Social worker, recreation programmer, vocational counselor available.
Area Served: Washington DC metropolitan area.

Rehabilitation: Independent living skills; personal management; orientation and mobility.
Computer Training: Access and training on computer aids/devices.
Low Vision: Evaluation and referral.
Low Vision Aids: On-site training. Provided on loan for trial purpose at no charge.
Low Vision Follow-up: Varies according to patient.

Georgetown University Medical Center
Center for Sight
3800 Reservoir Road
Washington, DC 20007
(202) 687-4448
FAX: (202) 687-4978
Dr. Howard Cupples, Chairman

Funded by: Client fees.
Hours of Operation: By appointment.
Staff: Ophthalmologist; ophthalmology residents.

Eligibility: Physician referral.
Area Served: Unlimited.

Low Vision Follow-up: By return appointment.

George Washington University Medical Center
Department of Ophthalmology
2150 Pennsylvania Avenue, N.W.
Floor 2A
Washington, DC 20037
(202) 994-4048
FAX: (202) 994-4065
Dr. John Zacharia, Chairman

Hours of Operation: Mon.-Fri. 8:30 AM-4:00 PM.
Staff: Ophthalmologist; ophthalmology residents.
Eligibility: None.
Area Served: Unlimited.

Low Vision Aids: Provided on loan for trial purposes; no rental fee charged; on-site training provided.
Low Vision Follow-up: By return appointment in 4 months.

Walter Reed Army Medical Center
Ophthalmology Service
Georgia Avenue and Fern Street
Washington, DC 20307-5001
(202) 782-6964
FAX: (202) 782-6156
Kenyon K. Kramer, M.D., Chief, Ophthalmology Service

County/District Where Located: District of Columbia.
Funded by: Federal government.
Hours of Operation: Mon.-Fri. 7:30AM-4:30 PM.
Staff: Ophthalmologist; ophthalmology residents; ophthalmic assistant/technician.
Eligibility: Active or retired military; authorized veterans; authorized dependents.
Area Served: Unlimited.

Low Vision: Ophthalmology services, evaluations.

Low Vision Aids: Provided on loan for trial purposes; no rental fee charged; on-site training provided.

◆ *Aging Services*

STATE UNITS ON AGING

Office on Aging

One Judiciary Square
441 Fourth Street, NW
Ninth Floor
Washington, DC 20001
(202) 724-5622
FAX: (202) 724-4979
Jearline Williams, Executive Director

Provides referrals to Area Agencies on Aging and information on other local aging services.

INDEPENDENT LIVING PROGRAMS

District of Columbia Department of Human Services

800 Ninth Street S.W.
Washington, DC 20024
(202) 645-5703
Wayne Casey, Director

Provides independent living services for persons age 55 and over. For further information, contact the Project Director or general phone number listed.

FLORIDA

♦ *Educational Services*

STATE SERVICES

Bureau of Instructional Support and Community Services
Florida Department of Education
Suite 614
Florida Education Center
Tallahassee, FL 32399-0400
(904) 488-1570
FAX: (904) 487-2194
David Mosrie, Deputy Department Director
Shan Goff, Bureau Chief
Carol Allman, Consultant, Visually Impaired Programs

Type of Agency: State.
Mission: Provides consultative services for the establishment and operation of school programs for visually impaired students. Provides assistance for in-service teacher training through state or regional workshops or technical assistance to individual programs. The Bureau also monitors public school districts and residential programs.
Funded by: Public funds; federal funds.
Hours of Operation: Mon.-Fri. 8:00 AM - 5:00 PM.
Area Served: Florida.

Educational: Has a clearinghouse of materials available on request, related to the education of persons with disabilities.
Professional Training: Teacher recertification provided through workshops.
Residential: Associated with the Florida School for the Deaf and the Blind, St. Augustine, Florida.

Rehabilitation: Interagency cooperation with the Division of Blind Services.
Computer Training: Access, training on computer aids and devices varies among school districts.
Low Vision: Materials available on request.

EARLY INTERVENTION COORDINATION

Children's Medical Services
Building 6
1323 Winewood Boulevard
Tallahassee, FL 32301
(904) 488-6005
FAX: (904) 921-5241
Fran Wilbur, Part H Early Childhood Coordinator

Office of Early Intervention and School Readiness
Florida Division of Public Schools/Department of Education
325 West Gaines Street
Suite 325
Tallahassee, FL 32399-0400
(904) 488-6830
FAX: (904) 487-0946
Patty Ball Thomas, Acting Director
Bessie Felton-Joseph, Program Specialist

SCHOOLS

Florida School for the Deaf and Blind
207 North San Marco Avenue
St. Augustine, FL 32084
(904) 823-4000
FAX: (904) 823-4018 or (904) 823-4203
URL: http://www.fsdb.k12.fl.us
Robert T. Dawson, President
Gerald W. Stewart, Principal of the Blind Department
Elmer Dillingham, Principal of the Deaf Department

Type of Agency: Public.
Mission: To provide an education for eligible visually impaired children grades pre-K through 12.
Funded by: Public funds.
Staff: 620 full time including all departments, 100 full time in the Department for the Blind.
History/Date: Est. 1885.
Eligibility: 20/70 in best eye after correction; special needs with the exception of children whose disabilities include the categories of trainable mental handicapped, profound mental handicapped, severe emotional disturbance, autism or homebound/hospitalized, or suffer severe medical problems beyond the School's resources to manage.
Area Served: Statewide.
Transportation: Y.
Age Requirements: From 3 to 21 years of age.

Health: Occupational, physical and speech therapy; diagnosis and evaluation of eye health; general medical services; dental services.
Counseling/Social Work/Self-Help: Social evaluations; psychological testing and evaluations; individual, group and family/parent counseling; linkage with other agencies and community services.
Educational: Grades K through 12; programs for college prep; general academic, and vocational/skill development. Cooperative school programs with the Division of Blind Services and St. Johns County School District.
Preschools: Preschool provided for 3 and 4 year olds.
Professional Training: In-service training program; tuition waivers to state universities; internship/practicum placement for student teachers in specific or general education areas.

Reading: Talking book record players and cassette players; talking book records and cassettes; large-print books; braille books and magazines; recorded magazines; access to regional talking book library, magnification copier; closed-circuit television; Optacon; Kurzweil Reading Machine.

Residential: Girls' and boys' elementary dormitories; multihandicapped dormitory; high school dormitories designed to enhance daily living skills progressively. Independent living apartments for high school students. Sequential dormitory curriculum covering toileting / personal hygiene, grooming / dressing; eating skills / food preparation; housekeeping skills / clothing care; health and safety; family life / interpersonal relationships; social and emotional skills / etiquette; indoor / outdoor recreation; leisure time activities; money management / time skills; calendar / telephone skills; career awareness / work habits and attitudes.

Rehabilitation: Personal management; activities of daily living; orientation / mobility; braille; typing; individual and group counseling; listening skills; use of video magnification and other low vision aids; remedial education.

Recreational: Afterschool recreation programs; active and leisure activities; arts and crafts; individual and team activities; clubs and hobby groups; swimming and wrestling teams; cheerleaders; scouting.

Employment: Prevocational / vocational evaluation; career and skill counseling; vocational work-study program; cooperative career planning with Division of Blind Services-Vocational Rehabilitation.

Computer Training: Extensive computer lab. Computers in classrooms. Training in use of computers, adaptive aids, and devices. Full access for practical and professional use.

Low Vision: Low vision clinic.

Low Vision Aids: Provided on loan.

Visually Impaired Program
Hillsborough County Schools

1202 East Palm Avenue
Tampa, FL 33602
(813) 273-7035
FAX: (813) 273-7301
Laura C. Brown, Coordinator

County/District Where Located: Hillsborough County.

Eligibility: Must meet state Department of Education rules regarding visual impairment.

Area Served: Hillsborough County.

Age Requirements: 0-21.

Educational: Itinerant, resource room and special class placements for visually impaired students, preschool-grade 12, with or without other impairments. Provides instruction in daily living skills, orientation / mobility, academic instruction, listening skills, specialized skills (braille, Nemeth Code).

Computer Training: Access to computers adapted for visually impaired persons. Variety of support services available on referral.

INFANT AND PRESCHOOL

Debbie School
Mailman Center for Child Development

1601 N.W. 12th Avenue
Miami, FL 33136
(305) 547-6961
Janet Dacharme, Principal

Type of Agency: Private.

County/District Where Located: Dade County.

Funded by: P.L. 89-313, private donations, state funds.

Staff: 20 full time, 2 part time, uses volunteers. Has advisory board.

History/Date: Est. 1975.

Area Served: Dade County and Miami.

Transportation: Y.

Health: Adaptive equipment; genetic counseling.

Counseling/Social Work/Self-Help: Parent counseling. Variety of support and related services available by consultation or referral. Provides neonatal, psychosocial, and educational intervention.

Educational: Provides direct instruction in all developmental areas. Home- and center-based programs for visually impaired, multiply disabled, and nondisabled children, 0-5 years.

Division of Blind Services
Florida Department of Labor

2551 Executive Center Circle
Tallahassee, FL 32399
(904) 488-1330
Whit Springfield, Director

Type of Agency: State.

Funded by: Gifts and donations, state funds, Title XX funds.

Staff: Social workers, rehabilitation teachers.

History/Date: Est. 1941.

Transportation: Y.

Age Requirements: 0-5 years.

Health: Adaptive equipment; genetic counseling. Visual and other health services referred to children's medical services or other agencies.

Counseling/Social Work/Self-Help: Parent counseling, with referrals to other facilities as needed.

Educational: Provides direct instruction. Home- and center-based programs for visually handicapped children, with or without other handicaps.

Preschools: Co-sponsors with Florida Lions Club twice yearly Camp Achievement, a preschool camp for the visually handicapped and their parents.

For Local Offices, see individual listings under Rehabilitation Services, State Services.

Merrick Educational Center
39 Zamora Avenue
Coral Gables, FL 33134
(305) 460-2909
FAX: (305) 444-2855
Michael Exelbert, Principal

Type of Agency: Public school program for visually handicapped, hearing impaired, and deaf-blind infants.
County/District Where Located: Dade County.
Staff: 4 full time (teacher of visually handicapped and hearing-impaired children).
History/Date: Est. 1983.
Area Served: Dade County.
Age Requirements: Birth-2 years.

Counseling/Social Work/Self-Help: Parent counseling, genetic counseling.
Low Vision: Low vision exams.

Home-based. Provides instruction in all developmental areas; immunizations available on referral.

INSTRUCTIONAL MATERIALS CENTERS

Florida Instructional Materials Center for the Visually Handicapped
5002 North Lois Avenue
Tampa, FL 33614
(813) 872-5281 or toll-free in Florida (800) 282-9193
FAX: (813) 872-5284
E-mail: daltons@mail.firn.edu
Suzanne A. Dalton, Supervisor

County/District Where Located: Hillsborough County.
Funded by: Public funds.
Area Served: Florida.
Groups Served: Up to 21 years of age.

Types/Content: Textbooks.
Media Formats: Braille books, talking books/cassettes, large print books.
Title Listings: Printed at no charge.

Serves as an instructional materials center, coordinating procurement, storage, and distribution of educational materials needed by students with visual disabilities. Operates clearinghouse depository and production center for braille, large-print, and recorded text books. Provides training and ongoing technical assistance to instructional, support personnel and other appropriate groups, including students and parents, in the areas of materials production, technological applications, and instructional strategies as they relate to students with visual disabilities. Organizes volunteers (statewide) for materials production. Houses Assistive Technology Educational Network of Florida, Regional Lab #4, serving students, parents, and professional staff in west central Florida. Provides information, print resources, assessment training, workshops, equipment display/preview, product demonstrations and short-term loan of assistive devices.

UNIVERSITY TRAINING PROGRAMS

Florida State University Visual Impairments
College of Education
209 Education Building
Tallahassee, FL 32306-3024
(904) 644-4880
FAX: (904) 644-8715
E-mail: lewis@mail.coe.fsu.edu
URL: http://www.fsu.edu./~spec-ed/spedvipr.html
Dr. Sandra Lewis, Visually Handicapped
Purvis Ponder, Orientation and Mobility

Programs Offered: Undergraduate and graduate (master's, doctoral) programs for teachers of students with visual impairments including multiple disabilities; master's programs for dual competency teachers of students with visual impairments/orientation and mobility specialists and rehabilitation teachers/orientation and mobility specialists.
Distance Education: Y.

◆ *Information Services*

LIBRARIES

Brevard County Library System Talking Books Library
308 Forrest Avenue
Cocoa, FL 32922-7781
(407) 633-1810 or (407) 633-1811
FAX: (407) 633-1790
Kay Briley, Librarian

Subregional library.

Broward County Talking Book Library
100 South Andrews Avenue

Ft. Lauderdale, FL 33301
(305) 357-7555 or (305) 357-7413
FAX: (305) 357-7413
Joann Block, Librarian

Subregional library.

Bureau of Braille and Talking Book Services
420 Platt Street
Daytona Beach, FL 32114
(904) 239-6000 or toll-free in
Florida (800) 226-6075
FAX: (904) 239-6069
E-mail: weberd@mail.firn.edu
Donald John Weber, Chief

Type of Agency: A bureau of the State of Florida Department of Education, Division of Labor.
County/District Where Located: Volusia County.
Mission: To provide books and magazines in braille and on disk and cassette to Florida residents unable to use conventional printed materials.
Funded by: Public funds.
Budget: $802,000.
Hours of Operation: Mon.-Fri. 8:00 AM-5:00 PM.
Program Accessibility: Building in compliance with ADA. Special cassette and record players can be adapted.
History/Date: Est. 1950.
Number of Clients Served: 40,000.
Eligibility: Inability to read conventional-size print for an extended period of time; inability to hold a book or turn the pages of a book or newspaper; reading disabilities such as dyslexia, with a doctor's certification.
Area Served: Florida.

Educational: Assistance in locating textbooks; volunteers braille college textbooks for students in Florida colleges and universities.

Reading: Books and magazines on cassette and disk and in braille.
Computer Training: Access.
Low Vision Aids: Sends catalogs only; does not sell items.

Dade County Talking Book Library
Miami-Dade Public Library System
150 N.E. 79th Street
Miami, FL 33138
(305) 751-8687 or TDD (305) 758-6599 or toll-free in Florida
(800) 451-9544
Barbara L. Moyer, Coordinator

Subregional library.

Hillsborough County Talking Book Library
Tampa-Hillsborough County
Public Library System
900 North Ashley Drive
Tampa, FL 33602-3788
(813) 223-8349 or (813) 223-8858
FAX: (813) 223-8278
Suzanne M. Bell, Librarian

Subregional library.

Lee County Subregional Library for the Blind and Physically Handicapped
13240 North Cleveland Avenue, #5-6
North Ft. Myers, FL 33903-4855
(813) 995-2665
Barbara Ferris, Librarian

Subregional library.

Talking Book Library Jacksonville Public Libraries
1755 Edgewood Avenue West
Suite 1
Jacksonville, FL 32208-7206
(904) 765-5588 or TDD (904) 630-2740
FAX: (904) 768-7404
Susan V. Arthur, Librarian

Subregional library.

Talking Books Palm Beach County Library Annex
7950 Central Industrial Drive
Suite 104
Riviera Beach, FL 33404-9947
(407) 845-4600
Pat Mistretta, Librarian

Subregional library.

Talking Book Service
Manatee Public Library System
1301 Barcarrota Boulevard
West Bradenton, FL 34205-7599
(813) 749-7114 or TDD (813) 749-7113
FAX: (813) 749-7191
Frederick Duda, Librarian

Subregional library.

West Florida Regional Library Subregional Talking Book Library
200 West Gregory Street
Pensacola, FL 32501
(904) 435-1760
FAX: (904) 432-9582
Martha L. Lazor, Librarian

Subregional library.

MEDIA PRODUCTION SERVICES
Escambia County School District
30 East Texar Drive
P.O. Box 1470
Pensacola, FL 32503
(904) 469-5524
Paul Fetsko, Coordinator

County/District Where Located: Escambia County.
Groups Served: Public school day program, enrolled students, birth through high school graduation or age 21.

Types/Content: Textbooks.
Media Formats: Braille books, talking books/cassettes, large print books.

Exceptional Student Education
2757 West Pensacola Street
Tallahassee, FL 32304
(904) 487-7155
Beverley Blanton, Area Leader

County/District Where Located: Leon County.
Groups Served: Birth-12.

Types/Content: Textbooks, worksheets.
Media Formats: Braille/large print books.

Palm Beach County Schools
3378 Forest Hill Boulevard
Suite A 201
West Palm Beach, FL 33406
(407) 434-8000
Ray Davis, Director

County/District Where Located: Palm Beach County.
Area Served: School district.
Groups Served: K-12.

Types/Content: Textbooks, recreational, Braille and Speak.
Media Formats: Braille books, talking books/cassettes, large print books.
Title Listings: Printed at no charge.

Pinellas County Schools
301 Fourth Street, S.W.
Administration Building
P.O. Box 2942
Largo, FL 33770
(813) 588-6030
FAX: (813) 588-6441
Noreen Murphy Price, Supervisor

Area Served: Pinellas County.
Groups Served: Preschool-12.

Types/Content: Textbooks, recreational, career/vocational.
Media Formats: Braille books, talking books/cassettes, large-print books.
Title Listings: No title listings available.

Recording for the Blind and Dyslexic
Florida Unit
6704 S.W. 80th Street
Miami, FL 33143
(305) 666-0552 or (800) 535-0552
FAX: (305) 667-2505
Christine McCarthy, Executive Director
Kathleen F. Craynock, Studio Director

County/District Where Located: Dade County.

See Recording for the Blind and Dyslexic in U.S. national listings.

Temple Sisterhood Braille Group
8727 San Jose Boulevard
Jacksonville, FL 32217
(904) 733-7078
Joan Madden, Chairperson

County/District Where Located: Duval County.
Groups Served: K-12, college students, other adults.

Types/Content: Recreational, career/vocational.
Media Formats: Braille books.
Title Listings: No title listings available.

RADIO READING

WGCU Radio Reading Service
Florida Gulf Coast University
8111 College Parkway - Areca 216

Ft. Myers, FL 33919
(941) 432-5581
FAX: (941) 432-5586
E-mail: gsabatka@fgcu.edu
URL: http://www.fgcu.edu
Glenn Sabatka, Manager

County/District Where Located: Lee County.
Funded by: Department of Education; donations.
Hours of Operation: Office: 24 hours a day.
History/Date: Est. 1985.
Area Served: Lee, Collier, Charlotte, Glades and Hendry Counties.
Age Requirements: None.

WLRN Radio Reading Service
172 N.E. 15th Street, #222
Miami, FL 33132
(305) 995-2218
Becky Trantlem, Volunteer Coordinator

County/District Where Located: Dade County.
Hours of Operation: Mon.-Fri. 8:00 AM-4:00 PM.
History/Date: Est. 1982.
Area Served: Dade, Broward and Palm Beach counties.

WMFE Radio Reading Service
11510 East Colonial Drive
Orlando, FL 32817
(407) 273-1519
Renae Neiberlein, Reading Service Manager

County/District Where Located: Orange County.
Hours of Operation: Mon.-Fri. 7:00 AM-11:00PM, Sat.-Sun. 8:00AM-11:00PM.
History/Date: Est. 1963.
Area Served: Orange, Osceola, Flagler, Vousia Lake, Seminole and Breuard Counties.
Age Requirements: None.

WUSF Radio Reading Service
University of South Florida, WRB 209
4202 E. Fowler Avenue
Tampa, FL 33620
(813) 974-4193
FAX: (813) 974-5016
JoAnn Urofsky, Director/Manager

County/District Where Located: Hillsborough County.
Funded by: Florida DOE Grant, listener contributions.
Hours of Operation: 24 hours a day.
History/Date: Est. 1976.
Area Served: Tampa and 60-mile radius from the city.
Age Requirements: None.

INFORMATION AND REFERRAL

The Foundation Fighting Blindness
Central Florida Affiliate
10332 Yorkmere Court
Orlando, FL 32817
(407) 687-4163
Jed Berman, President
Brenda Schoonover, Contact Person, (407) 788-0500

See The Foundation Fighting Blindness in U.S. national listings.

The Foundation Fighting Blindness
North Florida Affiliate
8149 Crosswind Road
Jacksonville, FL 32244
(904) 779-7606
Barbara Libero, President

See The Foundation Fighting Blindness in U.S. national listings.

The Foundation Fighting Blindness
Ormond Beach Affiliate
3 Ellsworth Avenue
Ormond Beach, FL 32174
(904) 677-2870
Gladys B. Holton, Contact Person

See The Foundation Fighting Blindness in U.S. national listings.

The Foundation Fighting Blindness
South Florida Affiliate
1999 University Drive
Coral Springs, FL 33071
(305) 341-6041
Nick Fischler, Contact Person

See The Foundation Fighting Blindness in U.S. national listings.

Prevent Blindness Florida
3825 Henderson Boulevard
Suite 402
Tampa, FL 33629
(813) 874-2020
Sarah Jordan-Holmes, President

See Prevent Blindness America in U.S. national listings.

See also in national listings:

American Association of Certified Orthoptists

Bible Alliance

Braille International

Gospel Association for the Blind

United States Blind Golfers Association

♦ Rehabilitation Services

STATE SERVICES

Division of Blind Services
Florida Department of Labor
2551 Executive Center Circle
Tallahassee, FL 32399
(904) 488-1330
FAX: (904) 487-1804
Whit Springfield, Director

Type of Agency: State.
Mission: Services for totally blind; legally blind; visually impaired; deaf-blind.
Funded by: State, federal or private sources.
Budget: $25 million.
Hours of Operation: Mon.-Fri. 8:00 AM-5:00 PM.
Staff: 329 full time. Uses volunteers.
History/Date: Est. 1941.
Eligibility: Legally blind; pathology or injury threatening loss of vision in one or both eyes.
Area Served: State of Florida.
Transportation: Y.

Health: Contracts and refers for all health services.
Counseling/Social Work/Self-Help: Social evaluation; psychological testing and evaluation; individual, group, family/parent, couple counseling. Contracts, refers, and provides consultation to other agencies for other counseling/social work services.
Educational: Remedial education.
Professional Training: Sensory training; internship/fieldwork placement in orientation/mobility; rehabilitation counseling; social work; rehabilitation teaching. In-service and short-term or summer training open to enrollment from other agencies.
Reading: Lends talking book record players and cassette players; talking book records and cassettes; braille books; braille magazines; recorded magazines. Information and referral; special collection; transcription to braille; translation to other languages; tape recording services on demand.

Residential: Maintains a 54-bed residential rehabilitation center.
Rehabilitation: Rehabilitation teaching in client's home and community; orientation/mobility; contracts, refers, and provides consultation to other agencies for all rehabilitation services.
Recreational: Personal management; braille; handwriting; listening skills; Optacon; typing; video magnifier; home management.
Employment: Prevocational evaluation; career and skill counseling; occupational skill development; job retention; job training; vocational placement; vending facility training. Contracts, refers, and provides consultation to other agencies for employment-oriented services.
Computer Training: Access; training on computer aids and devices. Vocational training in computer applications.
Low Vision: Y.
Low Vision Aids: Y.
Low Vision Follow-up: Follow-up service.

Local Offices:

Bradenton: 5117 26th Street West, Suite A, Bradenton, FL 34207, (941) 751-7670.
Daytona Beach: Division of Blind Services, 1185 Dunn Avenue, Daytona Beach, FL 32014, (904) 254-3824.
Daytona Beach: Bureau of Braille and Talking Books, 420 Platt Street, Daytona Beach, FL 32114, (904) 239-6000.
Daytona Beach: Rehabilitation Center for the Blind, 1111 Willis Avenue, Daytona Beach, FL 32014, (904) 258-4444.
Fort Lauderdale: Division of Blind Services, 3075 West Oakland Park Boulevard, Suite 211, Fort Lauderdale, FL 33311, (954) 497-3360.

Fort Myers: Division of Blind Services, 2830 Winkler Avenue, Fort Myers, FL 33916, (813) 278-7130.
Gainesville: Division of Blind Services, 417 S.W. 8th Street, Gainesville, FL 32301, (352) 336-2075.
Jacksonville: Division of Blind Services, 1809 Art Museum Drive, Room 201, Jacksonville, FL 32207, (904) 348-2730.
Miami: Division of Blind Services, 401 N.W. 2nd Avenue, Room S-714, Miami, FL 33128, (305) 377-5339.
Orlando: Division of Blind Services, 400 West Robinson Street, Suite 102, Orlando, FL 32801, (407) 245-0700.
Panama City: Division of Blind Services, 2611 Jenks Avenue, Panama City, FL 32405, (904) 872-4181.
Pensacola: Division of Blind Services, 7200 North 9th Avenue, Suite A-11, Pensacola, FL 32504, (904) 484-5030.
St. Augustine: Division of Blind Services, P.O. Box 69, St. Augustine, FL 32085-0069, (904) 825-5084.
St. Petersburg: Division of Blind Services, 3637 Fourth Street, North, Suite 310, St. Petersburg, FL 33704-1335, (813) 893-2341.
Tallahassee: Division of Blind Services, 2003 Parkway Building, Room 201, Tallahassee, FL 32399, (813) 278-7130.
Tampa: Division of Blind Services, 415 South Armenia Avenue, Tampa, FL 33609, (813) 871-7190.
West Palm Beach: Division of Blind Services, Palm Beach County Regional Service Center, 111 Sapodilla Avenue, 1st Floor, West Palm Beach, FL 33901, (305) 837-5026.

REHABILITATION

Center for the Visually Impaired, Inc.
1187 Dunn Avenue
Daytona Beach, FL 32114
(904) 253-8879 or toll-free in Florida only (800) 227-1284
FAX: (904) 253-9178
E-mail: rehabone@msn.com
Robert M. Hodge, Executive Director

Type of Agency: Community rehabilition program.
County/District Where Located: Volusia County.
Mission: Provide independent living, adjustment to blindness, orientation and mobility, low vision and peer support services to the elderly legally blind.
Budget: FY1997: $317,228.
Hours of Operation: Mon. - Fri. 8:00AM - 5:00PM.
Program Accessibility: Complies with the Americans with Disabilities Act.
History/Date: Est. 1985, Inc. 1988.
Number of Clients Served: 494.
Eligibility: Any nonvocational adult who is legally blind or at risk of becoming legally blind.
Area Served: Serves Flagler, Putnam and Volusia County.
Transportation: Y.
Age Requirements: 55 years and older in the independent living program, working age adults and the elderly in the orientation and mobility program, and all ages in the low vision program.

Health: Classes for legally blind diabetics.
Counseling/Social Work/Self-Help: Adjustment to blindness counseling program and a self-help program.
Rehabilitation: Independent living training and orientation and mobility training.

Low Vision: Low vision specialist every Wednesday to provide comprehensive low vision evaluation.

Low Vision Aids: Comprehensive inventory of low vision aids and devices. CCTVs for sale.

Low Vision Follow-up: Y.

Publications: Brochures on independent living classes, adjustment to blindness and low vision. Quarterly newsletter, *Eye Opener.*

CITE (Center for Independence, Technology and Education)

8807 Airport Boulevard
Leesburg, FL 34788
(352) 365-1544 or (800) 353-1544
FAX: (352) 365-6970
Robert Atchley, Program Coordinator
Anita Mahan, Rehabilitation Supervisor

County/District Where Located: Lake County.

Mission: To promote independence and self-reliance in persons who are blind or visually impaired through instruction in independent living skills and counseling.

Funded by: United Way; Florida Division of Blind Services, grants.

Budget: 1995-6: $162,600.

Hours of Operation: Mon.-Fri. 8:00 AM-5:00 PM. Also special evening programs.

Program Accessibility: Wheelchair accessibility.

Staff: 2 full time, 6 part time. Uses volunteers.

History/Date: Est. 1989.

Number of Clients Served: 186.

Eligibility: Totally blind, legally blind, and visually impaired; adults; referrals from the Division of Blind Services; mentally/physically able to benefit from services.

Area Served: Lake and Sumter Counties.

Transportation: Y.

Age Requirements: 55 years of age and older.

Counseling/Social Work/Self-Help: Individual, group, and family counseling; peer counseling; refers for and provides consultation to other agencies for other counseling/social work.

Reading: Instruction, in braille, closed-circuit televisions, talking book cassette players and record players, and talking book cassettes and records. Transcription to braille and tape recording available upon request. Information and referral.

Rehabilitation: Training in personal and home management, communications, orientation and mobility, sensory awareness, and community resources. Instruction in class and in clients' homes as noncredit college curriculum.

Recreational: Training offered in arts and crafts, exercise, and games with emphasis on learning the skills at the center and using the skills in the home and community programs; also offers special interest programs and referral to existing community programs.

Computer Training: Voice-operated computers.

Low Vision Aids: Assistive low vision screening.

CITE (Center for Independence, Technology and Education)

215 East New Hampshire Street
Orlando, FL 32804
(407) 898-2483
FAX: (407) 895-5255
Carol Adams, Director

Type of Agency: Comprehensive rehabilitation and training center for blind adults and families with blind children.

County/District Where Located: Orange County.

Mission: Services for totally blind; legally blind; multidisabled.

Funded by: State; Division of Blind Services; United Way; private foundations; and individuals.

Budget: $800,000.

Hours of Operation: Mon.-Fri. 8:00 AM-5:00 PM.

Program Accessibility: ADA accessible.

Staff: 8 full time, 19 part time. Uses volunteers.

History/Date: Est. 1976.

Number of Clients Served: 300-500 annually.

Eligibility: Legal blindness.

Area Served: Orange, Seminole, Osceola, Lake and Sumter Counties. Others for short term training.

Transportation: Y.

Age Requirements: All ages.

Counseling/Social Work/Self-Help: Social evaluation; individual, group, family counseling; referral to community services. Refers for other counseling/social work services. Provides consultations to other agencies. Peer counseling and support.

Educational: Program for adult continuing education; training for parents of blind preschool childen. Support groups; Assistive Technology Resource Center; Vocational Training Placement.

Professional Training: Regular in-service training programs. Short-term or summer training. Internship/fieldwork in rehabilitation counseling.

Reading: Volunteer readers matched with clients.

Rehabilitation: Activities of daily living; braille; handwriting; typing; home management; orientation/mobility; rehabilitation teaching;

low vision computer access technology; software training.
Recreational: Arts and crafts; hobby groups; leisure activities.
Employment: Prevocational evaluation; career and skill counseling; refers to other employment services; word processing/data base training.
Computer Training: Training on computer aids and devices; screen reading software; magnification software.
Low Vision: Screening and examinations.
Low Vision Follow-up: Follow-up service.

Conklin Center for Multihandicapped Blind

405 White Street
Daytona Beach, FL 32114
(904) 258-3441
FAX: (904) 258-1155
E-mail: ed@conklincenter.org
URL: http://
www.conklincenter.org
Edward F. McCoy, Executive Director

Type of Agency: Private; non-profit.
Mission: Services for totally blind, legally blind, deaf-blind, learning disabled, mentally retarded clients and those with cerebral palsy, seizure disorders, orthopedic involvements, behavioral disorders and head injuries.
Funded by: Purchase of service agreement, donations, tuition and fees, investment income, grants.
Budget: 1996-97: $1,459,904.
Hours of Operation: 24 hours per day.
Program Accessibility: Buildings and apartments are barrier-free. Changes in progress meet ADA requirements.
Staff: 37 full time, 8 part time. Uses volunteers.

History/Date: Est. 1979.
Number of Clients Served: 1995-96: 65.
Eligibility: Visual impairment. Legally blind with secondary handicap; current audiological and psychological exam.
Area Served: Unlimited.
Transportation: Y.
Age Requirements: 12 years of age or older.

Health: Low vision services, general medical services, occupational therapy, physical therapy, speech therapy.
Counseling/Social Work/Self-Help: Social evaluations; individual, family counseling. Contracts for neuropsychiatric services.
Educational: Programs for adult continuing education; adult basic education; remedial education; vocational/skill development.
Preschools: Consultation services available.
Professional Training: Internship/field work placement in orientation and mobility, rehabilitation counseling, social work, rehabilitation teaching, and vocational rehabilitation.
Reading: Talking book record players; cassette tape players; CCTVs; Kurzweil Readers; talking book records and tapes; braille and large-print books; braille and recorded magazines. Transcription to braille; tape recording services on request.
Residential: Dormitory, on-site and off-site apartments and supported living services for adults who are multiply disabled.
Rehabilitation: Activities of daily living; braille; gesticulation; handwriting; Optacon; typing; video magnifier; electronic mobility aids; home management; orientation/mobility; rehabilitation teaching in client's

home and community; remedial education; sensory training; supported living; supported employment. Provides consultation to other agencies.
Recreational: Arts and crafts; hobby groups; adult continuing education; bowling, swimming, track. Integration into community resources.
Employment: Prevocational evaluation; career and skill counseling; occupational skill development; job retention; job retraining; vocational placement; supported employment, follow-along services. workshop services. Provides consultation to other agencies.
Computer Training: Training and computer aids and devices for personal use.
Low Vision: Evaluations and services, on-site training provided.
Low Vision Aids: Low vision aids and devices.
Low Vision Follow-up: Follow-up service.

Florida Association of Workers for the Blind (Miami Lighthouse)

601 S.W. Eighth Avenue
Miami, FL 33130
(305) 856-2288
FAX: (305) 285-6967
E-mail: miamilighthouse@the-directory.com
URL: http://www.the-directory.com/miamilighthouse
Vernon Metcalf, Executive Director
Elly du Pré, DPA, Associate Executive Director
Frances Applebaum, Rehabilitation Coordinator

Type of Agency: Private; non-profit.
County/District Where Located: Dade County.
Mission: Services for totally blind, legally blind, visually impaired,

deaf-blind, learning disabled, and mentally retarded persons.

Funded by: Fees, contributions, grants.

Budget: 1997: $1,719.000.

Hours of Operation: Mon. - Thurs. 8:30 AM - 4:30 PM; Fri. 8:00 AM - 4:00 PM. Vocational Training Unit: flexible hours.

Program Accessibility: Accessible to disabled persons.

Staff: 35 full time, 1 part time. Uses volunteers.

History/Date: Est. 1931.

Number of Clients Served: 1995: 350.

Eligibility: Severe visual problem interfering with lifestyle.

Area Served: Dade County.

Transportation: Y.

Counseling/Social Work/Self-Help: Social evaluation; psychological testing and evaluation; self defense; peer counseling; diabetes education; individual, group, family/parent, couple counseling; placement in training; referral to community services. Contracts, refers and provides consultation to other agencies for other counseling/social work services.

Educational: Non-graded. Accepts deaf-blind; emotionally disturbed; learning disabled; mentally retarded; orthopedically disabled; anyone on evaluation basis. Programs: adult continuing education; personal adjustment training; computer training; paraprofessional training; summer children's program; job clinic.

Preschools: Counseling guidance and training of parents for child management and training.

Professional Training: Orientation/mobility; rehabilitation counseling; social work; special education; vocational rehabilitation; regular in-service training programs. Open to enrollment from other agencies. Paraprofessional training with staff serving as adjunct professors at Miami Dade Community College; Rehabilitation Engineering - consult to individuals and corporations.

Reading: Talking book record players and cassette players; talking book records and cassettes; braille books; braille magazines; recorded magazines; information and referral; transcription to braille and other languages.

Rehabilitation: Personal management; braille; gesticulation; handwriting; listening skills; typing; video magnifier; home management; orientation/mobility; rehabilitation teaching in client's home and community; computer training; remedial education; sensory training. "Store" outlet sells aids and appliances.

Recreational: Arts and crafts; special programs for elderly; sailing; "u-pick" and other field trips.

Employment: Prevocational evaluation; career and skill counseling; provides consultation for and refers to other agencies for employment-oriented services. Rehabilitation Engineering services for clients/employers.

Computer Training: Wide range of training available.

Low Vision Aids: Provided at cost.

Low Vision Follow-up: Follow-up service for regular clients.

Local Offices:

Miami: SW Seven Court, Vocational Training Unit, Miami, FL 33130, (305) 856-3347.

Florida Center for the Blind Incorporated

7651 SW Highway 200
Suite 502
Ocala, FL 34476-3869
(352) 873-4700
FAX: (352) 873-4751
Marilyn Womble, Director

Type of Agency: Non-profit; educational.

County/District Where Located: Marion County.

Mission: To develop and administer programs for persons who are blind (total/partial), oriented toward rehabilitation and assistance for such persons in adjusting to their environment. This will be accomplished through educational instruction, training in avocations, activities involving physical and social interaction, and emotional adaptive counseling, so as to promote the enhancement of such persons' independence, welfare, lifestyles and individual citizenship productivity.

Funded by: United Way; public funds.

Budget: $350,480.

Hours of Operation: Mon.-Fri. 8:00 AM-4:30 PM.

Program Accessibility: ADA compliant.

Staff: 7.

History/Date: Est. 1987.

Number of Clients Served: 324.

Eligibility: Blind or near blind.

Area Served: Statewide.

Age Requirements: None.

Health: Clients must be able to handle their own personal needs.

Counseling/Social Work/Self-Help: Support groups and adaptive counseling for the blind and their companions.

Rehabilitation: Assistance for the blind in adjusting to their environment, including independant living skills, mobility (use of the white cane), Braille, and use of adaptive aids and appliances.

Employment: Job skills training such as typing, computers with speech, employability and electronic communications skills are offered.

Computer Training: Speech and screen magnification software, scanners, Type-N-Speak and Braille-N-Speak, etc.

Low Vision: Evaluation and referral.

Low Vision Aids: Large display area and hands-on demonstrations of the latest in adaptive aids and appliances for the blind.

Professional Training: Training for FCB volunteers and staff, health care professionals, special education teachers, prison social workers, etc.

Independence for the Blind

7201 North Ninth, Suite A-8
Pensacola, FL 32504
(904) 477-2663
FAX: (904) 479-4025
Dick Cloutier, Executive Director

Type of Agency: Private; non-profit.

County/District Where Located: Escambia County.

Mission: Services for totally blind, legally blind, deaf-blind, multiple handicapped.

Staff: 4 full-time, 2 part-time. Uses volunteers.

History/Date: Est. 1980.

Eligibility: Legally blind; referral through Division of Blind Services.

Transportation: Y.

Health: Refers to other health services.

Educational: Accepts deaf-blind; emotionally disturbed; learning disabled; including those with wheelchairs.

Professional Training: Orientation/mobility.

Reading: Talking book record player; cassette tape player; talking book records and tapes; braille and recorded magazines. Lends braille and large print books.

Rehabilitation: Activities of daily living; braille; gesticulation; handwriting; typing; video magnifier; home management; orientation/mobility; rehabilitation teaching in client's home and community; sensory training.

Recreational: Arts and crafts; special programs for elderly. Refers for other recreation services. Provides consultation to other agencies.

Employment: Assistance in job placement.

Low Vision Aids: Low vision aids and devices.

Independence for the Blind

1278 Paul Russell Road
Tallahassee, FL 32301
(904) 942-3658
FAX: (904) 942-4518
E-mail: blind@noblestar.net
URL: http://www.noblestar.net/~blind
Skip Koch, Executive Director

Type of Agency: Private; non-profit.

County/District Where Located: Leon County.

Mission: Independent living services, vocational services, Assistive Technology.

Funded by: Donations, state contracts, earned income.

Budget: $400,000.

Hours of Operation: Mon.-Fri. 8:00 AM - 5:00 PM.

Program Accessibility: All materials are provided in accessible format; facility is fully accessible.

Staff: 12. Uses volunteers.

History/Date: Est. 1983.

Number of Clients Served: 325.

Eligibility: Legally blind; desire to improve independent living skills and vocational skills.

Area Served: 11 counties of north central Florida.

Age Requirements: 18 years or older.

Health: Referrals for medical services.

Counseling/Social Work/Self-Help: Social evaluation; counseling for individual/group/couples, support groups.

Educational: Adult continuing education; college prep; vocational/skill development.

Professional Training: Speakers Bureau.

Reading: Book selection services; information and referrals; tape recording as requested; closed circuit television, talking computers, large print.

Rehabilitation: Daily living; communication skills; orientation/mobility, on- and off-site, vocational skills.

Recreational: Hobby groups; special programs for the elderly; referrals.

Employment: Career/skill counseling; occupational skill development; refers for placement. Supported employment on-site.

Computer Training: On-site training provided.

Low Vision: Assistive low vision screening.

Low Vision Aids: Sells, lends, rents.

Publications: Annual report and brochures in print, braille, and cassette format.

Independent Living for Adult Blind (ILAB)

c/o Florida Community College at Jacksonville
101 West State Street
Jacksonville, FL 32202
(904) 633-8220
FAX: (904) 632-5107
Rebecca Simpson, Director

Type of Agency: Rehabilitation facility.

Mission: To provide instruction in adjustment to blindness skills to visually impaired adults who wish to improve their level of independence and/or return to work.

Funded by: Florida Division of Blind Services, City of Jacksonville; Florida Community College at Jacksonville; donations.

Budget: $233,000.

Hours of Operation: 8:00 AM - 5:00 PM.

Staff: 4 full time, 6 part time. Uses volunteers.

History/Date: Est. 1971.

Number of Clients Served: 180 annually.

Eligibility: Legal or total blindness; visually impaired; deaf-blind.

Area Served: Duval, Nassua, St. Johns Counties.

Transportation: Y.

Age Requirements: 16 years and older.

Counseling/Social Work/Self-Help: Individual, group and family counseling; referral service.

Rehabilitation: Personal management; orientation/mobility; communications skills; home management. Instruction provided as noncredit supplemental course.

Computer Training: Access training, which includes speech and magnified display software for IBM or compatibles. Offered as noncredit supplemental course.

Low Vision: Low vision screening for nonprescriptive assistive devices.

Lighthouse for the Blind of the Palm Beaches

7810 South Dixie Highway
West Palm Beach, FL 33405
(561) 586-5600
FAX: (561) 586-5630
William S. Thompson, President
Dawn Clemons, Director, Development and Community Relations

Type of Agency: Private; non-profit.

County/District Where Located: Palm Beach County.

Mission: To assist visually impaired persons to develop their capabilities to the fullest.

Funded by: Private donations, including bequests; government grants and fees; sale of products in Industrial Center Program; fee schedule for select services.

Budget: $2.8 million.

Hours of Operation: Mon.-Fri. 8:00 AM - 4:30 PM.

Program Accessibility: Meets accessibility standards.

Staff: 30 full time, 1 part time. Uses volunteers.

History/Date: Est. 1946.

Number of Clients Served: 1995: 6,000.

Eligibility: Blind or visually impaired.

Area Served: Coastal region of Palm Beach, Martin, St. Lucie, Indian River and Okeechobee Counties.

Age Requirements: All ages served; eligibility for some services based on age.

Health: Refers to appropriate health services.

Counseling/Social Work/Self-Help: Individual, family, and group counseling available.; Support groups available.

Preschools: Comprehensive, full-time early intervention and preschool services for blind, visually impaired, and multiply disabled blind children from birth to age 5.

Professional Training: Field work, observations and internships in orientation and mobility, rehabilitation teaching, social work, and special education; public education programs including speaker's bureau, films, demonstrations.

Reading: Refer to talking book, large-print, and braille resources; provides direct instructions in braille and adaptive technology and equipment for reading.

Rehabilitation: Training for persons 55 years and older in home or on-site; personal management, communications skills, orientation/mobility. Information and referral service provided.

Employment: Work evaluations; training, and job placement for Industrial Center, which provides permanent, full-time employment for adults in manufacturing plant. Referral to other job training and placement sites.

Computer Training: Computer skills assessment and computer training; adaptive hardware and software.

Low Vision: Comprehensive low vision evaluation, training, and follow-up.

Low Vision Aids: Prescribed and fitted; training; return policy.

Low Vision Follow-up: By return appointment as needed for further assessment, training, and adjustments.

Lighthouse for the Visually Impaired and Blind

8610 Galen Wilson Boulevard
Port Richey, FL 34668
(813) 815-0303
FAX: (813) 815-0203
Roxann Mayros, Executive Director

Type of Agency: Private; non-profit.

County/District Where Located:
Pasco County.
Mission: Comprehensive rehabilitation.
Funded by: United Way, Board of County Supervisors, Florida Division of Blind Services.
Budget: 1996-97: $400,000.
Hours of Operation: Mon.-Fri. 8:00 AM - 4:30 PM.
Staff: 12; uses volunteers.
History/Date: Est. 1983.
Eligibility: Legally blind; or with a condition leading to blindness.
Area Served: Pasco and Hernando Counties.
Transportation: Y.
Age Requirements: Adults: 14 years and up. Children: 0-5 years.

Counseling/Social Work/Self-Help: Counseling for individuals/groups; refers for school/training placement and community services.
Professional Training: In-service training programs for human services personnel, summer classes, open enrollment, job preparation and transition to workplace.
Rehabilitation: Daily living/communication skills; sensory training.
Recreational: Arts/crafts; hobby groups; programs for elderly; bowling.
Employment: Occupational skill development; supported employment; consultant to other agencies for vocational placement.
Computer Training: Y.
Low Vision: Refers to low vision clinics and services.
Low Vision Aids: Optician works with magnifiers and low vision aids.
Low Vision Follow-up: Training in use of low vision aids.

Local Offices:

Spring Hill: Rehabilitation Center, 7505 Forest Oaks Boulevard, Spring Hill, FL 34606, (352) 666-7007.

Lighthouse of Broward County

650 North Andrews Avenue
Ft. Lauderdale, FL 33311
(954) 463-4217
FAX: (954) 764-3825
Vicki Hersen, Executive Director

Type of Agency: Private; non-profit.
County/District Where Located: Broward County.
Mission: To provide services for totally blind; legally blind; learning disabled blind; mentally retarded blind. To train and rehabilitate persons with vision loss to lead safe, useful, productive, and independent lives.
Funded by: United Way; state Division of Blind Services and county funds; donations.
Budget: 1996: $540,000.
Hours of Operation: Mon.-Fri. 8:00 AM-4:30 PM.
Staff: 14 full time, 2 part time; uses volunteers.
History/Date: Est. 1973.
Number of Clients Served: 1996: 1,866.
Eligibility: Legally blind or impending blindness within 5 years.
Area Served: Broward County.
Transportation: Y.
Age Requirements: Children's camp and outreach: 12 years and under. Week day rehab program: 18 years and up.

Health: Refers for medical services.
Counseling/Social Work/Self-Help: Social evaluation; peer support groups; individual, group, and couple counseling; training placement; referral to community services. Refers for other counseling/social work services.
Educational: Vocational/skill development for persons with vision impairment of all abilities.
Professional Training: Regular in-service training.
Reading: Book selection service; information and referral; transcription to braille; tape recording on demand.
Rehabilitation: Personal management; braille; handwriting; typing; electronic mobility aids; home management; orientation/mobility; rehabilitation teaching in client's home and community; summer youth program.
Recreational: Arts and crafts; hobby groups; special programs for elderly; bowling. Refers for other recreational/leisure services.
Employment: Prevocational evaluation; career and skill counseling; occupational skill development; vocational placement.

Mana-Sota Lighthouse for the Blind

7318 North Tamiami Trail
Sarasota, FL 34243
(941) 359-1404
FAX: (941) 359-2373
E-mail: lighthse2@aol.com
Kathy L. Handra, Director

Type of Agency: Non-profit.
County/District Where Located: Manatee County.
Mission: Services to blind and visually impaired youth and adults.
Funded by: Florida Division of Blind Services, Manatee and Sarasota Counties, and other donations.
Hours of Operation: Mon.-Fri. 8:00 AM to 4:30 PM.
Staff: 8.
History/Date: Est. 1985.

Number of Clients Served: 167 adults, 35 children in 1996.
Eligibility: Legally blind, visually impaired.
Area Served: Sarasota and Manatee Counties.
Transportation: Y.
Age Requirements: None.

Educational: Transitioning into local schools.
Rehabilitation: Instruction in independent living skills and orientation/mobility.
Employment: Vocational evaluation.
Low Vision Aids: For demonstration purposes; none for purchase.

Pinellas Center for the Visually Impaired, Inc. (PCVI)
6925 112th Circle
Suite 103
Largo, FL 33773
(813) 544-4433
FAX: (813) 544-5511
Stephen S. Barrett, Executive Director

Type of Agency: Private; non-profit.
Mission: Services for totally blind, legally blind, and visually impaired persons.
Funded by: State and local contracts, private resources and PCVI Foundation.
Hours of Operation: Mon. - Fri. 8:00 AM - 4:30 PM.
Staff: 35.
Number of Clients Served: 1996: 1,762.
Area Served: Pinellas County.
Transportation: Y.

Counseling/Social Work/Self-Help: Group, individual and family counseling. Support groups. Referrals to community agencies.
Educational: In-service training available to other agencies and

nursing homes. Speakers available for public education.
Reading: Information and referrals for talking record players and cassette players, talking book records and cassettes, large-print books, braille books, closed-circuit TVs. Radio reading service.
Rehabilitation: Personal and home management, braille, handwriting, typing, orientation and mobility training. Services provided at center and in home. Low vision services. KIDS program: early intervention and training, parent education, and counseling.
Recreational: Arts and crafts, social group, speakers and special event activities.
Employment: Vocational services coordinated with local office of the Division of Blind Services. Job placement services.
Low Vision: Low vision clinic providing screening, optometric examinations, training in use of low vision aids and devices.

Tampa Lighthouse for the Blind
1106 West Platt Street
Tampa, FL 33606
(813) 251-2407
FAX: (813) 254-4305
C. E. Olstrom, Executive Director

Type of Agency: Private; non-profit.
Mission: To maximize independence and provide employment opportunities for persons who are blind or visually impaired.
Funded by: State of Florida, purchase of services agreement, industry sales, United Way, contributions.
Budget: 1996: $3,815,000.
Hours of Operation: Mon.-Fri. 8:00 AM - 4:30 PM.
Staff: 30 full-time, 1 part-time. Volunteers.

History/Date: Est. 1940.
Number of Clients Served: 1996: 602.
Eligibility: Adults only; totally blind, legally blind, visually impaired, and multiply impaired blind or visually impaired persons.
Area Served: Primarily Hillsborough and Polk Counties; some surrounding counties.
Transportation: Y.
Age Requirements: 18 and over.

Counseling/Social Work/Self-Help: Social evaluations; counseling: individual, group, family/parent, couple; placement in training; referral to community services. Refers for and provides consultation to other agencies for other counseling/social work.
Rehabilitation: Personal management; braille; handwriting; listening skills; kitchen skills; typing; video magnifier; home management; orientation/mobility; sensory training. Refers for electronic mobility aids. Center-based and community-based instruction.
Recreational: Recreation therapy.
Employment: Prevocational evaluation; career and skill counseling; on-the-job training program; industry program; vocational placement.
Low Vision: Screening; optometric examination; training in use of special aids and devices.
Low Vision Follow-up: Available.

Local Offices:

Lakeland: Lighthouse for the Blind, 3204 Winter Lake Road, Unit 6, Lakeland, FL 33803, (813) 667-1717, FAX (813) 665-4767, Al Garrett, Production Manager, Industries Program.

Winter Haven: Lighthouse for the Blind, 198 Avenue E., N.W., Winter Haven, FL 33881, (941) 299-3633, FAX (241) 299-3559, Robin Whiteley, Supervisor, Rehabilitation Program and Low Vision Clinic.

Visually Impaired Persons of Southwest Florida

P.O. Box 3464
North Ft. Myers, FL 33918-3464
(941) 997-7797
FAX: (941) 997-8462
E-mail: wardol@peganet.com
Marian M. Geiger, Executive Director

Type of Agency: Private; non-profit.
County/District Where Located: Lee County.
Mission: Services for totally blind, legally blind, and visually impaired persons.
Funded by: State grant; county contract; United Way; community funding; private contributions.
Budget: 1996-97: $401,790.
Hours of Operation: Mon.-Thurs. 7:30 AM - 5:00 PM, Fri. 8:30 AM - 12:30 PM.
Staff: 5 full time, 11 part time. Uses volunteers.
History/Date: Est. 1974.
Number of Clients Served: 725.
Eligibility: Severe visual impairment.
Area Served: Southwest Florida.
Transportation: Y.
Age Requirements: Adults.

Health: Recreational therapy. Refers and contracts for other health services. Provides consultation to other agencies.
Counseling/Social Work/Self-Help: Social evaluation; individual, group, family counseling. Refers for other counseling/social work services.

Professional Training: Internship/fieldwork placement; regular in-service program. Public education program, including films, demonstrations, and speakers.
Reading: Lends braille and large-print books; braille and recorded magazines; descriptive videos and recorded books. Book selection service; information and referral; transcription to braille; tape recording services on request; closed circuit television.
Rehabilitation: Activities of daily living; braille; typing; handwriting; remedial education; home management; orientation/mobility; sensory training. Services provided primarily at the center. Refers and provides consultation to other agencies for rehabilitation services.
Recreational: Arts & crafts programs; special interest events; speakers and activities; trips. Weekend programs.
Employment: Job development for computer students.
Computer Training: Training on computer aids and devices. Rehabilitation engineering assistance available.
Low Vision: Low vision clinic providing screening, examination, and training.
Low Vision Aids: Spectacles and low vision aids and devices.
Low Vision Follow-up: Provided as needed.

COMPUTER TRAINING CENTERS

CITE (Center for Independence, Technology and Education)

215 East New Hampshire Street
Orlando, FL 32804
(407) 898-2483
Carol Adams, Director

County/District Where Located: Orange County.

Computer Training: Speech output systems; screen magnification systems; braille access systems; closed-circuit television systems; word processing; database software; computer operating systems.

Training available for both children and adults; wide variety of training for visually impaired and multiply disabled children available.

Division of Blind Services Florida Department of Labor and Employment Security

401 Platt Street
Daytona Beach, FL 32114
(904) 254-3856
FAX: (904) 252-3800
Jerry Little, Supervisor

County/District Where Located: Volusia County.

Computer Training: 2 full-time instructors; training duration: 6 months.

Florida Association of Workers for the Blind

601 S.W. Eighth Avenue
Miami, FL 33130
(305) 856-2288
FAX: (305) 285-6967
E-mail: ellydu@dcfreenet.seflin.lib.fl.us
URL: http://www.the-directory.com/miamilighthouse
Elly du Pré, DPA, Coordinator

County/District Where Located: Dade County.

Computer Training: Speech output systems; screen magnification systems; braille access systems; closed-circuit television systems; word processing; computer operating systems.

Works in conjunction with other training programs for disabled or mainstream persons for additional software training and placement.

Independence for the Blind
1278 Paul Russell Road
Tallahassee, FL 32301
(904) 942-3658
FAX: (904) 942-4518
E-mail: blind@noblestar.net
URL: http://www.noblestar.net/~blind
Jim Breen, Assistive Technology Instructor

County/District Where Located: Leon County.

Computer Training: Speech output systems; screen magnification systems; braille access systems; optical character recognition systems; closed-circuit television systems; word processing; database software; computer operating systems.

Lighthouse for the Blind of the Palm Beaches
7810 South Dixie Highway
West Palm Beach, FL 33405
(407) 586-5600
FAX: (407) 586-5604
Kim Smith, Director of Rehabilitation

County/District Where Located: Palm Beach County.

Computer Training: Training in adaptive hardware and software. Speech output, magnifiers, braille access systems.

Tampa Lighthouse for the Blind
1106 West Platt Street
Tampa, FL 33606
(813) 251-2407
FAX: (813) 254-4305
Sheryl Brown, Supervisor

Computer Training: Speech output systems; screen magnification systems; braille access systems; word processing; database software; computer operating systems.

DOG GUIDE SCHOOLS
Southeastern Guide Dogs, Inc.
4210 77th Street East
Palmetto, FL 34221
(941) 729-5665
FAX: (941) 729-6646
R. Michael Sergeant, Executive Director

Type of Agency: Non-profit.
County/District Where Located: Manatee County.
Mission: Training of dogs and blind individuals for mobility purposes.
Funded by: Private donations, business groups, foundations.
Budget: 1997: $1,000,400.
Hours of Operation: Mon. - Fri. 8:30 AM - 4:30 PM.
Staff: 26 full-time, 13 part-time, plus volunteers.
History/Date: Est. 1982.
Number of Clients Served: Approximately 120 annually.
Eligibility: Blind; good physical health; financial competence to care for a dog.
Area Served: Southeastern U.S.
Age Requirements: 17 years or older.

Reading: Talking book records/tapes; large-print books; braille/recorded magazines; tape recording services on demand.
Rehabilitation: Orientation/mobility; follow-up services/with graduate in home or office area.
Publications: Newsletter printed four times a year.

◆ Low Vision Services

EYE CARE SOCIETIES
Florida Society of Ophthalmology
1133 West Morse Boulevard
Winter Park, FL 32789
(407) 647-8839
Marjorie Stealey, Executive Director

Florida Optometric Association
P.O. Box 13429
Tallahassee, FL 32317
(904) 877-4697
Mark Landreth

LOW VISION CENTERS
Bascom Palmer Eye Institute
Anne Bates Leach Eye Hospital
P.O. Box 016880
Miami, FL 33101
(800) 329-7000 or (305) 326-6136
FAX: (305) 326-6417
Dr. Charles J. Pappas, Director of Optometric Services

Type of Agency: Non-profit.
County/District Where Located: Dade and Palm Beach Counties.
Mission: Improvement of visual function with optical and non-optical devices.
Funded by: Client fees.
Hours of Operation: Mon.-Fri. 8:00 AM-4:30 PM.
Staff: Optometrists; low vision technician.
History/Date: Est. 1976.
Number of Clients Served: 1,200 annually.
Eligibility: Ophthalmology referral.
Area Served: Unlimited.
Transportation: Y.
Age Requirements: None.

Counseling/Social Work/Self-Help: State representative available on premises.
Low Vision Aids: Provided on loan for trial purposes; no rental fee; on-site training provided.
Low Vision Follow-up: By return appointment as necessary, generally 2 weeks follow-up recommended on loaned aids.

Local Offices:

Palm Beach Gardens: Eye Institute, 7108 Fairway Drive, Suite 340, Palm Beach Gardens, FL 33148, (561) 515-1500.

CITE (Center for Independence, Technology and Education) Low Vision Screening and Education Clinic

215 East New Hampshire Street
Orlando, FL 32804
(407) 898-2483
FAX: (407) 895-5255
Carol Adams, Director

Type of Agency: Non-profit.
County/District Where Located: Orange County.
Mission: To provide quality services, education, and training to the community to enhance the lives of people with visual impairments, blindness and multiple disabilities.
Funded by: Federal and public funds, private donations.
Budget: $305,615.
Hours of Operation: Mon.-Fri. 8:00 AM-5:00 PM.
Program Accessibility: ADA compliant.
Staff: Adaptive technology specialist; orientation/mobility instructor; optometrist; rehabilitation counselor; social worker; special educator; recreation programmer.
History/Date: Est. 1976.
Number of Clients Served: 1,043.

Eligibility: Referral; current ophthalmological or optometric report.
Area Served: Unlimited for technology program. Central Florida for independent living skills program for adults who are blind.
Transportation: Y.
Age Requirements: None.

Reading: Mail- and newspaper-reading service.
Rehabilitation: 15-week training program for adults who are blind/visually impaired.
Recreational: Leisure activities training program.
Employment: Limited assistance with preemployment skills.
Computer Training: Access; training; assistive technology.
Low Vision: Screening and clinic.
Low Vision Aids: Provided on loan for trial purpose at no charge; on-site, in-home or office training provided.
Low Vision Follow-up: Varies according to patient.

Halifax Hospital Medical Center Eye Clinic

303 North Clyde Morris Boulevard
Suite 100
Daytona Beach, FL 32114
(904) 254-4103
James W. Clower, M.D.
Margaret Davis, Orthopist

County/District Where Located: Volusia County.
Mission: To provide complete work-ups including specialized testing in an attempt to aid the patient with various high-powered telescopic lenses, microscopic lenses, prisms, high plus lenses, stand and hand magnifiers, closed circuit TV readers.
Funded by: Client fees.
Hours of Operation: Mon.-Fri. 8:00 AM-4:00 PM, By appointment.

Staff: Ophthalmologist; orthoptist, RNs.
Eligibility: Referred by an ophthalmologic report.
Area Served: Unlimited.

Counseling/Social Work/Self-Help: Social workers available in the medical center. Assistance, counseling, and training in the use of the low vision aids is given.
Low Vision: Comprehensive services.
Low Vision Aids: Provided on loan for trial purposes; on-site training provided.
Low Vision Follow-up: Immediate and as needed.

Hope Haven Children's Clinic Low Vision Clinic

4600 Beach Boulevard
P.O. Box 17607
Jacksonville, FL 32207
(904) 346-5100
Thomas Quinlan, Director
Jean Brightwell, Administrative Coordinator

Type of Agency: Non-profit.
County/District Where Located: Duval County.
Funded by: Client fees; foundations.
Eligibility: All ages, children through 18; generally visual acuity of 20/70 or less; opthalmological exam within the last year.
Area Served: Unlimited.

Financial assistance available to children.

Lighthouse for the Blind of the Palm Beaches

7810 South Dixie Highway
West Palm Beach, FL 33405
(561) 586-5600
FAX: (561) 586-5604
Michelle DeJisi, Low Vision Counselor

Type of Agency: Private; non-profit.
Mission: To assist blind and visually impaired persons to develop their capabilities to the fullest.
Funded by: Private donations, including bequests; government grants and fees; sale of products provided in Industries Program; and fee schedule for select services.
Budget: 1995: $1.6 million.
Hours of Operation: Mon.-Fri. 8:00 AM-4:30 PM.
Program Accessibility: Meets accessibility standards.
Staff: Low vision counselor and optometrist.
History/Date: Est. 1988.
Number of Clients Served: 1995: 972.
Eligibility: Blind or visually impaired.
Area Served: 5 counties; Palm Beach, Martin, Indian River, Okeechobee and St. Lucie.

Counseling/Social Work/Self-Help: Individual and family.
Professional Training: Internships, field study, in-service training.
Rehabilitation: Vision rehabilitation, referral, and coordination to other rehabilitation services, including orientation and mobility, and rehabilitation teaching.
Employment: Coordination with job placement counselor.
Low Vision: Comprehensive low vision evaluation, training, and follow-up.
Low Vision Aids: Prescribed and fitted; training; return policy.
Low Vision Follow-up: By return appointment as needed for further assessment, training, and adjustments.

Low Vision Center
Tampa Lighthouse for the Blind
1106 West Platt Street
Tampa, FL 33606
(813) 251-2407
FAX: (813) 254-4305
Sheryl Brown, Supervisor

Type of Agency: Non-profit.
County/District Where Located: Hillsborough County.
Mission: To maximize independence and provide employment opportunities for persons who are blind of visually impaired.
Funded by: Division of Blind Services, United Way, and contributions.
Hours of Operation: 8:00 AM-5:00 PM.
Staff: Optometrists; low vision technician.
Age Requirements: None.

Low Vision: Screening; optometric examinations; training in the use of special aids and devices.
Low Vision Aids: Available for sale.
Low Vision Follow-up: Available.

University of Florida
Eye Center, Low Vision Service
Box 100284, JHMHC
University of Florida College of Medicine
Gainesville, FL 32610
(352) 392-3451
G. M. Hope, Ph.D., Director, Low Vision Services

County/District Where Located: Alachua County.
Funded by: Client fees, state government.
Hours of Operation: Tues. and Thurs.
Staff: Department of Ophthalmology.
Eligibility: Referrals.

Area Served: Unlimited.

Low Vision Aids: On-site training in low-vision devices.
Low Vision Follow-up: Varies.

Veterans Administration Hospital
Low Vision Service, Eye Clinic
13000 Bruce B. Downs Boulevard
Tampa, FL 33612
(813) 972-7674
FAX: (813) 822-7570
Ken Tayant, Coordinator

County/District Where Located: Hillsborough County.
Mission: Veteran health and eye care.
Funded by: Federal government.
Hours of Operation: 2 days per month, by appointment only.
Staff: Ophthalmologist; ophthalmology resident; social worker; orientation/mobility instructor; rehabilitation teacher; special educator; occupational therapist; psychologist/counselor; rehabilitation counselor; audiologist.
Eligibility: Veteran; referral only.

Low Vision Aids: On loan for trial purposes; no rental charges; on-site training provided.
Low Vision Follow-up: By return appointment as needed.

◆ *Aging Services*

STATE UNITS ON AGING

Florida Department of Elder Affairs
4040 Esplanade Way
Building B, Suite 152
Tallahassee, FL 32399
(904) 414-2000
FAX: (904) 414-2002
Bentley Lipscomb, Secretary

Provides referrals to Area Agencies on Aging and information on other local aging services.

INDEPENDENT LIVING PROGRAMS

Florida Division of Blind Services

2551 Executive Center Circle
Tallahassee, FL 32399
(904) 488-1330 or (800) 342-1828
Marie Beauford, Bureau Chief

Provides independent living services for persons age 55 and over. For further information, contact the Project Director or general phone number listed.

GEORGIA

◆ *Educational Services*

STATE SERVICES

Georgia State Department of Education
Division of Exceptional Students
1870 Twin Towers East
Atlanta, GA 30334-5040
(404) 656-6317
Paulette Bragg, Director, Division for Exceptional Students,
(404) 656-3963
Marlene Bryar, Coordinator, Low Incidence
Ron Colarusso, Director of Special Education, Georgia State University, Urban Life Plaza, Atlanta, GA 30303, (404) 658-2310
Mary Phagan, Consultant
Toni Waylor-Bowen, Consultant, Pre-School

Type of Agency: State Department of Education.
County/District Where Located: Fulton County.
Mission: Provides consultation on educational services for local schools.
Funded by: Public funds.
History/Date: Est. 1951.
Area Served: Georgia.

Purchases and distributes braille and large-type books and materials.

Contact local school superintendent for program availability.

EARLY INTERVENTION COORDINATION

Early Intervention Programs
Division of Public Health
Georgia Department of Human Resources
Two Peachtree Street
Room 7-315
Atlanta, GA 30303
(404) 657-2727
FAX: (404) 657-2763
Eve Bogan, Director
Wendy Sanders, Early Childhood Coordinator

County/District Where Located: Fulton County.

SCHOOLS

Georgia Academy for the Blind
2895 Vineville Avenue
Macon, GA 31204
(912) 751-6083
FAX: (912) 751-6659
E-mail: gablib@mindscreen.com
Richard E. Hyer, Jr., Superintendent

Type of Agency: State.
County/District Where Located: Bibb County.
Mission: To provide educational opportunities to visually impaired and multiply disabled school age students.
Funded by: State and federal funding.
Hours of Operation: 24 hours a day.
Program Accessibility: Fully accessible.
Staff: 132 full time. Uses volunteers.
History/Date: Est. 1852.
Number of Clients Served: 175.
Eligibility: Resident of Georgia; legally blind or legally blind-multiply disabled; mentally impaired; hearing impaired.
Area Served: Georgia.

Transportation: Y.
Age Requirements: 3-21 years.
Health: Spectacles or low vision aids or devices. General medical services; occupational and physical therapy; speech therapy. Refers for other health services.
Counseling/Social Work/Self-Help: Social evaluation; psychological testing and evaluation; individual, group, family/parent counseling; placement in school. Provides consultation to other agencies. Refers to community services.
Educational: Grades K through 12. Accepts the visually impaired and visually impaired-multiply disabled. Programs for college prep; general academic; vocational/skill development.
Preschools: For children aged 3 and 4.
Professional Training: Internship/fieldwork placement in orientation/mobility; rehabilitation counseling; social work; special education; vocational rehabilitation.
Reading: Talking book record players and cassette players; talking book records and cassettes; braille books; large-print books; braille magazines; recorded magazines. Transcription to braille; book selection services; Optacon and Kurzweil Reading Machine.
Residential: Dormitories are available for students.
Rehabilitation: Personal management; handwriting; listening skills; typing; home management; orientation/mobility; remedial education; sensory training.
Recreational: Afterschool programs; arts and crafts; bowling; swimming; track; wrestling; softball; indoor games; cheerleading; intramural sports; scouting.

Employment: Prevocational and vocational evaluation; career counseling; occupational skill development; vocational placement. Refers for noncompetitive settings through rehabilitation services.
Computer Training: Y.
Low Vision: Y.
Low Vision Aids: Y.
Low Vision Follow-up: Y.

INFANT AND PRESCHOOL

**BEGIN
(Babies Early Growth
Intervention Network)
Center for the Visually Impaired**
763 Peachtree Street, N.E.
Atlanta, GA 30308
(404) 875-9011
FAX: (404) 607-0062
Anne McComiskey, Program
Director

Type of Agency: Full Service; rehabilitation.
County/District Where Located: Fulton County.
Mission: Support through information and skill development.
Funded by: Public and private monies.
Hours of Operation: Mon.-Fri. 8:00 AM-5:00 PM.
Staff: 3 full time, 5 part time. Uses volunteers.
History/Date: Est. 1985.
Eligibility: Blind or severely visually impaired.
Age Requirements: Birth to age 5.

Counseling/Social Work/Self-Help: Counseling, support, and information for parents and families.
Educational: Early intervention services for children designed to provide stimulation and growth in all developmental areas. Center-based and home-based services available.

Computer Training: Introduction to technology skills.
Low Vision: Low vision clinic.
Low Vision Aids: For sale and for loan.
Low Vision Follow-up: As needed.

STATEWIDE OUTREACH SERVICES

Georgia Academy for the Blind
2895 Vineville Avenue
Macon, GA 31204
(912) 751-6083
FAX: (912) 751-6659
E-mail: gablib@mindscreen.com
Faye Mullis Taylor, Contact Person

County/District Where Located: Bibb County.
Funded by: State and federal funds.
History/Date: Est. 1852.
Age Requirements: 3-22 years.

Assessment: Comprehensive psychoeducational evaluation for visually impaired students.
Consultation to Public Schools: Provides ongoing consultation/technical assistance to local school systems; an annual workshop for teachers of the visually impaired; quarterly newsletters to teachers of the visually impaired.
Direct Service: Educational placement; psychoeducational evaluations for students who attend schools in the local educational agency (LEA). All braille and large-print books for legally blind students in Georgia are ordered through the LEA Resource Center at the academy.
Parent Assistance: As needed or requested. Parents of academy students and of students in public school are provided information about technology for visually impaired, special parent workshops, summer camps, and educational programs.

Materials Production: For use by students enrolled at the academy; achievement tests are thermoformed and distributed to the LEA.
Professional Training: Teachers, instructional aides, and houseparents receive ongoing staff development to receive appropriate certification.

INSTRUCTIONAL MATERIALS CENTERS

LEA Resource Center
2895 Vineville Avenue
Macon, GA 31204
(912) 751-6096
FAX: (912) 751-6659
Marie Amerson, Teacher/Consultant

County/District Where Located: Bibb County.
Area Served: Georgia.
Groups Served: K-12.

Types/Content: Textbooks.
Media Formats: Braille books, large print books.
Title Listings: An inventory listing of braille and large-print textbooks is produced annually for titles available within the state.

Acts as a clearinghouse rather than a depository.

UNIVERSITY TRAINING PROGRAMS

Georgia State University
Department of Special Education
Atlanta, GA 30303
(404) 651-2310
Dr. Kathryn Heller, Project Director

County/District Where Located: Fulton County.

Programs Offered: Graduate (master's) program in visual impairment; add-on certification in visual impairment.

♦ Information Services

LIBRARIES

Albany Library for the Blind and Handicapped

Dougherty County Public Library
300 Pine Avenue
Albany, GA 31701
(912) 430-1920
FAX: (912) 430-4020
Kathryn R. Sinquefield, Librarian

Subregional library.

Bainbridge Subregional Library for the Blind and Physically Handicapped

301 South Monroe Street
Bainbridge, GA 31717
(912) 248-2665
FAX: (912) 248-2670
Lisa Reeves, Librarian

Subregional library.

La Fayette Subregional Library for the Blind and Physically Handicapped

P.O. Box 707
La Fayette, GA 30728
(706) 638-2992
FAX: (706) 638-4028
Lecia Eubanks, Librarian

Subregional library.

Georgia Regional Library for the Blind and Physically Handicapped

Georgia Department of Technical and Adult Education
1150 Murphy Avenue, S.W.
Atlanta, GA 30310
(404) 756-4619
FAX: (404) 756-4618
Linda Koldenhoven, Regional Librarian-Consultant

Mission: Provide general library service to eligible readers as part of the network of libraries

cooperating with the Library of Congess, National Library Service for the Blind and Physically Handicapped.
Funded by: Public funds.
Hours of Operation: Mon.-Fri. 8:00 AM-5:00 PM.
Staff: 5 full-time equivalents.
History/Date: Est. 1933.
Number of Clients Served: 2,200.
Eligibility: Requirements established by the National Library Service for the Blind and Physically Handicapped.
Area Served: Georgia.
Age Requirements: None.

Regional library supplying talking books, braille books, cassettes, taped books, talking book machines, and cassette machines. Coordinates talking book centers in 13 public libraries.

Library for the Blind and Physically Handicapped

Oconee Regional Library
P.O. Box 100
Dublin, GA 31021
(912) 272-5710
Patricia Fries, Librarian

Subregional library.

Library for the Blind and Physically Handicapped

127 Main Street N.W.
Gainsville, GA 30501
(770) 532-3311
FAX: (770) 532-4305
Sandra Whitmer, Librarian

Subregional library.

Macon Subregional Library for the Blind and Physically Handicapped

Washington Memorial Library
1180 Washington Avenue

Macon, GA 31201-1790
(912) 744-0850 or (912) 744-0877
FAX: (912) 744-0840
Rebecca Sherrill

Subregional library.

Rome Subregional Library for the Blind and Physically Handicapped

Sarah Hightower Regional Library
205 Riverside Parkway
Rome, GA 30161-2913
(706) 236-4609
FAX: (706) 236-4631
Diana Mills, Librarian

Subregional library.

Subregional Library for the Blind and Physically Handicapped

CEL Regional Library
2002 Bull Street
Savannah, GA 31499
(912) 652-3600
FAX: (912) 652-3638
Linda Stokes, Librarian

Subregional library.

Subregional Library for the Blind and Physically Handicapped

South Georgia Regional Library
300 Woodrow Wilson Drive
Valdosta, GA 31602-2592
(912) 333-5285
FAX: (912) 245-6483
Sharon Bernstein, Librarian

Type of Agency: Sub-regional branch of the National Library for the Blind and Physically Handicapped.
County/District Where Located: Lownds County.
Mission: To provide library services for persons unable to use standard print.
Funded by: Federal, state, and local governments.

Hours of Operation: Mon.-Thurs. 9:30 AM-6.00 PM, Fri. 9:30-5:30.
Staff: 1 full time, 1 part time.
Number of Clients Served: Approximately 500.
Eligibility: Inability to use standard print.
Area Served: 12 counties in central-southern Georgia.

Reading: Books and magazines on tape and record.

Subregional Library for the Blind and Physically Handicapped Talking Book Center

1120 Bradley Drive
Columbus, GA 31906
(706) 649-0780, ext. 22 or 23
FAX: (706) 649-1914
M. Holden-Head, Librarian

Subregional library.

Talking Book Center

Athens Regional Library
2025 Baxter Street
Atlanta, GA 30606
(706) 613-3650 or TDD (706) 613-3669
FAX: (706) 613-3660
Janet Wright, Librarian

Subregional library.

Talking Book Center

Augusta-Richmond County Public Library
902 Greene Street
Augusta, GA 30901
(706) 821-2600
FAX: (706) 724-5403
Gary Swint, Librarian

Subregional library.

Talking Book Center

Brunswick-Glynn County Regional Library
208 Gloucester Street
Brunswick, GA 31523
(912) 267-1212
Betty Ransom, Librarian

Subregional library.

MEDIA PRODUCTION SERVICES

Atlanta Braille Volunteers

5395 Laithbank Lane
Alpharetta, GA 30202
(770) 242-8424
Ruth Koloski

Groups Served: K-12; college students; other adults.

Types/Content: Textbooks; recreational; career/vocational; religious; menus; legal.
Media Formats: Braille books.

DeKalb County School System

Department of Special Services
Jim Cherry Center
2415-B North Druid Hills Road, N.E.
Atlanta, GA 30329
(404) 325-3011
FAX: (404) 633-7005
Phyllis Cole, Coordinator, Visually Impaired and Orthopedically Impaired Programs

County/District Where Located: DeKalb County.
Groups Served: Blind, visually impaired, and multiply disabled children whose visual impairment interferes with functioning in a regular school program.

Types/Content: None specified.
Media Formats: Braille books, talking books/cassettes, large-print books.
Title Listings: None specified.

Georgia Division of Rehabilitation Services

Two Peachtree Street, N.W.
35th Floor
Atlanta, GA 30303-3166
(404) 657-3071
FAX: (404) 657-3086
Peggy Rosser, Program Coordinator, Blind and Visually Impaired Program

County/District Where Located: Fulton County.
Area Served: Georgia.
Groups Served: Adults.

Types/Content: Vocational and independent living rehabilitation services.
Media Formats: None specified.
Title Listings: No title listings available.

NEGA RESA

375 Winter Street
Winterville, GA 30683
(706) 542-7675
FAX: (706) 742-8928
Raymond Akridge, Director

County/District Where Located: Clark County.
Area Served: 13 school systems in northeastern Georgia.
Groups Served: K-12.

Types/Content: Textbooks.
Media Formats: Braille books, talking books/cassettes, large-print books.
Title Listings: No title listings available.

Recording for the Blind and Dyslexic

120 Florida Avenue
Athens, GA 30605
(706) 549-1313
FAX: (706) 227-6161
Sandra Flowers, Executive Director
John Marshall, Studio Director

See Recording for the Blind and Dyslexic in U.S. national listings.

**Roosevelt Warm Springs
Institute for Rehabilitation**
P.O. Box 1000
Warm Springs, GA 31830
(706) 655-5001
FAX: (706) 655-5011
Frank C. Ruzycki, Director

County/District Where Located:
Meriwether County.
Groups Served: None specified.

Types/Content: None specified.
Media Formats: Braille books,
talking books/cassettes, large-
print books.
Title Listings: None specified.

Talking Book Center
2025 Baxter Street
Athens, GA 30606
(706) 613-3650
FAX: (706) 613-3660
Janet Wright, TBC Director

County/District Where Located:
Clarke County.
Area Served: 16 counties of
northeastern Georgia.
Groups Served: K-12; college
students; other adults.

Types/Content: Recreational;
career/vocational; religious;
general.
Media Formats: Talking books/
cassettes.
Title Listings: Print and braille
lists available at no charge.

RADIO READING

**Central Savannah River Area
Radio Reading Service, Inc.**
c/o WACG-FM, Augusta State
University
2500 Walton Way
Augusta, GA 30904-2200
(706) 737-1661
FAX: (706) 737-1773
Nancy Fominaya, Coordinator

County/District Where Located:
Richmond County.

Hours of Operation: Mon.-Fri.
9:00 AM-12:00 noon.
History/Date: Est. 1978.
Area Served: 90-mile radius from
Augusta.

**Georgia Radio Reading Service,
Inc.**
2581 Piedmont Road, N.E.
Suite C 1148
Atlanta, GA 30324
(404) 814-0222
Jim Cashin, Executive Director

Hours of Operation: 24 hours
daily.
History/Date: Est. 1980.
Area Served: Atlanta metropolitan
area: 100 miles to the south; 70
miles to the north and west; 30
miles to the east.

**Georgia Radio Reading Service,
Inc.**
409 East Liberty Street
Savannah, GA 31401
(912) 233-2822
Trish Coder, Director

Type of Agency: Private; non-
profit.
County/District Where Located:
Chatham County.
Funded by: Government grants,
private foundations, community
service organizations.
Hours of Operation: 8:00 AM -
12:30 PM; 6-8PM.
Staff: 2 full-time and 70
volunteers.
History/Date: Est. 1986.
Area Served: Coastal Georgia and
South Carolina.
Age Requirements: None.

INFORMATION AND REFERRAL

**American Foundation for the
Blind Southeast**
100 Peachtree Street
Suite 620

Atlanta, GA 30303
(404) 525-2303
FAX: (404) 659-6957
E-mail: atlanta@afb.org
URL: http://www.afb.org

See American Foundation for the
Blind in U.S. national listings.

**The Foundation Fighting
Blindness
Atlanta Affiliate**
4442 Dobbs Crossing
Marietta, GA 30068
(404) 885-9084 or (404) 889-9084
Judy Parker, President

See The Foundation Fighting
Blindness in U.S. national listings.

Prevent Blindness Georgia
455 East Paces Ferry Road/Suite
222
Atlanta, GA 30305
(404) 266-0071
FAX: (404) 266-0860
E-mail: 104708.1102@compuserve.
com
Jenny Pomeroy, Executive Director

County/District Where Located:
Fulton County.

See Prevent Blindness America in
U.S. national listings.

◆ Rehabilitation Services

STATE SERVICES

**Georgia Division of
Rehabilitation Services**
Two Peachtree Street, N.W.
35th Floor

Atlanta, GA 30303-3166
(404) 657-3000
FAX: (404) 657-3079
Peggy Rosser, Program
Coordinator, Blind and Visually
Impaired Program
Leon Parham, Resource
Development Representative

Type of Agency: State.
County/District Where Located:
Fulton County.
Mission: To help persons with
disabilities to find employment.
Funded by: Public funds.
Hours of Operation: Mon.-Fri.
8:00 AM-5:00 PM.
Area Served: Statewide.

Employment: Vocational
counseling, vocational training,
vocational placement, related
services.

Local Offices:

Albany: Office of Rehabilitation
Services, 110 Pine Avenue, P.O.
Box 1606, Albany, GA 31702,
(912) 430-4170.
Americus: Office of Rehabilitation
Services, 1604-C Vienna Highway,
Americus, GA 31709, (912) 931-
2516.
Athens: Office of Rehabilitation
Services, 125 Athens West
Parkway, Athens, GA 30606,
(706) 354-3900.
Atlanta: Office of Rehabilitation
Services, 1800 Peachtree Street,
N.W., Atlanta, GA 30309,
(404) 350-4700.
Augusta: Office of Rehabilitation
Services, 1727 Wrightsboro Road,
P.O. Box 12007, Augusta, GA
30914, (770) 737-1808.
Bainbridge: Office of
Rehabilitation Services, 502 West
Shotwell Street, Bainbridge, GA
31717, (912) 248-2480.
Baxley: 605-B South Main Street,
Baxley, GA 31513, (912) 367-9259.

Blairsville: 189 Rogers Street,
Blairsville, GA 30514, (706) 745-
5112.
Brunswick: Office of
Rehabilitation Services, 106
Shopper's Way, Brunswick, GA
31520, (912) 264-7287.
Canton: 3049 Marietta Highway,
Suite 130, Canton, GA 30114,
(770) 720-3570.
Carrollton: Office of
Rehabilitation Services, 1512 North
Highway 27, Carrollton, GA 30117,
(404) 836-6681.
Clarkesville: Office of
Rehabilitation Services, 103
Professional Park, P.O. Box 395,
Clarkesville, GA 30523, (706) 754-
6215.
Columbus: Office of
Rehabilitation Services, 233 12th
Street, Suite 700, P.O. Box 2863,
Columbus, GA 31902, (706) 649-
7400.
Dalton: Office of Rehabilitation
Services, 1615 Hickory Street,
Dalton, GA 30720, (706) 272-2303.
Decatur: Office of Rehabilitation
Services, New First National Bank
Building, Room 255, 315 West
Ponce de Leon Avenue, Decatur,
GA 30030, (404) 370-5140.
Douglasville: 4600 Timber Ridge
Drive, Room 319, Douglasville, GA
30135, (770) 489-3018.
Dublin: Office of Rehabilitation
Services, 904 Claxton Dairy Road,
P.O. Box 158, Dublin, GA 31040,
(912) 275-6519.
Eastman: 107 College Street,
Eastman, GA 31023, (912) 374-
6841.
East Point: 2801 R.N. Martin
Street, East Point, GA 30344,
(404) 669-3450.
Gainesville: Office of
Rehabilitation Services, 440 Enota
Drive, N.E., Gainesville, GA 30501,
(770) 535-5468.
Gracewood: P.O. Box 28,
Gracewood, GA 30812, (706) 790-
2105.

Griffin: Office of Rehabilitation
Services, 231-C South 10th Street,
Griffin, GA 30224, (770) 229-3140.
Hapeville: 3420 Norman Berry
Parkway, Hapeville, GA 30354,
(404) 669-3900.
Hinesville: P.O. Box 25,
Hinesville, GA 31313, (912) 876-
9338.
Jonesboro: 409 Arrowhead
Boulevard, Jonesboro, GA 30236,
(770) 473-2462.
Lafayette: P.O. Box 927, Lafayette,
GA 30728, (706) 638-5536.
LaGrange: 120-A Gordon
Commercial Drive, LaGrange, GA
30240, (706) 845-4025.
Macon: Office of Rehabilitation
Services, 711 Riverside Drive, P.O.
Box 6117, Macon, GA 31208,
(912) 751-6413.
Marietta: Office of Rehabilitation
Services, 2225 Northwest Parkway,
Marietta, GA 30067, (770) 916-2250.
Milledgeville: Office of
Rehabilitation Services, 2930
Heritage Place, Milledgeville, GA
31061, (912) 453-4781.
Newnan: Office of Rehabilitation
Services, 29 Farmer Industrial
Boulevard, Newnan, GA 30263,
(770) 254-7210.
Perry: 757 Carroll Street, Perry,
GA 31069, (912) 987-2286.
Reidsville: 108-B South Main
Street, Reidsville, GA 30453,
(912) 557-7558.
Rome: Office of Rehabilitation
Services, 404 South Broad Street,
Rome, GA 30161, (706) 295-6400.
Royston: 200 Bond Street,
Royston, GA 30662, (706) 245-7708.
Savannah: Office of Rehabilitation
Services, 420 Mall Boulevard, P.O.
Box 13427, Savannah, GA 31416,
(912) 356-2134.
Statesboro: 117 Savannah Avenue,
Statesboro, GA 30459, (912) 871-
1173.
Swainsboro: 536 South Main, P.O.
Box 660, Swainsboro, GA 30401,
(912) 237-7841.

Thomasville: Office of Rehabilitation Services, 1317 East Jackson Street, Thomasville, GA 31792, (912) 225-4045.

Tifton: 820 Love Avenue, Tifton, GA 31793, (912) 386-3522.

Valdosta: Office of Rehabilitation Services, 2517-A Bemiss Road, Valdosta, GA 31602, (912) 333-5248.

Waycross: Office of Rehabilitation Services, 2311 Knight Avenue, P.O. Box 2026, Waycross, GA 31502, (912) 285-6078.

REHABILITATION

Augusta Blind Rehabilitation Center
U. S. Department of Veterans Affairs

VA Medical Center
One Freedom Way
Augusta, GA 30904-6285
(706) 733-0188
FAX: (706) 481-6703
Penny Schuckers, Director

Type of Agency: Federal.
Mission: Provides residential rehabilitation services to eligible legally blind veterans.
Funded by: U. S. Department of Veterans Affairs.

Referral applications by Visual Impairment Services Programs located at VA Medical Centers and Outpatient Clinics in the geographical area served by the Blind Rehabilitation Center or Clinic.

See U. S. Department of Veterans Affairs in U. S. Federal Agencies listings.

Blind and Low Vision Services of North Georgia

3830 South Cobb Drive
Suite 125
Smyrna, GA 30080
(770) 432-7280
FAX: (770) 432-5457
Dr. Robert Crouse, Executive Director

Type of Agency: Private; non-profit.
County/District Where Located: Cobb County.
Mission: To assist persons who are blind or visually impaired to function independently in their environments.
Funded by: Public funds, United Way, grants, fees, and contributions.
Hours of Operation: 8:30 AM-4:30 PM.
Program Accessibility: Facility is totally accessible.
Staff: 5 staff and a large group of volunteers.
History/Date: Est. 1983.
Number of Clients Served: More than 250 annually.
Eligibility: Visual impairment; legally blind and totally blind.
Area Served: Primarily north Georgia; no geographic restrictions.
Transportation: Y.
Age Requirements: None; usually school age through senior citizens.

Health: Low vision clinic and training, activities coordinated with other health-related facilities.
Counseling/Social Work/Self-Help: Individual and family counseling provided. Coordination and consultation with mental health and social service agencies.
Educational: Remedial and basic education.
Reading: Reader services on request; information and referral.
Rehabilitation: Orientation/mobility; personal management; communications; independent living skills (services are provided at the center and in community environments).

Recreational: Coordinate activities with other agencies.
Employment: Counseling and coordination with Division of Rehabilitation services; prevocational training and vocational evaluation.
Computer Training: Access to and training on computer aids and devices.
Low Vision: Comprehensive low vision clinic.
Low Vision Aids: Prescriptions, dispensing and training.
Low Vision Follow-up: As needed, at least semi-annually.

Center for the Visually Impaired

763 Peachtree Street, N.E.
Atlanta, GA 30308
(404) 875-9011
FAX: (404) 607-0062
Scott McCall, Executive Director

Type of Agency: Private; non-profit.
County/District Where Located: Fulton County.
Mission: Independence with dignity.
Funded by: United Way, public funds, fees and foundation grants.
Budget: $2.5 million.
Hours of Operation: 8:00 AM-4:30 PM.
Staff: 40 full time, 10 part time.
History/Date: Est. 1973.
Number of Clients Served: 1995-96 fiscal year: 1,467 Information and referral calls: 1,669.
Eligibility: Legally blind or severely visually impaired.
Area Served: Statewide.
Age Requirements: None.

Health: Low vision clinic and training services.
Counseling/Social Work/Self-Help: Consultation and referral services; individual, group, and family counseling.

Educational: Remedial education; high school equivalency.
Preschools: "Begin" program for preschool children.
Reading: Reader services; tape recording on request; information and referral.
Rehabilitation: Orientation/ mobility; personal management; communications; community-based rehabilitation program for older persons and home-bound blind persons.
Recreational: Arts, crafts, games, physical conditioning.
Employment: Vocational evaluation; prevocational training; work adjustment program; job development and placement.
Computer Training: Access; training on computer aids and devices.
Low Vision: Comprehensive low vision services.
Low Vision Aids: Optical and nonoptical aids.
Low Vision Follow-up: Y.

Georgia Industries for the Blind

P.O. Box 218
Bainbridge, GA 31718-0218
(912) 248-2666
FAX: (912) 248-2669
Lane Whitley, Executive Director

Type of Agency: State.
Mission: Provide employment opportunities to severely visually impaired individuals.
Funded by: Sales of products.
Staff: 30 full time.
History/Date: Est. 1949.
Eligibility: Legally blind. Under 18 must be cleared by school superintendent. Services for totally blind, legally blind, deaf-blind clients.
Transportation: Y.
Health: Refers for health services.

Counseling/Social Work/Self-Help: Refers for counseling/social work.
Rehabilitation: Refers for rehabilitation services.
Recreational: Arts and crafts, hobby groups. Contracts for other recreational services.
Employment: Sheltered workshop.

Local Offices:

Atlanta: Georgia Industries for the Blind, 1080 Sylvan Road, Atlanta, GA 30310, (404) 756-4485.
Bainbridge: Georgia Industries for the Blind, P.O. Box 218, Bainbridge, GA 31717, Jim Turknett, Plant Manager, (912) 248-2666.
Griffin: Georgia Industries for the Blind, Emlet Drive, P.O. Box 98, Griffin, GA 30224, (770) 228-7221, FAX (770) 229-3311, Al Hardy, Plant Manager, (770) 288-7221.
Savannah: Georgia Industries for the Blind, 100 Aberdeen Street, P.O. Box 3672, Savannah, GA 31414, (912) 234-8220.

Georgia Lions Lighthouse Foundation, Inc.

1775 Clairmont Road
Decatur, GA 30033-4005
(404) 325-3630
FAX: (404) 636-5549
Linda Bassett, Executive Director

Type of Agency: Non-profit.
Mission: Provides eye examinations, eye treatments, eye surgery, eyeglasses, and hearing aids to needy residents of Georgia. Also provides information and referral.
Funded by: Contributions from the Lions Clubs of the state of Georgia, public donations, memorial contributions.
Budget: $750,000.
Hours of Operation: Mon.-Fri. 8:30 AM - 4:30 PM.

Staff: 5 full time, 1 part time.
History/Date: Inc. 1949.
Number of Clients Served: 5,000 annually.
Eligibility: Residents of Georgia.
Area Served: Georgia.

Goodwill Industries of the Coastal Empire, Inc.

7220 Sallie Mood Drive
P.O. Box 15007
Savannah, GA 31416
(912) 354-6611
FAX: (912) 354-3787
Robert A. Lapsley, President
Brian C. Reynolds, Director of Rehabilitation

Type of Agency: Private; non-profit.
County/District Where Located: Chatham County.
Mission: Services for totally blind, legally blind, visually impaired, learning disabled, mentally retarded, physically and emotionally disabled.
Funded by: United Way; self-generated revenue.
Budget: $4.5 million.
Hours of Operation: 8:00 AM - 5:00 PM.
Program Accessibility: Fully accessible.
Staff: 25 full time.
History/Date: Est. 1965.
Number of Clients Served: 500 annually.
Eligibility: 16 years or older; able to care for self.
Area Served: 29 counties of southeast Georgia and 3 in South Carolina.
Age Requirements: 16 years of age and older.

Counseling/Social Work/Self-Help: Social evaluations; individual counseling; referrals to community services; referrals to other counseling/social work services.

Educational: Literacy training.
Reading: Talking book record player and cassette player; talking book records and cassettes.
Rehabilitation: Vocational assessments; work-habit training; job placement.
Employment: Prevocational evaluation; career and skill counseling; occupational skill development; job retention; job retraining; sheltered workshops; vocational placement; follow-up service; refers for vending stand training.

Helen Keller National Center for Deaf-Blind Youths and Adults Southeast Region Office
1005 Virginia Avenue
Suite 104
Atlanta, GA 30354
(404) 766-9625 or TDD (404) 766-2320
FAX: (404) 766-3447
Susan Brooks, Regional Representative

County/District Where Located: Fulton County.
Eligibility: Deafblindness or significant vision and hearing loss.
Area Served: Southeast United States.
Age Requirements: Transition age or older.

See Helen Keller National Center for Deaf-Blind Youths and Adults in U.S. national listings.

Mobility Services, Inc.
761 Peachtree Street, N.E.
Atlanta, GA 30308
(404) 876-2636
FAX: (404) 872-5255
E-mail: msi-inc@mindspring.com
Belen B. Hickman, President

Type of Agency: Private.
County/District Where Located: Fulton County.

Mission: To provide services and goods to improve physical and intellectual independence of challenged persons.
Funded by: Private donations.
Hours of Operation: Mon.-Fri. 8:30AM-5:00PM.
Program Accessibility: Fully accessible.
Staff: 9.
History/Date: Est. 1986.
Number of Clients Served: 200.
Area Served: Statewide.
Age Requirements: None.

Counseling/Social Work/Self-Help: Coordination and referral service.
Rehabilitation: Orientation and mobility; rehabilitation teaching.
Recreational: Coordinate with other organizations.
Computer Training: Sales of adaptive hardware and software; training on products.
Low Vision: Informal assessment, referral to low vision clinics.
Low Vision Aids: Optical and nonoptical aids.
Professional Training: Student internship in orientation and mobility.

Savannah Association for the Blind, Inc.
214 Drayton Street
Savannah, GA 31401-4021
(912) 236-4473
Walt Simmons, Executive Director

Type of Agency: Private; non-profit.
County/District Where Located: Chatham County.
Mission: Ongoing provision of programs and services designed to help blind and visually impaired persons adjust and cope with their vision loss.
Funded by: Federal block grants, Chatham County, United Way, private donations.

Budget: $535,000.
Hours of Operation: Mon.-Fri. 8:30 AM-5:00 PM.
Staff: 14 full time.
History/Date: Est. 1963.
Number of Clients Served: 360.
Eligibility: Legally blind, visually impaired, of all ages.

Health: Refers for health services.
Counseling/Social Work/Self-Help: Social evaluations; individual, group, family/parent, couple counseling; referral to community services; refers for other counseling/social work services.
Educational: Refers for vocational and educational services.
Preschools: Visually impaired preschool services: serves children from birth to 5 years; in-home and family support services; transition to day care and preschool settings; consultation for workers in other preschool programs.
Professional Training: Internship/field work placement in social work and rehabilitation training; regular in-service training program.
Reading: Refers for reading materials.
Rehabilitation: Activities of daily living, communication skills, orientation and mobility, therapeutic skills development.
Recreational: Adult day care services; leisure education; refers for recreational activities; consultation to other recreation providers.
Employment: Refers for employment-oriented services.
Low Vision: Coastal low vision services; serves southeastern Georgia and coastal South Carolina.
Low Vision Aids: As prescribed by clinician, for non-fee-paying clients.

Low Vision Follow-up: Up to 6 months after the low vision examination.

Sensory Program Rehabilitation Research and Development Center (151 R) U.S. Department of Veterans Affairs
1670 Clairmont Road
Decatur, GA 30033
(404) 728-5064
FAX: (404) 728-7731
Bruce B. Blasch, Research Health Scientist
Wiliam R. Del'Aune, Research Psychologist
Gale R. Watson, Research Health Scientist

Type of Agency: Federal.
Mission: Conducts applied research to identify the needs of blind and visually impaired persons and to study problems relating to vision and aging. Develops and tests effectiveness of new devices and techniques in rehabilitation. Focus is on research in aging and mobility.
Funded by: U.S. Department of Veterans Affairs.
Budget: $1 million.
Hours of Operation: Mon.-Fri. 8:00 AM-4:30 PM.
Staff: Center staff includes 30 full time, including engineers, computer scientists, mobility specialists, and rehabilitation researchers.
History/Date: Est. 1983.

COMPUTER TRAINING CENTERS

Georgia Academy for the Blind
2895 Vineville Avenue
Macon, GA 31204
(912) 751-6088
FAX: (912) 751-6659
Thomas Ridgeway, Contact Person

County/District Where Located: Bibb County.

Computer Training: Screen magnification systems; braille access systems; closed-circuit television systems; word processing; database software; training for instructors.

Savannah Association for the Blind Communications Department, Inc
214 Drayton Street
Savannah, GA 31401-4021
(912) 236-4473
Walt Simmons, Director

County/District Where Located: Chatham County.

Computer Training: Speech output system; screen magnification system; closed-circuit television systems; word processing.

◆ Low Vision Services

EYE CARE SOCIETIES

Georgia Society of Ophthalmology
938 Peachtree Street, N.E.
Atlanta, GA 30309
(404) 881-5092
Vickie Staley, Executive Director

Georgia Optometric Association
1000 Corporate Center Drive
Suite 240
Morrow, GA 30260
(770) 961-9866 or (800) 949-0060
Georgianne Bearden, Executive Director

LOW VISION CENTERS

Blind and Low Vision Services of North Georgia
3830 South Cobb Drive
Suite 125
Smyrna, GA 30080
(770) 432-7280
FAX: (770) 432-5457
Sandra Coleman, Low Vision Clinic

County/District Where Located: Cobb County.
Staff: Optometrists specializing in low vision; low vision assistants.

Low Vision: Comprehensive examinations, adjustment services, training in use of devices in various environments.
Low Vision Aids: Prescribed by physician.
Low Vision Follow-up: Semiannual follow-ups or more often, depending on condition.

Eye Clinic Grady Memorial Hospital
80 Butler Street, S.E.
Atlanta, GA 30335
(404) 616-4671
Elizabeth Prophet-Jones, Unit Manager

County/District Where Located: Fulton County.
Hours of Operation: Mon.-Fri. 8:30 AM - 5:30 PM.
Area Served: All Fulton and Dekalb County residents.

Low Vision Follow-up: As appropriate.

Maxwell Low Vision Clinic Center for the Visually Impaired
763 Peachtree Street, N.E.

Atlanta, GA 30308
(404) 875-9011
Scott McCall, Executive Director
Anne Stewart, Low Vision
Manager
Debra Hudson, Client Services
Manager

Type of Agency: Non-profit.
County/District Where Located:
Fulton County.
Mission: To provide
independence with dignity for the
visually impaired.
Funded by: Division of
Rehabilitation Services, United
Way, grants and client fees.
Hours of Operation: Low vision
clinic: Mon. and Fri. 8:00 AM-
4:30 PM; low vision training:
Mon. - Fri. 8:00 AM-4:30 PM.
Staff: Ophthalmologist;
optometrist; social worker; low
vision rehabilitation specialist.
Other rehabilitation personnel
available within the agency.
Number of Clients Served: 895.
Eligibility: Functional visual
impairment; ophthalmological
report no more than one year old.
Area Served: Unlimited.

Computer Training: Access,
training on computer aids and
devices.
Low Vision Aids: Provided on
loan for trial purposes; training
provided.
Low Vision Follow-up: Training
and return appointments
scheduled as needed.

Medical College of Georgia Low Vision Clinic

Department of Ophthalmology
School of Medicine
1120 15th Street
Augusta, GA 30912-3400
(706) 721-2020
FAX: (706) 721-1156
Malcolm N. Luxenberg, Chairman

Type of Agency: Medical school.
County/District Where Located:
Richmond County.
Funded by: State funds.
Hours of Operation: Alternate
Wed. mornings.
Staff: Ophthalmologists;
ophthalmology residents;
ophthalmic technologist.
Number of Clients Served: 8 per
month.
Eligibility: Recent
ophthalmological examination
with report and referral or an exam
in the medical college clinic.
Area Served: Georgia and South
Carolina primarily; no restriction
on referrals.

Low Vision Aids: Prescribed; on-
site training provided.
Low Vision Follow-up: As
needed.

◆ *Aging Services*

STATE UNITS ON AGING

Office of Aging

Two Peachtree Street, N.E.
18th floor
Atlanta, GA 30303
(404) 657-5258 or High Care
Hotline (800) 657-5334
FAX: (404) 657-5285
Judy Hagebak, Director

Provides referrals to Area Agencies
on Aging and information on other
local aging services.

**INDEPENDENT LIVING
PROGRAMS**

Georgia Department of Human Resources Division of Rehabilitation Services

Two Peachtree Street N.W.
Atlanta, GA 30303
(404) 657-3005
Karen Boyer, Manager

Provides independent living
services for persons age 55 and
over. For further information,
contact the Project Director or
general phone number listed.

GUAM

◆ Educational Services

STATE SERVICES

Guam Department of Education
P.O. Box DE
Agana, GU 96932
(671) 475-0495
FAX: (671) 475-9666
Ronald Taimanglo, Director

Mission: Provides special classes and mobility instruction for totally blind, partially sighted, deaf, and hard of hearing students at the Guam School for the Deaf and the Blind. Has academic and prevocational programs for partially sighted students.
Funded by: Public funds.

EARLY INTERVENTION COORDINATION

Guam Department of Education Division of Special Education
P.O. Box DE
Agana, GU 96932
(671) 475-0534
FAX: (671) 475-0562
Leilani T. Nishimura, Director

◆ Information Services

LIBRARIES

Guam Public Library for the Blind and Physically Handicapped
254 Martyr Street
Agana, GU 96910
(671) 475-4753
FAX: (671) 477-9777
E-mail: csctsmth@kuentos.guam.net
Christine K. Scott-Smith, Director

Mission: Subregional library of the Hawaii Library for the Blind and Physically Handicapped. Serves as sublending agency for machines; circulates cassette books.
Funded by: United States Department of Education, Title III.
Budget: $19,197.
Hours of Operation: Mon., Wed., Fri. 9:30 AM - 6:00 PM. Tues., Thurs. 9:30 - 8:00 PM. Sat. 10:00 - 4:00 PM. Sun. 12:00 - 4:00 PM.
Area Served: Guam and the Mariana Islands.

◆ Rehabilitation Services

STATE SERVICES

Guam Department of Vocational Rehabilitation
1313 Central Avenue
Tiyuan, GU 96913
(671) 475-4645
FAX: (671) 477-2892
E-mail: dvrcam@ite.net
Joseph Artero-Cameron, State Director

Mission: To enable qualified individuals with disabilities, especially with severe disabilities, to achieve employment and community independence.
Funded by: Public funds.
Budget: $1.8 million.
Hours of Operation: Mon.-Fri. 8:00 AM - 5:00 PM.
Staff: 31.
History/Date: Est. 1958.
Eligibility: Physically and mentally disabled.
Age Requirements: 18 years and older.

Health: Diagnosis and evaluation of eye health.
Counseling/Social Work/Self-Help: Social evaluation; psychological testing and evaluation.
Rehabilitation: Personal management.
Employment: Prevocational evaluation; prevocational training; vocational training; vocational placement; follow-up service; vending stand training.

◆ Aging Services

STATE UNITS ON AGING

Division of Senior Citizens Guam Department of Public Health and Social Services
P.O. Box 2816
Agana, GU 96910
(671) 475-0263
FAX: (671) 477-2930
Florence P. Shimizu, Administrator

Provides referrals to Area Agencies on Aging and information on other local aging services.

INDEPENDENT LIVING PROGRAMS

Guam Department of Vocational Rehabilitation
1313 Central Avenue
Tiyuan, GU 96913
(671) 475-4646
Mildred Campbell, Vision Administrator

Provides independent living services for persons age 55 and over. For further information, contact the Project Director or general phone number listed.

HAWAII

◆ *Educational Services*

STATE SERVICES

Hawaii Department of Education Hawaii Center for the Deaf and the Blind
3440 Leahi Avenue
Honolulu, HI 96815
(808) 733-4999 (voice / TDD)
FAX: (808) 733-4824
Dr. Jeanne G. Prickett,
Administrator
Robert Campell, Office of
Instructional Services, Special
Education Section

Mission: Provides special
materials and consultation for local
schools. Offers testing and
evaluation. Maintains resource
room.
Funded by: Public funds.
Hours of Operation: Mon.-Fri.
8:00AM-3:00PM.
History/Date: Est. 1914.
Eligibility: Visually impaired.
Area Served: Hawaii.

Contact local school
superintendent for program
information and additional
services, or Hawaii Center for the
Deaf and the Blind.

EARLY INTERVENTION COORDINATION

Zero to 3 Hawaii Project
Pan American Building
1600 Kapiolani Boulevard
Suite 1401
Honolulu, HI 96814
(808) 957-0066
FAX: (808) 946-5222
Jean Johnson, Project Coordinator

All services required under
Hawaii's State Plan for Early
Intervention Part H services.

SCHOOLS

Hawaii Center for the Deaf and Blind
3440 Leahi Avenue
Honolulu, HI 96815
(808) 733-4999 (voice/TDD)
FAX: (808) 733-4824
E-mail: jeanne@hcdb.kiz.hi.us
Dr. Jean Glidden Prickett,
Administrator
Margi Flora, Resource Teacher for
the Visually Impaired

Type of Agency: Public.
County/District Where Located:
Honolulu County.
Mission: Services for blind, deaf/
blind, and deaf students from 3-20
years.
Funded by: Public funds.
Hours of Operation: Mon.-Fri.
7:00 AM-5:00 PM.
Staff: 10 teachers, 1 counselor, 7
diagnostic personnel, 10
educational assistants, 21 support
staff.
History/Date: Est. 1914.
Number of Clients Served: 67
on-site. Varies annually for
diagnostics, materials provision.
Eligibility: All students statewide
for whom placement is
appropriate, based on diagnostic
recommendation.
Area Served: All of Hawaiian
Islands.
Transportation: Y.
Age Requirements: Preschool
through 20.

Health: Services available.
Counseling/Social Work/Self-Help: Services available.
Educational: Technical assistance
for braille, orientation and
mobility, and other special skills
blind children need to function in
public schools. Provision of

educational materials for inclusion
programs.
Residential: For outer island
students only.

STATEWIDE OUTREACH SERVICES

Hawaii Center for the Deaf and Blind
3440 Leahi Avenue
Honolulu, HI 96815
(808) 733-4999
FAX: (808) 733-4824
Dr. Jeanne G. Prickett,
Administrator

County/District Where Located:
Honolulu County.
Funded by: Department of
Education; public funds.
History/Date: Est. 1914.
Age Requirements: 3-21 years.

Assessment: By diagnostic team:
psychologist, social worker, family
educator, teacher for visually
impaired students, orientation and
mobility instructor, teacher for
hearing impaired students, speech
pathologist, audiologist.
Consultation to Public Schools:
For visually and hearing impaired
students.
Direct Service: Classroom
instruction.
Materials Production:
Coordinates statewide ordering of
large-print braille, and special
material for visually impaired
students.

◆ *Information Services*

LIBRARIES

Hawaii Library for the Blind and Physically Handicapped
402 Kapahulu Avenue

Honolulu, HI 96815
(808) 733-8444 (voice/TDD)
FAX: (808) 733-8449
E-mail: olbcirc@lib.state.hi.
us
Fusako Miyashiro, Librarian

Type of Agency: A division of the Hawaii State Public Library System and a regional library in the network of the National Library Service for the Blind and Physically Handicapped.
Mission: Provides free, modern library service for people who need library material in a special format. Provides library advisory service to state-supported residential institutions.
Funded by: Public funds and contributions.
Hours of Operation: Mon.-Sat. 9:30 AM - 4:30 PM.
Staff: 12.
History/Date: Est. 1931.
Eligibility: For NLS collection, must meet requirements of Public Law 89-522. Large-type books available to all holders of Hawaii State public library service card.
Area Served: Hawaii and U.S. Pacific Islands.

Regional library providing braille, disks, cassettes and large-type books; inkprint books about various disabilities; transcribing services in braille, large-type, and disabled recorded cassette. Serves as machine lending agency. Serves other disabled persons requiring audio-visual materials. Houses Hawaii State Public Library system's large-type collection. Provides Radio Reading services; DVT (descriptive videotape).

Subregional library in Guam. Machine sublending agencies in Hilo, Kahului and Lihue.

MEDIA PRODUCTION SERVICES

Hawaii Library for the Blind and Physically Handicapped
402 Kapahulu Avenue
Honolulu, HI 96815
(808) 733-8444 (voice/TDD)
FAX: (808) 733-8449
E-mail: olbcirc@lib.state.hi.
us
Fusako Miyashiro, Director

Area Served: State of Hawaii, United States, Pacific Islands.
Groups Served: K-12; college students; other adults; must be certified as eligible for National Library Service for Blind and Physically Handicapped service.

Types/Content: Textbooks; recreational.
Media Formats: Braille books; recorded cassette books, large-print books, Radio Reading service; DVT (descriptive videotapes).
Title Listings: Title listings available on request.

INFORMATION AND REFERRAL

The Foundation Fighting Blindness
Hawaii Affiliate
45-573 Awanene Way
Kaneohe, HI 96744
(808) 247-0970
Caroline Lim, Contact Person

See The Foundation Fighting Blindness in U.S. national listings.

♦ Rehabilitation Services

STATE SERVICES

Ho'opono Services for the Blind
Hawaii Department of Human Services
Vocational Rehabilitation and Services for the Blind Division
1901 Bachelot Street
Honolulu, HI 96817
(808) 586-5266
FAX: (808) 586-5288
David Eveland, Administrator

Type of Agency: State.
Mission: To improve the standard of living and quality of life of persons with blindness or visual impairments residing in the State of Hawaii.
Funded by: Federal and state grants.
Hours of Operation: 7:45 AM - 4:30 PM.
Staff: 29 full time. Uses volunteers.
History/Date: Est. 1935.
Number of Clients Served: 1,214.
Eligibility: Visual impairment that interferes with ability to function personally, socially, vocationally. Services for totally blind, legally blind, visually impaired, and deaf-blind persons.
Area Served: Statewide.
Transportation: Y.

Health: Low vision clinic or service; low vision aids. Refers for other health services.
Counseling/Social Work/Self-Help: Social evaluation; arranges psychological testing and evaluation; individual, couple counseling; placement in training; referral to community services. Refers for and provides consultation to other agencies for other counseling/social work services.

Professional Training:
Internship / fieldwork placement in occupational therapy, mobility.
Rehabilitation: Personal management; braille; handwriting; typing; electronic mobility aids; home management; occupational therapy; orientation / mobility skills; rehabilitation teaching in client's home and community; sensory training; orientation to adaptive equipment.
Recreational: Arts and crafts; hobby groups; special programs for elderly; bowling; swimming. Refers for other recreational services.
Employment: Prevocational evaluation; career and skill counseling; referrals for occupational skill development; job retention; job retraining; sheltered workshops; vocational placement; follow-up service; vending stand training.
Computer Training: As related to use of adaptive equipment.
Low Vision: Conducts low vision evaluations.
Low Vision Follow-up: Limited follow-up.

Local Offices:

Hilo: Hawaii Branch, 75 Aupuni, Hilo, HI 96720, (808) 961-7331.
Lihue: Kauai Branch, P.O. Box 1028, Lihue, HI 96766, (808) 245-4333.
Wailuku: Maui Branch, P.O. Box RRR, Wailuku, HI 96793, (808) 244-4291.

REHABILITATION

Ho'opono Workshop for the Blind
1901 Bachelot Street
Honolulu, HI 96817
(808) 586-5286
FAX: (808) 586-5288
Jon L. Koki, Manager

Type of Agency: Workshop for blind persons.
Funded by: State funds.
Hours of Operation: Mon.-Fri. 8:00 AM-4:00 PM.
Staff: 2.
History/Date: Est. 1962.
Number of Clients Served: 40.
Eligibility: Legally blind or visually and hearing impaired persons.
Area Served: Island of Oahu, Hawaii.
Transportation: Y.
Age Requirements: 18 years and older.

Employment: Sheltered workshop employment.

DOG GUIDE SCHOOLS

Eye of the Pacific Guide Dogs and Mobility Services, Inc.
747 Amana Street, #407
Honolulu, HI 96814
(808) 941-1088
FAX: (808) 941-1088
Victoria Cozloff, Executive Secretary
Joseph Sunderland, President

Type of Agency: Non-profit.
Mission: Supplies dog guides and electronic mobility aids to blind persons.
Funded by: United Funds and service organizations.
Budget: $40,000.
Hours of Operation: One day per week.
Staff: 1 part-time.
History/Date: Est. 1955 and Inc. 1957.
Number of Clients Served: 61.
Eligibility: Six months of residency in Hawaii, Guam, or Alaska. Candidates must be evaluated and have a doctor's endorsement.
Area Served: Hawaii and Guam, and Alaska.

Age Requirements: 18 years or older.

Rehabilitation: Training with guide dogs and use of electronic aids.
Low Vision Aids: Electronic aids provided.

◆ Low Vision Services

EYE CARE SOCIETIES

Hawaii Ophthalmological Society
1300 Lusitana Street
Honolulu, HI 96813
(808) 528-5333
FAX: (808) 545-7236
Jon M. Portis, M.D., President

Hawaii Optometric Association
49-955 Kamehameha Highway
Honolulu, HI 96744
(808) 247-7888
Bryan Sakka, Executive Director

LOW VISION CENTERS

Low Vision Clinic
Ho'opono Rehabilitation Center for the Blind and Visually Impaired
1901 Bachelot Street
Honolulu, HI 96817
(808) 586-5276
FAX: (808) 586-5288
Lillian Kaneshiro, Social Worker
Bryon Wong, M.D., Staff Ophthalmologist
Harry Terada, O.D., Optometrist

Type of Agency: State.
Funded by: State funds.
Hours of Operation: Wed. 9:00 AM-4:30 PM.
Staff: Optometrist; social worker; ophthalmologist; refers as needed for services of orientation / mobility instructor, rehabilitation

teacher,vocational rehabilitation counselor, and social group worker.
History/Date: Est. 1964.
Eligibility: Ophthalmologist's or optometrist's report.
Area Served: Statewide.

Low Vision: Examination by optometrist specializing in low vision.
Low Vision Aids: Provided on loan for trial purposes; no rental fee; on-site training provided.
Low Vision Follow-up: By home visit 1st or 2nd month; phone interviews are conducted in 2 or 3 months.

♦ Aging Services

STATE UNITS ON AGING

Executive Office on Aging
Office of the Governor
One Capitol District
250 South Hotel Street, Suite 107
Honolulu, HI 96813
(808) 586-0100 or Information & Referral In State (800) 468-4644
FAX: (808) 586-0185
Mariyan Seely, Director

Provides referrals to Area Agencies on Aging and information on other local aging services.

INDEPENDENT LIVING PROGRAMS

Division of Vocational Rehabilitation
Hawaii Department of Human Services
Bishop Trust Building
1000 Bishop Street, Room 615
Honolulu, HI 96813
(808) 586-5366
Neil Shim, Acting Administrator

Provides independent living services for persons age 55 and over. For further information, contact the Project Director or general phone number listed.

IDAHO

♦ Educational Services

STATE SERVICES

Idaho State Department of Education
650 West State Street
Len B. Jordon Building, Room 150
Boise, ID 83702
(208) 332-6800
FAX: (208) 334-2228
Dr. Anne C. Fox, Superintendent of Public Instruction
Nolene Weaver, State Director of Special Education

Type of Agency: State.
County/District Where Located: Ada County.
Funded by: Public funds.
Hours of Operation: 8:00 AM - 5:00 PM.
Area Served: Idaho.

For information about local facilities, consult the superintendent of schools in the area.

EARLY INTERVENTION COORDINATION

Bureau of Developmental Disabilities
Idaho Department of Health and Welfare
450 West State Street
P.O. Box 83720
Boise, ID 83720-0036
(208) 334-5523
FAX: (208) 334-6664
Mary Jones, Manager, Infant Toddler Programs

County/District Where Located: Statewide.

Administers program of early intervention services.

SCHOOLS

Idaho School for the Deaf and the Blind
1450 Main Street
Gooding, ID 83330
(208) 934-4457
FAX: (208) 934-8352
E-mail: rdarcy@isdb.state.id.us
Ron Darcy, Superintendent

Type of Agency: State.
County/District Where Located: Gooding County.
Mission: Counseling, vocational evaluation, orientation/mobility, residential services. Audiological and special pathology services.
Funded by: State residential school.
Hours of Operation: 8:00 AM-5:00 PM.
Program Accessibility: School provides dormitory living situations and transportation to and from home on weekends. Daily busing program available for day students within 50-mile radius of the school.
Staff: 135 full time. Uses volunteers.
History/Date: Est. 1906.
Number of Clients Served: 115.
Eligibility: Visually and/or hearing impaired, deaf-blind, or multiply disabled persons.
Area Served: State of Idaho.
Transportation: Y.
Age Requirements: 3-21 years.

Health: Nurses on duty to provide general medical services.
Counseling/Social Work/Self-Help: Trained counselors on site; summer camp provides psychological programs.
Educational: Academic programs for children, preschool through high school; career-oriented vocational program for nonacademic students; home-bound preschool program. Itinerant instructions for students attending public school programs.
Preschools: Regional statewide in-house programs for children age 0-3. For children age 3-kindergarten consultation services to public schools.
Professional Training: Professional internships in special education or related fields.
Reading: Media center for providing braille, large-print, other aids.
Residential: Residential component for blind, deaf, or multiply disabled clients.
Recreational: Recreational specialist coordinates after-school activities. Extracurricular activities provided: soccer, basketball, swimming, volleyball, track, gym, group activities.
Computer Training: Individual instruction depending on needs. Consultation to schools.
Low Vision: Contracts for assessments.
Low Vision Aids: Workshops for school districts.
Low Vision Follow-up: Y.

Contact local school superintendent for program information.

INFANT AND PRESCHOOL

Idaho School for the Deaf and the Blind
1450 Main Street
Gooding, ID 83330
(208) 934-4457
FAX: (208) 934-8352
E-mail: rdarcy@isdb.state.id.us
Ron Darcy, Superintendent

Type of Agency: Residential school.
County/District Where Located: Gooding County.
Mission: Serve educational needs of children.

Funded by: State funds and grants.

Hours of Operation: 8:00 AM - 5:00 PM.

Staff: 6 full time. Various therapists available as consultants. Has advisory board for overall program, including a parent member.

History/Date: Est. 1906.

Eligibility: Visually impaired/ multiply disabled; resident of Idaho.

Area Served: State of Idaho.

Age Requirements: Birth - kindergarten.

Health: Adaptive equipment; other health services.

Counseling/Social Work/Self-Help: Home-based programs and consultant services to other programs. Perceptual development and parent counseling available on consultant or referral basis.

Educational: Provides instruction in all developmental areas.

Preschools: Itinerant teachers work with agencies and with parents at home, statewide; preschool classroom for children 3 years-kindergarten.

Professional Training: Workshops for itinerant teachers and for regular education teachers in public schools.

Low Vision Aids: Devices available on loan.

STATEWIDE OUTREACH SERVICES

Idaho School for the Deaf and the Blind
1450 Main Street
Gooding, ID 83330
(208) 934-4457
FAX: (208) 934-8352
E-mail: rdarcy@isdb.state.id. us
Ron Darcy, Superintendent

County/District Where Located: Gooding County.

Funded by: State funds; foundation grants.

Located at: Gooding, with regional offices throughout the state.

Age Requirements: 0-21 years.

Assessment: Evaluation and referral.

Parent Assistance: Counseling.

Materials Production: Large print.

INSTRUCTIONAL MATERIALS CENTERS

Idaho School for the Deaf and the Blind
1450 Main Street
Gooding, ID 83330
(208) 934-4457
FAX: (208) 934-8352
Shirley Cobble, Media Supervisor

County/District Where Located: Gooding County.

Area Served: Idaho.

Groups Served: Preschool - grade 12.

Types/Content: Textbooks.

Media Formats: Large-print books; Braille books.

Title Listings: No title listings available.

♦ Information Services

LIBRARIES

Idaho State Library Services for Blind and Physically Handicapped
325 West State Street

Boise, ID 83702
(208) 334-2117 or toll-free in Idaho (800) 233-4931
FAX: (208) 334-2194
E-mail: ksalmon@isl.state.id. us
Kay H. Salmon, Librarian

Type of Agency: Part of the Library of Congress network.

Mission: To provide library materials and information to print-disabled residents of the state of Idaho in formats that are appropriate for their use.

Funded by: State and federal monies.

Hours of Operation: Mon.-Fri. 8:00 AM - 5:00 PM.

Staff: 12.

History/Date: Est. 1973. Prior to 1973, services provided by Utah under the auspices of Idaho state library.

Number of Clients Served: 3,700.

Eligibility: Visually impaired persons and disabled persons who cannot use printed materials.

Area Served: Idaho.

Lending library for Idaho and distributor of talking book machines for the blind and physically handicapped.

MEDIA PRODUCTION SERVICES

Boise Public Schools
1207 Fort Street
Boise, ID 83702
(208) 338-3456
FAX: (208) 338-3477
Mike Anderson, Director of Communication Disorders

Area Served: Boise City.

Groups Served: Preschool - grade 12.

Types/Content: Textbooks.

Media Formats: Braille/large-print books.

Title Listings: Printed at no charge.

Idaho State Library Services for Blind and Physically Handicapped

325 West State Street
Boise, ID 83702
(208) 334-2117 or toll-free in Idaho (800) 233-4931
FAX: (208) 334-2194
E-mail: ksalmon@isl.state.id.us
Kay H. Salmon, Director

Area Served: Statewide.
Groups Served: Visually impaired and physically disabled persons.

Types/Content: Books, magazines, and DVS.
Media Formats: Cassettes, recorded disks, braille, large-print.

RADIO READING

Idaho Radio Reading Service

P.O. Box 83720
Boise, ID 83702-0012
(208) 334-3220
Brett Winchester, Director

County/District Where Located: Ada County.
Hours of Operation: Seven days, 8:00 AM-2:00 AM.
History/Date: Est. 1977.
Area Served: Treasure Valley and southwest area of Idaho, plus a small portion of eastern Oregon and northern Nevada.

◆ Rehabilitation Services

STATE SERVICES

Idaho Commission for the Blind and Visually Impaired

341 West Washington Street
Boise, ID 83720-6000
(208) 334-3220
FAX: (208) 334-2963
E-mail: blackaller@icbvi.state.id.us
Mike Blackaller, Rehabilitation Services Chief
Jim Monroe, Administrator

Type of Agency: State.
County/District Where Located: Ada County.
Mission: Services for functionally blind, legally blind, deaf-blind.
Funded by: State appropriated funds, federal matching funds.
Budget: $4 million.
Hours of Operation: Mon.-Fri. 8:00AM - 5:00PM.
Staff: 45 full time.
History/Date: Est. 1967.
Number of Clients Served: 900 annually.
Eligibility: Legally blind, functionally blind.

Health: Refers for health services.
Counseling/Social Work/Self-Help: Individual, family/parent, couple counseling.
Professional Training: Regular in-service, short-term or summer training open for enrollment to other agencies in subjects requested by agencies.
Reading: Talking book record players and cassette players; braille books; large print books; braille magazines; recorded magazines.
Residential: Orientation and adjustment center for adults.
Rehabilitation: Personal management; braille; typing; home management; cane travel; rehabilitation teaching in client's home and community. Job training and placement.
Recreational: Refers for recreational services.
Employment: Prevocational evaluation; career and skill counseling; occupational skill development; vocational placement; vending stand training; on-the-job training.
Local Offices:

Coeur d'Alene: Coeur d'Alene Regional Office, Coeur d'Alene, ID 83814, (208) 667-8494.
Lewiston: Lewiston Regional Office, Lewiston, ID 83501, (208) 746-3241, ext. 298.
Pocatello: Pocatello Regional Office, 427 North Main Street, Suite J, Pocatello, ID 83204, (208) 233-7171.

◆ Low Vision Services

EYE CARE SOCIETIES

Idaho Society of Ophthalmology

526-H Shoup Avenue West
Twin Falls, ID 83301
(208) 733-2400
FAX: (208) 634-0343
Robert C. Welch, M.D., President

Idaho Optometric Association

9077 Maple Hill Drive
Boise, ID 83709
(208) 378-7700
Larry Benton, Executive Director

◆ Aging Services

STATE UNITS ON AGING

Commission on Aging

700 West Jefferson, Room 108
P.O. Box 83720
Boise, ID 83720-0007
(208) 334-2423
FAX: (208) 334-3033
Arlene Davidson, Director

Provides referrals to Area Agencies on Aging and information on other local aging services.

INDEPENDENT LIVING PROGRAMS

Idaho Commission for the Blind and Visually Impaired
341 West Washington
Boise, ID 83702
(208) 334-3220
Mike Blackaller, Administrator

Provides independent living services for persons age 55 and over. For further information, contact the Project Director or general phone number listed.

ILLINOIS

◆ *Educational Services*

STATE SERVICES

Illinois State Board of Education
100 North First Street
Springfield, IL 62777
(217) 782-6601
FAX: (217) 782-0372
Paula Stadeker, Consultant

Type of Agency: State.
County/District Where Located: Sangamon County.
Mission: Provides adapted materials. Offers reader services as needed. Cooperates with the Illinois State Board of Education Program Service Teams in offering technical assistance to local programs.
Funded by: Public funds. Administers supplemental state and federal funds.
Hours of Operation: 8:00 AM - 5:00 PM.
Eligibility: Visually impaired students in local schools and residential schools.
Area Served: Illinois.
Age Requirements: Birth - 21 years of age.

Educational: Programs for students aged 3-21.
Preschools: Programs for children aged 0-3.

EARLY INTERVENTION COORDINATION

Early Childhood Division
Illinois State Board of Education
100 West Randolph, C14-300
Chicago, IL 60601
(312) 814-5560
FAX: (312) 814-2282
Audrey Witzman, Principal Consultant and Part H Coordinator

Early intervention services for children aged 0-5.

SCHOOLS

The Hope School
50 Hazel Lane
Springfield, IL 62716
(217) 786-3350
FAX: (217) 786-3356
Shawn E. Jeffers, Executive Director
Joan Shea-Rogers, Principal

Type of Agency: Private; non-profit; residential school.
County/District Where Located: Sangamon County.
Mission: Services for children who are totally blind, legally blind, visually impaired, deaf-blind, learning disabled, mentally retarded, physically handicapped.
Funded by: Fees, private contributions.
Hours of Operation: 24 hours, 7 days.
Staff: Nearly 300. Uses volunteers.
History/Date: Est. 1957.
Number of Clients Served: 117.
Eligibility: Non-ambulatory, ambulatory, controlled seizures.
Transportation: Y.
Age Requirements: 5-21 years.

Health: General medical services. Contracts for other medical, dental and vision health services.
Counseling/Social Work/Self-Help: Social evaluation; individual, family counseling; placement in school.
Educational: Non-graded.
Professional Training: Internship/supervised fieldwork placement in special education.
Regular in-service/short term training programs.
Reading: Talking book record player and cassette player; talking book records and cassettes; braille books; large print books; braille magazines; information and referral system.
Residential: Dormitory beds for children with multiple disabilities.
Rehabilitation: Personal management; braille; gesticulation; handwriting; listening skills; orientation/mobility.
Recreational: Arts and crafts; hobby groups; therapeutic recreation.
Employment: Contracts for sheltered workshops.
Low Vision: MTI Photoscreener.

Licensed by the Illinois Department of Family Services and accredited by the North Central Association of Colleges and Schools as a Special Function School.

Illinois School for the Visually Impaired

658 East State Street
Jacksonville, IL 62650
(217) 479-4400
FAX: (217) 479-4479
Dorothy Arensman, Superintendent
Eric Emberg, Assistant Superintendent

Type of Agency: State.
Mission: Services for visually impaired, deaf-blind, multiply disabled blind students.
Funded by: State funds.
Hours of Operation: 24 hours per day, 7 days per week, during the academic school year and at other times as dictated by programs.
Program Accessibility: All aspects of the program are/will be in compliance with ADA requirements.

Staff: 143 full time. Uses volunteers.
History/Date: Est. 1849.
Number of Clients Served: 110 students during the academic year and 42 infants birth through 5 years old, each year.
Eligibility: Resident of Illinois with visual impairment who is between the ages of birth through 21.
Area Served: State of Illinois.
Transportation: Y.
Age Requirements: Birth through 5 for Parent Infant; 4 through 21 for other programs.

Health: Evaluation of eye health; treatment of eye conditions; audiology therapy; general medical services; speech therapy. Contracts, refers, and provides consultation to other agencies for other health services.
Counseling/Social Work/Self-Help: Social evaluation; psychological testing and evaluation; individual, group counseling. Refers for other counseling/social work services.
Educational: Grades K through 12. Programs for college prep; general academic; prevocational/vocational/living skill development.
Professional Training: Internship/fieldwork placement in special education. Regular in-service training programs.
Reading: Talking book records and cassettes; braille; large-print books; information and referral; special collection; transcription to braille.
Residential: Dormitories.
Recreational: Afterschool programs; arts and crafts; hobby groups; swimming; music; drama; track; wrestling. Refers for and provides consultation to other agencies for other recreational services.

Employment: Career and skill counseling; occupational skill development; job retention. Refers for and provides consultation to other agencies for other employment-oriented services.
Computer Training: Provided via computer lab exposure/training approach.
Low Vision: Services provided via clinics sponsored by state Lions organization and ongoing activities.
Low Vision Aids: Prescription of spectacles or aids.
Low Vision Follow-up: Evaluation of eye treatment or prescription.

Contact local school superintendent for program availability, or Department of Special Education, Illinois State Board of Education, 100 North First Street, Springfield, IL 62777, (217) 782-6601.

Philip J. Rock Center and School

818 DuPage Boulevard
Glen Ellyn, IL 60137
(630) 790-2474
FAX: (630) 790-4893
Christine D. Dorsey, C.A.S., Chief Administrator

Type of Agency: State.
County/District Where Located: DuPage County.
Mission: Services for children who are deaf-blind.
Funded by: Illinois State Board of Education.
Budget: $2,000,000.
Hours of Operation: 24 hours a day.
Staff: 63 full time, 15 part time. Uses volunteers.
History/Date: Est. 1978.
Number of Clients Served: 21 in residential school; 463 served by the service center.

Eligibility: Auditory and visual impairment.
Area Served: Illinois.
Transportation: Y.
Age Requirements: 0-21 years.

Health: Audiology; general medical services; occupational therapy; physical therapy; speech therapy. Refers for and contracts for other medical services.
Counseling/Social Work/Self-Help: School and training placement. Refers and contracts for other counseling/social work services.
Educational: Prevocational; daily living skills; community-based education; leisure and recreation.
Professional Training: Regular in-service training, open to enrollment from other agencies. Sponsors conferences on a quarterly basis.
Reading: Cassette tape players; large-print books; information and referral; transcription to braille.
Residential: Dormitory.
Rehabilitation: Personal management; braille; gesticulation; handwriting; home management; orientation/mobility; sensory training.
Recreational: Afterschool programs; arts and crafts; residential summer camp; swimming; track. Evening and weekend programs.
Employment: Supported employment training opportunities.
Computer Training: 5 Apple computers for students' use.
Low Vision: Evaluations and training available.
Low Vision Aids: Will supply aids to meet individual students needs.
Low Vision Follow-up: Evaluation of eye treatment or prescription.

INFANT AND PRESCHOOL

Chicago Lighthouse for People Who Are Blind or Visually Impaired
Development Center

1850 West Roosevelt Road
Chicago, IL 60608
(312) 666-1331 or TDD (312) 666-8874
FAX: (312) 243-8539
Mary Zabelski, Director of Educational Services

Type of Agency: Private; non-profit.
County/District Where Located: Cook County.
Mission: To create opportunities for blind and visually impaired people, including those who are multiply disabled. To develop and promote effective programs that maximize the potential for independent living, assist in achieving economic self-support, and prevent unnecessary institutionalization.
Funded by: Preschool program supported by tuition from local school boards. Infant program funded by United Way and Department of Mental Health grants.
Hours of Operation: 8:45 AM-5:00 PM throughout the year.
Program Accessibility: Fully accessible.
Staff: 23 full time; 10 part time.
History/Date: Est. 1969.
Number of Clients Served: 40 (day school); 120 (infant and pre-school).
Eligibility: Blind or visually impaired.
Area Served: Chicago area and collar suburbs.
Transportation: Y.
Age Requirements: 3 years and under.

Health: Low vision exams; occupational, physical, speech therapy; medical consultation available.
Counseling/Social Work/Self-Help: Parent counseling; psychological consultation available; referrals to other agencies.
Educational: Provides instruction in all developmental areas; orientation/mobility.

Preschool program serves 3-5 year olds in multiply disabled classroom. Infant program serves 0-3 year olds at home.

Approved as nonpublic education facility for disabled children by State of Illinois.

DuPage/West Cook Regional Special Education Association

1500 South Grace
Lombard, IL 60148
(630) 629-7272
Joan Allison, Director

Type of Agency: Public school program.
Funded by: P.L. 94-142 monies and state funds.
Staff: 13 full time (early childhood/teachers of visually impaired children, orientation/mobility instructors, therapists).
History/Date: Est. 1970.
Area Served: DuPage and western Cook counties.
Transportation: Y.
Age Requirements: 0-5 years.

Health: Adaptive equipment.
Counseling/Social Work/Self-Help: Parent counseling; social work services.
Educational: Provides direct instruction in all developmental areas.
Low Vision: Exams available on referral basis.

Center-based with home component for visually impaired children, with or without other disabilities, 0-3 years. Classes for visually impaired, multiply disabled children, resource rooms, and consultant services to other programs for children 3-5 years. Itinerant vision services to public schools.

Illinois School for the Visually Impaired

658 East State Street
Jacksonville, IL 62650
(217) 479-4400
FAX: (217) 479-4479
Dorothy Arensman, Superintendent

Type of Agency: State funds.
Mission: Services for visually impaired, deaf-blind, and multiply disabled blind students.
Funded by: State funds.
Hours of Operation: 24 hours per day, 7 days per week during academic school year and at other times as dictated by programs.
Program Accessibility: All aspects of the program are/will be in compliance with ADA requirements.
Staff: 143 full time for total program. Has advisory board, including parent members.
History/Date: Est. 1849.
Number of Clients Served: 110 students during the academic year and 42 infants birth through 5 years old each year.
Eligibility: Resident of Illinois with visual impairment.
Area Served: Entire state.
Transportation: Y.
Age Requirements: Birth through 5 for Parent Infant.

Consultant, evaluation, and referral services for visually impaired, multiply disabled, and deaf-blind children, 0-5 years, are provided on request to parents and other programs via an annual institute and outreach services as needed and requested.

LICA-NSSEO Infant Vision Program

799 West Kensington Road
Mount Prospect, IL 60056
(847) 577-7749
FAX: (847) 577-0357
Dr. Alice Epstein,
Superintendent/Director, NSSEO
Terri Mertz, LICA-NSSEO Vision
Coordinator

Type of Agency: Intermediate education program.
County/District Where Located: Cook County.
Mission: Services for visually impaired children with or without other impairments.
Funded by: 94-142 monies, private donations, and state funds.
Staff: 2 full time (teacher of visually impaired children), 1 part time, variety of other staff available for consultation. Has advisory board, including parent members.
Age Requirements: 0-5 years.

Health: Various health services available on referral.
Counseling/Social Work/Self-Help: Parent education groups, parent support groups, and parent counseling.
Educational: Provides instruction in all developmental areas, speech/language and communication.
Rehabilitation: Orientation/mobility; daily living skills; physical therapy; occupational therapy.

Home-based program with center component for 0-3 year olds; multiply disabled and non-categorical classes for 3-5 year olds. Infant and multiply disabled vision clinic provided monthly by optometrist.

STATEWIDE OUTREACH SERVICES

Illinois School for the Visually Impaired

658 East State Street
Jacksonville, IL 62650
(217) 479-4400
FAX: (217) 479-4479
Dorothy Arensman,
Superintendent
Eric Emberg, Assistant
Superintendent

Funded by: State funds.
History/Date: Est. 1847.
Age Requirements: None.

Consultation to Public Schools: As needed or requested.
Direct Service: Assessments, including components of case studies.
Parent Assistance: As needed or requested.
Materials Production: Provided along with technical assistance/consultation by computer lab.
Professional Training: Programs presented, as requested.

INSTRUCTIONAL MATERIALS CENTERS

Illinois Industrial Materials

3031 Stanton Center
Springfield, IL 62703
(217) 525-3300
FAX: (217) 525-3029
Alice Post, Contact Person

Area Served: Illinois.
Groups Served: Students (ages 0-adult) with visual impairments enrolled in a formal educational program.

Types/Content: Educational materials.
Media Formats: Braille books, tangible aids, adaptive computer equipment.
Title Listings: Braille masters stored in the depository are listed in the American Printing House for the Blind's central catalog under the acronym SEIMC.

Southern Will County Cooperative

707 West Jefferson Street, Suite K
Sherwood, IL 60431
(815) 741-7777
FAX: (915) 741-7779
Patricia M. Hall, Coordinator,
Visually Impaired Programs

Area Served: Grundy, Will, Kendall, Kankakee, and LaSalle Counties.
Groups Served: 3-12.

Coordinates services to visually impaired students in school districts.

UNIVERSITY TRAINING PROGRAMS

Illinois State University

University Laboratory Schools,
Elementary/Secondary Programs
for the Visually Handicapped
533 DeGarmo Hall
P.O. Box 5910
Normal, IL 61790-5910
(309) 438-5419
Paula Smith, Chairperson,
Specialist Education
Norma DeMario, Instructor

County/District Where Located: McLean County.

Programs Offered: Undergraduate and graduate (master's, doctoral) programs for teachers of the visually handicapped and multihandicapped.

Northern Illinois University

Programs in Vision
Faculty of Special Education

DeKalb, IL 60115
(815) 753-8459
FAX: (815) 753-9250
E-mail: vision@niu.edu
Dr. Gaylen Kapperman,
Coordinator, (815) 753-8453
Dr. Toni Heinze, Teacher of
Visually Impaired Children
Ms. Brucie Hawkins, Orientation
and Mobility Teacher

Programs Offered: Undergraduate
and graduate programs for
teachers of visually impaired and
multiply disabled children, for
rehabilitation teachers, and for
orientation and mobility
instructors.

Southern Illinois University

Rehabilitation Institute
Rehn Hall 317
Carbondale, IL 62901-4609
(618) 536-7704
FAX: (618) 453-8271
Dr. Darrell Taylor, Associate
Professor

County/District Where Located:
Jackson County.

Programs Offered: Special course
in job development and placement
for employed rehabilitation
professionals offered at both
undergraduate and graduate
levels.

◆ Information Services

LIBRARIES

Chicago Public Library Illinois Regional Library for the Blind and Physically Handicapped

1055 West Roosevelt Road
Chicago, IL 60608
(312) 746-9210
FAX: (312) 746-9192
Barbara Perkis, Acting Director

Type of Agency: Regional library
for the blind and physically
handicapped.
County/District Where Located:
Cook County.
Funded by: Public funds.
Budget: $669,713 (library).
Hours of Operation: Mon.-Fri.
9:00AM-5:00PM.
Staff: 3 librarians; 1
paraprofessional; 10 support staff.
History/Date: Est. 1893.
Number of Clients Served:
22,000.
Eligibility: Blind, visually
impaired, or physically disabled
according to National Library
Service guidelines.
Area Served: Illinois. Also
provides braille reader service for
Wisconsin.
Age Requirements: None.

Professional Training: Limited.
Reference/reader advisor
assistance available.
Reading: General; career/
vocational: fiction.
Low Vision Aids: By request.

Chicago Public Library Talking Book Center

400 South State Street
Chicago, IL 60605
(312) 747-4001
FAX: (312) 747-1609
Mamie Grady, Librarian

Subregional library.

Heart of Illinois Talking Book Center

Illinois Valley Library System
845 Brenkman Drive
Pekin, IL 61554
(309) 353-4110 or toll-free in Illinois
(800) 426-0709
FAX: (309) 353-8281
Valerie Wilford, Librarian

Subregional library.

Mid-Illinois Talking Book Center

Great River Library System
515 York
Quincy, IL 62301
(217) 224-6619 or toll-free in Illinois
(800) 537-1274 or TDD (217) 224-6619
Eileen Sheppard, Librarian

Subregional library.

Southern Illinois Talking Book Center

Shawnee Library System
607 Greenbriar Road
Carterville, IL 62918-1600
(618) 985-8375 or toll-free in Illinois
(800) 458-0475 or TDD (618) 985-8375
FAX: (618) 985-4211
Kristi Gordon, Librarian

Subregional library.

Talking Book Center of Northwest Illinois

P.O. Box 125
Coal Valley, IL 61240
(309) 799-3137 or toll-free in Illinois
(800) 747-3137
FAX: (309) 799-7916
Karen Odean, Librarian

Subregional library.

MEDIA PRODUCTION SERVICES

Braille Transcribers Club of Illinois

7240 North Overhill
Chicago, IL 60631-4206
(773) 774-6638
Martha E. Williams, Contact
Chairperson
Elaine L. Peterson, President

County/District Where Located:
Cook County.
Groups Served: K-12; college
students; other adults.

Types/Content: Textbooks;
recreational; career/vocational;

religious; foreign languages (French, Spanish, German).
Media Formats: Braille books.
Title Listings: No title listings available.

Central Blind Rehabilitation Center

Edward Hines, Jr. VA Hospital
P.O. Box 5000 (EH)
Hines, IL 60141
(708) 216-2272
FAX: (708) 531-7949
Charles Brancheau, Supervisor, Living Skills

Area Served: Midwest.
Groups Served: Adults.

Types/Content: Notes; learning aids.
Media Formats: Braille books, talking books/cassettes, large-print books.
Title Listings: No title listings available.

Chicago Public Library Illinois Regional Library for the Blind and Physically Handicapped

1055 West Roosevelt Road
Chicago, IL 60608
(312) 746-9210
FAX: (312) 746-9192
Barbara Perkis, Acting Director

County/District Where Located: Cook County.
Area Served: Statewide.
Groups Served: K-12; college students; other adults.

Types/Content: Recreational, informational and educational.
Media Formats: Braille/cassette books.
Title Listings: No title listings available.

Guild for the Blind

180 North Michigan Avenue
Suite 1700
Chicago, IL 60601-7463
(312) 236-8569
FAX: (312) 236-8128
David M. McGowan, CFRE, Executive Director
Denise M. Butera, Director of Services

Area Served: Unlimited.
Groups Served: K-12; college students; adults; senior citizens.

Types/Content: Recreational, career/vocational, and religious publications.
Media Formats: Braille and large print material, talking books/ cassettes.
Title Listings: Large-print, braille and audio lists available at no charge.
Free tape-lending library; audio, large print and audio transcription; braille, computer and Tae Kwon Do instruction; devotional material and self help books in large print, braille and audio cassette; education seminars for children and adults; phonote (a daily recording of retail and grocery stores ads); Consumer Product Center offering sensory and low vision aids; monthly newsletter, *Guild Briefs*.

Horizons for the Blind

16-A Meadowdale Shopping Center
Carpentersville, IL 60114
(847) 836-1400 (voice/TDD)
FAX: (847) 836-1443
Camille Caffarelli, Director

County/District Where Located: Kane County.
Area Served: Nationwide.
Groups Served: K-12; college students; other adults.

Types/Content: Recreational; menus; employment-related

documents for organizations and corporations.
Media Formats: Braille books; talking books/cassettes; large-print books.
Title Listings: Supplied in print and braille forms with and without a charge.

Illinois Instructional Materials Center

3031 Stanton
Springfield, IL 62703-4316
(217) 525-3300
FAX: (217) 525-7916
E-mail: ampost@springfield.kiz.il.us
Alice M. Post, Manager

County/District Where Located: Sangemon County.
Area Served: Illinois.
Groups Served: Blind and visually impaired people, children through adults.

Types/Content: Primarily instructional materials.
Media Formats: Braille and large print.

Illinois School for the Visually Impaired

658 East State Street
Jacksonville, IL 62650
(217) 479-4400
FAX: (217) 479-4479
Dorothy Arensman, Superintendent
Eric Emberg, Assistant Superintendent

Area Served: State of Illinois.
Groups Served: K-12.

Types/Content: None specified.
Media Formats: Braille books, talking books/cassettes, large print books.
Title Listings: None specified.

Johanna Bureau for the Blind and Physically Handicapped, Inc.

8 South Michigan Avenue
Suite 300
Chicago, IL 60603
(312) 332-6076
FAX: (312) 332-0780
Edith Weiner, Executive Chairman

Area Served: United States.
Groups Served: K-12; college students; other adults.

Types/Content: Textbooks; recreational.
Media Formats: Braille and tape.

LICA-NSSEO Vision East

1131 South Dee Road
Park Ridge, IL 60068
(847) 696-3600 or (800) 696-3600
FAX: (847) 696-3254
Gary Lieder, Special Education Director

County/District Where Located: Cook County.
Area Served: Chicago.
Groups Served: K-12.

Types/Content: Textbooks, recreational, career/vocational.
Media Formats: Braille books, talking books/cassettes, large print books.
Title Listings: Printed with and without a charge.

LICA-NSSEO Vision West

1855 Mount Prospect Road
Des Plaines, IL 60018
(847) 803-9444
FAX: (847) 803-9480
E-mail: jkimellica@worldnet.att. net
Jacqueline Kimel, Agency Administrator

County/District Where Located: Cook County.
Area Served: Northwest suburban Chicago.

Groups Served: Birth through age 21.

Types/Content: Textbooks, recreational, career/vocational.
Media Formats: Braille books, talking books/cassettes, large print books.
Title Listings: Printed with and without a charge.

Naperville Area Transcribing for the Blind

25 South Washington
Naperville, IL 60540
(630) 357-9464
FAX: (630) 357-9464
Gloria K. Buntrock, Coordinator

Groups Served: K-12 and adults.

Types/Content: Textbooks, recreational, career/vocational.
Media Formats: Braille books.
Title Listings: None specified.

Peoria Area Blind People's Center, Inc.

2905 West Garden Street
Peoria, IL 61605
(309) 637-3693
Shirley Harlan, Executive Director

Area Served: 40-mile radius of Peoria county courthouse.
Groups Served: Visually impaired and blind.

Types/Content: None specified.
Media Formats: Braille books, talking books/cassettes, large-print books.

Recording for the Blind and Dyslexic

Chicago Unit
18 South Michigan
Room 806
Chicago, IL 60603
(312) 236-8715
FAX: (312) 236-8719
E-mail: chicago@rfbd.org
Jill Bulinski, Director

County/District Where Located: Cook County.

See Recording for the Blind and Dyslexic in U.S. national listings.

Recording for the Blind and Dyslexic

University of Chicago
Hinds Building, Room 59-B
5734 South Ellis Avenue
Chicago, IL 60637
(773) 288-7077
Brenda Smith, Director
Maria Ahlstrom, Director

See Recording for the Blind and Dyslexic in U.S. national listings.

Recording for the Blind and Dyslexic

North Central College
30 North Brainard Street
Naperville, IL 60540
(630) 420-0722
Katherine Fuhrman, Director

County/District Where Located: Dupage County.

See Recording for the Blind and Dystexic in U.S. national listings.

Recording for the Blind and Dyslexic

708 Oak Street
P.O. Box 204
Winnetka, IL 60093
(847) 446-3338
FAX: (847) 446-9062
Barbara Gass, Director

County/District Where Located: Cook County.

See Recording for the Blind and Dyslexic in U.S. national listings.

Southern Illinois University

Rehabilitation Institute
Rehn Hall 317

Carbondale, IL 62901-4609
(618) 536-7704
FAX: (618) 453-8271
Dr. Darrell Taylor, Associate
Professor

County/District Where Located:
Jackson County.
Groups Served: College students,
other adults.

Types/Content: Textbooks,
career/vocational.
Media Formats: Braille books,
talking books/cassettes.
Title Listings: No title listings
available.

University of Illinois at Urbana-Champaign
Division of Rehabilitation Education Services

1207 South Oak Street
Champaign, IL 61820
(217) 333-4604
FAX: (217) 333-0248
Bryan McMurray, Supervisor,
Services for Sensory
Accommodations

County/District Where Located:
Champaign County.
Groups Served: College students,
other adults.

Types/Content: Textbooks,
recreational.
Media Formats: Braille books,
talking books/cassettes, large-
print books.
Title Listings: No title listings
available.

RADIO READING

APRIS
c/o WVIK
Augustana College
639 38th Street
Rock Island, IL 61201
(309) 794-7500
FAX: (309) 794-1236
Diane Stokeld, Director

Hours of Operation: Mon.-Fri.
8:00 AM - 5:00 PM.
History/Date: Est. 1989.
Area Served: 60 miles WVIK/40
miles APRIS.

Chicagoland Radio Information Service, Inc.
77 East Randolph
Pedestrian Walkway
Chicago, IL 60601
(312) 541-8400
FAX: (312) 541-8312
Bonnie Miller-Barnes, General
Manager

County/District Where Located:
Cook County.
Hours of Operation: 24 hours a
day, seven days a week.
Staff: 9.
History/Date: Est. 1980; est. 1996:
Dial-in News Reading Service.
Area Served: Chicago
Metropolitan area.

Illinois Radio Reader
59 East Armory
Champaign, IL 61820
(217) 333-6503
E-mail: dgeiken@uiuc.edu
Deane Geiken, Coordinator

Funded by: Illinois state library.
Hours of Operation: Mon.-Fri.
7:00 AM-12:00 PM; Sat.-Sun.
8:00 AM-11:00 PM; local
programming presented
11:00 AM-11:00 PM weekdays,
11:00 AM-12:00 PM weekends.
Contact the reading service for
exact schedule.
History/Date: Est. 1978.
Area Served: 80-mile radius from
Monticello, Illinois (transmitter
site).

Northern Illinois Radio Information Services/WNIJ
711 North Main Street

Rockford, IL 61103
(815) 961-8000
Ann McHale, Director

County/District Where Located:
Winnebago County.

Northern Illinois Radio Information Services/WNIU-FM
Northern Illinois University
DeKalb, IL 60115
(815) 753-0074
Ann McHale, Director

County/District Where Located:
DeKalb County.
Hours of Operation: 24 hours, 7
days.
History/Date: Est. 1979.
Area Served: 60-mile radius from
DeKalb in northern Illinois.

Radio Information Service
Wabash Valley College
2200 College Drive
Mt. Carmel, IL 62863
(618) 262-8641, ext. 253
Glenda Raber, Program Director
Jerry Bayne, Coordinator

County/District Where Located:
Wabash County.
Hours of Operation: Mon.-Sun.
6:00 AM-12:00 midnight.
History/Date: Est. 1977.
Area Served: 45-mile radius from
Mt. Carmel, including portions of
Indiana.

Radio Information Service for Blind and Print Handicapped
9541 Church Circle Drive
Belleville, IL 62223
(618) 397-6700, ext. 2221 or in St.
Louis area, (314) 241-3400
Joseph E. Kasperek, Executive
Director

County/District Where Located:
St. Claire County.
Hours of Operation: Mon.-Fri.
7:00 AM-12:00 PM; Sat.-Sun.
8:00 AM-11:00 PM.

History/Date: Est. 1973.
Area Served: Greater St. Louis metropolitan area.

Southern Illinois Radio Information Service

P.O. Box 1056
Carbondale, IL 62903
(618) 549-5604
FAX: (618) 453-6186
E-mail: bill_gilmore@wsiu.pbs.org
Bill Gilmore, Manager

County/District Where Located: Jackson County.
Hours of Operation: Mon.-Sun. 5:00 AM-1:00 AM.
History/Date: Est. 1984.
Area Served: Southern Illinois, Missouri, Kentucky.
Age Requirements: None.

Radio reading service for the blind and physically impaired.

WCBU Radio Information Service

1501 West Bradley Avenue
Peoria, IL 61625
(309) 677-3690
Keith Berry, General Manager
Louis Grayer, Volunteer Coordinator

Hours of Operation: Mon.-Fri. 7:30 AM-4:00 PM.
History/Date: Est. 1981.
Area Served: 40-mile radius from Peoria.

WIUM/WIUW Radio Information Service

Western Illinois University
504 Memorial Hall
Macomb, IL 61455
(309) 298-2403
FAX: (309) 298-2133
E-mail: carol_dennhardt@ccmail.wiu.edu
Carol Dennhardt, Director
Ken Zahnle, Programming

County/District Where Located: McDonough County.
Funded by: School of Continuing Education at WIU, Illinois State Library, and local United Ways.
Hours of Operation: 24 hours a day. Local programming: Mon.-Fri. 8:00 AM-11:00 PM; Sat.-Sun. 8:00 AM-11:30 PM.
History/Date: Est. 1978.
Area Served: All or parts of a 20-county area in west central Illinois, southeast Iowa, and northeast Missouri.
Age Requirements: None.

WUIS/WIPA Radio Information Service

University of Illinois at Springfield
Springfield, IL 62794-9243
(217) 786-6516
FAX: (217) 786-6527
E-mail: kearneytrish@uis.edu
URL: http://www.uis.edu/~wuis/wuis2.htm
Trish Kearney, Coordinator/Director

County/District Where Located: Sangamon County.
Funded by: Illinois State Library, University of Illinois at Springfield, WUIS/WIPA civic organizations, listeners; volunteers.
Hours of Operation: Mon.-Fri. 5:00 AM-12:00 AM; Sat. 6:00 AM-12:00 AM; Sun. 6:00 AM-12:00 AM, 4:30 PM-6:00 PM.
History/Date: Est. 1981.
Area Served: 40-mile radius of Springfield, Illinois, and 40-mile radius of Pittsfield, Illinois.
Age Requirements: None.

INFORMATION AND REFERRAL

American Foundation for the Blind Midwest

401 North Michigan Avenue
Suite 308

Chicago, IL 60611
(312) 245-9961
FAX: (312) 245-9965
E-mail: chicago@afb.org
URL: http://www.afb.org

See American Foundation for the Blind in U.S. national listings.

The Foundation Fighting Blindness Chicago Affiliate

1011 South Waiola
La Grange, IL 60525
(708) 354-8108
FAX: (708) 354-8108
Ann Rasch, Contact Person

See The Foundation Fighting Blindness in U.S. national listings.

Illinois Society for the Prevention of Blindness

407 South Dearborn Street
Suite 1000
Chicago, IL 60605
(312) 922-8710
E-mail: ispb@aol.com
James A. McKechnie, Jr.

Type of Agency: Non-profit.
County/District Where Located: Cook County.
Mission: To prevent needless blindness through education and information.
Funded by: Individual contributions, bequests, corporate & foundation grants.
Hours of Operation: Mon.-Fri. 8:30AM - 4:30PM.

Promotes eye health/safety via public/professional education programs.

Prevent Blindness America

500 East Remington Road

Schaumburg, IL 60173
(847) 843-2020 or PBA Center for
Sight (800) 331-2020 or (800) 221-
3004
FAX: (847) 843-8458
E-mail: preventblindness
@compuserve.com
URL: http://www.prevent-
blindness.org
Ricahrd T. Hellner, President and
CEO.

See Prevent Blindness America in
U.S. national listings. Local and
affiliate offices are listed in their
respective states.

See also in national listings:

**American Blind Skiing
Foundation**

**American Society for
Contemporary Ophthalmology**

Hadley School for the Blind

Knights Templar Eye Foundation

Lions Clubs International

Myasthenia Gravis Foundation

National Easter Seals Society

**National Eye Research
Foundation (Optometry)**

Prevent Blindness America

♦ Rehabilitation Services

STATE SERVICES

**Illinois Department of
Rehabilitation Services**

623 East Adams Street
P.O. Box 19429
Springfield, IL 62794-9429
(217) 782-2093 or TDD (217) 782-
5734 or (800) 275-3677
FAX: (217) 785-5753
Audrey McCrimon, Director
Glenn Crawford, Deputy Director

Type of Agency: State.
County/District Where Located:
Sangamon County.
Funded by: Public funds.
Eligibility: One of the following:
Adults who have a severe visual
impairment and require assistance
in adjusting to their loss of vision;
persons below age 60 whose
disability places them in danger of
long-term institutionalization and
for whom the cost of home
services would be reasonably
related to the cost of institutional
care (need not have a vocational
goal); severely disabled school-age
children and youths (blind, deaf,
and/or orthopedically disabled)
who would benefit from a
residential school setting and who
cannot be served appropriately by
local resources.

Rehabilitation: Directly provides
rehabilitation counseling,
guidance, some testing, job
placement services, rehabilitation
teaching and orientation/mobility
instruction in a community-based
or residential setting. Other
necessary services are purchased
in whole or in part (depending
upon similar benefits and other
resources) by the department.

Local Offices:

Aurora: Illinois Department of
Rehabilitation Services, 888 South
Edgelawn, Suite 1771, Aurora, IL
60505, (630) 892-7417 (voice) or
(TDD) (630) 892-7702.
Belleville: Illinois Department of
Rehabilitation Services, 601 South
High Street, Belleville, IL 62220,
(618) 235-5300 (voice/TDD).
Carbondale: Illinois Department
of Rehabilitation Services, 309 East
Jackson, P.O. Box 2348,
Carbondale, IL 62902-2348,
(618) 457-2107 (voice/ TDD).

Champaign: Illinois Department
of Rehabilitation Services, 510
Devonshire, Champaign, IL 61820,
(217) 333-5707 or (TDD) (217) 333-
5716.
Chicago: Illinois Department of
Rehabilitation Services, 100 West
Randolph, Suite 8-100, Chicago, IL
60601, (312) 814-2934 (voice) or
(TDD) (312) 814-5000.
Chicago: Illinois Department of
Rehabilitation Services, 8840 South
Stony Island, Chicago, IL 60617,
(773) 768-6700 (voice/TDD).
Chicago: Illinois Department of
Rehabilitation Services, 6200 N.
Hiawatha, 3rd floor, Chicago, IL
60646, (312) 794-4800 (voice/TDD).
Chicago: Illinois Department of
Rehabilitation Services, 3710 North
Kedzie, Chicago, IL 60618-4504,
(773) 509-1070 or (TDD) (773) 509-
1058.
Chicago: Illinois Center for
Rehabilitation and Education, 1151
South Wood Street, Chicago, IL
60612, (312) 633-3520 (voice) or
(TDD) (312) 633-3524.
Chicago: Illinois Department of
Rehabilitation Services, 3556 South
Ashland Avenue, Chicago, IL
60608, (773) 650-4640 (voice/TDD).
Chicago Heights: Illinois
Department of Rehabilitation
Services, 1010 Dixie Highway, 4th
flr, Chicago Heights, IL 60411,
(708) 709-3333 (voice) or
(TDD) (708) 709-3337.
Decatur: Illinois Department of
Rehabilitation Services, 1065 West
Pershing Road, Decatur, IL 62526,
(217) 875-4866 (voice/TDD).
Downers Grove: Illinois
Department of Rehabilitation
Services, 2901 Finley Road, Suite
109, Downers Grove, IL 60515,
(630) 495-0500 (voice) or (TDD)
(630) 495-2294.

Evergreen Park: Illinois Department of Rehabilitation Services, 9730 South Western Avenue, Room 612, Evergreen Park, IL 60805-2814, (708) 857-2350 or (TDD) (708) 857-2359.

Granite City: Illinois Department of Rehabilitation Services, 3675 Nameoki Road, Granite City, IL 62040, (618) 877-0753 (voice/TDD).

Jacksonville: Illinois Department of Rehabilitation Services, 1429 South Main, Jacksonville, IL 62650, (217) 245-9585 (voice/TDD).

Mt. Vernon: Illinois Department of Rehabilitation Services, 4 Doctors Park Road, Mt. Vernon, IL 62864, (618) 244-0331 (voice) or (TDD) (618) 244-0339.

Peoria: Illinois Department of Rehabilitation Services, 4808 North Sheridan Road, Peoria, IL 61614, (309) 686-6000 or (TDD) (309) 686-6088.

Rockford: Illinois Department of Rehabilitation Services, 615 North Longwood, Rockford, IL 61107, (815) 964-0360 (voice/TDD).

Rock Island: Illinois Department of Rehabilitation Services, 4711 44th Street, Suite #3, Rock Island, IL 61201, (309) 786-6468 or (TDD) (309) 786-6460.

Rolling Meadows: Illinois Department of Rehabilitation Services, 5340 Keystone Court, Rolling Meadows, IL 60008, (847) 253-6200 (voice) or (TDD) (847) 253-1362.

Springfield: Illinois Department of Rehabilitation Services, 1124 North Walnut Street, Springfield, IL 62702, (217) 782-4830 (voice/TDD).

REHABILITATION

Blind Service Association

22 West Monroe
11th Floor
Chicago, IL 60603-2501
(312) 236-0808
FAX: (312) 236-8679
Anna Perlberg, Executive Director

Type of Agency: Private; non-profit.
Mission: Services to help blind and visually impaired people achieve and maintain independence.
Funded by: Private contributions.
Hours of Operation: Mon.-Thurs. 9:00 AM-8:00 PM; Fri. 9:00 AM-5:00 PM.
Staff: 7 full-time equivalents.
History/Date: Est. 1924.
Number of Clients Served: 1,000.
Eligibility: Legal blindness or reading disability.
Area Served: Chicago and five surrounding counties.

Health: Refers for diagnosis and evaluation of eye health.
Counseling/Social Work/Self-Help: Self-help and support groups for young adults, seminars, "mid-lifers", job seekers.
Educational: Summer transition programs for high school students; variety of school-year programs for blind and visually impaired students in Chicago public schools.
Reading: Tape recording of college textbooks, personal, professional and business material; one-to-one reading services in organization's office, five public library satellite programs and clients' offices and homes.
Recreational: Variety of outings and parties.
Computer Training: Peer training, workshops, consultation.
Low Vision: Non-medical low vision consultation.
Low Vision Aids: Assistance with ordering, as part of low vision consultation.

Center for Sight and Hearing Impaired

625 Adams Street
Rockford, IL 61107
(815) 965-4454 (voice/TTD)
FAX: (815) 965-6023
Diane Jones, Director of Professional Services
Linda O'Reilly, Instructor of Sensory Impaired

Type of Agency: Non-profit.
County/District Where Located: Winnebago County.
Mission: To provide services to assist persons born with or affected by a sight or hearing loss in reaching their maximum potential and full community integration.
Funded by: Client fees; vocational rehabilitation funds; donations.
Hours of Operation: Mon.-Fri. 8:00 AM - 4:30 PM and Thurs. 8:00 AM-12:30 PM low vision services.
Staff: 8 full-time; 11 part-time.
History/Date: Founded visually inpaired center in 1962; hearing impaired services added in 1984.
Number of Clients Served: 550.
Eligibility: 18 years and older with documentation of a vision or hearing impairment.
Area Served: Northern Illinois and southern Wisconsin.
Transportation: Y.
Age Requirements: Adults for rehabilitation program; children-adults for low vision clinic.

Health: Agency serves persons for whom visual impairment is the primary disability.
Counseling/Social Work/Self-Help: Support group for consumers.
Counseling/Social Work/Self-Help: Support group for consumers.
Professional Training: Internships in rehabilitation teaching; rehabilitation counseling specialization.

Rehabilitation: Personal management; home management; communication skills, in center or in clients' homes.
Recreational: Regularly scheduled social/recreational activities for adults with visual disabilities.
Computer Training: Access and training available.
Low Vision: Low vision clinic. On-site training provided.
Low Vision Aids: Loan/purchase.
Low Vision Follow-up: Return appointment; home visit; phone interviews.

Central Blind Rehabilitation Center
U.S. Department of Veterans Affairs

Edward Hines, Jr. VA Hospital
P.O. Box 5000
Hines, IL 60141
(708) 216-2272
FAX: (708) 531-7949
J. J. Whitehead, Director

Type of Agency: Federal.
County/District Where Located: Cook County.
Mission: Provides residential rehabilitation services to eligible legally blind veterans.
Funded by: Department of Veteran Affairs.
Hours of Operation: Mon.-Fri. 7:30 AM-4:00 PM.
History/Date: Est. 1948.
Number of Clients Served: 30-bed inpatient capacity.
Area Served: Midwest states.
Age Requirements: None.

Health: Staffed by part time physician and 24-hour nursing coverage.
Counseling/Social Work/Self-Help: Counseling provided by psychologist and social worker.
Professional Training: Intern site for graduate students in

rehabilitation teaching and orientation and mobility.
Reading: Teach braille and use of low vision aids, plus reading machines.
Rehabilitation: Provides a comprehensive blind rehabilitation training program.
Recreational: Limited.
Employment: Prevocational counseling and testing provided.
Computer Training: Access training on computer aids and reading machines.
Low Vision: Full scope of low vision instruction.
Low Vision Aids: Issued to eligible blinded veterans.
Low Vision Follow-up: By phone interview and questionnaire in 2-3 months.

Referral applications by Visual Impairment Services programs located at Medical Centers and Outpatient Clinics in the geographical area served by the Blind Rehabilitation Center or Clinic.

See U.S. Department of Veterans Affairs in U.S. Federal Agencies listings.

Central Illinois Sight Center
TCRC Sight Center

117 East Washington Street
East Peoria, IL 61611
(309) 698-4001
FAX: (309) 698-9227
Tina Probyn, Executive Vice President of Rehabilitation Services

Type of Agency: Private; non-profit.
County/District Where Located: Tazewell County.
Mission: To provide a broad range of services designed to meet critical, unmet needs of persons throughout central Illinois who are blind or partially sighted.

Funded by: Client fees; grants; donations.
Hours of Operation: Mon.- Fri. 8:30 AM - 5:00 PM.
Staff: 4 full time. Uses volunteers.
History/Date: Est. 1986 as outgrowth and expansion of former Central Illinois Low Vision Aids Clinic.
Eligibility: Blind or visually impaired.
Area Served: All of central Illinois without geographic restriction.

Counseling/Social Work/Self-Help: Support services, case management, and referral services.
Rehabilitation: Orientation and mobility; independent living services.
Recreational: Games and recreational aids available for purchase.
Low Vision: Clinic.
Low Vision Aids: Aids and appliances center has wide assortment of independent living aids available for demonstration and purchase. Includes electronic aids; health aids; lamps; household, kitchen, and sewing aids; writing aids; large-print bibles and reference books; recreation aids. Low vision clinic recommends and dispenses optical aids.
Low Vision Follow-up: Provided as needed, by phone or in person.

Chicago Lighthouse for People Who Are Blind or Visually Impaired

1850 West Roosevelt Road
Chicago, IL 60608
(312) 666-1331 or TDD (312) 666-8874
FAX: (312) 243-8539
James Kesteloot, Executive Director

Type of Agency: Private; non-profit.

County/District Where Located:
Cook County.
Mission: To create opportunities for blind and visually impaired people, including those who are multiply disabled. To develop and promote effective programs that maximize the potential for independent living, assist in achieving economic self-support, and prevent unnecessary institutionalization.
Funded by: Fees; United Way; grants; workshop sales; capital income; legacies and bequests; rehabilitation training fees.
Hours of Operation: 8:45 AM-5:00 PM.
Program Accessibility: Fully accessible building and grounds.
Staff: 115 full time. Uses volunteers.
History/Date: Est. 1906.
Eligibility: Visually impaired. Does not accept persons with uncontrolled seizures.
Area Served: Chicago and metropolitan area.
Transportation: Y.

Health: Evaluation of eye health; treatment of eye conditions; prescription of spectacles or aids. Refers for other health services.
Counseling/Social Work/Self-Help: Limited psychological testing and evaluation; individual, group, family/parent, couple counseling; placement in training. Refers for other counseling/social work services. Provides consultation to other agencies.
Educational: Accepts deaf-blind, emotionally disturbed, learning disabled, and mentally retarded persons. Programs: birth-3, preschool, vocational skill development, high school equivalency.
Preschools: Child development program.

Professional Training:
Internship/fieldwork placement in low vision, rehabilitation counseling, special education. In-service training programs. Short-term or summer training. Programs open to enrollment from other agencies.
Rehabilitation: Handwriting; typing; video magnifiers; orientation/mobility; remedial education; sensory training. Refers for other rehabilitation services.
Recreational: Refers for recreational services.
Employment: Prevocational evaluation; vocational evaluation; career and skill counseling; occupational skill development; job retention; job retraining; rehabilitation workshop; vocational placement; supported employment. Follow-up service. Refers for other employment-oriented services.
Computer Training: Training available, with focus on employment applications of computer and other sensory aids.
Low Vision: Clinic, two satellite programs.
Low Vision Aids: Aids and equipment lending program.
Low Vision Follow-up: Follow-up evaluation of eye treatment or prescription.

Helen Keller National Center for Deaf-Blind Youths and Adults North Central Region Office
205 West Wacker Drive
Suite 919
Chicago, IL 60606-1212
(312) 726-2090 (voice) or TDD
(312) 726-2810
FAX: (312) 726-3503
Catherine Klein, Secretary
Laura Thomas Roebal, Regional Representative

County/District Where Located:
Cook County.

Mission: To facilitate a national, coordinated effort to meet the social, rehabilitative and independent living needs of Americans who are deaf-blind.
Funded by: Federal funds.
Budget: $7.4 million.
Hours of Operation: Mon.-Fri. 9:00AM - 5:00AM.
Area Served: Northcentral states.
Age Requirements: 16 years and older.

Health: Must be in good health & free of communicable diseases.
Employment: Work experience and on-the-job training.

See Helen Keller National Center for Deaf-Blind Youths and Adults in U.S. national listings.

Kagan Home for the Blind
3525 West Foster Avenue
Chicago, IL 60625
(773) 478-7040
FAX: (773) 478-4762
Robert Lieberman, Executive Director

Type of Agency: Private; non-profit; sheltered care home.
County/District Where Located:
Cook County.
Mission: Services for totally blind, legally blind, visually impaired.
Budget: $910,000.
Hours of Operation: 24 hours, 7 days a week.
Staff: Uses volunteers.
History/Date: Est. 1944.
Number of Clients Served: 50 residents.
Eligibility: Blind or legally blind.
Area Served: Chicago metropolitan area.
Transportation: Y.
Age Requirements: 17 years and over.

Counseling/Social Work/Self-Help: Individual, family/parent, couple counseling.

Educational: College-level classes in cooperation with City College of Chicago.
Reading: Lends talking book record players and cassette players; talking book records and cassettes; braille books; large print books; braille magazines; recorded magazines; information and referral.
Residential: Room and board for blind and visually handicapped 15 years of age and up. Must be ambulatory and continent.
Rehabilitation: Referrals for physical, occupational and speech therapy.
Employment: Training programs and workshops.
Computer Training: Referrals.
Low Vision: Referrals to oustide clinics.
Low Vision Follow-up: Y.

Mary Bryant Home for the Blind

2960 Stanton
Springfield, IL 62703
(217) 529-1611
FAX: (217) 529-6975
Monica J. Lederbrand, Administrator

Type of Agency: Private; non-profit.
Mission: Residential facility for visually impaired/blind individuals.
Funded by: Dues; donations; resident's income.
Hours of Operation: Mon.-Fri. 9:00 AM - 5:00 PM.
Staff: 18 full time. Uses volunteers.
Number of Clients Served: 46.
Eligibility: Legally blind; able to care for self.
Area Served: Nationwide.
Transportation: Y.
Age Requirements: 18 years and older.

Professional Training: Regular in-service programs.
Residential: Assisted living for adults.
Recreational: Recrectional, religious, and community-service activities and educational programs.

Peoria Area Blind People's Center, Inc.

2905 West Garden Street
Peoria, IL 61605
(309) 637-3693
Shirley Harlan, Executive Director

Type of Agency: Private; non-profit.
Mission: Services for visually handicapped of central Illinois.
Funded by: Special events, contributions, United Way, grants, capital income, legacies and bequests, activity fees.
Hours of Operation: Mon.-Fri. 8:00 AM-4:30 PM.
Staff: 2 full time, 2 part time. Uses volunteers.
History/Date: Est. 1956.
Area Served: 40 mile radius of Peoria.
Transportation: Y.

Health: Nutrition class.
Counseling/Social Work/Self-Help: Needs assessment; individual and family counseling; support network; peer counseling; information and referral service to other agencies.
Reading: Parent education; braille; handwriting skills; braille and large print materials; library and radio reader services.
Rehabilitation: Referral services and consultation to other agencies; volunteer opportunities for clients.
Low Vision Aids: Available through director.

Services for Sensory Accommodations
University of Illinois at Urbana-Champaign
Division of Rehabilitation Education Services

1207 South Oak Street
Champaign, IL 68120
(217) 333-4604
FAX: (217) 333-0248
Paul Leung, Director
Paul Reinert, Supervisor

Mission: To provide technical support to persons who use adapted computer technologies and services for students with disabilities.
Funded by: University of Illinois; private contributions.
Hours of Operation: Mon.-Fri. 8:00 AM-5:00 PM.
Staff: 1.5 full-time equivalent. Professionals in physical therapy, recreation, athletics, counseling, and sensory impairment. Uses volunteers.
History/Date: Est. 1947.
Eligibility: Students attending the University of Illinois at Urbana-Champaign receive first priority for services.
Age Requirements: School aged; post-secondary school aged; and adults.

Counseling/Social Work/Self-Help: Referral services; casework; group work; and psychological testing.
Educational: Post-high school.
Reading: Talking book record player and cassette player; talking book records and cassettes; braille books; large print books.
Rehabilitation: Personal management; braille; gesticulation; handwriting; listening skills; Optacon; typing; video magnifier; orientation/mobility; remedial education; sensory training.
Recreational: Bowling; swimming.

Computer Training: Provide computer assessments/evaluations; one-on-one training on adapted computer technologies for individuals who are visually impaired.

COMPUTER TRAINING CENTERS

Central Blind Rehabilitation Center

Edward Hines, Jr. VA Hospital
P.O. Box 5000 (EH)
Hines, IL 60141
(708) 343-7200
FAX: (708) 531-7927
Leonard Mowinski, Computer Training

Computer Training: Speech output systems; screen magnification systems; braille access systems; optical character recognition systems; closed-circuit television systems; word processing; database software; computer operating systems.

Chicago Lighthouse for People Who Are Blind or Visually Impaired

1850 West Roosevelt Road
Chicago, IL 60608
(312) 666-1331 or TDD (312) 666-8874
FAX: (312) 243-8539
James Kesteloot, Director

County/District Where Located: Cook County.

Computer Training: Speech output systems; screen magnification systems; braille access systems; optical character recognition systems; closed-circuit television systems; word processing; database software; computer operating systems; training for instructors.

Equipment loans and employer services also available.

Illinois Department of Rehabilitation Services Bureau of Blind Services

622 East Washington Street
P.O. Box 19429
Springfield, IL 62794-9429
(217) 785-3887
FAX: (217) 524-1235
Alex J. Jones, Management Systems Specialist

Computer Training: Speech output systems; screen magnification systems; braille access systems; optical character recognition systems; closed-circuit television systems; word processing; computer operating systems.

Illinois School for the Visually Impaired

658 East State Street
Jacksonville, IL 62650-2183
(217) 479-4400
FAX: (217) 479-4479
URL: http://www.dors.state.il.us/isvi
Brian Fay, Assitive Technology Specialist
Patricia Langdon, Low Vision Coordinator

Computer Training: Evaluations and training of assistive technologies including computer screen magnification, speech input/output, reading systems, and stand alone products. Most major vendor products are used including GW Micro, Telesensory, HumanWave, Henter-Joyce, AFB, APH, ABP, AI-squared, Micro System Internat'l, DecTalk, RCSystems, Automated Functions, Blazie Engineering, and others.

◆ Low Vision Services

EYE CARE SOCIETIES

Illinois Association of Ophthalmology

Metro Square One
Ten West Phillips Road
Vernon Hills, IL 60061-1730
(847) 680-1666
FAX: (847) 680-1682
E-mail: ileyedocs@aol.com
Rich Paul, Executive Director
John Hanlon M.D., President

County/District Where Located: Lake County.

Illinois Optometric Association

304 West Washington Street
Springfield, IL 62701
(217) 525-8012
Michael G. Horstman, President

LOW VISION CENTERS

Central Blind Rehabilitation Center

Edward Hines, Jr. VA Hospital
P.O. Box 5000 (EH)
Hines, IL 60141
(708) 216-2124
FAX: (708) 531-7949
Dr. Joan Stelmark, Director

Type of Agency: Federal.
Mission: To provide blind rehabilitation training.
Funded by: Federal government.
Hours of Operation: Mon.-Fri. 7:30 AM-4.00 PM.
Staff: Optometrist; low vision specialist; social worker; orientation/mobility instructor; rehabilitation teacher; psychologist.
History/Date: Est. 1948.
Eligibility: Legally blind veterans only; ophthalmologic report required.

Area Served: Midwest.

Computer Training: Access; training on computer aids and devices.

Low Vision Aids: Provided on loan for trial purposes; no fee charged; on-site training provided.

Low Vision Follow-up: By phone interview and questionnaire in 3 months; occasionally by return appointment; home visit after 9 months and visit to place of employment.

Chicago Lighthouse for People Who Are Blind or Visually Impaired

1850 West Roosevelt Road
Chicago, IL 60608
(312) 666-1331 or TDD (312) 666-8874
FAX: (312) 243-8539
Marge Miller, Director of Clinical Services
A. A. Rosenbloom, O.D.
Gerald Fishman, M.D.

Type of Agency: Private; non-profit.

County/District Where Located: Cook County.

Mission: To create opportunities for blind and visually impaired people, including those who are multiply disabled. To develop and promote effective programs that maximize the potential for independent living, assist in achieving economic self-support, and prevent unnecessary institutionalization.

Funded by: Client fees; Department of Rehabilitation Services funding.

Budget: $269,782.

Hours of Operation: Mon.-Fri; hours vary.

Staff: Ophthalmologist; optometrist; optometry student/resident; ophthalmology resident; ophthalmic assistant/technician; low vision assistant; rehabilitation counselor; social worker; orientation/mobility instructor; special educator; psychologist/counselor; audiologist.

History/Date: Est. 1957.

Number of Clients Served: More than 700.

Eligibility: Prior ophthalmological exam.

Area Served: Unlimited.

Age Requirements: None.

Counseling/Social Work/Self-Help: Available.

Rehabilitation: Referrals.

Computer Training: Y.

Low Vision Aids: Provided on loan for trial purposes; no rental fee; on-site training provided.

Low Vision Follow-up: By phone interview in 6 months and return appointment at that time by patient's request; 2-year review questionnaire.

Deicke Center for Visual Rehabilitation

219 East Cole Avenue
Wheaton, IL 60187
(630) 690-7115
FAX: (630) 690-9037
E-mail: tech center: eyetec@interaccess.com
R. Tracy Williams, O.D., Executive Director

Type of Agency: Non-profit.

County/District Where Located: Du Page County.

Mission: To help people with visual impairments become as independent as possible through comprehensive visual rehabilitation.

Funded by: Client fees, foundation grants, private donations.

Budget: $543,995.

Hours of Operation: Mon. - Fri. 9:00 AM - 4:30 PM.

Staff: 6 full time, 5 part-time; low vision assistants; optometrist.

History/Date: Est. 1985.

Number of Clients Served: 5,000 to date.

Eligibility: Doctor or rehabilitation referral or current ophthalmology report.

Area Served: Statewide.

Age Requirements: 6 years and up.

Counseling/Social Work/Self-Help: Individual, group and family counseling.

Professional Training: Supervision/training programs in gerontology, low vision, optometry, social work.

Reading: Large print-books.

Rehabilitation: Training in activities of daily living and use of optical devices and high tech.

Computer Training: Computers with speech capability and enlargement software.

Low Vision: On-site training provided.

Low Vision Aids: Prescribed/fitted for purchase; trial period.

Low Vision Follow-up: Return appointment; phone interviews.

Eye Clinic, Children's Memorial Hospital

2300 Children's Plaza
Chicago, IL 60614
(773) 880-4532
Mark Greenwald, Head, Division of Ophthalmology

Type of Agency: Non-profit.

County/District Where Located: Cook County.

Funded by: Client fees.

Hours of Operation: By appointment only.

Staff: Ophthalmology residents.

Area Served: Chicago metropolitan area.

Age Requirements: Under 16 years.

Illinois Center for Rehabilitation and Education

1151 South Wood Street
Chicago, IL 60612
(312) 633-3520
Betty Odem Davis, Director

Type of Agency: Part of Illinois Department of Rehabilitation Services, Bureau of Blind Services.
County/District Where Located: Cook County.
Funded by: State.
Hours of Operation: Mon., Tues. 1:00PM - 4:30PM; Wed. 9:00AM - 12 noon.
Staff: Optometrist; rehabilitation teacher; orientation/mobility specialist, vocational counselor, adjustment counselor.
Eligibility: Visual impairment interfering with work or independence.
Area Served: Illinois.
Age Requirements: 18 years and older.

Educational: GED program.
Reading: Braille and tape instruction.
Employment: Vocational counseling.
Computer Training: Orientation; some advanced classes.
Low Vision: Clinical services.
Low Vision Aids: Available on case basis.
Low Vision Follow-up: Yes.

Illinois Eye Institute/Illinois College of Optometry

3241 South Michigan Avenue
Chicago, IL 60616
(312) 949-7255
John Rimkus O.D., Vision Rehabilitation Services
Dennis Siemsen O.D., Chief

Type of Agency: Non-profit.
County/District Where Located: Cook County.

Mission: To provide a wide range of quality services to blind and visually impaired children, adults and seniors. As a clinical facility, we have a dual mission to train the next generation of eye health professionals.
Funded by: Patient fees; foundation grants.
Hours of Operation: Mon. - Sat. by appointment.
Staff: Low vision specialists, optometrists; ophthalmologist; opticians.
History/Date: Est. 1872.
Eligibility: None.
Area Served: Unlimited.

Health: Optometry, ophthalmology, and internal medicine services available on site.
Counseling/Social Work/Self-Help: On-site.
Rehabilitation: Daily living activities; orientation and mobility; referrals.
Computer Training: Large-print computer programs available; training referrals.
Low Vision: Full variety of low vision services provided.
Low Vision Aids: Wide variety of low vision aids available for trial purposes; on-site training provided.
Low Vision Follow-up: By telephone or in person.

Loyola University Medical Center
Department of Ophthalmology

2160 South First Avenue
Maywood, IL 60153
(708) 216-3789
FAX: (708) 216-3557
Walter Jay, Chairman
Peggy Squires, COA

County/District Where Located: Cook County.
Mission: Provides vision aids and training in their use to visually impaired persons and refer patients for advanced services and equipment as necessary.
Funded by: Medical School.
Hours of Operation: By appointment.
Program Accessibility: Wheelchair accessibility.
Staff: Ophthalmologist.
History/Date: Est. 1978.
Number of Clients Served: About 120 new patients per year.
Eligibility: None.
Area Served: Unlimited.

Counseling/Social Work/Self-Help: Referrals to appropriate local agencies and self-help groups.
Low Vision Follow-up: By appointment.

Northwestern Medical Faculty Foundation

645 North Michigan Avenue
Chicago, IL 60611
(312) 943-4272
Carol Barron, O.D., Director, Low Vision

Type of Agency: Non-profit.
County/District Where Located: Cook County.
Funded by: Client fees, private donations.
Hours of Operation: Mon. - Fri. 8:00 AM - 5:00 PM.
Staff: Low vision assistant; ophthalmology resident/assistant; optometrist; optician.
Area Served: Unlimited.

Low Vision: On-site training provided.
Low Vision Aids: Loaned at no cost; can be purchased; prescribed; fitted.
Low Vision Follow-up: Return appointment.

**Veterans Administration
West Side Medical Center
VICTORS Program**
820 South Damen
Chicago, IL 60612
(312) 666-6500, ext. 3501
FAX: (312) 633-2148
E-mail: stelmack.t@chicago-west.va.gov
Thomas R. Stelmack, O.D., Chief,
Optometry Service and Director,
VICTORS

Type of Agency: Non-profit.
County/District Where Located:
Cook County.
Mission: To provide
comprehensive multidisciplinary
low vision rehabilitation services
to partially sighted veterans in a
manner allowing training with
devices prescribed and dispensed
during program.
Funded by: Federal government.
Hours of Operation: 7:30 AM-
7:00 PM.
Staff: Ophthalmologist;
optometrist; low vision assistant;
occupational therapist on
consulting basis. One person
trained in orientation and mobility
and low vision training functions
as low vision training specialist,
psychologist and medical social
worker. Audiologist.
History/Date: Est. 1996.
Number of Clients Served: 100
per year.
Eligibility: Visually impaired
veterans.
Area Served: Midwest/north
central United States.

**Counseling/Social Work/Self-
Help:** Social worker, psychologist
routinely see patients.
Professional Training: Teaching
program with residents and
students.
Rehabilitation: Intensive 4-day
residential rehabilitation program
for partially sighted veterans.

Computer Training: Computer
access provided.
Low Vision: On-site training
provided.
Low Vision Aids: Prescriptions at
no charge.
Low Vision Follow-up: Return
appointment; phone interviews.

◆ *Aging Services*

STATE UNITS ON AGING

Illinois Department on Aging
421 East Capitol Avenue
Springfield, IL 62701
(217) 785-2870 or Information &
Referral In State (800) 252-8966
FAX: (217) 785-4477
Maralee Lindley, Acting Director

Provides referrals to Area Agencies
on Aging and information on other
local aging services.

INDEPENDENT LIVING PROGRAMS

**Illinois Department of
Rehabilitation Services**
623 East Adams Street
P.O. Box 19429
Springfield, IL 62794-9429
(217) 782-2093 or (800) 275-3677
FAX: (217) 524-1234
Andrey McCrimon, Director
Linda Krueger, Public Service
Administrator

Provides independent living
services for persons age 55 and
over. For further information,
contact the Project Director or
general phone number listed.

INDIANA

◆ *Educational Services*

STATE SERVICES

Indiana Department of Education
Division of Special Education
Room 229, State House
Indianapolis, IN 46204-2798
(317) 232-0581
FAX: (317) 232-0589
E-mail: knoths@speced.state.in.us
Sharon Knoth, Consultant, Visually Impaired
Leslie C. Durst, Resource Coordinator for Indiana Educational Resource Center

Type of Agency: State.
Mission: Administers supplemental state aid for visually impaired children in local public schools. Provides consultation on educational programs. Maintains lending library of braille and large-type textbooks.
Funded by: Public funds.
Hours of Operation: 8:00 AM - 4:30 PM.
Staff: 31.
History/Date: Est. 1947.
Eligibility: Determined pursuant to P.L. 101-476.
Area Served: Indiana.
Age Requirements: 3 - 21 years.

For information about local facilities, consult the superintendent of schools in the area, or Sharon Knoth at the above address.

EARLY INTERVENTION COORDINATION

First Steps
Family and Social Services Administration
402 West Washington Street
W-386
Indianapolis, IN 46204
(317) 232-2429
FAX: (317) 232-7948
Maureen Greer, Director

County/District Where Located: Marion County.

Implements a statewide system of early intervention services in Indiana for infants and toddlers (birth through age 2) with delays, disabilities, or at risk of substantial delays, and their families. Provides information and referral to assist in identifying a local referral contact for early intervention services.

SCHOOLS

Indiana School for the Blind
7725 North College Avenue
Indianapolis, IN 46240
(317) 253-1481
FAX: (317) 251-6511
E-mail: michael_bina@inspeced.ccmail.compuserve.com
Dr. Michael Bina, Superintendent

Type of Agency: Public.
Mission: To ensure that each student enters adulthood adequately prepared for further education, work, and independent living. Has both on- and off-campus programs for school-age residents of the state who have visual impairments.
Funded by: Public funds.
Budget: $8 million.
Staff: 255.
History/Date: Est. 1847.
Number of Clients Served: 200 on campus; 150 through outreach programs.

Eligibility: School-age residents of the state who are blind and visually impaired.
Area Served: State of Indiana.
Transportation: Y.
Age Requirements: 0 - 21 years.

Health: General medical, psychiatric, neurological, physical therapy; occupational therapy, dental, low vision services; genetic counseling; ophthalmologic services.
Counseling/Social Work/Self-Help: Comprehensive services available in meeting student's individual needs.
Educational: Preschool through 12th grade. Programs are adapted per students' individual needs.
Preschools: Consultation and direct services to preschool children and parents.
Residential: Independent and semi-independent living homes are available in addition to dormitories.
Rehabilitation: Personal management; orientation/mobility; home economics; independent living.
Recreational: Afterschool programs in bowling, swimming, wrestling, track, cheerleading, scouting, intramural sports, forensics, community activities.
Employment: Evaluation; prevocational and career preparation training.
Computer Training: Comprehensive program available.
Low Vision: Evaluation, training, and follow-up service.
Low Vision Aids: Aids are available, including training in effective use of them.

INFANT AND PRESCHOOL

Gary Community Public Schools Corporation

Lew Wallace Building, Suite B122
415 West 45th Avenue
Gary, IN 46408
(219) 980-6305
Bashir A. Masoodi, Special
Education Coordinator

Type of Agency: Public school program.
Mission: Serve blind and visually impaired children and youths in a mainstream setting.
Funded by: P.L. 89-313, Handicapped Children's Early Education Program, private donations, P.L. 94-142, state funds, and local property taxes.
Hours of Operation: Mon.-Fri. 8:00 AM - 4:00 PM.
Staff: 12 full time (dually certified teachers and teachers of visually impaired children); 5 paraprofessionals; 3 part time; various specialists available as consultants. Has advisory board (parent members) for overall program. Uses volunteers.
History/Date: Est. 1974.
Eligibility: Visually impaired infants, children and youths, with or without other disabilities.
Area Served: Gary School District and nearby communities.
Transportation: Y.
Age Requirements: Preschool age - postschool age.

Health: Refers for genetic counseling, immunizations. Blood tests available on consultant or referral basis.
Counseling/Social Work/Self-Help: Parent counseling; student counseling and guidance; family counseling.
Educational: Provides instruction in all developmental areas. Bilingual instruction; home teaching; visually impaired and multiply disabled classes; resource rooms; itinerant program for preschool children, 3-5 years. Provides computer literacy instruction, assistance with regular class subjects.
Preschools: Provides instruction for infants and preschoolers.
Reading: Provides textbooks, educational materials in braille, large- print, cassette tapes and on computer disks.
Rehabilitation: Refers to rehabilitation agencies.
Recreational: Refers to camps, local recreational facilities; provides adaptive aquatics and recreation.
Employment: Assists students in securing summer and afterschool employment with local businesses. Provides computer training and exposure to technology.
Low Vision: Assessments, opticals, training, and follow-up in cooperation with Indiana University. Each student is evaluated every 3 years and provided with necessary opticals and aids free of charge.
Low Vision Aids: Provides closed-circuit televisions, magnifiers, and other aids for school work.

Consultant services to other programs for visually impaired /multiply disabled infants, 0-3 years and to students ages 3-21, transitional services and vocational and career guidance.

STATEWIDE OUTREACH SERVICES

Indiana School for the Blind

7725 North College Avenue
Indianapolis, IN 46240
(317) 253-1481
FAX: (317) 251-6511
E-mail: judy_whyte@isbmail.
ccmail.compuserve.com
Judith Whyte, Contact Person

County/District Where Located: Marion County.
Funded by: State funds.
History/Date: Est. 1847.
Age Requirements: 0-21 years.

Assessment: Psychoeducational, orientation and mobility, low vision, literacy assessment, functional vision assessment, computer skills, and preschool assessments.
Consultation to Public Schools: In all academic and skill areas.
Direct Service: In all academic and skill areas, depending upon staff availability.
Parent Assistance: Consultations, direct service, and training.
Materials Production: Braille and large print instructional aids.
Professional Training: Workshops for parents and professionals.

INSTRUCTIONAL MATERIALS CENTERS

Indiana Educational Resource Center
Indiana School for the Blind

7725 North College Avenue
Indianapolis, IN 46240
(317) 232-0587
FAX: (317) 475-9181
Leslie C. Durst, Outreach Resource Coordinator

Area Served: State of Indiana.
Groups Served: Students preschool-12th grade.

Types/Content: Textbooks.
Media Formats: Large-print, braille, print.

Provides adapted classroom materials to students through a statewide centralized depository.

◆ *Information Services*

LIBRARIES

Bartholomew County Public Library

536 Fifth Street
Columbus, IN 47201
(812) 379-1277
Wilma J. Perry, Coordinator

Subregional library.

Blind and Physically Handicapped Services

Elkhart Public Library
300 South Second
Elkhart, IN 46516-3184
(219) 522-2665, ext. 46
Pat Ciancio, Librarian

Subregional library.

Indiana State Library Special Services Division

140 North State Avenue
Indianapolis, IN 46204
(317) 232-3684 or toll-free in
Indiana (800) 622-4970 or TDD
(317) 232-7763
FAX: (317) 232-3728
E-mail: lbph@statelib.lib.in.
us
URL: http://
www.statelib.lib.in.us
Lissa Shanahan, Regional Librarian

Type of Agency: State.
County/District Where Located:
Marion County.
Funded by: Public funds.
Hours of Operation: Mon.-Fri.
8:00 AM - 4:30 PM.
Program Accessibility: Primarily
telephone and mail service.
Staff: 13.
History/Date: Est. 1905.
Number of Clients Served:
13,000.
Eligibility: Anyone prevented
from reading a standard print book

due to a visual or physical
disability.
Area Served: Indiana.

National Library Service for the
Blind and Physically Handicapped
Regional Library provides braille,
large-type and recorded books and
magazines and the equipment
needed to play the recorded books.
Free library service for anyone
who qualifies.

Northwest Indiana Subregional Library for the Blind and Physically Handicapped

Lake County Public Library
1919 West 81st Avenue
Merrillville, IN 46410
(219) 769-3541, ext. 237 or
(219) 769-3541
Joanne Pansasuk, Coordinator

Subregional library.

Readers' Services Department

Allen County Public Library
P.O. Box 2270
Fort Wayne, IN 46801
(219) 424-7241, ext. 2215
Joyce Misner, Librarian

Subregional library.

Talking Book Services

Evansville-Vanderburgh County
Public Library
22 S.E. Fifth Street
Evansville, IN 47708
(812) 428-8235
Barbara Shanks, Librarian

Subregional library.

TALKING BOOK MACHINE DISTRIBUTORS

Indiana State Library Special Services Division

140 North State Avenue

Indianapolis, IN 46204
(317) 232-3684 or (800) 622-4970
FAX: (317) 232-3728
E-mail: lbph@statelib.lib.in.
us
URL: http://
www.statelib.lib.in.us/www/
lbph/lvph0.hrml
Lissa Shanahan, Indiana Regional
Librarian

Type of Agency: State.
County/District Where Located:
Marion County.
Funded by: Public funds.
Hours of Operation: Mon-Fri,
8:00AM - 4:30PM.
Staff: 13.
Number of Clients Served:
13,000.
Eligibility: Anyone unable to read
a standard print book due to a
visual or physical disability.
Area Served: Statewide.

National Library Service for the
Blind and Physically Handicapped
Regional Library provides braille,
large-type and recorded books and
the equipment needed to play the
recorded books. Free library
service for anyone who qualifies.

MEDIA PRODUCTION SERVICES

Gary Public Schools, V.I.P. Resource Center

Lew Wallace Building, Suite B122
415 West 45th Avenue
Gary, IN 46408
(219) 980-6305
Bashir A. Masoodi, Special
Education Coordinator

Groups Served: K-12, college
students, other adults,
preschoolers.

Types/Content: Textbooks,
recreational, career/vocational,
counseling, career planning.

Media Formats: Braille books, talking books/cassettes, large-print books.
Title Listings: Print and braille lists available.

RADIO READING

Central Indiana Radio Reading, Inc.

1401 North Meridian Street
Indianapolis, IN 46202
(317) 636-2020, ext. 2003
FAX: (317) 633-7418
E-mail: bill_franzmann@wfyi.pbs.org
Bill Franzmann, Director
Jennifer Evans, Volunteer Manager

County/District Where Located: Marion County.
Funded by: Central Indiana Radio Reading, Inc.
Hours of Operation: 24 hours a day, seven days a week.
History/Date: Est. 1983.
Area Served: 35-40-mile radius from Indianapolis.
Age Requirements: None.

North Eastern Indiana Radio Reading Service, Inc. (NEIRRS)

920 Florence Avenue
Fort Wayne, IN 46808
(219) 422-8230
FAX: (219) 423-6191
Cynthia Smyth-Wartzok, Executive Director

County/District Where Located: Allen County.
Funded by: Voluntary contributions.
Hours of Operation: Mon.-Fri. 8:00 AM-4:00 PM.
Staff: 2 full time, 5 part time.
History/Date: Est. 1979.
Area Served: Northeastern Indiana and small portion of northwestern Ohio.

WNIN Radio Reading Service

405 Carpenter
Evansville, IN 47708
(812) 423-2973
FAX: (812) 428-7548
E-mail: jnoyes@wnindsmtp.usi.edu
Jean Noyes, Station Manager
Joan Cooper, Volunteer Coordinator

County/District Where Located: Vanderburgh County.
Hours of Operation: Mon.-Sun. 8:00 AM - 12 Noon; In Touch: 24 hours per day.
Staff: Volunteers.
History/Date: Est. 1972.
Area Served: Tri-state area.
Age Requirements: None.

INFORMATION AND REFERRAL

Prevent Blindness Indiana

911 East 86th Street
Suite 102
Indianapolis, IN 46240
(317) 257-2020
FAX: (317) 259-8175
E-mail: 104706.1103@compuserve.com
John Pratt, Executive Director

See Prevent Blindness America in U.S. national listings.

See also in national listings:

Association of Visual Science Librarians

Christian Mission for the Blind

◆ Rehabilitation Services

STATE SERVICES

Blind and Visually Impaired Services
Indiana Family and Social Services Administration
Indiana Government Center
402 West Washington Street
P.O. Box 7083
Indianapolis, IN 46207-7083
(317) 232-1433
FAX: (317) 232-6478
Richard Parrish, Deputy Director
Bobby Conner, Director, Division of Disability, Aging and Rehabilitative Services

Type of Agency: State.
Mission: To assist Indiana citizens who are blind/visually impaired in achieving vocational and personal independence by providing and supporting coordinated, effective, and efficient services and advocacy statewide.
Funded by: Public funds.
Hours of Operation: 8:00 AM-4:30 PM.
Staff: 33.
History/Date: Est. 1915.
Eligibility: A visual impairment that results in the inability to obtain or maintain suitable employment.
Age Requirements: Employment age.
Health: Public education about visual impairments.
Counseling/Social Work/Self-Help: Consultation and referral services.
Rehabilitation: Personal management; orientation/mobility; home mechanics; home economics; communications. (Provided by the Bosma Rehabilitation Center and the Itinerant Rehabilitation Teaching Program).

Employment: Evaluation; prevocational training; vending stand training and placement.
Computer Training: Computer literacy and exposure to technology. Sensory aid assessments to determine and recommend needs of clients for sensory aids for training and/or employment.
Low Vision: Resource and referral services.
Low Vision Follow-up: Conducted by the Itinerant Rehabilitation Teaching Program at 2, 6, and 12 months to determine effectiveness of prescribed low vision aids.

Local Offices:

Clarksville: Vocational Rehabilitation Services, 1452 Vaxter Avenue, P.O. Box 2517, Clarksville, IN 47131, (812) 288-8261.
Evansville: Vocational Rehabilitation Services, Evansville Area Office, 2305 West Michigan, Evansville, IN 47712, (812) 425-4545.
Fort Wayne: Vocational Rehabilitation Services, Fort Wayne Area Office, 702 Commerce Building, 219 West Wayne Street, Fort Wayne, IN 46802, (219) 426-9781.
Gary: Vocational Rehabilitation Services, Gary Area Office, 504 Broadway, Suite 444, Gary, IN 46402, (219) 881-6746.
Indianapolis: Randolph-sheppard Vending Training Program, 402 West Washington Street, W453, Indianapolis, IN 46207-7083.
Indianapolis: Vocational Rehabilitation Services, 2506 Willowbrook Parkway, Suite 320, Indianapolis, IN 46205, (317) 254-6700.

Indianapolis: Bosma Rehabilitation Center, 445 North Pennsylvania Street, Indianapolis, IN 46204.
Indianapolis: Adaptive Technology Lab, 445 North Pennsylvania Street, Indianapolis, IN 46204.
Indianapolis: Randolph-Sheppard Vending Training Program, 445 North Pennsylvania Street, Indianapolis, IN 46204.
Lafayette: Vocational Rehabilitation Services, Lafayette Area Office, 323 Columbia Street, Suite 2A, Lafayette, IN 47901-1315, (317) 423-2276.
Muncie: Vocational Rehabilitation Services, 201 East Charles Street, Suite 130, Muncie, IN 47305, (317) 282-9863.
South Bend: Vocational Rehabilitation Services, South Bend Area Office, 221 West Wayne Street, South Bend, IN 46601, (219) 232-4861.

REHABILITATION

Bosma Industries for the Blind
59 South State Avenue
Indianapolis, IN 46201-3876
(317) 684-0600
FAX: (317) 684-1946
Barry Graves, Director

Type of Agency: Manufacturing plant employing blind and visually impaired workers.
County/District Where Located: Marion County.
Mission: To provide vocational training and employment opportunities to individuals who are blind or visually impaired.
Funded by: Sale of products, fees for service, and donations.
Budget: $2 million.
Hours of Operation: 7:30 AM-4:00 PM.
Staff: 9.

History/Date: State operated 1915-1988; private corporation since 1988.
Number of Clients Served: 95-100 annually.
Eligibility: Blind or visually impaired.
Area Served: Indiana.
Age Requirements: 18 years or older.

Educational: Vocational training program and job placement.
Employment: Sheltered, transitional, and competitive.

Evansville Association for the Blind, Inc.
500 Second Avenue
P.O. Box 6445
Evansville, IN 47712
(812) 422-1181
FAX: (812) 424-3154
E-mail: eabcdc@evansville.net
Frank E. Kern, Executive Director

Type of Agency: Private; non-profit.
County/District Where Located: Vandenburgh County.
Mission: Services for totally blind, legally blind, visually impaired, deaf-blind, learning disabled, mentally retarded, physically and emotionally impaired persons.
Funded by: Fees; janitorial product sales; sub-contracts; capital funds; donations; trusts.
Budget: 1997: $3,399.500.
Hours of Operation: 7:00 AM - 5:00 PM.
Program Accessibility: Fully accessible.
Staff: 23 full time.
History/Date: Est. 1918; inc. 1923.
Number of Clients Served: 700.
Eligibility: Disability and need the Association can meet.
Area Served: Southwestern Indiana, southern Illinois, and western Kentucky.

Age Requirements: None.

Health: Refers for some health services.

Counseling/Social Work/Self-Help: Evaluations; psychological testing and evaluations; individual, group, family/parent, couple counseling; placement in school, training, institution; referral to community services.

Educational: Summer on-campus college program.

Preschools: Referrals to other agencies only.

Professional Training: Internship/fieldwork placement in orientation/mobility; rehabilitation counseling; special education. Regular in-service training programs conducted for staffs of health care facilities.

Rehabilitation: Personal management; braille; handwriting; listening skills; typing; home management; orientation/mobility; rehabilitation teaching in client's home and community; remedial education.

Recreational: Special programs for persons over 55.

Employment: Vocational evaluation; career and skill counseling; occupational skill development; sheltered workshops; placement; follow-up service.

Computer Training: Adaptive technology available as well as clerical vocational skills training.

Low Vision Aids: Y.

Low Vision Follow-up: Y.

League for the Blind and Disabled, Inc.

5800 Fairfield Avenue
Suite 210
Fort Wayne, IN 46807
(219) 745-5491 or (800) 889-3443
FAX: (219) 744-2202
David A. Nelson, Executive Director
Julie Garshwiler, Program Director

Type of Agency: Private; non-profit.

County/District Where Located: Allen County.

Funded by: Donations and bequests, grants, vocational rehabilitation contracts.

Hours of Operation: 8:00 AM-5:00 PM.

Program Accessibility: Fully accessible.

Staff: 8 full time, 1 part time. Uses volunteers.

History/Date: Est. 1950.

Number of Clients Served: 260.

Eligibility: Totally blind, legally blind, print impaired.

Area Served: Northeastern Indiana.

Transportation: Y.

Counseling/Social Work/Self-Help: Individual/family counseling; peer support/groups.

Reading: Volunteer reading services; braille transcription; large-print reproduction; cassette duplication.

Rehabilitation: Orientation/mobility; personal management; communications; low vision technology; computer technology; household management; Job Accommodation Center; information/referral.

Recreational: Sports and social activities organized.

Employment: Job Accommodation Center. Provides technical assistance to employees and employers concerning the Americans with Disabilities Act.

Computer Training: Individual instruction in speech synthesis, magnification systems, word processing, and databases.

Low Vision: Adaptive/low vision aids for sale or loan.

Northern Indiana Independent Living Service ADEC Resources for Independence

702 Williams Street
Elkhart, IN 46516
(219) 293-7509
FAX: (219) 293-8783
James E. Grice, Executive Director
Cary Kelsey, Department Director

Type of Agency: Private; non-profit.

Mission: Services for totally blind, legally blind, visually impaired, deaf-blind persons. Provides services for school-age children, vocational rehabilitation services for working-age adults, and independent living services for older persons.

Funded by: Fees set by state; grants.

Budget: 1992: $350,000.

Hours of Operation: Mon.-Fri. 8:00 AM-4:30 PM.

Program Accessibility: Center-based facility is accessible. Also provide itinerant services in clients' homes or neighborhoods.

Staff: 6 full time, 2 part time. Uses volunteers.

History/Date: Est. 1968.

Number of Clients Served: 1996: 360.

Eligibility: 20/60 or less or field restriction of 20 degrees or less for traditional vocational rehabilitation referral. Newsprint disability for persons served through independent living program.

Area Served: All of northern Indiana for vocational rehabilitation and public school referrals. Elkhart, La Porte, St. Joseph, Marshall, and Kosciusko Counties only for independent living program.

Transportation: Y.
Age Requirements: Independent living program, age 55 and over.

Counseling/Social Work/Self-Help: Social evaluations; individual, family/parent, couple counseling. Contracts for other counseling/social work services.
Professional Training: Internship/fieldwork placement in rehabilitation teaching.
Reading: Talking book record players and cassette players; talking book records and cassettes; braille books; large-print books; braille magazines; recorded magazines; information and referral.
Residential: On-site residential services for youths and adults.
Rehabilitation: Personal management; braille; handwriting; listening skills; typing; home management; orientation/mobility; rehabilitation teaching in client's home and community; sensory training; low vision training.
Recreational: Arts and crafts; bowling; evening activities; beep ball; goal ball.
Employment: Prevocational evaluations; career and skill counseling; sheltered workshops. Assists with job development and job coaching for vocational rehabilitation referrals. Accepts emotionally disturbed, learning disabled, mentally impaired, orthopedically disabled, other multiply disabled persons. Programs for vocational skill development.
Computer Training: Computer lab with IBM hardware and various software applications. Voice synthesis zoom text, and screen reader available.
Low Vision: Referrals.
Low Vision Follow-up: Y.

Program for Visually Impaired Adults
Family Service Association

615 North Alabama
Foundation Building, Room 220
Indianapolis, IN 46204
(317) 634-6341
Anita Osborne, Program Manager

Type of Agency: Private; non-profit.
County/District Where Located: Marion County.
Funded by: United Way; Rotary Foundation of Indianapolis; and private donations.
Hours of Operation: 8:30 AM - 5:00 PM.
Staff: 2.
History/Date: Est. 1975.
Eligibility: Resident of Marion County over 18 years of age; blind or visually impaired.
Age Requirements: 18 years or older.

Counseling/Social Work/Self-Help: Social evaluation; individual and group counseling; referral to community services.
Educational: Skill development; eye diseases and related topics; information and referral.
Professional Training: Internship/fieldwork placement in social work. Short-term training.
Reading: Braille books. Takes applications for Talking Book Division of State Library.
Rehabilitation: Personal management; braille; home management; rehabilitation teaching in client's home and community.
Recreational: Special programs for elderly persons; training in leisure time activities; volunteer opportunities for clients.
Low Vision Aids: Lends aids and appliances.

Trade Winds Rehabilitation Center

5901 West Seventh Avenue
P.O. Box 6308
Gary, IN 46406-0308
(219) 949-4000 or (800) 694-4242, ext. 202
FAX: (219) 944-8134
Marianne Randjelovic, Executive Director

Type of Agency: Non-profit vocational rehabilitation.
County/District Where Located: Lake County.
Mission: To enhance the lives of children and adults with disabilities and special challenges.
Funded by: United Way; Vocational Rehabilitation; First Steps; Medicaid; Veterans Administration.
Hours of Operation: Mon.-Fri. 8:00 AM-5:00 PM.
Program Accessibility: Community-based and site-based transporation available.
Staff: 220.
History/Date: Est. 1946.
Number of Clients Served: 1,000 annually.
Eligibility: Any person with a visual impairment.
Area Served: Primarily northwest Indiana, statewide available.
Transportation: Y.
Age Requirements: None.

Health: No special requirements.
Counseling/Social Work/Self-Help: Support group.
Preschools: Day child care services available.
Reading: Braille and verbal to cassette tape available.
Rehabilitation: Personal management; home mechanics; daily living skills (cooking, cleaning, personal care, etc.); communications (braille and cassette tape); orientation/

mobility; social services to individual and family.

Recreational: Community outings with support group.

Employment: Vocational evaluation; work adjustment; vocational placement; workshop program; vocational skills training; supported employment; follow-up services; psychological testing.

Computer Training: Screen reader software, voice synthesis, braille translation, and alternative computer access.

Low Vision: Referral available.

Low Vision Aids: Assistive technology and adaptive aids for sale.

Low Vision Follow-up: Referral available.

COMPUTER TRAINING CENTERS

ADEC Resources for Independence

702 Williams Street
Elkhart, IN 46516
(219) 293-7509
FAX: (219) 293-8783
Charlie Adams, Contact Person

County/District Where Located: Elkhart County.

Computer Training: Speech output systems; word processing.

Also works with spreadsheets, database applications, DOS functions, magnification systems, braille output, Braille 'n Speak. Does on-job-site consultation.

Crossroads Rehabilitation Center

4740 Kingsway Drive

Indianapolis, IN 46205
(317) 466-2013
FAX: (317) 466-2000
E-mail: xroadsatc@iquest.net
URL: http://www.iquest.net/crossroads
Thomas Blackman, Manager, Assistive Technology Center and Central Indiana Technology Resource & Information Center

County/District Where Located: Marion County.

Computer Training: Speech output systems; screen magnification systems; braille access systems; optical character recognition systems; closed-circuit television systems; word processing; database software; computer operating systems; training for instructors.

Equipment loan and demonstration center.

League for the Blind and Disabled

5800 Fairfield Aveneue, Suite 210
Fort Wayne, IN 46807
(219) 745-5491 (voice/TTD) or (800) 889-3443
FAX: (219) 744-2202
E-mail: lbfw@ct/net.com
David A. Nelson, Executive Director
John Gulngrich, Program Director

County/District Where Located: Allen County.

Computer Training: Speech output systems; screen magnification systems; braille access systems; optical character recognition systems; closed-circuit television systems; word processing; database software; computer operating systems.

◆ Low Vision Services

EYE CARE SOCIETIES

Indiana Academy of Ophthalmology

5920 Castleway West Drive
Suite 210
Indianapolis, IN 46250
(317) 577-3062
FAX: (317) 577-3061
Joy Newby, Executive Director

Indiana Optometric Association

201 North Illinois Street
Suite 1920
Indianapolis, IN 46204-4236
(317) 237-3560
Ronald W. Wuensch, Executive Director

LOW VISION CENTERS

Indianapolis Eye Care Center Indiana University School of Optometry

501 Indiana
Suite 100
Indianapolis, IN 46202
(317) 321-1470
FAX: (317) 321-1475
Debra McConnaha, Low Vision Service Chief

County/District Where Located: Marion County.
Funded by: Client fees.
Hours of Operation: Mon.-Fri. 8:30 AM-5:00 PM.
Program Accessibility: Accessible to disabled persons.
Staff: Optometrist; optometry interns; optometric assistant/technician.
Eligibility: None.
Area Served: Unlimited.

Low Vision Aids: On-site training provided.
Low Vision Follow-up: By return appointment as indicated.

◆ *Aging Services*

STATE UNITS ON AGING

Bureau of Aging
In-Home Services
402 West Washington Street
#E-431
Indianapolis, IN 46207-7083
(317) 232-7020 or Information &
Referral in state (800) 545-7763
FAX: (317) 232-7867
Geneva Shedd, Director

Provides referrals to Area Agencies
on Aging and information on other
local aging services.

INDEPENDENT LIVING PROGRAMS

Family and Social Services
Administration
Disability, Aging and
Rehabilitation Services
402 West Washington Street
Indianapolis, IN 46207
(317) 232-6478
Kary Kelsey, Director

Provides independent living
services for persons age 55 and
over. For further information,
contact the Project Director or
general phone number listed.

IOWA

♦ Educational Services

STATE SERVICES

Iowa Department of Education
Grimes State Office Building
Des Moines, IA 50319-0146
(515) 281-4030
FAX: (515) 242-5988
Ted Stilwill, Director
Nancy Brees, Administrative
Secretary, Special Education
Division
Ian Stewart, Consultant, Visual
Disabilities

County/District Where Located:
Polk County.
Mission: Administers
supplemental state funds for
visually impaired children
attending local schools.
Funded by: Public funds.
Area Served: Iowa.

Health: Offers psychological
testing and eye health public
education program.
Educational: Provides
consultation on educational
programs.
Reading: Distributes braille and
large-type textbooks, tapes, and
tape recorders.

For information about local
facilities, consult the Bureau of
Special Education of the
Department of Education.

EARLY INTERVENTION COORDINATION

**Bureau of Special Education
Iowa State Department of
Education**
Grimes State Office Building

Des Moines, IA 50319-0146
(515) 281-5433
FAX: (515) 242-6019
Mary Schertz, Coordinator

County/District Where Located:
Polk County.

SCHOOLS

**Iowa Braille and Sight Saving
School**
1002 G Avenue
Vinton, IA 52349
(319) 472-5221
FAX: (319) 472-4371
Dennis Thurman, Superintendent

Type of Agency: Public.
Mission: To serve Iowa students
of all ability levels who are
visually impaired and to prepare
them to function as independently
as possible in all aspects of adult
life.
Funded by: Public funds.
Budget: $4.2 million.
Staff: 90 full-time equivalents;
uses volunteers; various therapists
and specialists available as
consultants.
History/Date: Est. 1853.
Number of Clients Served: 55 in
residential program; 350 in
outreach programs.
Eligibility: Blind and partially
sighted students with or without
additional disabilities.
Area Served: Iowa.
Transportation: Y.
Age Requirements: 5-21 years.

Health: Medical services are
available.
**Counseling/Social Work/Self-
Help:** Parent counseling;
consultant services; orientation/
mobility consultation.
Educational: Provides instruction
in all developmental areas. K
through 12th grade; resource
services; educational evaluations.

Preschools: Through outreach
program.
Reading: Large-print materials;
materials loan; and media services.
Residential: Y.
Recreational: Full line of
recreational activities, including
athletics, forensics, music, and
overseas trips.
Employment: Transition planning;
vocational work experience
placements.
Computer Training: Access,
training on computer aids and
devices; state depository for high
technology equipment and
learning aids.
Low Vision: Low vision and
ophthalmology exams available on
consultant or referral basis; low
vision clinics; state vision
consultant.
Low Vision Aids: Provided as
part of the school's low vision
clinics.
Low Vision Follow-up: Through
low vision clinics.

Materials and consultant services
to parents of visually impaired
children and to the public schools.

Contact area education agency for
program information.

STATEWIDE OUTREACH SERVICES

**Iowa Braille and Sight Saving
School**
1002 G Avenue
Vinton, IA 52349
(319) 472-5221
FAX: (319) 472-4371
E-mail: d.stock@www.mebbs.com
Ian Stewart, Director, Outreach
Services

Funded by: State funds; and fee
for service.
Age Requirements: 0-21.

Assessment: Field or center-based educational and functional skills assessments and low vision clinics.
Consultation to Public Schools: Y.
Direct Service: Orientation and mobility, itinerant teachers, low vision clinic follow-up.
Parent Assistance: Y.
Materials Production: Large-print, braille, tactile adaptations.
Professional Training: Workshops and in-service training.

INSTRUCTIONAL MATERIALS CENTERS

Iowa Braille and Sight Saving School
1002 G Avenue
Vinton, IA 52349
(319) 472-5221, ext. 1233
FAX: (319) 472-4371
E-mail: d.hassman@mebbs.com
Dotta J. Hassman, Coordinator

Groups Served: K-12.

Types/Content: Textbooks, recreational, career/vocational.
Media Formats: Braille books, talking books/cassettes, large-print books.
Title Listings: No title listings available.

◆ Information Services

LIBRARIES

Iowa Library for the Blind and Physically Handicapped
Iowa Department for the Blind
524 Fourth Street
Des Moines, IA 50309-2364
(515) 281-1333 or toll-free in Iowa (800) 362-2587 or TDD (515) 281-1355
FAX: (515) 281-1378
Catherine Ford, Program Manager/Librarian

Type of Agency: Public library for the blind and physically handicapped.
Funded by: Public funds.
Staff: 26.
History/Date: Est. 1960.
Number of Clients Served: 9,100.
Eligibility: Inability to use standard print with ease because of blindness, visual impairment, physical disabilities, or reading disabilities based on organic dysfunctions.
Area Served: Iowa.

Produces and supplies talking books, braille books, large-type books and cassette machines.

MEDIA PRODUCTION SERVICES

Iowa Department for the Blind
524 Fourth Street
Des Moines, IA 50309-2364
(515) 281-1333 or TDD (515) 281-1355
FAX: (515) 281-1378
Carol Eckey, Librarian
Karen Paloma, Librarian

Area Served: Iowa.
Groups Served: K-12, college students, other adults.

Types/Content: Textbooks; career, vocational materials; leisure.
Media Formats: Braille, cassette, recorded disk, large-type, computer disk.
Title Listings: 89,000 titles, catalogs of media and genre available.

RADIO READING

Iowa Radio Reading Information Service (IRIS)
100 East Euclid Avenue
Des Moines, IA 50313
(515) 243-6833
Laurie Nelson-Hood, Director

History/Date: Est. 1989.
Area Served: 60 mile radius around both Des Moines and Fort Dodge.

INFORMATION AND REFERRAL

The Foundation Fighting Blindness
Iowa Affiliate
P.O. Box 1213
Cedar Falls, IA 50613
(319) 236-2830
Jack Johns, Contact Person

See The Foundation Fighting Blindness in U.S. national listings.

Prevent Blindness Iowa
1111 Ninth Street, Suite 250
Des Moines, IA 50314
(515) 244-4341
FAX: (515) 244-4718
E-mail: 104706.2025@compuserve.com
Jeanne Burmeister, Executive Director

County/District Where Located: Polk County.

See Prevent Blindness America in U.S. national listings.

◆ Rehabilitation Services

STATE SERVICES

Iowa Department for the Blind
524 Fourth Street
Des Moines, IA 50309-2364
(515) 281-1333 or toll-free in Iowa (800) 362-2587 or TDD (515) 281-1355
FAX: (515) 281-1263
E-mail: creigs@blind.state.ia.us
R. Creig Slayton, Director

Type of Agency: State.

Mission: To work with Iowans who are blind in support of their rights and aspirations to participate fully, productively, and equally as first-class citizens with society.

Funded by: Public funds.

Hours of Operation: Mon.-Fri. 8:00 AM-5:00 PM.

Program Accessibility: Building and facilities are accessible. Information is provided in alternative media.

Staff: 95 full time. Uses volunteers.

History/Date: Est. 1926.

Number of Clients Served: Approximately 10,000.

Eligibility: For most purposes, any Iowan who is considered blind or deaf-blind.

Area Served: Iowa.

Counseling/Social Work/Self-Help: Consultation and referral service.

Reading: Talking book record players and cassette players; talking book records and cassettes; braille books; large print books. Reader service.

Residential: Adult orientation and adjustment training center.

Rehabilitation: Personal management; orientation/ mobility; industrial arts; home economics; communications; independent living deaf-blindness services; guidance and counseling; training and information.

Employment: Evaluation; prevocational and vocational training; vocational placement; follow-up service; vending facility training.

Computer Training: Training on computer aids and devices.

Low Vision Aids: As warranted on a case-by-case basis.

Local Offices:

Cedar Rapids: Department for the Blind, 118 Third Avenue S.E., Cedar Rapids, IA 52401, (319) 365-9111.

Waterloo: Department for the Blind, First National Building, Suite 400, Waterloo, IA 50703, (319) 235-1403.

COMPUTER TRAINING CENTERS

Iowa Department for the Blind

524 Fourth Street
Des Moines, IA 50309-2364
(515) 281-1309 or TDD (515) 281-1355
FAX: (515) 281-1263
Doris Moritz, Assistive Technology Clerk

Computer Training: Speech output systems; screen magnification systems; braille access systems; optical character recognition systems; closed-circuit television systems; word processing; computer operating systems.

♦ Low Vision Services

EYE CARE SOCIETIES

Iowa Academy of Ophthalmology

Ten West Phillips Road
Metro Square One, Suite 120
Vernon Hills, IL 60061
(847) 680-1666
Richard H. Paul, Executive Director

Iowa Optometric Association

1454 30th Street
Suite 204
West Des Moines, IA 50266-1312
(515) 222-5679
Virgil Deering, Executive Director

LOW VISION CENTERS

Low Vision Clinic Department of Ophthalmology, University of Iowa Hospitals and Clinics

200 Hawkins Drive
Iowa City, IA 52242
(319) 356-2215
FAX: (319) 353-7699
Christine W. Sindt, O.D., Director, Low Vision Service

Type of Agency: Non-profit.

County/District Where Located: Johnson County.

Mission: To provide comprehensive vision rehabilitation and counseling.

Funded by: Client fees.

Hours of Operation: Mon.-Fri. 8:00 AM - 5:00PM.

Staff: Optometrist, low vision assistant, ophthalmologist, opthalmology resident, optician, social worker, genetic counselor.

Number of Clients Served: 500/year.

Eligibility: Referral.

Area Served: Unlimited.

Rehabilitation: Provide counseling for activities of daily living.

Low Vision Aids: Prescribed and provided for purchase; provides for trial use at no charge.

Low Vision Follow-up: Return appointments are given if necessary.

Low Vision/Contact Lens Service

The University of Iowa Hospitals and Clinics
Department of Ophthalmology
200 Hawkins Drive

Iowa City, IA 52242-1091
(319) 356-2861
FAX: (319) 356-0363
E-mail: william-mathers@uiowa.
edu
URL: http://www.uiowa.edu
William Mathers, Director of
Contact Lens

County/District Where Located:
Johnson County.
Funded by: State funds.

Vision Rehabilitation Institute
Genesis Medical Center

1351 West Central Park
Suite 3700
Davenport, IA 52804
(319) 421-1587 or (800) 383-1298
E-mail: mewilkin@netexpress.net
Mark E. Wilkinson, O.D.,
Optometric Director
Julie Yoerger, Low Vision Educator

Type of Agency: Non-profit.
Mission: To improve the quality
of life of all individuals with visual
impairments.
Funded by: Client fees,
foundation grants.
Hours of Operation: Mon.- Fri.
8:00 AM - 4:30 PM.
Program Accessibility: Fully
accessible.
Staff: Audiologist; low vision
assistant; occupational therapist;
ophthalmologist; optometrist.
History/Date: Est. 1986.
Number of Clients Served: 450.
Eligibility: All visually impaired
individuals. No referral required.
Area Served: Unlimited; primary
areas: eastern Iowa and western
Illinois.
Age Requirements: None.
Health: None.
**Counseling/Social Work/Self-
Help:** Counselor/social worker/
vocational evaluator, psychiatrist
available.

Rehabilitation: Counselors/
orientation and mobility
instructors available.
Recreational: Programmer/
coordinator available.
Computer Training: Access and
training provided through
Telesensory.
Low Vision: On-site training
provided.
Low Vision Aids: Loan/purchase;
prescriptions filled.
Low Vision Follow-up: Return
appointment; phone interviews;
mail.

◆ Aging Services

STATE UNITS ON AGING

Iowa Department of Elder Affairs
200 Tenth Street
Clemens Building, Third Floor
Des Moines, IA 50309-3609
(515) 281-5187
FAX: (515) 281-4036
Betty Grandquist, Executive
Director

Provides referrals to Area Agencies
on Aging and information on other
local aging services.

INDEPENDENT LIVING PROGRAMS

Iowa Department for the Blind
524 Fourth Street
Des Moines, IA 50309-2364
(515) 281-1333 or TDD (515) 281-
1355 or (800) 362-2587
R. Creig Slayton, Director
Becky Criswell, Project Director,
(515) 281-1299

Provides independent living
services for persons age 55 and
over. For further information,
contact the Project Director or
general phone number listed.

KANSAS

♦ *Educational Services*

STATE SERVICES

Kansas State Department of Education
Student Support Services
120 Southeast Tenth Avenue
Topeka, KS 66612-1182
(913) 291-3097
FAX: (913) 296-1413
Betty Weithers, Team Leader for Special Education
Michael Remus, Team Leader Student Support Services

Type of Agency: A division of the State Board of Education.
County/District Where Located: Shawnee County.
Mission: Administers special education program in public schools.
Funded by: Public funds.
Hours of Operation: Mon.- Fri. 7:30 A.M.- 5:30.
History/Date: Est. 1949.
Area Served: Kansas.

EARLY INTERVENTION COORDINATION

Kansas Department of Health and Environment
Landon State Office Building
900 S.W. Jackson
Tenth Floor
Topeka, KS 66612-1290
(913) 296-6135
FAX: (913) 296-8626
Lori Michel, Director, Children's Developmental Services

County/District Where Located: Shawnee County.

Part H (Idea) systems development for Kansas technical assistance to early intervention networks statewide.

SCHOOLS

Kansas State School for the Blind
1100 State Avenue
Kansas City, KS 66102
(913) 281-3308
FAX: (913) 281-3104
E-mail: suptksb@tyrell.net
William Daugherty, Superintendent
Madeline Burkindine, Principal

Type of Agency: State.
Mission: To serve all blind and visually impaired Kansans, aged 0-21.
Funded by: State of Kansas.
Hours of Operation: 24 hours/day; receptionist on duty Mon. - Fri. 7:00 PM - 9:00 PM.
Program Accessibility: Fully accessible.
Staff: 93 full time. Uses volunteers.
History/Date: Est. 1867.
Number of Clients Served: 1996: campus 60; outreach 500.
Eligibility: Visually impaired, blind, deaf-blind, emotionally disturbed, including students with multiple disabilities.
Area Served: State of Kansas.
Transportation: Y.
Age Requirements: 0 to 21 years.

Health: General medical services. Refers for other health services.
Counseling/Social Work/Self-Help: Psychological testing, licensed clincial social work, and evaluation; individual, group, family/parent, counseling; referral to community services. Refers and provides consultation to other agencies for other counseling/social work services.
Educational: Placement in school, preschool through 12; programs for general academics, vocational/skill development, life skills.
Preschools: 3 - 5 years.
Professional Training: Internships/fieldwork placement. Regular in-service training programs and short-term or summer training programs.
Residential: Dormitories.
Recreational: Afterschool programs; arts and crafts; hobby groups; bowling; swimming; track; wrestling; goal ball. Provides consultation to other agencies for some recreation services.
Employment: Prevocational evaluation; career and skill development; refers for vocational placement, follow-up service.
Computer Training: Access; training on computer aids and devices.
Low Vision: Provided statewide through contract with Kansas University Medical Center.
Low Vision Follow-up: Provided by school staff.

Contact local school superintendent for program availability.

INFANT AND PRESCHOOL

Early Education Center Training and Evaluation Center of Hutchinson
303 East Bigger
P.O. Box 399
Hutchinson, KS 67504-0399
(316) 663-2671 or (316) 663-1596
FAX: (316) 663-1293
Maurice F. Cummings, President/CEO
KaAnn Graham, Early Education Director

Type of Agency: Cooperative public-private education program.
County/District Where Located: Reno County.
Mission: To integrate disabled persons into society in the least

restrictive manner, providing programs in preschool, residential, and employment deployment.
Funded by: P.L. 100-297 monies, private donations, state educational funds, United Way, county mill levy, P.L. 99-457.
Budget: $1.1 million.
Hours of Operation: Mon.-Fri. 8:30 AM-4:00 PM.
Staff: 11 full time.
History/Date: Est. 1975.
Number of Clients Served: 250 children with disabilities or at risk; 64 age-appropriate children.
Eligibility: Twenty-five percent developed on 1.5 SD below mean in one area of development; specific diagnosis.
Area Served: Reno County school districts.
Transportation: Y.
Age Requirements: 0-5 years.

Health: Adaptive equipment. Hearing tests, other support services available on referral basis.
Counseling/Social Work/Self-Help: Parent counseling and social work.
Educational: Provides instruction in most developmental areas. Home-based program for visually impaired and other disabled infants, 0-3 years. Multiply disabled and noncategorical classes, consultant services to other programs for 3-5 year olds in an integrated, community-based setting.
Low Vision: Exams.

Tri-Valley Developmental Services

13 South National
Fort Scott, KS 66701
(316) 223-3990
FAX: (316) 223-3997
Alene Jolly, Program Director

Type of Agency: Interagency cooperative program, public school and private agency.
County/District Where Located: Bourbon County.
Funded by: P.L. 89-313 and 94-142 monies, private donations, state funds, United Way, county mill levy.
Staff: 3 full time; psychologist, various therapists, orientation/mobility specialist available on consultation basis. Uses volunteers. Advisory board with parent members.
Area Served: Bourbon County.
Age Requirements: 18 or older.

Counseling/Social Work/Self-Help: Parent counseling.
Educational: Provides instruction in most developmental areas. Orientation/mobility and various related services available on referral basis.

STATEWIDE OUTREACH SERVICES

Kansas State School for the Blind

1100 State Avenue
Kansas City, KS 66102
(913) 281-3308
FAX: (913) 281-3104
Virgene Martin, Contact Person

Age Requirements: 0-21 years old.

Consultation to Public Schools: Consultations & evaluations provided across the state to students who are visually impaired or blind.
Direct Service: Some direct service is available.
Professional Training: Regular inservice training programs.

INSTRUCTIONAL MATERIALS CENTERS

Kansas Instructional Resource Center for the Blind and Visually Impaired

1100 State Avenue
Kansas City, KS 66102-4486
(913) 281-3308 or toll-free in Kansas (800) 572-5463
FAX: (913) 281-3104
E-mail: jcdkirc@tyrell.net
Jacqueline Denk, Coordinator

Area Served: Kansas.
Groups Served: K-12; ages 0-21.

Types/Content: Textbooks, recreational books, educational aids.
Media Formats: Braille books; large-print books; cassettes.
Title Listings: No listings available.

Coordinates, catalogs, produces, stores, and distributes educational materials needed by children who are blind/visually impaired. Also provides information and support for teachers.

◆ Information Services

LIBRARIES

Kansas City, Kansas Public Library
Kansas Braille Library

625 Minnesota Avenue
Kansas City, KS 66101
(913) 621-3073, ext. 228 or toll-free in Kansas (800) 279-6645
FAX: (913) 621-0963
Joan Gandert, Librarian

Subregional library lending braille materials only.

**Kansas Talking Book Service
Kansas State Library**
Emporia State University
Memorial Union
1200 Commercial
Emporia, KS 66801
(316) 343-7124 or toll-free in
Kansas (800) 362-0699
FAX: (316) 343-7124
Patti Lang, Librarian

Type of Agency: Library for the
blind and physically disabled.
Funded by: Public funds.
Hours of Operation: 8:00 AM -
5:00 PM.
Eligibility: Anyone who, because
of a physical disability, is unable to
use normal print.
Area Served: Kansas.

Provides talking books on
cassettes, records and braille.

Manhattan Public Library
Juliette and Poyntz Streets
Manhattan, KS 66502
(913) 776-4741 or toll-free in
Kansas (800) 432-2796
FAX: (913) 776-1545
Marion Rice, Librarian

Subregional library.

**Northwest Kansas Library
System
Talking Books**
P.O. Box 446
Norton, KS 67654
(913) 877-5148 or toll-free in
Kansas (800) 432-2858
FAX: (913) 877-5697
Clarice Howard, Librarian

Subregional library.

**South Central Kansas Library
System
Talking Book Division**
901 North Main Street

Hutchinson, KS 67501
(316) 663-5441 or toll-free in
Kansas (800) 234-0529
FAX: (316) 663-1215
Karen Socha, Librarian

Subregional library.

Talking Books
Topeka and Shawnee Counties
1515 Southwest Tenth Avenue
Topeka, KS 66604
(913) 233-2040 or toll-free in
Kansas (800) 432-2925
FAX: (913) 233-2055
Susan Bundy, Librarian

Subregional library.

Talking Books Department
Wichita Public Library
223 South Main
Wichita, KS 67202
(316) 262-0611 or toll-free in
Kansas (800) 362-2869 or TDD
(316) 262-3972
FAX: (316) 262-2552
Betty C. Spriggs, Librarian

Subregional library.

**Talking Book Service
Library for the Blind and
Physically Handicapped**
1409 Williams
Great Bend, KS 67530
(316) 792-2393 or toll-free in
Kansas (800) 362-2642
FAX: (316) 792-5495
Juanita Doll, Librarian

Subregional library.

MEDIA PRODUCTION SERVICES

**American Red Cross
Midway-Kansas Chapter**
707 North Main

Wichita, KS 67203-3669
(316) 683-6706
FAX: (316) 268-0888
E-mail: eulertv@usa.red-cross.
org
Von E. Eulert, Chairperson, Braille
Service

Area Served: National.
Groups Served: K-12; college
students; other adults.

Types/Content: Textbooks;
recreational; career/vocational;
religious.
Media Formats: Braille books.
Title Listings: Available on
request. All titles listed with the
American Printing House for the
Blind.

Braille Association of Kansas
P.O. Box 17032
Wichita, KS 67217
(316) 265-6504
Mary Ann Oblinger, Workshop
Manager

Area Served: Sedgwick County
and surrounding counties; will do
work for outside areas, time and
volunteers permitting.
Groups Served: All ages.

Media Formats: Braille or taped
(cassette) material.

**Kansas Rehabilitation Center for
the Blind**
2516 S.W. Sixth Avenue
Topeka, KS 66606-1703
(913) 296-3311
Suzannah Erhart, Administrator

County/District Where Located:
Shawnee County.
Groups Served: College students,
other adults.

Types/Content: Textbooks.
Media Formats: Braille books,
talking books/cassettes.
Title Listings: No title listings
available.

RADIO READING

Audio Reader of Cloud County

P.O. Box 629
Concordia, KS 66901
(913) 243-1414
Joe Jindra, Station Manager

Hours of Operation: Mon.-Sat.
6:00 AM - 11:00 PM; Sun.
7:00 AM-11:00 PM.
History/Date: Est. 1954.
Area Served: North central
Kansas.

Kansas Audio-Reader Network

University of Kansas
P.O. Box 847
Lawrence, KS 66044
(913) 864-4600
Janet Campbell, Director

County/District Where Located:
Douglas County.
Hours of Operation: Office:
Mon.-Fri. 8:00 AM-5:00 PM;
Broadcast services 24 hours a day.
History/Date: Est. 1971.
Area Served: Kansas and Western
Missouri; other radio reading
services via satellite.

Reading Radio Service

815 North Walnut
Suite 300
Hutchinson, KS 67501
(316) 665-3555
Rose Fragoza, Director

Hours of Operation: Mon.-Fri.
6:00 AM-12:00 midnight; Sat.-Sun.
8:00 AM-6:00 PM.
History/Date: Est. 1979.
Area Served: 80-mile radius from
Hutchinson.

University of Kansas Audio Reader Network

P.O. Box 847

Lawrence, KS 66044
(913) 864-4600
FAX: (913) 864-4053
URL: http://www.ukans.edu/
~arnet
Janet Campbell, Director

County/District Where Located:
Douglas County.
Hours of Operation: Mon.-Sat. 24
hours a day; sign-off midnight Sun.
to 6:00 AM Mon.
History/Date: Est. 1971.
Area Served: Statewide.

Wichita Radio Reading Service

1751 North Fairmount
Wichita, KS 67208
(316) 978-6600
Pat V. Hayes, Program Supervisor

County/District Where Located:
Sedgwick County.
Hours of Operation: 18 hours a
day, 365 days a year.
Staff: Wichita State University
students.
History/Date: Est. 1975.
Area Served: 60-mile radius
centered on Wichita, covering
south central Kansas.

◆ Rehabilitation Services

STATE SERVICES

Kansas Division of Services for the Blind

300 S.W. Oakley
Topeka, KS 66606
(913) 296-4454
FAX: (913) 368-6200
Suzanne A. Erhart, Director

Type of Agency: State.
Mission: Services for totally blind,
legally blind, visually impaired,
deaf-blind.
Funded by: State and federal tax
funds.

Budget: $5.8 million.
Staff: 68 full time. Uses
volunteers.
History/Date: Est. 1937.
Number of Clients Served: 1,800
annually.
Eligibility: Blind, visually
impaired, or deaf-blind persons.
Area Served: Kansas.
Transportation: Y.

Health: Evaluation of eye
treatment or prescription.
Contracts for other health services.
**Counseling/Social Work/Self-
Help:** Social evaluation;
vocational evaluation; counseling,
individual, family/parent;
placement in training. Contracts,
refers for, provides consultation to
other agencies for counseling/
social work services.
Professional Training:
Internship/fieldwork placement in
rehabilitation counseling. Regular
training programs open to other
agencies.
Residential: Dormitory for adults
at Rehabilitation Center for the
Blind.
Rehabilitation: Personal
management; braille; handwriting;
listening skills; Optacon; typing;
video magnifier; home
management; orientation/
mobility; rehabilitation teaching in
client's home and community;
sensory training. Refers and
provides consultation to other
agencies for other rehabilitation
services.
Recreational: Arts and crafts;
bowling; swimming. Refers and
provides consultation for other
recreational services.
Employment: Prevocational
evaluation; career and skill
counseling; occupational skill
development; sheltered
workshops; vocational placement;
follow-up service; vending facility

training. Contracts for other employment-oriented services.

Field Offices:

Chanute: 1500 West Seventh Street, P.O. Box 708, Chanute, KS 66720, (316) 431-5000.

Garden City: 907 Zerr Road, P.O. Box 1078, Garden City, KS 67846, (316) 272-5920.

Hays: 3000 Broadway, P.O. Box 549, Hays, KS 67601, (913) 625-3489.

Kansas City: 1119 North 5th Street, P.O. Box 171248, Kansas City, KS 66117, (913) 371-6700.

Manhattan: 445 E Poyntz, Manhattan, KS 66502, (913) 539-5804.

Salina: 901 Westchester Drive, P.O. Box 6200, Salina, KS 67401, (913) 826-8035.

Topeka: 235 Kansas Avenue, P.O. Box 1424, Topeka, KS 66601, (913) 296-4424.

Wichita: 238 East William, P.O. Box 518, Wichita, KS 67201, (316) 337-7230.

Local Offices:

Topeka: Rehabilitation Center for the Blind, 2516 S.W. Sixth Avenue, Topeka, KS 66606, (913) 296-3311.

Topeka: Kansas Industries for the Blind, 425 MacVicar, Topeka, KS 66606, (913) 296-3211.

REHABILITATION

Helen Keller National Center for Deaf-Blind Youths and Adults Great Plains Region Office

4330 Shawnee Mission Parkway
Suite 108
Shawnee Mission, KS 66205-3522
(913) 677-4562 (voice and TDD)
FAX: (913) 677-1544
Beth A. Jordan, Regional Representative

County/District Where Located: Johnson County.

Mission: To provide information and advocacy to deafblind individuals and their families; consultation to the agencies / organizations who serve this population.

Hours of Operation: Mon.-Fri. 8:30AM - 4:30PM.

Eligibility: Person must have both a vision and hearing loss.

See Helen Keller National Center for Deaf-Blind Youths and Adults in U.S. national listings.

Kansas Industries for the Blind

425 MacVicar Street
Topeka, KS 66606
(913) 296-3211
FAX: (913) 296-0728
Eric Boling, General Manager

Type of Agency: State.

County/District Where Located: Shawnee County.

Mission: Serve totally blind, visually impaired, and blind multiply disabled persons.

Funded by: Fees, product sales (government contracts, public and private sales).

Hours of Operation: Mon.-Fri. 8:00 AM-4:00 PM.

Staff: 5 on management team.

Eligibility: Blind or visually impaired.

Counseling/Social Work/Self-Help: Social evaluation; individual counseling; placement in training.

Employment: Employment transition program.

Wichita Industries and Services for the Blind

801 East Lincoln
Wichita, KS 67211
(316) 267-2244
FAX: (316) 267-4312
Linda Merrill, President

Type of Agency: Private; non-profit.

County/District Where Located: Sedgwick County.

Mission: To enhance the personal independence of individuals whose blindness, often accompanied by other disabilities, impacts their opportunities for employment, success, and integration into community life.

Funded by: Sales and contributions.

Budget: $10,000,000.

Hours of Operation: Mon. - Fri. 8:00 AM - 5:00 PM.

Staff: 16 full time.

History/Date: Est. 1931.

Number of Clients Served: 1,234.

Eligibility: Totally blind, legally blind, visually impaired, deaf-blind, learning disabled, mentally retarded, emotionally disturbed, cerebral palsy. Preference given to visual impairment over other disabilities.

Area Served: Kansas and surrounding areas.

Transportation: Y.

Age Requirements: 16 years and older.

Counseling/Social Work/Self-Help: Resources and referrals, orientation and mobility, independent living skills, assistive technology.

Rehabilitation: Work adjustment.

Employment: Occupational skill development; employment; placement.

Low Vision Aids: White Canes and More Retail Store, 530 North Lorraine, Wichita, KS (316) 681-0870.

Local Offices:

Kansas City: Industries for the Blind, 925 Sunshine Road, Kansas City, KS 66115, (913) 281-0710, FAX (913) 281-2450, Don Chippeaux, Plant Manager.

Pittsburg: Industries for the Blind, 1600 North Walnut, Pittsburg, KS 66762, (316) 231-8600, FAX (316) 231-8620, Dave Burr, Plant Manager.

COMPUTER TRAINING CENTERS

Kansas Rehabilitation Center for the Blind

2516 S.W. Sixth Avenue
Topeka, KS 66606-1703
(913) 296-3311
FAX: (913) 291-3138
Ann Byington

County/District Where Located: Shawnee County.

Computer Training: Speech output systems; screen magnification systems; braille access systems; optical character recognition systems; closed-circuit television systems; word processing; database software; computer operating systems.

Special Education Technology Center

1800 Pflumm Road
Olathe, KS 66062
(913) 780-7679
FAX: (913) 780-8007
J. Daniel Magrone, Coordinator

County/District Where Located: Johnson County.

Computer Training: Speech output systems; screen magnification systems; braille access systems; word processing; computer operating systems; training for instructors.

DOG GUIDE SCHOOLS

Kansas Specialty Dog Service

124 West Seventh
P.O. Box 216

Washington, KS 66968
(913) 325-2256
FAX: (913) 325-2258
Bill Acree

Type of Agency: Non-profit.
Mission: Canine assistance; guide dogs for blind and visually impaired persons; service dogs for physically disabled persons.
Funded by: Charitable contributions and donations.
Hours of Operation: Mon.-Fri. 8:00 AM-5:00 PM.
Staff: 7.
History/Date: Est. 1990.
Number of Clients Served: 1992: 16.
Area Served: Primarily Kansas, Colorado, Missouri, Iowa, Oklahoma, Texas, North Dakota, South Dakota. Other states served, as needed.
Age Requirements: Children and adults considered.

◆ Low Vision Services

EYE CARE SOCIETIES

Kansas State Ophthalmological Society

P.O. Box 4842
Topeka, KS 66604
(913) 234-9719
FAX: (913) 234-9718
Rebecca S. Rice, Executive Director

Kansas Optometric Association

1266 S.W. Topeka Boulevard
Topeka, KS 66612
(913) 232-0225
Gary Robbins, C.A.E.

LOW VISION CENTERS

Kansas Eye Center
University of Kansas Medical Center
Low Vision Rehabilitation Service

3901 Rainbow Boulevard
Kansas City, KS 66160-7379
(913) 588-6609
FAX: (913) 588-6615
Joseph Maino, O.D., Director, Low Vision Rehabilitation Service
Dirk Dittemore O.D., Low Vision Specialist
Janette E. Sanders-Reh, Patient Counselor

Type of Agency: Medical facility.
County/District Where Located: Wyandotte County.
Mission: To help low vision patients live with visual impairment more successfully.
Funded by: Client fees and state funds.
Hours of Operation: By appointment only.
Program Accessibility: Fully accessible.
Staff: Ophthalmologist; ophthalmology resident; optometrist; optician; rehabilitation counselor.
History/Date: Est.1966.
Number of Clients Served: 8-10 weekly.
Eligibility: Referral by ophthalmologist, optometrist, or agency with medical report.
Area Served: Unlimited.

Counseling/Social Work/Self-Help: Referral to appropriate agencies.
Educational: Referrals made to appropriate agencies.
Preschools: Referrals made to appropriate agencies.
Professional Training: Referrals made to appropriate agencies.

Reading: Training in use of hand-held aids and closed-circuit televisions.

Rehabilitation: Referral to state agencies.

Recreational: Referral to state agencies.

Employment: Assist patient to obtain employment aids by referral to state agencies.

Computer Training: Evaluation only; training is performed in state agencies.

Low Vision: Evaluations available.

Low Vision Aids: Provided for purchase; limited trial loan of some aids available; on-site training provided.

Low Vision Follow-up: By return appointment or telephone, as needed.

Vision Rehabilitation Center

530 North Lorraine, Suite 5
Wichita, KS 67214
(316) 682-4646
FAX: (316) 682-4747
Geri McFadden, Coordinator

Type of Agency: Non-profit.
County/District Where Located: Sedgwick County.
Funded by: Client fees.
Hours of Operation: Mon.-Fri. 8:00 AM-5:00 PM.
Staff: 10.
History/Date: Est. 1996.
Number of Clients Served: 700 annually.
Area Served: Unlimited.
Transportation: Y.
Age Requirements: 5 years and up.

Low Vision: Evaluation and assessment; rehabilitation program.
Low Vision Aids: Provided on loan for trial purposes; no rental fee charged; on-site training provided.

Low Vision Follow-up: Y.

♦ Aging Services

STATE UNITS ON AGING

Kansas Department on Aging

Docking State Office Building
915 S.W. Harrison
Topeka, KS 66612-1500
(913) 296-4986 or Information & Referral in state (800) 432-3535
FAX: (913) 296-0256
Thelma Hunter Gordon, Director

Provides referrals to Area Agencies on Aging and information on other local aging services.

INDEPENDENT LIVING PROGRAMS

Rehabilitation Center for the Blind
Kansas Department of Social Services

2516 S.W. Sixth Avenue
Topeka, KS 66606
(913) 296-3311
Suzannah Erhart, Director

Provides independent living services for persons age 55 and over. For further information, contact the Project Director or general phone number listed.

KENTUCKY

◆ *Educational Services*

STATE SERVICES

Kentucky Department of Education
Division of Exceptional Children Services
500 Mero Street
Capital Plaza Towers, Room 805
Frankfort, KY 40601
(502) 564-4970
FAX: (502) 564-6721
Mike Armstrong, Director

Type of Agency: A division of the Department of Education.
County/District Where Located: Franklin County.
Funded by: Public funds.
Area Served: Kentucky.

Counseling/Social Work/Self-Help: Services for parents, local agencies, and schools on educational programs.
Educational: Assists school personnel in appraising the needs of visually handicapped children and in developing the appropriate education programs for these children.
Professional Training: Conducts in-service training for teachers.
Computer Training: Access; training on computer aids and devices.

EARLY INTERVENTION COORDINATION

Infant-Toddler Program
Kentucky Department of Mental Health and Mental Retardation Services
275 East Main Street
Frankfort, KY 40621
(502) 564-7722
FAX: (502) 564-3844
Jim Henson, Part H Early Childhood Coordinator

County/District Where Located: Franklin County.

SCHOOLS

Kentucky School for the Blind
1867 Frankfort Avenue
Louisville, KY 40206
(502) 897-1583
FAX: (502) 897-1583
Ralph E. Bartley, Ph.D., Superintendent

Type of Agency: Public.
Mission: To affect transformation of education of the blind and visually impaired by the use of exemplary practices; to create superior learning environments.
Funded by: Public funds.
Staff: 45.
History/Date: Est. 1842.
Eligibility: Blind and visually impaired school-age children who are residents of Kentucky.

Health: General care.
Educational: K through 12.
Professional Training: Fieldwork opportunities.
Reading: Lends braille and large-print textbooks and educational aids to Kentucky school districts that serve blind and visually impaired students.
Residential: Supervised living areas for students.
Rehabilitation: Personal management; orientation/mobility; independent living; job skills; transition activities.
Recreational: Afterschool activities. Leisure counseling and training in recreational skills.

Provides consultations, technical assistance and educational assessments for local schools in Kentucky.

Contact local school superintendent for program availability.

University of Kentucky Deafblind Project
229 Taylor Education Building
University of Kentucky
Lexington, KY 40506-0001
(606) 257-3730 or (502) 897-1583, ext. 258
FAX: (502) 897-1583
E-mail: sandilbb@aol.com
Sandi Baker, State Coordinator for Services to Deafblind Children
Diane Haynes, Training Coordinator
Carol McCraken, Transition Coordinator

Type of Agency: State.
Mission: Provide consultation and technical assistance to families of and educational programs for infants, children, and youth (birth to 22 years) who are deafblind.
Funded by: Title VI-C.
Hours of Operation: Mon.-Fri. 8:00 AM-4:30 PM.
Staff: 3 full time, 1 part time. Various therapists, medical specialists, teachers of visually impaired children, orientation/mobility specialists available as consultants. Advisory board with parent members.
History/Date: Est. 1976.
Number of Clients Served: 170.
Eligibility: All individuals on the Kentucky Deafblind Census must have vision and hearing impairments (in combination).
Area Served: Kentucky.
Age Requirements: 0-21 years.

Educational: Intensive consultant services for early childhood and transition-age students.
Professional Training: Faculty seminars; summer institute.

Local Offices:

Louisville: Kentucky Deafblind Project, 1867 Frankfort Avenue, Louisville, KY 40206, (502) 897-1583.

A wide variety of services and instruction delivered on consultant or referral basis. Training is delivered on site.

INFANT AND PRESCHOOL

Visually Impaired Preschool Services (VIPS)

1229 Garvin Place
Louisville, KY 40203
(502) 636-3207
FAX: (502) 636-0024
URL: http://www.vips.org
Sharon Bensinger, Executive Director

Type of Agency: Private; non-profit.
County/District Where Located: Jefferson County.
Mission: To offer appropriate services to visually impaired children from birth to school age and their families; to maximize each child's developmental potential through direct services, advocacy and community education.
Funded by: Private donations, local fundraising efforts.
Budget: $400,000 (1995-96).
Hours of Operation: Mon.-Fri. 8:30 AM-4:30 PM.
Program Accessibility: Totally accessible.
Staff: 9 full time, 6 part time.
History/Date: Est. 1984.
Number of Clients Served: 142 (direct), 65 (outreach).
Eligibility: Blind, visually impaired, multiply handicapped.
Area Served: 50-mile radius of Louisville (including southern Indiana). VIPS-Central Kentucky services Lexington and

surrounding counties, outreach services to other parts of the state.
Age Requirements: 0-5 years.

Counseling/Social Work/Self-Help: Parent education and support.
Educational: Parent/infant classes; in-home early intervention; day care/preschool consultation; parent support group; bi-monthly parent newsletter.
Professional Training: "Can Do!" video series.
Reading: Small lending library of books, tapes, and video tapes for families in program.
Recreational: Family retreat weekend; family outings, field trips.
Consultant services to other programs also available throughout Kentucky on a limited basis.

Local Offices:

Lexington: VIPS-Central Kentucky, 343 Walter Avenue, #303, Lexington, KY 40504, (606) 254-5519.

STATEWIDE OUTREACH SERVICES

Kentucky School for the Blind

1867 Frankfort Avenue
Louisville, KY 40206
(502) 897-1583
FAX: (502) 897-1583
Barbara Bunuan, Contact Person

Funded by: State funds.
Age Requirements: 0-21.

Assessment: Conducted according to the needs of the individual student.
Consultation to Public Schools: Available statewide.
Parent Assistance: Parent resource center and annual conference.

INSTRUCTIONAL MATERIALS CENTERS

Kentucky Instructional Materials Resource Center

1867 Frankfort Avenue
Louisville, KY 40206
(502) 897-1583, ext. 213
FAX: (502) 897-1583
Adam Ruschival, Manager

County/District Where Located: Jefferson County.
Area Served: State of Kentucky.
Groups Served: K-12, adults.

Types/Content: Textbooks and other instructional materials.
Media Formats: Braille books and large print books.
Title Listings: Print and braille lists available at no charge.

UNIVERSITY TRAINING PROGRAMS

University of Louisville School of Education

Department of Special Education
Louisville, KY 40292
(502) 852-6421
FAX: (502) 852-0570
URL: http://www.louisville.edu/edu.edsp/distance/dedge
Dr. Ed Berlá, Coordinator, Visual Impairment Program

County/District Where Located: Jefferson County.

Programs Offered: Undergraduate and graduate (master's, doctoral) programs for teachers of visually impaired students. Refer to WWW site.
Distance Education: Y.

◆ *Information Services*

LIBRARIES

Kentucky Library for the Blind and Physically Handicapped

300 Coffee Tree Road
P.O. Box 818
Frankfort, KY 40602
(502) 564-8300 or toll-free in
Kentucky (800) 372-2968
FAX: (502) 564-5773
E-mail: rfeindel@ctr.kdlo.state.
ky.us
URL: http://
www.kdlo.state.ky.us
Richard Feindel, Librarian

Type of Agency: Library.
Mission: Provides books and
magazines recorded on tapes and
records and in braille.
Funded by: Public funds.
Budget: $320,000.
Hours of Operation: Mon.-Fri.
8:00 AM-4:30 PM.
Program Accessibility: Fully
accessible.
Staff: 10.5 full-time equivalents.
History/Date: Est. 1968.
Number of Clients Served: 5,500.
Eligibility: Print handicapped
(blind; physically handicapped and
unable to hold a book or turn its
pages; or learning disabled).
Area Served: Kentucky.

Northern Kentucky Talking Book Library

502 Scott Street
Covington, KY 41011
(606) 491-7610
Alice Manchikes, Librarian

Subregional library.

Talking Book Library

Louisville Free Public Library
301 West York Street
Louisville, KY 40203
(502) 574-1625 or TDD (502) 561-
8621
FAX: (502) 561-8657
Maxine Harris, Librarian

Subregional library.

MEDIA PRODUCTION SERVICES

Jefferson County Public Schools

P.O. Box 34020
Louisville, KY 40232-4020
(502) 485-3011
FAX: (502) 485-3776
Jan Moseley, Specialist, Visually
Impaired

County/District Where Located:
Jefferson County.
Groups Served: K-12.

Types/Content: Textbooks.
Media Formats: Braille books,
talking books/cassettes, large-
print books.
Title Listings: No title listings
available.

Owensboro Recording Unit

450 Griffith Avenue
Owensboro, KY 42301
(502) 684-0212
FAX: (502) 685-0914
Liz Gray, Coordinator

Area Served: Initial recordings
accepted only from within the
state of Kentucky. Books already
in our library may be available to
anyone qualifying for the service.
Groups Served: K-12; college
students; other adults.

Types/Content: Textbooks,
career/vocational.
Media Formats: Talking books/
cassettes.
Title Listings: No title listings
available.

Recording for the Blind and Dyslexic

240 Haldeman Avenue
Louisville, KY 40206
(502) 895-9068
FAX: (502) 897-1145
Mark Stewart, Executive Director
Douglas Trusner, Studio Director

County/District Where Located:
Jefferson County.

See Recording for the Blind and
Dyslexic in U.S. national listings.

RADIO READING

Central Kentucky Radio Eye

1541 Beacon Hill
Lexington, KY 40504
(606) 257-2702
Al Crabb, President

County/District Where Located:
Lexington County.
Funded by: Gifts and grants.
Hours of Operation: Mon.-Fri
8:00 AM - 1:00 PM; Weekends
8:00 AM - 12:00 noon.
Staff: Uses volunteers.
History/Date: Est. 1990.
Area Served: Central Kentucky.
Age Requirements: None.

INFORMATION AND REFERRAL

The Foundation Fighting Blindness
Eastern Kentucky Affiliate

HC 71, Box 363
Jeremiah, KY 41826
(606) 633-5498
Hassie Helton, President

See The Foundation Fighting
Blindness in U.S. national listings.

Prevent Blindness Kentucky

101 West Chestnut Street
Louisville, KY 40202
(502) 584-6127
FAX: (502) 584-0828
Fred Wright, Program Director

County/District Where Located: Jefferson County.

See Prevent Blindness America in U.S. national listings.

See also in national listings:

American Printing House for the Blind, Inc.

Audio Studio for the Reading Impaired

National Association to Promote the Use of Braille

♦ *Rehabilitation Services*

STATE SERVICES

Kentucky Department for the Blind
P.O. Box 757
Frankfort, KY 40602
(502) 564-4754
FAX: (502) 564-2951
Denise Placido, Commissioner

Type of Agency: State.
Mission: To provide opportunities to persons with visual disabilities to enable them to become more independent and productive in the community and workplace.
Funded by: Public funds.
Budget: $9,302,200.
Hours of Operation: Mon. - Fri. 8:00 AM - 4:30 PM.
Staff: 129 full time, 47 part time.
Number of Clients Served: 1,100.
Eligibility: Legally blind or visually impaired.
Area Served: Kentucky.
Age Requirements: 16 and older for job placement; any age for independent living services.

Counseling/Social Work/Self-Help: Rehabilitation counseling staff.
Residential: Charles W. McDowell Rehabilitation Center.
Rehabilitation: Aids and mobility training.
Employment: Evaluation; prevocational and vocational training; vocational placement; follow-up services.
Computer Training: Access; training on computer aids and devices.
Low Vision: Available for purchase.
Low Vision Aids: Available for purchase.

Local Offices:

Ashland: Department for the Blind, 1405 Greenup Avenue, Ashland, KY 41101, (606) 920-2000.
Bowling Green: Center for Independent Living, 300 Chestnut Bldg., 604 Fairview Court, Bowling Green, KY 42101, (502) 746-7479.
Bowling Green: Department for the Blind, 300 Chestnut Bldg., Fairview Court, Bowling Green, KY 42101, (502) 746-7479.
Elizabethtown: Department for the Blind, 409 North Miles Street, Elizabethtown, KY 42701, (502) 766-5126.
Florence: Department for the Blind, 7410 U.S. 42, Suite 112, Florence, KY 41042, (606) 371-3380.
Lexington: Department for the Blind, 153 Patchen Drive, Suite 21, Lexington, KY 40517, (606) 246-2111.
Louisville: Charles W. McDowell Rehabilitation Center, Center for Independent Living, 8412 Westport Road, Louisville, KY 40242, (502) 327-6010 or (800) 346-2115 (tollfree).
Murray: Center for Independent Living, 104 North Fifth Street, Suite 203, Murray, KY 42071, (502) 759-9227.

Owensboro: Department for the Blind, 3000 Alvey Park Dr., West, Owensboro, KY 42303, (502) 687-7306.
Paducah: Department for the Blind, 220 North Eighth Street, Suite E, Paducah, KY 42001, (502) 575-7315.
Prestonsburg: Department for the Blind, 2565 South Lake Drive, Prestonsburg, KY 41653, (606) 886-2730.
Somerset: Department for the Blind, 650 North Main Street, Gateway Center, Suite 240, Somerset, KY 42501, (606) 677-4045.

REHABILITATION

Kentucky Industries for the Blind
1900 Brownsboro Road
Louisville, KY 40206
(502) 893-0211
FAX: (502) 893-3885
Jim Sparks, Director

Type of Agency: A division of Kentucky Department for the Blind.
Mission: To provide training and long-term employment opportunities for blind and visually impaired residents of Kentucky.
Funded by: Workshop sales and fees.
Budget: $1,500,000.
Hours of Operation: 8:00 AM - 4:30 PM.
Program Accessibility: In compliance with ADA guidelines.
Staff: 10 full time. Uses volunteers.
History/Date: Est. 1918.
Number of Clients Served: 35-50 annually.
Eligibility: Legally blind or visually impaired.
Area Served: Kentucky.

Age Requirements: 18 and above.

Counseling/Social Work/Self-Help: Provided by Division of Client Services.

Employment: Sub-assembly trainees, janitorial training and outplacement, and sheltered employment in a factory setting.

COMPUTER TRAINING CENTERS

Assistive Technology Services Kentucky Department for the Blind

8412 Westport Road
Louisville, KY 40242
(502) 327-6010
FAX: (502) 327-9620
Jenny Tyree, Supervisor

County/District Where Located: Jefferson County.

Computer Training: Speech output systems; screen magnification systems; braille access systems; optical character recognition systems; closed-circuit television systems; word processing; database software; computer operating systems.

♦ Low Vision Services

EYE CARE SOCIETIES

Kentucky Academy of Eye Physicians and Surgeons
P.O. Box 1690
Lexington, KY 40592
(606) 254-3412
FAX: (606) 288-4282
Judith Taylor, Executive Director

Kentucky Optometric Association
P. O. Box 572

Frankfort, KY 40602
(502) 875-3516
FAX: (502) 875-3782
E-mail: koainfo@mis.net
Darlene Eakin, CAE, Executive Director

LOW VISION CENTERS

**Kentucky Clinic
University of Kentucky
Department of Ophthalmology**
Chandler Medical Center
Lexington, KY 40536-0284
(606) 233-6649 or (606) 233-5867
FAX: (606) 257-6718
E-mail: crutcho@pop.uky.edu
Barbara K. Crutchfield, O.D., F.A.A.O., Director, Low Vision Service, Department of Ophthalmology

Type of Agency: Ophthalmology clinic.
Funded by: Client fees, state funds.
Hours of Operation: Mon.-Fri. 8:00 AM-5:00 PM.
Staff: Ophthalmologists; ophthalmology residents; optometrist; ophthalmic technicians.
Number of Clients Served: Approximately 5-10 patients weekly.
Eligibility: None.
Area Served: Unlimited.
Age Requirements: None.

Low Vision Aids: Not provided on loan.
Low Vision Follow-up: By return appointment as needed.

**Kentucky Lions Eye Center, Low Vision Clinic
University of Louisville
Department of Ophthalmology**
301 East Muhammad Ali Boulevard

Louisville, KY 40202
(502) 583-0564
FAX: (502) 852-6596
Kay Lutz, Director

Type of Agency: Ophthalmology clinic.
County/District Where Located: Jefferson County.
Mission: Direct service to visually impaired persons.
Funded by: Client fees, state funds, donations.
Hours of Operation: By appointment only through the Eye Clinic.
Staff: Ophthalmologist; ophthalmology resident. Optician available locally.
Eligibility: Referral from eye care specialist or state agency.
Area Served: Unlimited.
Age Requirements: Generally do not serve infants.

Professional Training: For residents and ophthalmic technicians.
Low Vision Aids: Provided for demonstration; procured for patient at cost.
Low Vision Follow-up: As needed by patient.

Low Vision Service of Jessamine Optometric Association
506 North Main Street
Nicholasville, KY 40356
(606) 887-2441
FAX: (606) 885-3323
E-mail: musick1@sprintmail.com
John E. Musick, O.D.,F.A.A.O., Clinical Director

County/District Where Located: Jessamine County.
Funded by: Client fees.
Hours of Operation: Mon.-Fri. 8:30 AM - 5:00 PM.
Staff: Counselor; low vision assistant; ophthalmologist; optician; optometrist.

Area Served: Unlimited.
Age Requirements: None.

Counseling/Social Work/Self-Help: Counseling available.
Rehabilitation: Rehabilitation counselor, occupational therapist and orientation/mobility instructor available.
Low Vision: On-site training provided.
Low Vision Aids: Lend/purchase; sold at cost. Prescriptions filled.
Low Vision Follow-up: Return appointment.

Local Offices:

Lexington: Insight Low Vision Rehabilitation Service, St. Joseph Hospital, One St. Joseph Drive, Lexington, KY 40503, (606) 278-3436.
Louisville: McDowell Center for the Blind, 8412 Westport Road, Louisville, KY 40242, (502) 327-6010.

Low Vision Services of Kentucky

120 North Eagle Creek, Suite 501
Lexington, KY 40509
(606) 263-3757
FAX: (606) 263-3757
William J. Wood, M.D., Clinical Director
Rick D. Isernhagen, Clinical Director
Jeanne VanArsdall, Director

Type of Agency: Private; non-profit.
County/District Where Located: Fayette County.
Funded by: Client fees.
Hours of Operation: Mon.-Fri. 8:30 AM-5:00 PM.
Staff: Ophthalmologists; ophthalmic assistant/technician; low vision assistant/specialist; registered nurse. Available for consultation or referral: social

worker, rehabilitation counselor, audiologist.
History/Date: Est. 1987.
Eligibility: Ophthalmology/optometry referral.
Area Served: Unlimited.

Low Vision Aids: Provided for evaluation and loan for trial purposes; on-site training provided.
Low Vision Follow-up: By return appointment or home visit as necessary.

♦ Aging Services

STATE UNITS ON AGING

Division of Aging Services Cabinet for Human Resources
CHR Building, Sixth West
275 East Main Street
Frankfort, KY 40621
(502) 564-6930
FAX: (502) 564-4595
Jerry Whitley, Director

Provides referrals to Area Agencies on Aging and information on other local aging services.

INDEPENDENT LIVING PROGRAMS

Kentucky Department for the Blind
8412 Westport Road
Louisville, KY 40242
(502) 327-6010 or (800) 346-2115
LuAnne Qualls, Administrator

Provides independent living services for persons age 55 and over. For further information, contact the Project Director or general phone number listed.

LOUISIANA

◆ *Educational Services*

STATE SERVICES

Louisiana Learning Resources System
Louisiana State Department of Education
2758-C Brightside Lane
Baton Rouge, LA 70820-3507
(504) 763-5431
FAX: (504) 763-3937
E-mail: bvaccaro@mail.doe.state.la.us
Carol Wines, Program Director

Type of Agency: Resource Center.
County/District Where Located: Baton Rouge Parish.
Mission: Provides consultation on educational services to local schools and agencies. Acts as a clearinghouse and depository for large print and braille textbooks for visually impaired and blind students in Louisiana.
Funded by: State and federal funds.
Hours of Operation: Mon.-Fri. 8:00AM-5:00PM.
Staff: 6.
Number of Clients Served: 867.
Eligibility: Visual impairment.
Area Served: Louisiana.

For further information, contact Office of Special Education Services, Louisiana State Department of Education, P.O. Box 94064, Baton Rouge, LA 90804-9064, (514) 342-6118, Joyce E. Russo, Supervisor of Visually Impaired Services.

For information about local facilities, consult the superintendent of schools in the area.

EARLY INTERVENTION COORDINATION

Office of Special Education Services
P.O. Box 94064
Baton Rouge, LA 70804-9064
(504) 763-3552
FAX: (504) 763-3553
E-mail: sbatson@mail.doe.state.la.us
URL: http://www.doe.state.la.us/
Susan Wagley Batson, Director

State administration of early intervention and early childhood special education programs. Also provides in-service training and technical assistance programs to school systems, parent organizations, and any other public or private agencies.

SCHOOLS

Louisiana School for the Visually Impaired
P.O. Box 4328
Baton Rouge, LA 70821-4328
(504) 342-8694
FAX: (504) 342-1885
Richard N. Day, Superintendent

Type of Agency: State.
Mission: Services for totally blind and legally blind.
Funded by: Public funds.
Budget: $3.8 million.
Staff: 90 full time; 3 part time.
History/Date: Est. 1897.
Number of Clients Served: 1997: 50, plus field services.
Eligibility: Educable, ambulatory, visually impaired, resident of Louisiana, under 22 years.
Area Served: Statewide.
Transportation: Y.
Age Requirements: 3-21 years.

Health: Diagnosis and evaluation of eye health; treatment of eye condition; prescription of spectacles or aids; follow-up evaluation of eye treatment or prescription; general medical services; speech therapy.
Counseling/Social Work/Self-Help: Individual, group, family/parent, couple counseling; placement in school.
Educational: Grades K through 12. Programs for college prep; general academic; vocational/skill development.
Preschools: Limited to daily commuters.
Professional Training: Regular in-service training programs, open to enrollment from other agencies.
Reading: Talking book record players and cassette players; talking book records and cassettes; braille books; large-print books; braille magazines; recorded magazines.
Residential: Dormitories.
Rehabilitation: Personal management; braille; handwriting; typing; home management; orientation/mobility; remedial education; sensory training; speech therapy; physical therapy.
Recreational: Afterschool programs; arts and crafts; bowling; swimming; track; wrestling; modified football; softball; tandem biking.
Employment: Transition planning; vocational training.
Computer Training: Speech output systems, screen magnifiers, braille access systems, computer-assisted instruction.
Low Vision: Biweekly on-site clinic.
Low Vision Aids: As needed.
Low Vision Follow-up: Not less than annual.

Contact local school superintendent for program information or Special School District #1, Louisiana State Department of Education, P.O. Box

94064, Baton Rouge, LA 70804
(504) 342-1508.

STATEWIDE OUTREACH SERVICES

Louisiana School for the Visually Impaired
1120 Government Street
Baton Rouge, LA 70802-4897
(504) 342-4756 or (504) 342-5144
FAX: (504) 342-1885
Mitzi Jones, Director of Support and Field Services
Warren Figueiredo, Resources Specialist, Braille Technology Center

Funded by: State and federal funds.
History/Date: Est. 1994.
Age Requirements: Under 22 years.

Professional Training: Workshops and conferences.
Assessment: Multidisciplinary evaluation.
Consultation to Public Schools: On request, on-site consultation regarding programming and delivery of services.
Direct Service: Technical assistance to local personnel.
Parent Assistance: Training; lending library; resources and information; support groups.
Materials Production: Limited braille and large print assistance; tacticle adaptations.

INSTRUCTIONAL MATERIALS CENTERS

Louisiana Learning Resources System
Louisiana State Department of Education
2758-C Brightside Lane

Baton Rouge, LA 70821-3507
(504) 763-5430
FAX: (504) 763-3937
E-mail: cwines@mail.doe.state.la.us
Carol Wines, Program Manager

County/District Where Located: East Baton Rouge Parish.
Area Served: Louisiana.
Groups Served: Blind and visually impaired students.

Media Formats: Large-print and braille textbooks.

Acts as clearinghouse and depository for large-print and braille textbooks. Maintains additional instructional materials.

◆ Information Services

LIBRARIES

Louisiana State Library Section for the Blind and Physically Handicapped
260 North Third
Baton Rouge, LA 70802-5232
(504) 342-4944 or (504) 342-4943
FAX: (504) 342-3547
Jennifer Anjier, Librarian
Michael Acosta, Machine Lending Information

Funded by: Public funds.
Hours of Operation: Mon. - Fri. 8:00 AM - 4:30 PM.
History/Date: Est. 1958.
Area Served: Louisiana.

Regional library supplying talking books, braille, large type books, cassettes, and play-back equipment.

MEDIA PRODUCTION SERVICES

Louisiana School for the Visually Impaired
P.O. Box 4328
Baton Rouge, LA 70821-4328
(504) 342-5244
FAX: (504) 342-1885
E-mail: warrendfic@aol.com
Warren Figueiredo, Director

Area Served: Statewide.
Groups Served: K-12.

Types/Content: Educational material.
Media Formats: Braille books; large-print books.
Title Listings: No title listings available.

RADIO READING

WRBH-FM/Radio for the Blind
3606 Magazine
New Orleans, LA 70115
(504) 899-1144
FAX: (504) 899-1165
Randy Savoy, News Director

County/District Where Located: Orleans Parish.
Hours of Operation: 24 hours a day.
History/Date: Est. 1982.
Area Served: 75-mile radius from New Orleans.

INFORMATION AND REFERRAL

Louisiana Council for the Blind
1894 Dallas Drive
Suite B
Baton Rouge, LA 70806
(504) 925-1635
Sydney Ishee, Office Manager

Type of Agency: Non-profit consumer organization.
County/District Where Located: East Baton Rouge Parish.
Mission: Provides information in braille and large-print and on

cassette to the visually impaired population on matters affecting this segment of the population. Provides information on aids and appliances. Makes other appropriate referrals.

Funded by: Contributions & grants.

Hours of Operation: Mon.-Fri. 9:00 AM-4:30 PM.

Staff: 1.

Number of Clients Served: 8.000: 1996.

Eligibility: All visually impaired.

Area Served: Louisiana.

Age Requirements: 18 years or older.

Members are available to discuss common problems of visual impairment.

See also in national listings:

Contact Lens Association of Ophthalmologists

Randolph-Sheppard Vendors of America

◆ Rehabilitation Services

STATE SERVICES

Louisiana Rehabilitation Services

8225 Florida Boulevard
Baton Rouge, LA 70806-4834
(504) 925-4131
FAX: (504) 925-4184
May Nelson, Director
Susan Mitchell, Blind Services

Type of Agency: State.

Mission: To provide opportunities for employment and independence to individuals with handicapping disabilities through vocational and other rehabilitation services.

Funded by: State funds; federal funds.

Hours of Operation: Mon.-Fri. 8:00 AM-4:30 PM.

Staff: 470 full-time staff; 11 counselors for the blind.

Eligibility: The presence of a physical and/or mental disability that constitutes or results in a substantial handicap to employment; and a reasonable expectation that vocational rehabilitation services will benefit the individual in terms of employability.

Area Served: Louisiana.

Transportation: Y.

Age Requirements: Based on the eligibility criteria an individual would need to be at or near an age that such services in a reasonable time frame would render the individual employable.

Health: Preliminary diagnostic evaluation; some physical restoration and surgical procedures based on the agency guidelines; and other health services as needed and allowable under agency guidelines health services.

Counseling/Social Work/Self-Help: Social evaluation; individual counseling; referral to community services; contracts for other counseling/social work; independent living services.

Educational: Assistance with college training; work and other training programs as appropriate.

Professional Training: Vending facility programs, on-the-job training, on-site training and job coaching.

Reading: Aids can be provided for eligible clients if aids are determined necessary.

Rehabilitation: Personal management; braille; orientation/mobility; teaching in client's home

and community. Contracts for other rehabilitation services.

Employment: Prevocational evaluation; career and skill counseling; vocational training; job retention; vocational placement; follow-up service; vending stand training.

Computer Training: Training, aids and devices provided for eligible clients if assistance is determined necessary.

Low Vision: Services purchased for the client if need is determined.

Low Vision Aids: Provided for eligible clients if prescribed.

Low Vision Follow-up: Provided for eligible clients if prescribed.

Local Offices:

Alexandria: 900 Murray Street, Room H-100, Alexandria, LA 71301-7699, (318) 487-5335.

Baton Rouge: 2097 Beaumont Drive, Baton Rouge, LA 70806, (504) 925-4985.

Hammond: 130 Robin Hood Drive, Hammond, LA 70403-5763, (504) 543-4040.

Houma: P.O. Box Drawer 469, Houma, LA 70361, (504) 857-3652.

Lafayette: 825 Kaliste Saloom Road, Building VI, Suite 350, Lafayette, LA 70508, (318) 265-5353.

Lake Charles: 3616 Kirkman Street, Lake Charles, LA 70605-3006, (318) 475-8038.

Monroe: 122 St. John Street, State Office Building, Third Floor, Monroe, LA 71201, (318) 362-3232.

New Orleans: 2026 St. Charles Street, Second Floor, New Orleans, LA 70130-5300, (504) 568-8815.

Shreveport: 1525 Fairfield Avenue, 708 State Office Building, Shreveport, LA 71101-4388, (318) 676-7155.

REHABILITATION

Lighthouse for the Blind in New Orleans

123 State Street
New Orleans, LA 70118
(504) 899-4501
FAX: (504) 895-4162
William Price, President

Type of Agency: Non-profit.
County/District Where Located: Orleans Parish.
Mission: To enable blind and visually impaired persons to maintain and achieve independence through employment, rehabilitation, services, and recreation activities.
Funded by: Contributions, workshop sales, sub-contracts and endowment.
Budget: 1996: $4.5 million.
Hours of Operation: Mon.-Fri. 7:45 AM-4:15 PM.
Program Accessibility: Architecturally barrier-free.
Staff: 16 full time.
History/Date: Est. 1913.
Eligibility: Legally blind.
Area Served: Greater New Orleans and surrounding area.
Age Requirements: Except for STARS program (teens), minimum age is 18.

Health: Eye health public education program.
Counseling/Social Work/Self-Help: Consultation and referral services.
Rehabilitation: Adjustment-to-blindness program (comprehensive 3-6 month skills training program directed toward independence); orientation and mobility training; braille training; job evaluations.
Recreational: Senior social group; STARS (Students Together Acquiring Recreational Skills) for teens.

Employment: Manufacturing of products and commodities.

Louisiana Association for the Blind

1750 Claiborne Avenue
Shreveport, LA 71103
(318) 635-6471
FAX: (318) 635-8902
James Bowen, Jr., Executive Director

Type of Agency: Private; non-profit.
County/District Where Located: Caddo Parish.
Mission: Services for totally blind, legally blind, visually impaired, deaf-blind.
Staff: 60 full time.
Eligibility: Legally or totally blind.

Health: Refers for health services to the state.
Counseling/Social Work/Self-Help: Personal adjustment and vocational counseling, psychological testing.
Educational: Vocational/skill development.
Reading: Talking book record player and cassette player; talking book records and cassettes; braille books; large print books. Lends braille and recorded books.
Residential: Provides housing for out of town clients while going through evaluation.
Rehabilitation: Personal management; braille; communication skills; home management; orientation/mobility; remedial education.
Recreational: Bowling; seasonal activities.
Employment: Prevocational evaluation; career and skill counseling; occupational skill development; sheltered workshops; job placement service; school-to-work transition program.

Local Offices:

Shreveport: Louisiana Association for the Blind, 1107 Burt Street, Shreveport, LA 71103, (318) 227-2869, Doug Young, Manager.

Louisiana Center for the Blind

101 South Trenton Street
Ruston, LA 71270
(318) 251-2891 or (800) 234-4166
FAX: (318) 251-0109
Joann Wilson, Director

Type of Agency: Residential rehabilitation agency for blind and visually impaired adults; summer programs for children and teenagers.
County/District Where Located: Lincoln Parish.
Mission: To help blind persons fully participate in the economic, social and spiritual lives of their communities.
Funded by: Grants and fees for services.
Budget: Approximately $500,000.
Hours of Operation: Mon.-Fri. 8:00 AM-5:00 PM.
Program Accessibility: Wheelchair accessible.
Staff: 15 full time; 3 part time.
History/Date: Est. 1985.
Number of Clients Served: 400 to date.
Eligibility: Legally blind adults and children.
Area Served: United States, primarily Louisiana.
Transportation: Y.
Age Requirements: 18 years and older. Summer programs for 8-12 years and 13-17 years old.

Counseling/Social Work/Self-Help: Available.
Educational: 6-9 month program offering training in cane travel, braille, keyboarding, computer literacy, and home economics, independent living skills, mobility and industrial arts.

Reading: Braille classes.
Residential: Apartments available for students.
Rehabilitation: Orientation and adjustment; employment assistance.
Recreational: Twice weekly participation in a health/recreational facility is mandatory.
Employment: Occasional volunteerism for on-the-job training. Assistance in job placement following services and training.
Computer Training: A full range of adaptive technology.

COMPUTER TRAINING CENTERS

Affiliated Blind of Louisiana, Inc.
409 W. St. Mary Boulevard
Lafayette, LA 70506
(318) 234-6492
FAX: (318) 232-4244
John Lemairie, Executive Director
Judy Lejeune, Program Director

Computer Training: Training in keyboarding, DOS, Windows, speech and large print programs, Wordperfect, Lotus 1-2-3, braille output devices (KTS), scanners, notetaking devices, and braille printers. Some training in D-base and Quicken also available.

◆ Low Vision Services

EYE CARE SOCIETIES

Louisiana Ophthalmological Association
2820 Napoleon Avenue
New Orleans, LA 70115
(504) 895-5959
William F. Rachal, M.D., President

Louisiana State Association of Optometrists
P.O. Box 13451
Alexandria, LA 71315-3451
(318) 449-9467
Susan Jong, O.D., Executive Director

LOW VISION CENTERS

Louisiana State University Eye Center
Low Vision Clinic
2020 Gravier Street
Suite B
New Orleans, LA 70112
(504) 568-6700
Dr. Mandi Conway, M.D., Director of Medical Retina Services
Cathy Edwards, Clinic Director

County/District Where Located: Orleans Parish.
Funded by: State funds, fees charged to private patients.
Staff: Ophthalmologist; optometrist.
Area Served: Louisiana and Gulf Coast of Mississippi.

Low Vision Follow-up: By return appointment in 1 month if needed.

Low Vision Clinic
Schumpert Eye and Laser Center
1801 Fairfield, Suite 106
Shreveport, LA 71101
(318) 681-6669 or (800) 527-3709
FAX: (318) 681-6780
Charlotte Alford, Manager

Type of Agency: Non-profit, hospital-based, full-service diagnostic and surgical eye center.
Mission: To provide state-of-the-art service to the region, to detect disease and preserve and enhance sight.
Funded by: Sisters of Charity of the Incarnate World.
Hours of Operation: Mon., Thurs., 2:00 PM-4:30 PM.

Program Accessibility: Fully accessible.
Staff: Optometrist with low vision training; 16 ophthamologists; registered nurses; ophthalmic technicians.
History/Date: Low Vision Center opened as a component of the Eye Center in 1986.
Number of Clients Served: Approximately 6 per week.
Eligibility: Referral by a physician on staff.
Area Served: 170 mile radius.
Age Requirements: None.

Counseling/Social Work/Self-Help: Available through other hospital departments and in local community.
Educational: Only in low vision use.
Low Vision: Y.
Low Vision Aids: Y.
Low Vision Follow-up: Y.

Tulane Medical Center Hospital and Clinic
1415 Tulane Avenue
New Orleans, LA 70112
(504) 588-5312 or toll-free in Louisiana (800) 654-5935 or toll-free in other southern states (800) 233-8967
FAX: (504) 584-1681
Delmar R. Caldwell, M.D.
Dr. Joseph Rummage, Low Vision Coordinator

Type of Agency: For-profit hospital.
County/District Where Located: Orleans Parish.
Funded by: Client fees.
Hours of Operation: Mon.-Fri. 8:00 AM-5:00 PM.
Staff: Low vision coordinator; occupational therapist; ophthalmic resident assistant; ophthalmologist.
Number of Clients Served: 350 per year.

Eligibility: Legally blind. Referral and current ophthalmological report.
Area Served: Louisiana, Mississippi, northern Florida.
Transportation: Y.
Age Requirements: 4 years and older.

Counseling/Social Work/Self-Help: Counselor, psychologist and social workers available.
Low Vision: On-site training provided.
Low Vision Aids: Loaned at no cost for 1-2 weeks. Sold at cost.
Low Vision Follow-up: Return appointment, phone interviews.

♦ *Aging Services*

STATE UNITS ON AGING

Office of Elderly Affairs
412 North Fourth Street
Baton Rouge, LA 70802
(504) 342-7100
FAX: (504) 342-8409
Richard Collins, Executive Director

Provides referrals to Area Agencies on Aging and information on other local aging services.

INDEPENDENT LIVING PROGRAMS

Louisiana Rehabilitation Services
Department of Social Services
8225 Florida Boulevard
Baton Rouge, LA 70806
(504) 925-3594 or (800) 737-2958
Suzanne Mitchell, Director

Provides independent living services for persons age 55 and over. For further information, contact the Project Director or general phone number listed.

MAINE

♦ Educational Services

STATE SERVICES

Division for the Blind and Visually Impaired
Maine Department of Human Services
35 Anthony Avenue
State House Station #150
Augusta, ME 04330-0150
(207) 624-5323
Harold Lewis, Director

Type of Agency: State.
County/District Where Located: Kennebec County.
Mission: To support the education of blind children.
Funded by: State funds.
Budget: $1,500,000.
Staff: 9 full-time equivalents (plus 14 contract itinerant teachers). Various therapists available as needed; medical personnel available on consultant basis; advisory board with parent members for overall program.
Number of Clients Served: 500.
Eligibility: Visually impaired with functional limitations which interfere with regular classroom education.
Area Served: Maine.
Age Requirements: Birth to 21 years.

Counseling/Social Work/Self-Help: Parent counseling; genetic counseling; other social and health services available on referral basis.
Educational: Adaptive equipment; assessment, consultation and instruction in orientation and mobility, and all developmental areas.

EARLY INTERVENTION COORDINATION

Interdepartmental Coordinating Council on Early Intervention Child Development Services
State House Station ɥ46
Augusta, ME 04333
(207) 287-3272
FAX: (207) 289-5900
Joanne Holmes, Part H Early Childhood Coordinator

County/District Where Located: Kennebec County.

Early intervention services to children aged 0-5.

INSTRUCTIONAL MATERIALS CENTERS

Instructional Materials Center for the Blind
123 Free Street
Portland, ME 04101
(207) 871-7440, ext. 141
FAX: (207) 871-1243
Youngok Raymond, Manager

Area Served: Maine.
Groups Served: Preschool-12th grade.

Types/Content: Textbooks and instructional materials.
Media Formats: Braille, large print.

Also supplies instructional tools and other materials.

♦ Information Services

LIBRARIES

Maine State Library
Library Services for the Blind and Physically Handicapped
State House Station #64
Augusta, ME 04333
(207) 289-5650 or (207) 947-8336 or toll-free in Maine (800) 452-8793
FAX: (207) 287-5624
E-mail: benitad@ursus1.ursus.maine.edu
Benita Davis, Librarian

Type of Agency: State library.
County/District Where Located: Kennebec County.
Funded by: State funds.
Hours of Operation: Mon.-Fri., 7:30 AM-4:00 PM.
History/Date: Est. 1971.
Number of Clients Served: 4,000.
Area Served: Statewide.

Provides talking books, large print books, reference service, and volunteer-produced material.

MEDIA PRODUCTION SERVICES

Maine Division for the Blind and Visually Impaired
State House Station #150
Augusta, ME 04330-0150
(207) 624-5323
FAX: (207) 624-5302
Harold Lewis, Director

County/District Where Located: Kennebec County.
Area Served: Maine.
Groups Served: K-12, college students, other adults.

Types/Content: Textbooks, career/vocational.
Media Formats: Braille/large-print books.
Title Listings: Print, braille, computer disk listings free of charge.

INFORMATION AND REFERRAL

The Foundation Fighting Blindness
Maine Affiliate
136 Knox Lane

Millinocket, ME 04462
(207) 723-4338
Ellen Pelkey, Contact Person

See The Foundation Fighting
Blindness in U.S. national listings.

◆ *Rehabilitation Services*

STATE SERVICES

**Division for the Blind and
Visually Impaired
Maine Department of Labor**
35 Anthony Avenue
State House Station #150
Augusta, ME 04333-0150
(207) 624-5323
FAX: (207) 624-5302
Harold Lewis, Director

Type of Agency: State.
County/District Where Located:
Kennebec County.
Mission: Administers the federal-
state vocational rehabilitation
program and independent living
program. Provides case
management, direct instruction,
and orientation and mobility
services; employs under contract
all teachers of the blind/visually
impaired in Maine. Services for
totally blind, legally blind, visually
impaired, deaf-blind, and multiply
disabled persons.
Funded by: Federal and state
appropriations.
Budget: 1996: $3,500,000.
Hours of Operation: Mon.-Fri.
8:00 AM-5:00 PM.
Staff: 31 full time.
History/Date: Est. 1941.
Number of Clients Served: 1996:
1,200.
Eligibility: Severe visual disability
that results in functional
limitations.
Area Served: Maine.

Transportation: Y.
Health: Contracts, refers and
provides consultation to other
agencies for health services.
**Counseling/Social Work/Self-
Help:** Vocational counseling;
referral to community services.
Contracts, refers and provides
consultation to other agencies for
other counseling/social work
services.
Educational: Preschool to 12th
grade, age 21. Accepts deaf-blind,
emotionally disturbed, learning
disabled, mentally retarded, and
orthopedically disabled persons.
Professional Training:
Internship/fieldwork placement in
low vision; orientation and
mobility; vocational rehabilitation.
Regular in-service training
programs, short-term or summer
programs open for enrollment to
other agencies.
Reading: Braille books, large print
books, information and referral;
transcription to braille and tape
recording services on demand for
clients. Library services provided
by state library.
Rehabilitation: Personal
management; communication;
home management; orientation/
mobility; all skills training in home
and community; contracts, refers
and provides consultation to other
agencies for other rehabilitation
services.
Recreational: Contracts, refers
and provides consultation to other
agencies for recreation services.
Employment: Career and skill
counseling; vocational placement;
follow-up service; vending stand
training. Contracts, refers and
provides consultation to other
agencies for other employment-
oriented services.
Computer Training: Training on
computer; access and software.
Low Vision: Contracts and refers
for low vision services.

Low Vision Aids: Y.
Low Vision Follow-up: Y.

Local Offices:

Augusta: Division for the Blind
and Visually Impaired, 73 State
House Station, Augusta, ME 04330,
(207) 287-6702.
Bangor: Division for the Blind and
Visually Impaired, 396 Griffin
Road, Bangor, ME 04401,
(207) 561-4374.
Caribou: Division for the Blind
and Visually Impaired, RR2 Box
8700, Caribou, ME 04736,
(207) 493-4120.
Ellsworth: Division for the Blind
and Visually Impaired, P.O. Box
737, Plaka Mall, Ellsworth, ME
04605, (207) 667-5361.
Lewiston: Division for the Blind
and Visually Impaired, 200 Main
Street, Lewiston, ME 04240,
(207) 795-4421.
Portland: Division for the Blind
and Visually Impaired, 105 Elm
Street, Portland, ME 04104,
(207) 822-0400.
Rockland: Division for the Blind
and Visually Impaired, 279 Main
Street, Rockland, ME 04841,
(207) 594-1834.

REHABILITATION

**Maine Center for the Blind and
Visually Impaired**
189 Park Avenue
Portland, ME 04102
(207) 774-6273
FAX: (207) 774-0679
Steven Obremeski, Executive
Director

Type of Agency: Private; non-
profit.
Funded by: Fees, state of Maine,
donations, product sales.
Hours of Operation: 8:00 AM-
4:00 PM.
Program Accessibility: Y.

Staff: Over 50 full time and part time.

History/Date: Est. 1905.

Number of Clients Served: Over 800 per year.

Eligibility: Legally blind or severe vision loss affecting life functions.

Area Served: Maine.

Counseling/Social Work/Self-Help: Consultation and referral services.

Residential: State-licensed residence.

Rehabilitation: Mobility; vocational evaluation; rehabilitation teaching in homes state-wide.

Recreational: Recreation services for residents; sports and recreation program for interested participants.

Employment: Work adjustment and training; extended employment.

Computer Training: Comprehensive computer access program.

Low Vision: Sells aids and appliances; low vision service.

Local Offices:

Bangor: Department of Human Services, 396 Griffin Road, P.O. Box 445, Bangor, ME 04402-0445, (207) 947-0511, Sue Martin, Rehabilitation Teacher.

Caribou: Department of Human Services, RR 2, Caribou, ME 04736, (207) 498-8151, Kristy Swallow, Rehabilitation Teacher.

Lewiston: Department of Human Services, 200 Main Street, Lewiston, ME 04240, (207) 795-4400, Gerald Kewley, Rehabilitation Teacher.

Saco: Kimball Health Center, 333 Lincoln Street, Saco, ME 04072, (207) 284-4081, Laura Marletta, Rehabilitation Teacher.

COMPUTER TRAINING CENTERS

Maine Center for the Blind and Visually Impaired
189 Park Avenue
Portland, ME 04102
(207) 774-6273
FAX: (207) 774-0679
E-mail: mbwalsh@ime.net
Mary Beth Walsh, Computer Specialist

Computer Training: Speech output systems; screen magnification systems; braille access systems; optical character recognition systems; closed-circuit television systems; word processing; database software; computer operating systems.

◆ Low Vision Services

EYE CARE SOCIETIES

Maine Society of Eye Physicians and Surgeons
Association Drive
P.O. Box 190
Manchester, ME 04351
(207) 622-3374
FAX: (207) 622-3332
Gordon H. Smith, Esq., President

Maine Optometric Association, Inc.
RR #1, Box 2675
Litchfield, ME 04350-9730
(207) 582-9910
Nan-Elizabeth B. Reynolds, Executive Director

◆ Aging Services

STATE UNITS ON AGING

Bureau of Elder and Adult Services
Maine Department of Human Services
35 Anthony Avenue
State House Station #11
Augusta, ME 04333-0011
(207) 624-5335 or (800) 262-2232
FAX: (207) 624-5361
Christine Gianopoulos, Director

Provides referrals to Area Agencies on Aging and information on other local aging services.

INDEPENDENT LIVING PROGRAMS

Division for the Blind and Visually Impaired
Bureau of Rehabilitation Services
Department of Labor
State House Station #150
Augusta, ME 04333-0150
(207) 624-5323
FAX: (207) 624-5302
Harold Lewis, Director

Provides independent living services for persons age 55 and over. For further information, contact the Project Director or general phone number listed.

MARYLAND

♦ *Educational Services*

STATE SERVICES

Maryland State Department of Education
200 West Baltimore Street
Baltimore, MD 21201
(410) 767-0238
FAX: (410) 333-8165
Nancy S. Grassmick, State Superintendent of Schools
Richard Steinke, Deputy State Superintendent, Office of School Improvement
Carol Ann Baglin, Assistant State Superintendent, Division of Special Education

Mission: Administers supplemental state and federal funds for visually handicapped children attending local school systems. Provides consultation for local schools and the Maryland School for the Blind.
Funded by: Public funds.
Area Served: Maryland.

For information about local programs and facilities, consult the superintendent of schools in the area.

EARLY INTERVENTION COORDINATION

Baltimore Infants and Toddlers Program
10 West Eager Street
Baltimore, MD 21201
(410) 396-1666
FAX: (410) 547-8292
E-mail: rezchaz@adl.com
Charles Baugh, Director

Early intervention services for infants age birth to 3 years and their families.

SCHOOLS

Maryland School for the Blind
3501 Taylor Avenue
Baltimore, MD 21236-4499
(410) 444-5000
FAX: (410) 426-4807
Louis M. Tutt, President

Type of Agency: Private; non-profit.
Mission: Services for totally blind, legally blind, and visually impaired students, as well as for those whose blindness and visual impairment are complicated by deafness, learning disabilities, mental retardation, emotional problems, or orthopedic disabilities.
Funded by: State appropriation, private funding sources.
Budget: 1998: $10,284,031.
Hours of Operation: Offices: 8:00 AM - 4:30 PM.
Program Accessibility: Complies with ADA requirements.
Staff: 310 full time; 30 part time. Uses volunteers.
History/Date: Est. 1853.
Number of Clients Served: 1996: 500.
Eligibility: Visually impaired; must be referred by student's local school system.
Area Served: Maryland.
Transportation: Y.
Age Requirements: 2-21 years.

Health: Diagnosis and evaluation of eye health; treatment of eye condition; prescription of spectacles or aids; audiology; occupational therapy; physical therapy; speech therapy. On-campus medical specialty clinics.
Counseling/Social Work/Self-Help: Social evaluation; psychological testing and evaluation; individual counseling; placement in school, training, institution.

Educational: Grades K through 12 and nongraded. Programs for pre-school; general academic; vocational/skill development; infants and toddlers; community-based instruction.
Professional Training: Internship/fieldwork placement in special education; social work; speech pathology; orientation/mobility; psychology; occupational therapy; physical therapy; recreation; in-service training programs for staff and for other agencies.
Reading: Talking book record players and cassette players; talking book records and cassettes; braille books; large-print books; braille magazines; recorded magazines; Optacon; Kurzweil Reading Machine; various other computers; assistive technology devices.
Residential: Dormitories, cottages, on-site apartments for advanced students; residential programming focuses on social development and living skills.
Rehabilitation: Personal management; braille; handwriting; typing; video magnifier; home management; orientation/mobility.
Recreational: Afterschool programs; arts and crafts; hobby groups; bowling; swimming; track; wrestling; skiing; roller skating; off-campus trips; community-based recreation.
Employment: Prevocational evaluation; career and skill counseling; occupational skill development; vending stand training. Provides consultation to other organizations.
Computer Training: Training on computer aids and devices.
Low Vision: Low vision specialist provides training.
Low Vision Aids: Provided on loan for trial purposes.

Prescription for spectacles and low vision aids.

Low Vision Follow-up: Provided as needed.

Outreach services to visually impaired students in local schools and to recent graduates seeking community placement.

INFANT AND PRESCHOOL

Vision Services
Early Childhood Learning Center
Montgomery County Public Schools
Rock View Elementary School
3901 Denfeld Avenue
Kensington, MD 20895
(301) 929-2006 or (301) 649-8151
Anthony Caetano, Supervisor

Type of Agency: Public school program.
County/District Where Located: Montgomery County.
Funded by: Federal, state and community funds.
Staff: Full-time staff includes teachers of visually impaired students holding additional certification, social worker, supervisor, and paraprofessionals. Part-time staff includes dually certified teacher, occupational therapists, physical therapists, speech therapists, orientation/mobility specialist. Psychologist available on consultant basis. Uses volunteers. Has parent task force for overall program.
History/Date: Est. 1954.
Area Served: Montgomery County.
Transportation: Y.
Age Requirements: 0-5 years.

Health: Health services available from Montgomery County Health Department and private providers.
Counseling/Social Work/Self-Help: Parent counseling; parent education and support group;

sibling group; personal and family counseling.
Educational: Provides instruction in all developmental areas. Home-based program for visually impaired persons, with or without other impairments. Visually impaired and multiply disabled classes.

Consultant services to other programs, for children 0-5 years old.

STATEWIDE OUTREACH SERVICES

Maryland School for the Blind
3501 Taylor Avenue
Baltimore, MD 21236-4499
(410) 444-5000 or toll-free in Maryland (800) 400-4915
FAX: (410) 426-2590
Ruth Ann Robinson, Contact Person

Funded by: State grants; endowments; private donations.
History/Date: Est. 1853. Outreach services since 1985.
Age Requirements: 22 years of age and under.

Assessment: Through the Diagnostic Services Program, assessments are available in the following areas: low vision, occupational and physical therapy, speech language, psychology, social work, vocational education, audiology, braille, therapeutic recreation, living skills, and health review. Assessment of students residing outside of Maryland is available on a fee-for-service basis.
Consultation to Public Schools: Provided by the Educational Consultant and/or other specialists.
Direct Service: Provided through short-term attendance at main campus program, students in grades 6-12 are eligible for a four-week summer program experience.

Parent Assistance: provided through parent training opportunities, access to information, and referral to appropriate local agencies.
Materials Production: Available through Resource Services Program and includes braille production, textbook and materials searches and loan of available items.
Professional Training: In-service programs are offered on a requested basis.

INSTRUCTIONAL MATERIALS CENTERS

Maryland School for the Blind
3501 Taylor Avenue
Baltimore, MD 21236
(410) 444-5000, ext. 250
FAX: (410) 426-3360
Robb Farrell, Contact Person

Area Served: Statewide.

Types/Content: Textbooks.
Media Formats: Braille; large print; audio; tactile media.

◆ Information Services

LIBRARIES

Maryland State Library for the Blind and Physically Handicapped
415 Park Avenue
Baltimore, MD 21201
(410) 333-2668 or toll-free in Maryland (800) 492-5627
FAX: (410) 333-2095
URL: http://www.msde.state.md.us/lbph/
Sharron McFarland, Director

Funded by: State and federal funds.
Budget: $600,000.

Hours of Operation: Mon. - Fri. 8:00 AM - 5:00 PM.
Staff: 14.
History/Date: Est. 1968.
Number of Clients Served: 10,000.
Eligibility: Application required.
Area Served: Maryland.

Regional library supplying talking books, large type books, books in braille, cassette, talking book machines, and information and referral services.

Special Needs Library
Montgomery County Department of Public Libraries
6400 Democracy Boulevard
Bethesda, MD 20817
(301) 493-2555 or TDD (301) 493-2554
FAX: (301) 530-8941

Subregional library.

Talking Book Center
Prince George's County Memorial Library
6530 Adelphi Road
Hyattsville, MD 20782
(301) 779-2570
Judy Walsh, Librarian

Subregional library.

MEDIA PRODUCTION SERVICES

Montgomery County Public Schools Vision Services Center
2600 Hayden Drive
Silver Spring, MD 20902-5400
(301) 649-8151
FAX: (301) 649-8061
Anthony Caetano, Supervisor

County/District Where Located: Montgomery County.
Groups Served: 0-21 years.

Types/Content: None specified.
Media Formats: Braille and large print textbooks.

Title Listings: No title listings available.

Volunteers for the Visually Handicapped
8720 Georgia Avenue
Suite 210
Silver Spring, MD 20910
(301) 589-0894
FAX: (301) 589-7281
Judy Rasmussen, Executive Director

Area Served: Washington, D.C. metropolitan area.
Groups Served: Blind and visually impaired adults.

Types/Content: None specified.
Media Formats: Braille books, talking books/cassettes, large-print books.
Title Listings: No title listings available.

RADIO READING

Eastern Shore Radio Reading Service
WESM-FM
University of Maryland/Eastern Shore
Princess Anne, MD 21853
(410) 651-6281
Robert Franklin, Director

County/District Where Located: Somerset County.
Hours of Operation: Mon.-Sun. 5:00 AM-2:00 AM.
Area Served: Counties in Maryland, Virginia, and Delaware encompassing the Delmarva Peninsula.

Metropolitan Washington Ear, Inc.
35 University Boulevard East

Silver Spring, MD 20901
(301) 681-6636
FAX: (301) 681-5227
E-mail: washear@his.com
Nancy Knauss, Administrative Director

Hours of Operation: Mon.-Fri. 8:00 AM-5:00 PM.
History/Date: Est. 1974.
Area Served: Greater Washington, D.C., area.

Trained Washington Ear volunteers provide audio description for the visually impaired at the Kennedy Center, Arena Stage, National and Ford theaters in Washington, D.C.; at the Tawes and Roundhouse theaters in suburban Maryland. Program notes for National Symphony Orchestra concert series are taped by volunteers at the Washington Ear Studios.

Radio Reading Network of Maryland
2901 Liberty Heights Avenue
Baltimore, MD 21215
(410) 462-8580
Lois Elliott, Office Manager
Mary Jo Pons, Executive Director

County/District Where Located: Baltimore County.
Funded by: Various subdivisions, foundations, corporations, and individuals.
History/Date: Est. 1979.
Area Served: State of Maryland.

PHONE-IN NEWSPAPERS

Dialing-In
Metropolitan Washington Ear
35 University Boulevard East
Silver Spring, MD 20901
(301) 681-6636
FAX: (301) 681-7188
E-mail: washear@his.com
Nancy Knauss, Administrative Director

County/District Where Located: Montgomery County.

Newspapers Read: *Washington Post, Wall Street Journal, Washingtonian* Magazine, *Time* Magazine.

INFORMATION AND REFERRAL

The Foundation Fighting Blindness Maryland Affiliate

8810 Sigrid Road
Randallstown, MD 21133
(410) 655-3884
David Nanney, President

See The Foundation Fighting Blindness in U.S. national listings.

The Foundation Fighting Blindness (National Retinitis Pigmentosa Foundation, Inc.)

11350 McCormick Road
Executive Plaza, Suite 800
Huntville, MD 21031-1014
(410) 785-1414 or TDD (410) 785-9687 or (888) 394-3937 or TDD (800) 683-3552
FAX: (410) 771-9470
URL: http://www.blindness.org
Jessica Beach, Outreach Program Coordinator

Local and affiliate offices are listed in their respective states.

See The Foundation Fighting Blindness (National Retinitis Pigmentosa Foundation, Inc.) in U.S. national listings.

Low Vision Information Center

7701 Woodmont Avenue
Suite 302
Bethesda, MD 20814
(301) 951-4444
FAX: (301) 951-0078
Sandra S. Eastep, Executive Director

Type of Agency: Non-profit.
County/District Where Located: Montgomery County.
Mission: Comprehensive resource center for people with low vision; public education seminars.
Funded by: Private foundation, grants, and donations.
Hours of Operation: Mon.-Fri. 9:00AM-5:00PM.
Program Accessibility: Wheelcahir accessible.
Staff: 2.
History/Date: Est. 1979.
Number of Clients Served: 1,400.
Area Served: Washington, D.C. metropolitan area.
Age Requirements: 18 years and older.

Low Vision: Free information and referral service.
Low Vision Aids: Extensive hands-on display for clients to try aids in the office.
Low Vision Follow-up: yes.

Maryland Society For Sight

1313 West Old Cold Spring Lane
Baltimore, MD 21209
(410) 243-2020
FAX: (410) 889-2505
Kathleen Curtin, Executive Director

Type of Agency: Private; non-profit.
Mission: To prevent blindness by providing consumer eye health and safety information, testing, counseling, and referral.
Funded by: Private donations; United Way.
Budget: $354,424.
Hours of Operation: Mon.-Fri. 9:00 AM-5:00 PM.
Staff: 2 full time, 4 part time eye health educators and one Director of Volunteers.
History/Date: Est. 1909.
Number of Clients Served: 30,000 per year.

Area Served: All of Maryland except Washington metro counties of Prince George and Montgomery.

Health: Information and screening services to those at-risk for potentially blinding eye conditions; eye safety information.
Counseling/Social Work/Self-Help: Information and referral with follow-up.
Educational: Counseling, talks, films, pamphlets, exhibits, posters.
Professional Training: Training of technicians, nurses, school personnel in eye screening techniques.
Low Vision: Information and referral.

See also in national listings:

American Association for the Deaf-Blind

The Association for Persons with Severe Handicaps (TASH)

Audio Description Metropolitan Washington Ear

The Foundation Fighting Blindness (National Retinitis Pigmentosa Foundation Inc.)

Guide Dog Users

Laurence-Moon Bardet-Biedl Syndrome Self-Help Support Network

National Federation of the Blind

National Glaucoma Research Program of the American Health Assistance Foundation

◆ *Rehabilitation Services*

STATE SERVICES

Maryland Division of Vocational Rehabilitation Services

2301 Argonne Drive
Baltimore, MD 21218
(410) 554-9405
Glen DiChiera, Staff Specialist

Type of Agency: State.
Funded by: Public funds.
History/Date: Est. 1929.

Counseling/Social Work/Self-Help: Consultation and referral.
Reading: Reader service.
Rehabilitation: Personal management; home management; orientation/mobility; communication.
Employment: Evaluation; prevocational and vocational training; placement; follow-up; vending facility program.

Regional Offices:

Annapolis: 2001 A Commerce Park Drive, Annapolis, MD 21401, (410) 974-6708.
Baltimore: 1515 West Mount Royal Avenue, Baltimore, MD 21217-4247, (410) 333-6119.
Baltimore: Unit for the Blind, Maryland Rehabilitation Center, 2301 Argonne Drive, Baltimore, MD 21218, (410) 554-3208.
Hagerstown: Professional Arts Building, Suite 311, Hagerstown, MD 21740-5583, (301) 791-4764.
Salisbury: District Court/Multiservice Center, Salisbury, MD 21801-4975, (410) 543-6906.
Towson: 17 West Pennsylvania Avenue, Towson, MD 21204, (410) 321-4042.

REHABILITATION

Blind Industries and Services of Maryland

2901 Strickland Street
Baltimore, MD 21223
(410) 233-4567
FAX: (410) 233-0544
Frederick J. Puente, President

County/District Where Located: Baltimore County.
Mission: Provides employment and training for travel and communication skills, housing, counseling, leisure management and cooking.
Funded by: Production and sales of products to government and industrial customers, public support, trust fund and appropriation from the Maryland General Assembly.
Budget: $14 million.
Hours of Operation: 8:00 AM - 4:30 PM.
History/Date: Est. 1908.
Area Served: Maryland.
Transportation: Y.
Age Requirements: Adults.

Counseling/Social Work/Self-Help: Offers consultation, information and referral, research, and demonstration services.
Educational: Offers prevocational and vocational training and employment.
Rehabilitation: Rehabilitation and industry division programs.
Employment: Operates vending facilities program.
Low Vision Aids: Sells aids and appliances at cost.

Blind Industries and Services of Maryland
Eastern Shore Division

2240 Northwood Drive
P.O. Box 2133
Salisbury, MD 21801
(410) 749-1366
FAX: (410) 548-5085
Jack Grizzel, Plant Manager

County/District Where Located: Wicomico County.

Employment: Employment opportunities and training.

Blind Industries and Services of Maryland
Western Maryland Division

322 Paca Street
Cumberland, MD 21502
(301) 724-4111
FAX: (301) 724-4116
Marion E. Leib, Plant Manager

Type of Agency: Sheltered workshop.
County/District Where Located: Allengheny County.

Employment: Employment opportunities and on-the-job training.

Helen Keller National Center for Deaf-Blind Youths and Adults East Central Region Office

6801 Kenilworth Avenue
Suite 100
Riverdale, MD 20737
(301) 699-6255 (voice/TDD)
FAX: (301) 699-8564
Cynthia L. Ingraham, Regional Representative

See Helen Keller National Center for Deaf-Blind Youths and Adults in U.S. national listings.

Volunteers for the Visually Handicapped

8720 Georgia Avenue
Suite 210
Silver Spring, MD 20910
(301) 589-0894
FAX: (301) 589-7281
Judy Rasmussen, Executive Director

Type of Agency: Private; non-profit.
County/District Where Located: Montgomery County.
Mission: Community services.
Funded by: United Fund; sub-contracts; capital funds; donations; dues.
Budget: 1996: $270,000.
Hours of Operation: Mon. - Fri. 9:00 AM - 4:00 PM.
Program Accessibility: Y.
Staff: 7.
History/Date: Est. 1969.
Number of Clients Served: 4,500.
Eligibility: Blind or visually impaired; print handicapped.
Area Served: Washington, D.C. metropolitan area.
Age Requirements: Visually impaired adults.

Counseling/Social Work/Self-Help: Individual counseling, also accepts family/parents. Refers for social evaluation, testing, vocation placement.
Professional Training: In-service training programs for health-care providers.
Reading: Provides volunteer readers; braille/large-print; information/referral; translation to braille; closed circuit television.
Rehabilitation: Provides daily living/braille/ handwriting skills, orientation/mobility.
Recreational: Refers for all forms; provides monthly/weekend activities, and provides transportation to these activities.
Employment: Refers for prevocational evaluation, occupational skill development, training, placement.
Low Vision: Refers to low vision clinics/services.
Low Vision Aids: Sells magnifiers and other low vision aids.

COMPUTER TRAINING CENTERS

Maryland Division of Vocational Rehabilitation Services
2301 Argonne Drive
Baltimore, MD 21218
(410) 554-9405
Glen DiChiera, Staff Specialist

Computer Training: Speech output systems; screen magnification systems; braille access systems; optical character recognition systems; closed-circuit television systems; word processing; computer operating systems.

Maryland School for the Blind
3501 Taylor Avenue
Baltimore, MD 21236-4499
(410) 444-5000
Margaret Reitz, Teacher

Computer Training: Speech output systems; screen magnification systems; braille access systems; closed-circuit television systems; word processing; training for instructors.

Ruth Parker Eason School
648 Old Mill Road
Millersville, MD 21108
(410) 222-3815
Julia Wright, Teacher

County/District Where Located: Anne Arundel County.

Computer Training: Speech output systems.

◆ Low Vision Services

EYE CARE SOCIETIES

Maryland Society of Eye Physicians and Surgeons
1211 Cathedral Street
Baltimore, MD 21201-5585
(410) 244-7320
FAX: (410) 545-4169
E-mail: msepseye@aol.com
Lorraine Wallace, Executive Director

Maryland Optometric Association, Inc.
720 Light Street
Baltimore, MD 21230
(410) 727-7800 or (800) 492-3925
Thomas C. Shaner, CAE, Executive Director

LOW VISION CENTERS

Lions Vision Research and Rehabilitation Center Wilmer Ophthalmological Institute
Johns Hopkins School of Medicine
550 North Broadway
Sixth Floor
Baltimore, MD 21205
(410) 955-0580
FAX: (410) 955-1829
Gislin Dagnelie, Ph.D., Director
Pat Luberecki, Coordinator

Type of Agency: Private; non-profit.
Mission: To provide low vision services and conduct low vision research.
Funded by: Clinical revenues, clinical research funds, and charitable donations.
Budget: $220,000.
Hours of Operation: Mon., Wed., & Thurs. 8:30 AM-4:30 PM.
Staff: Optometrists; social workers; ophthalmologists by referral, occupational therapists.
Number of Clients Served: 1,000/year.
Eligibility: Ophthalmologist's or optometrist's referral.
Area Served: Unlimited.

Counseling/Social Work/Self-Help: Counseling and social work services available.

Rehabilitation: Training provided by therapists; aims at adaptation of the environment, acquiring visual skills, and use of devices. Referral to other professionals as indicated.
Low Vision: Low vision rehabilitation and evalution by optometric low vision specialist, with recommendation/ prescription of devices and/or services. Referral to other professionals as indicated.
Low Vision Aids: Provided on loan for trial purposes; no rental fee; on-site training provided.
Low Vision Follow-up: As requested by ophthalmologist or patient.

National Naval Medical Center Ophthalmology Service

8901 Wisconsin Avenue
Bethesda, MD 20889
(301) 295-1339
FAX: (301) 295-1481
Dr. Marsha Krasicky, O.D.

County/District Where Located: Montgomery County.
Funded by: Federal funds.
Staff: Ophthalmologist; ophthalmology residents; optometrist.
Eligibility: Military, dependents, retired personnel; referral from O.D. or M.D.
Area Served: Unlimited.

Low Vision Aids: On-site training provided.
Low Vision Follow-up: By phone interview after 2 months.

Richard E. Hoover Services for Low Vision and Blindness Department of Ophthalmology Greater Baltimore Medical Center

6701 North Charles Street
Baltimore, MD 21204
(410) 828-2658
FAX: (410) 828-2303
Donna Reihl, Director

Type of Agency: Non-profit.
County/District Where Located: Baltimore County.
Funded by: Private endowments, private grants, and client fees.
Hours of Operation: Mon. 8:30 AM-5:00 PM. Evenings by appointment.
Staff: Ophthalmologist; ophthalmology residents; rehabilitation teachers; orientation and mobility specialists; low vision specialist.
Number of Clients Served: 550 new clients annually (approximately).
Eligibility: Referral; ophthalmologic report.
Area Served: Baltimore, Washington, D.C., and surrounding counties.
Transportation: Y.

Counseling/Social Work/Self-Help: Monthly support/interest group, monthly newsletter.
Professional Training: In-service and community education programs provided.
Rehabilitation: Training provided in patient's environment.
Recreational: Leisure education is available.
Employment: Yes, on site.
Computer Training: Available in addition to other technologies.
Low Vision: Evaluation in client's own environment. Clinical exams provided on campus.
Low Vision Aids: Provided on loan for trial purposes; available for purchase.
Low Vision Follow-up: Provided in patient's environment.

University of Maryland Department of Ophthalmology Low Vision Program

419 West Redwood Street
Suite 420
Baltimore, MD 21201
(410) 328-6533
FAX: (410) 328-6500
E-mail: cfox@umabnet.ab.umd.edu
Charles Fox, O.D., Ph.D., Director, Vision Rehabilitation

Type of Agency: Medical system.
County/District Where Located: Baltimore County.
Mission: To provide comprehensive vision rehabilitation.
Funded by: Client fees; private grants.
Hours of Operation: By appointment.
Staff: Rehabilitative optometrist; ophthalmologist; ophthalmology residents; optician; optometrist; orthoptist; low vision assistant; other specialists.
Eligibility: Current ophthalmological report.
Area Served: Unlimited.
Age Requirements: All ages.

Counseling/Social Work/Self-Help: By referral.
Educational: Lectures on all topics are available.
Professional Training: CME in various areas.
Rehabilitation: Full services available.
Employment: By referral.
Computer Training: By referral.
Low Vision: Provided by full-time rehabilitative optometrist.
Low Vision Aids: Provided for purchase; prescribed and fitted for variable charge; on-site training; custom designing.
Low Vision Follow-up: Return appointment.

Multiple offices in Greater Balitmore area.

♦ *Aging Services*

STATE UNITS ON AGING

Office on Aging
State Office Building
301 West Preston Street, Room #1004
Baltimore, MD 21201
(410) 767-1100 or Information and referral in-state (800) 243-3425
FAX: (410) 333-7943
Sue Ward, Director

Provides referrals to Area Agencies on Aging and information on other local aging services.

INDEPENDENT LIVING PROGRAMS

Maryland Division of Vocational Rehabilitation Services
Administrative Offices
2301 Argonne Drive
Baltimore, MD 21218
(410) 554-9405
FAX: (410) 554-9412
Robert Burns, Assistant Superintendent
Glenn DiChiera, Staff Specialist

Provides independent living services for persons age 55 and over. For further information, contact the Project Director or general phone number listed.

MAS-SACHUSETTS

♦ *Educational Services*

Massachusetts Department of Education
Educational Improvement Group
350 Main Street
Malden, MA 02148
(617) 388-3300
FAX: (617) 388-3394
Carole Thomson, Acting Associate Commissioner, (617) 388-3300, ext. 438
Marcia Mittnacht, State Director, Special Education, (617) 388-3300, ext. 461

Mission: Oversees services to children with disabilities and enforces federal and other regulations concerning those services. Maintains contact with local resource and itinerant specialists in terms of local program monitoring and evaluation, technical assistance, and resolution of individual pupils' programming. Approves state and federal aid to local cities and towns for special programs, services, educational materials and equipment.
Funded by: Public funds.
Area Served: Massachusetts.

For program information, contact local school superintendent.

EARLY INTERVENTION COORDINATION

Early Intervention Services
Massachusetts Department of Public Health
250 Washington Street

Boston, MA 02108
(617) 624-5969
FAX: (617) 624-5990
Ron Benham, Director

County/District Where Located: Suffolk County.

SCHOOLS

Boston Center for Blind Children
147 South Huntington Avenue
Boston, MA 02130
(617) 296-4232
Michael DeLalla, Executive Director

Type of Agency: Private; non-profit.
Mission: Special education.
Funded by: Tuition.
Budget: $2.4 million.
Hours of Operation: 24 hours a day, 365 days a year.
Program Accessibility: Fully accessible.
Staff: 80 full time.
History/Date: Est. 1901.
Number of Clients Served: 22.
Area Served: Primarily Massachusetts, other states.
Age Requirements: 6-22 years.

Counseling/Social Work/Self-Help: Parent counseling, information and referral, assistance/advocacy for parents in P.L. 94-142 process.
Educational: Provides instruction in most developmental areas.
Low Vision: Services available.

The Fernald Center
200 Trapella Road
P.O. Box 9108
Belmont, MA 02178
(617) 894-3600
Jacqueline Bouyea, Acting Director

Type of Agency: Public.
County/District Where Located: Middlesex County.

Mission: Services for developmentally disabled including blind of all ages.
Funded by: State funds.
History/Date: Est. 1848.

Educational: Education and training program for blind, multiply handicapped of all ages.
Computer Training: Training on computer aids and devices.

Northeast Vision Consultants
P.O. Box 486
Sharon, MA 02067
(617) 784-0642
FAX: (617) 784-0642
E-mail: nvc@sharon.k12.ma.us
Timothy Traut-Savino, Vice President

Type of Agency: Private.
Mission: Consultant services/orientation and mobility for visually impaired children and adults at home, at school, and at other agencies.
Funded by: Contracting services from public school systems, private agencies, and individuals.
Staff: 2 full time, 11 part time.
History/Date: Est. July 1984.
Eligibility: Legally blind or visually impaired.
Area Served: Eastern Massachusetts, southern New Hampshire.

Counseling/Social Work/Self-Help: Refers for psychological testing and evaluation, individual/group/family/couple counseling.
Educational: K-12; assessment; program planning; direct/indirect services.
Preschools: Nursery school.
Professional Training: Training/supervised fieldwork in low vision (BS/MA), orientation/mobility (MA), special education (MA).

Rehabilitation: Daily living; communication skills; orientation/mobility; on/off-site.
Recreational: Refers for afterschool programs.
Employment: Career/skill counseling; refers for prevocational evaluation, job retention/training, occupational skill development.

Perkins School for the Blind

175 North Beacon Street
Watertown, MA 02172
(617) 924-3434
FAX: (617) 926-2027
Kevin J. Lessard, Director

Type of Agency: Private; non-profit.
Mission: Services for blind, deaf-blind, visually impaired, and multi-impaired children, teenagers, and adults.
Funded by: Public funds, endowments, contributions, and tuition.
Budget: 1996: $31,000,000.
Hours of Operation: 8:00 AM - 5:00 PM.
Program Accessibility: Fully accessible.
Staff: 450 full time; 150 part time.
History/Date: Est. 1829.
Number of Clients Served: 180 on campus; hundreds off campus.
Eligibility: Diagnostic evaluation program available to determine program needs.
Area Served: Primarily serves New England; accepts students from all areas of the United States and overseas.
Transportation: Y.

Health: Comprehensive health services available.
Counseling/Social Work/Self-Help: Counseling and guidance; parent counseling; child advocacy services.

Educational: Grades: preschool through adult. Special programs for multi-impaired and deaf-blind. Summer school programs. Community-based outreach programs.
Professional Training: Internship/fieldwork program for local universities; in-service training program in sign language and child care.
Reading: Braille books; large-type and recorded materials; Optacon and Kurzweil Reading Machine. Braille and talking book library for Massachusetts. Howe Press of the Perkins School distributes the Perkins Brailler, brailling accessories, low vision aids, and other materials and equipment.
Residential: Cottages for students; independent apartment living program.
Rehabilitation: Home management; personal management; orientation/mobility; communications; vocational.
Recreational: Recreation services both on and off campus.
Employment: Evaluation, prevocational and vocational training. Programs for training in industry, business, food service, retail management, child care, vending stand, piano servicing, and work activities centers. Summer employment program.
Computer Training: Available to all students.
Low Vision: Low vision clinic on campus is available.
Low Vision Aids: Available from low vision center.
Low Vision Follow-up: Yes.

Regional Offices:

Bangkok, Thailand: 420 Rajavithi Road, Bangkok 10400, Thailand, (662) 246-0070, Kirk Horton, Regional Representative, Asia/Pacific Region.

Cordoba, Argentina: Instituto Helen Keller, Av. Velez, Sarfield 2100 CU, Aj, Postal Number 4, Cordoba 5000, Argentina, 54-51-605046, Graciela Ferioli, Regional Representative, Latin America.

Local Offices:

Hyannis: Perkins Outreach Satellite Program, 270 Communications Way, Suite 2D, Hyannis, MA 02601, Robert Steele, Coordinator, (508) 771-2101.
Northfield: Perkins Outreach Satellite Program, 168 Main Street, Northfield, MA 01360, Richard Ely, Coordinator, (413) 498-5358.

Coordinates funding of deaf-blind programs in New England for the U.S. Department of Health and Human Services through the New England Regional Center for Services to the Deaf-Blind. Innovative vocational models for deaf/blind youths.

Offers evaluation service to outside agencies and individuals; designed to assess a diverse special needs population that includes but is not limited to multi-impaired blind and deaf-blind.

INFANT AND PRESCHOOL

Perkins School for the Blind

175 North Beacon Street
Watertown, MA 02172
(617) 924-3434
FAX: (617) 923-8076
Kevin J. Lessard, Director
Tom Miller, Supervisor, Preschool Services

Type of Agency: Private; non-profit.
Funded by: Income from local education agencies and grants.
Staff: 14 full time/part time (includes early childhood/teachers of visually impaired and deaf-blind students); 6 part time (includes social worker/parent

counselor, psychologist, occupational/speech/physical therapists). Medical consultants available. Uses volunteers.

History/Date: Est. 1979.

Number of Clients Served: 230 (infants); 25 (preschool).

Area Served: Entire state.

Counseling/Social Work/Self-Help: Parent counseling. Various support and related services available on consultative or referral basis.

Educational: Provides instruction in all developmental areas. Home-based program with center component for visually impaired children, 0-3 years, with or without other impairments, including deaf-blindness. Home teaching, classrooms for multiply impaired students, and community-based vision and deaf-blindness services to local education authorities offered for children aged 3-6.

Consultative services to other programs offered at all age levels.

STATEWIDE OUTREACH SERVICES

**Outreach Services
Perkins School for the Blind**

175 North Beacon Street
Watertown, MA 02172
(617) 924-3434
FAX: (617) 926-2027
Mary Beth Caruso, Contact Person, ext. 7434

Funded by: Fees for service; tuition; and grants.

History/Date: Outreach services; est. 1980.

Age Requirements: Birth-22 years.

Assessment: Assessments of infants, preschoolers, and school-age children in school, at home, and in specialized programs.

Consultation to Public Schools: Consultation to teachers, aides, administrators, and related personnel individually and through in-service education.

Direct Service: Assessments and instruction in all developmental areas to assist student's integration in public and private schools.

Parent Assistance: Parent and teacher support groups facilitated; workshops for parents; annual parent/teacher conferences.

Materials Production: Production of braille and large-print materials.

Professional Training: Short-term workshops offered throughout the state; graduate-level summer institute.

INSTRUCTIONAL MATERIALS CENTERS

Vision Resources Library

3 Randolph Street
Baylies Lower Building
Canton, MA 02021
(617) 575-1843
FAX: (617) 575-9601
E-mail: 74731.210@compuserve.com
Carrie A. Meyers, Contact Person

Area Served: Statewide.

Types/Content: Textbooks, research materials.

Media Formats: Braille, large print.

UNIVERSITY TRAINING PROGRAMS

Boston College
Graduate School of Education

Department of Curriculum, Administration, and Special Education
Campion Hall 211

Chestnut Hill, MA 02167-3813
(617) 552-8429
FAX: (617) 552-0812
Dr. Richard M. Jackson, Director, Programs in Vision Studies and Low Incidence Disabilities Program
Barbara A. McLetchie, Coordinator of Teacher Preperation in Deaf-Blind and Multiple Disabilities

County/District Where Located: Suffolk County.

Programs Offered: Graduate (master's) level personnel preparation programs for teachers of visually impaired, deaf-blind, and multiply disabled students.

Northeastern University

Department of Counseling Psychology, Rehabilitation, and Special Education
203 Lake Hall
Boston, MA 02115
(617) 373-2485
FAX: (617) 373-8892
Dr. Louise Lafontaine, Severe Special Needs
Dr. Karen Lifter, Moderate Special Needs
Dr. James Scorzelli, Rehabilitation Education

County/District Where Located: Suffolk County.

Programs Offered: Undergraduate and graduate (master's) program for teachers of multiply disabled students. Master's program for rehabilitation counselors of deaf-blind persons.

University of Massachusetts at Boston

Graduate College of Education
Harbor Campus
Boston, MA 02125-3393
(617) 287-5709
William E. Kiernan, Ph.D.

County/District Where Located:
Suffolk County.

Programs Offered: Graduate
program in orientation and
mobility and master's program in
rehabilitation counseling or special
education.

◆ *Information Services*

LIBRARIES

Massachusetts Braille and Talking Book Library
Perkins School for the Blind
175 North Beacon Street
Watertown, MA 02172
(617) 924-3434, ext. 240 or
(617) 972-7240 or toll-free in
Massachusetts (800) 852-3133
FAX: (617) 926-2027
Patricia A. Kirk, Librarian

Mission: To provide quality
recreational and informational
library services to legally blind,
visually impaired, physically
disabled, and learning disabled
Massachusetts residents who are
unable to read conventional print.
Funded by: Public funds and
contributions.
Hours of Operation: Mon. - Fri.
8:30 AM - 5:00 PM.
Program Accessibility: Fully
accessible.
Staff: 22 full-time equivalents.
History/Date: Est. 1931.
Number of Clients Served:
15,000.
Area Served: Massachusetts.

Talking books, braille, and cassette
books and magazines; provides
braille books for Maine, New
Hampshire, Vermont, and Rhode
Island readers. Loans Library of
Congress talking book and cassette
book machines and accessories to
patrons.

Talking Book Library
Worcester Public Library
1 Salem Square
Worcester, MA 01608
(508) 799-1730 or (508) 799-1661 or
toll-free in Massachusetts
(800) 762-0085 or TDD (508) 799-
1731
FAX: (508) 799-1652
James Izatt, Librarian

Subregional library.

Vision Resources Library Massachusetts Department of Education
3 Randolph Street/Baylies Lower
Canton, MA 02021
(617) 575-1843
FAX: (617) 575-9601
Carrie Myers, Library Coordinator

Type of Agency: State.
County/District Where Located:
Norfolk County.
Funded by: State and federal
monies.
Hours of Operation: Mon.-Fri.
7:30 AM - 3:30 PM.
Staff: Coordinator; technicians.
History/Date: Est. 1965.
Number of Clients Served: 1,100.
Eligibility: Registration by
certified teacher/consultant of
visually impaired students.
Area Served: Massachusetts.
Age Requirements: 0-21 years.

Library center for research and
distribution of media and
materials for various curricula
offered to visually impaired
individuals. Maintains contact
with local resource and itinerant
specialists in terms of local
program monitoring and
evaluation, technical assistance,
in-service experiences, and
resolution of individual pupils'
problems.

TALKING BOOK MACHINE DISTRIBUTORS

Massachusetts Braille and Talking Book Library
Perkins School for the Blind
175 North Beacon Street
Watertown, MA 02172
(617) 972-7240 or toll-free in New
England (800) 852-3133
Vicki Vogt, Outreach Services
Librarian

Machine-lending agency for the
Library of Congress National
Library Service for the Blind and
Physically Handicapped. Other
machines are distributed by the
state regional libraries.

MEDIA PRODUCTION SERVICES

Massachusetts Association for the Blind
200 Ivy Street
Brookline, MA 02146
(617) 738-5110
FAX: (617) 738-1247
E-mail: mablind@tiac.net
URL: http://www.tiac.net/
users/mablind
Debby Smith, Contact Person

Area Served: Unlimited.
Groups Served: All groups, but
primarily adults.

Types/Content: Books and other
materials, including mathematics,
music, and computer-related
materials.
Media Formats: Braille,
thermoform, or cassette.

Recording for the Blind and Dyslexic
Bulfinch Square
43 Thorndike Street
Cambridge, MA 02141
(617) 577-1111
FAX: (617) 577-1113
Christina Dotti, Executive Director
Ted Washburn, Studio Director

County/District Where Located: Middlesex County.

See Recording for the Blind and Dyslexic in U.S. national listings.

Recording for the Blind and Dyslexic
12 Church Street
Lenox, MA 01240
(413) 637-0889
FAX: (413) 637-2214
Helen Gasparian, Director

County/District Where Located: Berkshire County.

See Recording for the Blind and Dyslexic in U.S. national listings.

Recording for the Blind and Dyslexic
5600 Rochester Road
Troy, MA 48098
(313) 879-0101
Jean Lowmaster, Contact Person

See Recording for the Blind and Dyslexic in U.S. national listings.

Recording for the Blind and Dyslexic
c/o Mt. Greylock Regional High School, 1781 Cold Spring Road
Williamstown, MA 01267
(413) 458-3641
FAX: (413) 458-3641
URL: http://www.rfbd.org
Gail M. Burns, Studio Director

County/District Where Located: Berkshire County.

See Recording for the Blind and Dyslexic in U.S. national listings.

Vision Resources Library
Massachusetts Department of Education
Three Randolph Street/Baylies Lower

Canton, MA 02121
(617) 575-1843
FAX: (617) 575-9601
Carrie Myers, Library Coordinator

Area Served: Massachusetts.
Groups Served: K-12.

Types/Content: Textbooks.
Media Formats: Large-print and braille.

RADIO READING

Audio Journal
172 Lincoln Street
Worcester, MA 01605
(508) 797-1117
FAX: (508) 792-4739
E-mail: ajournal@ziplink.net
URL: http://www.ziplink.net/~ajournal
Susan Wagner, Director

Funded by: Memorial Foundation for the Blind, Massachusetts Commission for the Blind, Worcester Commission on Elder Affairs.
Hours of Operation: Mon.-Fri. 9:00 AM-1:00 PM Office; 7:00AM-11:00PM Broadcast.
Staff: 6.
History/Date: Est. 1987.
Area Served: Central Massachusetts.
Age Requirements: None.

Radio Reading Service of Western New England
460 Main Street, #5
Indian Orchard, MA 01151-1222
(413) 543-8558
Kathleen G. Turnbull, Director

County/District Where Located: Hampden County.
Hours of Operation: 24 hours, 7 days.
History/Date: Est. 1983.
Area Served: Springfield and vicinity; western Massachusetts.

Talking Information Center
130 Enterprise Drive
P.O. Box 519
Marshfield, MA 02050
(617) 834-4400
FAX: (617) 834-7716
E-mail: talking@ultranet.com
URL: http://www.radioview.com/tic
Ron Bersani, Executive Director

Funded by: Massachusetts Commission for the Blind, Massachusetts Cultural Council, private contributions.
Hours of Operation: 24 hours.
Staff: 4.
History/Date: Est. 1978.
Area Served: All of Massachusetts and New Hampshire; parts of Connecticut, Vermont, Maine.
Age Requirements: None.

INFORMATION AND REFERRAL

The Foundation Fighting Blindness
Massachusetts Affiliate
P.O. Box 850139
Braintree, MA 01284
(617) 738-8890
Paul Saner, President

See The Foundation Fighting Blindness in U.S. national listings.

Prevent Blindness Massachusetts
375 Concord Avenue
Belmont, MA 02178
(617) 489-0007
FAX: (617) 489-3575
Laura Riedinger, Executive Director
Nancy Venator, Community Services

See Prevent Blindness America in U.S. national listings.

See also in national listings:

Braille Inc.

Christian Science Publishing Society

Descriptive Video Service WGBH-TV

Hilton/Perkins Program Perkins School for the Blind

Howe Press of Perkins School for the Blind

Joslin Diabetes Center

National Association for Parents of the Visually Impaired

National Birth Defects Center

National Braille Press

National Coalition on Deaf-Blindness

National Council of Private Agencies for the Blind

Resources for Rehabilitation

Schepens Eye Research Institute

Sight Line Productions

Wheeler Publishing, Inc.

◆ Rehabilitation Services

STATE SERVICES

Massachusetts State Commission for the Blind

88 Kingston Street
Boston, MA 02111-2227
(617) 727-5550, ext. 4503 or
(800) 392-6450
FAX: (617) 727-5960
E-mail: ccrawford@state.ma.us
Charles Crawford, Commissioner

Type of Agency: State.
County/District Where Located: Suffolk County.
Mission: Administers the federal-state vocational rehabilitation program, Title XX, Title XIX, and Supplemental Security Income for the blind. Provides services for totally blind, legally blind, multiply handicapped blind, children under 6 years old with vision impairment.
Funded by: State funding; fees.
Hours of Operation: Mon.-Fri. 8:45 AM-5:00 PM.
Staff: 250 full time, 16 part time.
History/Date: Est. 1906.
Eligibility: Legally blind.

Health: Contracts, refers for and provides consultation to other agencies on health services.
Counseling/Social Work/Self-Help: Social evaluation; individual, family/parent, couple counseling; placement in school, training. Contracts and refers for other counseling/social work services.
Reading: Lends talking book record player and cassette player.
Rehabilitation: Personal management; braille; handwriting; listening skills; Optacon; typing; electronic mobility aids; home management; orientation/mobility; rehabilitation teaching in client's home and community; sensory training. Contracts and provides consultation to other agencies for other rehabilitation services.
Recreational: Refers for and provides consultation to other agencies on recreation services.
Employment: Career and skill counseling; occupational skill development; job retention; job retraining; sheltered workshop; vocational placement; follow-up service; vending stand training. Contracts and provides consultation to other agencies for other employment services.
Computer Training: Training on computer aids and devices.

Local Offices:

New Bedford: 800 Purchase Street, New Bedford, MA 02740, (508) 993-6140.
Springfield: 1694 Main Street, Springfield, MA 01130, (413) 781-1290 or (800) 392-6450.
Worcester: 340 Main Street, Worcester, MA 01608, (508) 754-1148 or (800) 392-6450.

REHABILITATION

Boston Aid to the Blind

1980 Centre Street
P.O. Box 218
Boston, MA 02132-0002
(617) 323-5111
FAX: (617) 323-6687
Elliot Feldman, Executive Director

Type of Agency: Private; non-profit.
Mission: To enrich the lives of visually impaired adults, aged 50 and older, with a focus on aiding their adjustment to visual impairment; teach techniques of daily living, provide recreation and socialization programs, and serve as advocates in the broader community.
Funded by: Contributions, bequests, fund raising, membership dues, third-party reimbursements, and Medicaid.
Budget: $615,000.
Hours of Operation: Mon.-Fri. 8:00 AM-5:00 PM.
Program Accessibility: Wheelchair accessible.
Staff: 8 full time, 10 part time. Uses volunteers.
History/Date: Est. 1912.
Number of Clients Served: 1996: 200.
Eligibility: Ambulatory, legally blind, or severely visually impaired.
Area Served: Greater Boston.
Transportation: Y.

Age Requirements: 50 years and older.

Health: Preventive nursing care.

Counseling/Social Work/Self-Help: Individual and group counseling; information and referral; crisis intervention.

Professional Training: Internships and fieldwork placements.

Reading: Talking book record players and cassette players; talking book records and cassettes; braille books; large-print books; braille magazines.

Rehabilitation: Personal management; braille; typing; home management. For day program clients. A short-term training program is available.

Recreational: Arts therapy; summer day program; bowling; woodworking; dressmaking; music; cooking; drama; knitting; crocheting; physical education; cultural enrichment program; weaving; swimming.

Low Vision: Preliminary screening, referrals to low vision clinics.

Low Vision Aids: Training with optical devices and nonoptical aids.

Low Vision Follow-up: Periodic follow-up after training.

Boston Center for Blind Children

1235 Morton Street
Mattapan, MA 02120
(617) 296-4232
William McDevitt, III, Chairman of the Board

Type of Agency: Private; non-profit.

County/District Where Located: Suffolk County.

History/Date: Est. 1901.

Carroll Center for the Blind

770 Centre Street
Newton, MA 02158-2597
(617) 969-6200 or toll-free in Massachusetts (800) 852-3131
FAX: (617) 969-6204
Rachel Ethier Rosenbaum, President

Type of Agency: Private; non-profit.

Mission: Serves people who are visually impaired with rehabilitation and skills training, information, and opportunities to achieve independence, self-sufficiency, and self-fulfillment.

Funded by: Fees, fund raising, bequests.

Budget: $3,116,000.

Hours of Operation: 8:30 AM-5:00 PM. Some weekend and evening courses. Recreational programs on weekends.

Program Accessibility: Wheelchair accessible.

Staff: 29 full time, 16 part time, 20 itinerant teacher consultants and mobility instructors. Uses volunteers.

History/Date: Est. 1936.

Number of Clients Served: 1996: 787 in community programs; 318 in rehabilitation programs.

Eligibility: Legally blind, visually impaired.

Area Served: Primarily Massachusetts and New England, although some referrals are from other areas of the U.S. and international.

Age Requirements: Summer youth programs: 15-25 years; adult residential: 16 and over; Community: 3 and over. Other programs have no age requirement.

Health: Functional vision assessment and training in use of low vision aids; audiological screening; training in self-care for individuals with diabetes and visual impairment.

Counseling/Social Work/Self-Help: Individual, group and family sessions.

Educational: Itinerant school-based special education instruction and support services for ages 3-21.

Professional Training: University internships. Inservice and Staff Development network. Teacher education program, international candidates. Computer training for teachers on educational software. Workshops and seminars for allied health professionals. Training in technology.

Reading: Training in the use of talking book records and cassettes; braille books; large-print books; braille magazines; use of volunteer readers.

Residential: 22 beds, semi-private room facility.

Rehabilitation: 1 day, 1 week, or 2 week diagnostic evaluation; 4-16 week courses in independent living; skills include low vision training, personal management, braille, typing, handwriting, tape recording, orientation and mobility, and sensory development.

Recreational: Outdoor enrichment program for adults; skiing; skating; camping; sailing; bicycling; hiking.

Employment: Career and skill counseling; job training programs in medical transcription, customer service, telemarketing; assistance with job placement and retention. Job-site evaluation.

Computer Training: Training in use of adaptive devices for computers. Classes can be at the Center, school, or job site.

Low Vision: Functional vision assessment, clinical low vision examination, low vision training, vocational vision assessment. JCAHPO training site.

Low Vision Aids: Low vision devices on loan to clients within the training program. Provision of devices by doctors' prescriptions.
Low Vision Follow-up: Ongoing training during residential program.

Ferguson Industries for the Blind

173 Second Street
Cambridge, MA 02142
(617) 727-9840 or toll-free in Massachusetts (800) 392-6450, ext. 9840
Carol A. Sullivan, Director

Type of Agency: Sheltered employment workshop.
County/District Where Located: Middlesex County.
Mission: To employ blind and visually impaired people in the manufacture of various items.
Funded by: State funds.
Budget: $1.3 million.
Hours of Operation: 8:00 AM-4:00 PM.
Staff: 9.
History/Date: Est. 1906.
Number of Clients Served: 44.
Eligibility: Referral from Massachusetts Commission for the Blind.
Area Served: Massachusetts.

Ferguson Industries for the Blind

59 Howard Street
Springfield, MA 01105
(413) 737-5108
Earl L'Esperance, Supervisor

Type of Agency: Sheltered workshop.
County/District Where Located: Hamden County.

Helen Keller National Center for Deaf-Blind Youths and Adults New England Region Office

313 Washington Street
Newton Corners, MA 02158-1626
(617) 630-1580 (voice / TDD)
FAX: (617) 630-1579
Mary Ellen Barbiasz, Regional Representative

County/District Where Located: Middlesex County.

See Helen Keller National Center for Deaf-Blind Youths and Adults in U.S. national listings.

Lowell Association for the Blind Center for the Blind and Visually Impaired

174 Central Street
Lowell, MA 01852
(508) 454-5704
FAX: (508) 458-5563
Arthur R. Kelts, Executive Director

Type of Agency: Non-profit, community based.
County/District Where Located: Middlesex County.
Mission: To encourage and assist each consumer in gaining the confidence and independence necessary to function in a sighted world.
Funded by: United Way of Merrimack Valley, endowments, contributions, sustaining donations, and volunteers.
Budget: $230,000 annually.
Hours of Operation: Mon. - Fri. 8:30 AM - 4:30 PM.
Staff: 4 full time, 3 part-time.
History/Date: Est. 1923.; inc. 1928.
Number of Clients Served: 1995-1996: 468.
Eligibility: Legally blind or functionally blind; any visual difficulty.
Area Served: Greater Lowell area.
Transportation: Y.
Age Requirements: None.

Health: Referral services; aids and appliances; public education.
Counseling/Social Work/Self-Help: Advocacy; support groups; and referral services.
Educational: Itinerant vision teaching, birth-12th grade.
Reading: Volunteers, tapes, radio reading service.
Rehabilitation: Volunteer readers and drivers; shopping programs.
Recreational: Social and recreational activities for the elderly, working-age adults, and youth. Beep baseball, bowling, newsletters.
Employment: Job search assistance.
Computer Training: Word processing, speech synthesis.
Low Vision: Functional evaluations.
Low Vision Aids: Available on trial basis, assistance in selection.

Massachusetts Association for the Blind

200 Ivy Street
Brookline, MA 02146
(617) 738-5110 or toll-free in Massachusetts (800) 682-9200 or TDD (617) 731-6444
FAX: (617) 738-1247
E-mail: mablind@tiac.net
URL: http://www.tiac.net/users/mablind
Joseph Collins, Executive Director

Type of Agency: Private; non-profit.
Mission: As a multi-service, state-wide agency, provides a diverse range of programs and services to blind and visually impaired persons, multi-disabled adults and adolescents with brain injuries; fosters self-reliance, equal opportunity, and independence.
Funded by: Contributions; United Way; endowment; and fees.
Budget: 1997: $4,700,000.

Hours of Operation: Residential services: 24 hours a day; community services: Mon.-Thurs. 9:00 AM-5:00 PM.
Staff: 100. Uses volunteers.
History/Date: Est. 1903.
Number of Clients Served: 1997: 976.
Eligibility: Visual impairment or print handicap that can benefit from services.
Area Served: Massachusetts (agency's store and braille and recording services also serve persons in other states).
Age Requirements: Residential programs have specific age requirements; community services do not.

Health: Aids and appliances stores.
Counseling/Social Work/Self-Help: Provides community education; information and referral; 24-hour telephone tape.
Educational: School for adolescents with brain injuries.
Reading: Transcribes print materials into braille and tape.
Residential: Dormitories for students with brain injuries; residential apartments for adults.
Rehabilitation: Activity program for blind retarded adults. Activities of daily living, communications skills, mobility and prevocational skills.
Employment: Workshop employs and trains blind retarded adults.
Low Vision: Low vision center located at Springfield offfice.
Publications: Publishes aid and appliances catalog in large print, cassette, braille, and computer disk.

Local Offices:

Fitchburg: 76 Summer Street, Suite 110, Fitchburg, MA 01420, (508) 345-4411.

Springfield: 77 Maple Street, Springfield, MA 01105, (413) 734-7343.
Worcester: 51 Harvard Street, Worcester, MA 01609, (617) 791-8237.

Morgan Memorial Goodwill Industries, Inc.
1010 Harrison Avenue
Roxbury, MA 02119
(617) 445-1010
Debra Jacobson, Director of Employment and Career Services
Mary L. Reed, Vice President, Human Services

Type of Agency: Private; non-profit.
County/District Where Located: Suffolk County.
Mission: Services for totally blind, legally blind, visually impaired, deaf-blind, learning disabled, mentally retarded, emotionally disabled, physically disabled.
Funded by: Fees, workshop, sub-contracts, grants.
Staff: 45 full time, 3 part time.
Eligibility: Referred by state or private agency, minimal self care, mobility.
Age Requirements: 16 years or older.

Counseling/Social Work/Self-Help: Social evaluation; psychological testing and evaluation; individual counseling; placement training; referral to community services. Refers for other counseling/social work services.
Educational: Accepts deaf-blind; emotionally disturbed; learning disabled; mentally retarded; orthopedically handicapped; other multiply handicapped. Programs: vocational/skill development.
Professional Training: Internship/fieldwork placement in rehabilitation counseling;

vocational rehabilitation. Regular in-service training programs.
Rehabilitation: Refers for rehabilitation services.
Recreational: Overnight camp. Refers for adult continuing education.
Employment: Prevocational evaluation; career and skill counseling; occupational skill development; job retention; job retraining; sheltered workshops; vocational placement; follow-up service.

New England Home for the Deaf (Aged, Blind or Infirm)
154 Water Street
Danvers, MA 01923
(617) 774-0445
Judith Good, Acting Executive Director

Type of Agency: Non-profit.
County/District Where Located: Essex County.
Mission: Residential and health services for older deaf-blind adults.
Funded by: Endowment, contributions and state aid.
Budget: $750,000.
Staff: 26.
History/Date: Est. 1901.
Number of Clients Served: 30.
Eligibility: Deaf or deaf-blind.
Area Served: New England.
Transportation: Y.
Age Requirements: 50 years and older.

Health: Health services for residents.
Counseling/Social Work/Self-Help: For residents.
Residential: Facilities for aging deaf men and women. Also accepts deaf-blind persons.
Rehabilitation: Limited.
Recreational: Social and leisure activities.

Low Vision: Services for residents.
Low Vision Aids: Available on site.
Low Vision Follow-up: Y.

The Occupational Rehabilitation Group, Inc.
Harvard Square
P.O. Box 2937
Cambridge, MA 02238
(617) 661-5667
John Robichaud, Rehabilitation Engineer
Stephen Duclos, Vocational Rehabilitation Specialist

Type of Agency: Vocational rehabilitation agency serving disabled adults.
County/District Where Located: Middlesex County.
Funded by: Third parties, state and federal agencies.
Hours of Operation: Mon.-Fri. 9:00 AM-5:00 PM.
Program Accessibility: Services provided at the workplace or in client's home.
History/Date: Est. 1977.
Number of Clients Served: 200-250/year.
Eligibility: Must be eligible for state/federal VR services.
Area Served: New England.
Age Requirements: None.

Counseling/Social Work/Self-Help: Certified vocational rehabilitation counselor on staff.
Employment: Vocational evaluation and testing; rehabilitation engineering; job modification; job development; job placement.

Outreach Services to Elders Perkins School for the Blind
175 North Beacon Street

Watertown, MA 02172
(617) 924-3434
FAX: (617) 926-2027
Mary Beth Caruso, Contact Person, ext. 7434

Type of Agency: Private; non-profit.
Funded by: Fees for service and grants.
Staff: 3 full time.
History/Date: Est. 1992.
Eligibility: Legally blind.
Area Served: Greater Watertown area, Cape Cod, or the Islands.
Age Requirements: 60 years or older.

Counseling/Social Work/Self-Help: Adjustment training and referral to community services.
Reading: Talking book records and cassettes and players, braille books, large-print books, braille and recorded magazines, closed-circuit television systems, and volunteers.
Rehabilitation: Personal management, braille, communications, daily living skills, home management, community integration.
Recreational: Individual training in leisure and recreation. Referrals to community resources.
Low Vision: Prescription and provision of low vision aids; referral services; public education.

VISION Foundation
818 Mt. Auburn Street
Watertown, MA 02172
(617) 926-4232 or toll-free in Massachusetts (800) 852-3029
FAX: (617) 926-1412
Barbara R. Kibler, Executive Director

Type of Agency: Private; non-profit.
Mission: To provide practical and emotional support to individuals with vision loss.

Funded by: Sub-contracts; memberships; grants; individuals, corporations; foundations; sales; and United Way.
Budget: 1996: $439,229.
Hours of Operation: 9:00 AM-5:00 PM.
Staff: 4 full time, 10 part time. Uses volunteers.
History/Date: Inc. 1976.
Number of Clients Served: 1996: 6,000.
Eligibility: Visually impaired.
Area Served: Massachusetts primarily: information and services and publications available nationwide.
Age Requirements: Adults.

Health: Refers for medical services.
Counseling/Social Work/Self-Help: Peer counseling; buddy telephone system; referral to community services, other counseling/social work services.
Professional Training: In-service training for peer counselors, volunteers, staff.
Reading: Information and referral (database accessible in print, large-print and speech); telephone information tape; resources in special media.
Rehabilitation: Refers for vocational rehabilitation services. Provides rehabilitation teaching services to elders 60 years of age and older who are visually impaired but not legally blind.
Recreational: Refers for and provides consultation to other agencies on recreational/leisure services.
Employment: VIPEG (visually impaired persons employment group) volunteer placement. Refers for other employment orientation services.

Service for elders: Survival Skills training for visually impaired elders age 60 and over who are not legally blind; self-help groups for elders; outreach programs. Also serves ethnic minorities and linquistic minorities.

COMPUTER TRAINING CENTERS

Massachusetts State Commission for the Blind

88 Kingston Street
Boston, MA 02111-2227
(617) 727-5550
FAX: (617) 727-5960
E-mail: jlazzaro@state.ma.us
URL: http://magnet.state.ma.us/mcb
Joseph Lazzaro, Director

Computer Training: Speech output systems; screen magnification systems; braille access systems; optical character recognition systems; closed-circuit television systems.

Operates as part of federally funded and state-funded vocational rehabilitation program providing many forms of assistive technology for blind and visually impaired persons.

The Occupational Rehabilitation Group, Inc.

Harvard Square
P.O. Box 2937
Cambridge, MA 02238
(617) 661-5667
John Robichaud, Rehabilitation Engineer
Stephen Duclos, Vocational Rehabilitation Specialist

Computer Training: Speech output systems; braille access systems; optical character recognition systems; closed-circuit television systems; word processing; computer operating systems; training for instructors.

Project CABLE
Carroll Center for the Blind

770 Centre Street
Newton, MA 02158-2597
(617) 969-6200
FAX: (617) 969-6204
E-mail: carrollb@tiac.net
URL: http://www.tiac.carrollb.net
Dina Rosenbaum, Director

Computer Training: Speech output systems; screen magnification systems; braille access systems; optical character recognition systems; closed-circuit television systems; word processing; database software; computer operating systems; training for instructors.

Work with spreadsheets and job training programs also available.

◆ Low Vision Services

EYE CARE SOCIETIES

Massachusetts Society of Eye Physicians and Surgeons

P.O. Box 557
Sudbury, MA 01776
(617) 426-2020
FAX: (508) 443-5677
Joel Kraut, M.D., President

County/District Where Located: Middlesex County.

Massachusetts Society of Optometrists, Inc.

101 Tremont Street, Suite #600
Boston, MA 02108
(617) 542-9200
FAX: (617) 542-3696
Carmine A. Guida, O.D.

County/District Where Located: Suffolk County.

LOW VISION CENTERS

Boston Medical Center

University Eye Associates
720 Harrison Avenue
Boston, MA 02118
(617) 638-8350
FAX: (617) 638-8321
Gerald Friedman, Director

Type of Agency: Non-profit.
County/District Where Located: Middlesex County.
Funded by: Client fees.
Hours of Operation: Thurs., Fri. 8:00 AM-4:30 PM.
Staff: Ophthalmologist; ophthalmology resident; optometrist.
Eligibility: Ophthalmologic report.
Area Served: Unlimited.

Low Vision Aids: Provided on loan for trial; rental fee; on-site training provided.
Low Vision Follow-up: By return appointment and/or phone interview in 1 month; home visits made rarely.

Joslin Diabetes Center
William P. Beetham Eye Research and Treatment Unit

One Joslin Place
Boston, MA 02215
(617) 732-2552 (appointments) or
(617) 732-2554 (other information)
Lloyd M. Aiello, M.D., Director
Richard M. Calderon, O.D.
Robert A. Poole, O.D.
Jerry D. Cavallerano, O.D., Ph.D.
Phillip M. Silver, Optometrist

Type of Agency: Non-profit.
County/District Where Located: Suffolk County.
Funded by: Client fees and grants.
Hours of Operation: Mon.-Fri. 8:30 AM-5:00 PM.
Staff: Counselor; low vision assistant; ophthalmic photographer; ophthalmic

technician; ophthalmologist; optometrist; optometry students; optometry residents; nurse; special educator.
Eligibility: Diabetic or referred by ophthalmologist.
Area Served: Unlimited.

Low Vision Aids: Provided on loan or purchase; on-site training provided.

Low Vision Rehabilitation Center
Carroll Center for the Blind

770 Centre Street
Newton, MA 02158-2597
(617) 969-6200
FAX: (617) 969-6204
E-mail: carrollb@tiac.com
Robert McGillivray, Contact Person
Joanne Callahan, Ophthalmic Technician

Type of Agency: Non-profit.
County/District Where Located: Middlesex County.
Hours of Operation: As needed.
Staff: Optometrist; low vision assistant; social worker; orientation/mobility instructor; rehabilitation teacher; ophthalmologist; psychologist/counselor; occupational therapist; rehabilitation counselor.
History/Date: Founded 1979.
Eligibility: Legally blind, residents of Carroll Center Rehabilitation Program.
Area Served: Unlimited.
Transportation: N.

Employment: Work assessment program available.
Computer Training: Computer access assessments provided.
Low Vision: Functional vision assessments; clinical low vision examinations.
Low Vision Aids: Provided on loan for trial; no rental fee; on-site training provided.

Low Vision Follow-up: By return appointment in 2 months.

Low Vision Service
Perkins School for the Blind

175 North Beacon Street
Watertown, MA 02172
(617) 924-3434
FAX: (617) 926-2027
Mary Beth Caruso, Contact Person, ext. 7434

Type of Agency: Private; non-profit.
Funded by: Fees for service, tuition, and grants.
Hours of Operation: Tues. 8:30 AM-4:30 PM; Wed. 8:30 AM-4:30 PM (optometric exams); Mon.-Fri. 8:30 AM-4:30 PM (functional assessments); alternative times by arrangement.
Staff: Low vision optometrist with expertise in pediatric and rehabilitation optometry. Low vision specialists with expertise in orientation and mobility, special education, and rehabilitation teaching.
Area Served: New England.
Age Requirements: None.

Counseling/Social Work/Self-Help: Consultation to families, programs, and schools. Referral to local community, state, and national resources.
Low Vision: Functional vision assessments, clinical vision examinations, environmental evaluations, optical and nonoptical device assessments and prescriptions, sun wear evaluations, on-site visits to individual's home, job, school or program. Training in vision utilizations, use of optical and neoptical aids. In-service training.
Low Vision Aids: Loan of devices, materials, and equipment.
Low Vision Follow-up: Return appointments at clinic; follow-up

in the individual's home, job, school, or program.

Massachusetts Eye and Ear Infirmary
Vision Rehabilitation Services

243 Charles Street
Boston, MA 02114
(617) 573-4177
FAX: (617) 573-3350
E-mail: pat_mccabe@meei.harvard.edu
Patricia McCabe, MPH, PT, Director
Joel A. Kraut, M.D., FACS, Medical Director
Paulette D. Turco, O.D., FAAO, Associate Director

Type of Agency: Non-profit.
County/District Where Located: Middlesex County.
Mission: To help partially sighted people of all ages to learn to successfully use their remaining vision to be as independent as possible.
Funded by: Client fees; contributions.
Budget: $350,000.
Hours of Operation: Mon.- Fri. 8:30 AM - 5:00 PM.
Program Accessibility: Wheelchair accessible; interpreters provided for deaf persons.
Staff: Ophthalmologists; optometrist; social workers; occupational therapists; ophthalmic assistant. Uses volunteers.
History/Date: Vision rehabilitation service and vision care service for the deaf and hard of hearing since 1985; low vision services since 1970.
Area Served: Unlimited.
Age Requirements: None.

Counseling/Social Work/Self-Help: Clinical social workers provide counseling/support services.

Educational: Library and information services available.

Reading: Closed-circuit television evaluation available. Talking books and adaptive reading material in vision rehabilitation service library.

Rehabilitation: Referrals to community services and other rehabilitation services.

Employment: Referral to community resources.

Computer Training: Demonstrations of large print software.

Low Vision: Complete optical and nonoptical low vision evaluations and services.

Low Vision Aids: For trial, purchase; on-site training provided; personal reading machines.

Low Vision Follow-up: By return appointment, phone interview, and visits to home, school, and place of employment.

New England Eye Institute of the New England College of Optometry, Low Vision Clinic

1255 Boylston Street
Boston, MA 02215
(617) 262-2020, ext. 321
FAX: (617) 236-5144
Dr. Louis Frank, Low Vision Services

Type of Agency: Non-profit.
County/District Where Located: Suffolk County.
Funded by: Client fees.
Hours of Operation: Mon., Fri. 9:00 AM - 4:00 PM; Thurs. 9:00 AM-9:00 PM; Sat. 9:00 AM-3:00 PM.
Program Accessibility: Wheelchair accessible.
Staff: Optometrist; optometry student/resident; low vision assistant; ophthalmologist; optician; orientation/mobility instructor.
Eligibility: Referral.
Area Served: Unlimited.

Counseling/Social Work/Self-Help: Referrals.
Low Vision: Evaluation.
Low Vision Aids: Provided on loan for trial; no fee charged; on-site training provided.
Low Vision Follow-up: By return appointment, phone interview, questionnaire, school visit.

New England Medical Center New England Eye Center

750 Washington Street
Boston, MA 02111
(617) 956-5743
Eli Peli, O.D., Director of Vision Rehabilitation Service

Type of Agency: Outpatient.
Funded by: Client fees.
Hours of Operation: Mon. 9:00 AM - 5:00 PM; Fri. 9:00 AM - 1:00 PM and by appointment.
Program Accessibility: Fully accessible.
Staff: Ophthalmology resident; optometrist; ophthalmic assistant/technician; social worker; ophthalmologist; psychologist/counselor; genetic counselor; audiologist.
History/Date: Est. 1983.
Eligibility: None.
Area Served: Unlimited.
Age Requirements: None.

Low Vision: Information, evaluation, referrals.
Low Vision Aids: Provided on loan for trial; on-site training provided.
Low Vision Follow-up: By return appointment as needed.

Schepens Retina Associates Low Vision Rehabilitation Center

100 Charles River Plaza
Cambridge Street
Boston, MA 02114
(617) 523-7800
FAX: (617) 227-0996
E-mail: schepens_retina_associates@msn.com
URL: http://www.schepens.com
Marc Gucciardi, Controller
Stephanie Caruso, Marketing Coordinator

County/District Where Located: Suffolk County.
Funded by: Client fees.
Hours of Operation: Mon.-Fri. 9:00 AM-6:00 PM.
Staff: Ophthalmologist; ophthalmology residents; optometrist; optician; low vision assistant; social worker; orientation/mobility instructor; rehabilitation teacher; special educator; occupational therapist; psychologist/counselor; rehabilitation counselor; genetic counselor; audiologist; bioengineers; psychophysics Ph.D.
History/Date: Est. 1951.
Eligibility: Referral only.

Low Vision Aids: Provided on loan for trial purposes; no rental fees; on-site training provided.
Low Vision Follow-up: By return appointment, phone interview, questionnaire, home visit, school visit or visit to place of employment in 1 month.

◆ Aging Services

STATE UNITS ON AGING

Executive Office of Elder Affairs
1 Ashburton Place
Fifth Floor

Boston, MA 02108
(617) 727-7750 or Information and
referral in-state (800) 882-2003 or
TCY in-state only (800) 872-0166 or
Elder Abuse Hotline, in-state only
(800) 922-2275
FAX: (617) 727-6944
Franklin P. Ollivierre, Secretary

Provides referrals to Area Agencies
on Aging and information on other
local aging services.

INDEPENDENT LIVING PROGRAMS

Massachusetts Commission for the Blind

88 Kingston Street
Boston, MA 02111
(617) 727-5550 or (800) 392-6450
Cheryl Standley, Director

Provides independent living
services for persons age 55 and
over. For further information,
contact the Project Director or
general phone number listed.

MICHIGAN

♦ *Educational Services*

STATE SERVICES

Michigan Department of Education
Special Education Services
P.O. Box 30008
Lansing, MI 48909
(517) 373-9433
FAX: (517) 373-7504
Arthur E. Ellis, Superintendent of Public Instruction
Dr. Richard L. Baldwin, Director of Special Education

Type of Agency: State.
County/District Where Located: Ingham County.
Mission: Conducts statewide educational planning for disabled students in Michigan. Provides both guidelines and directives to intermediate and local districts for the purposes of publicizing and monitoring comprehensive continuum of services mandated for all disabled students aged 0-25. Also administers federal quota of American Printing House for the Blind resources for both residential and local school students through the state school system.
Funded by: State funds; foundation grants.

EARLY INTERVENTION COORDINATION

Early Childhood Education
Michigan Department of Education
P.O. Box 30008
Lansing, MI 48909
(517) 373-8483
FAX: (517) 373-1233
E-mail: thompjac@state.mi.us
Jacquelyn Thompson, Coordinator

Office of the Michigan State Coordinator for Part H of the Individuals with Disabilities Education Act (IDEA).

SCHOOLS

Michigan School for the Deaf and Blind
West Court and Miller Road
Flint, MI 48503
(810) 257-1400
FAX: (810) 238-1220
Kathleen Brown, Principal

Type of Agency: State.
Mission: Services for totally blind, legally blind, visually impaired, deaf-blind, learning disabled, physically disabled, emotionally disturbed, orthopedically disabled, and mentally retarded persons.
Funded by: State and local funds.
Budget: 1992: $5,000,000.
Hours of Operation: 7:30 AM-4:30 PM.
Staff: 82. Uses volunteers.
History/Date: Est. 1879.
Eligibility: Legally blind state resident, referred.
Area Served: Michigan.
Age Requirements: 0 to 25 years.

Health: Diagnosis and evaluation of eye health; treatment of eye condition; prescription of spectacles or aids; low vision service; low vision aids; occupational therapy; physical therapy; speech therapy. Contracts and provides consultation to other agencies for other health services.
Counseling/Social Work/Self-Help: Social evaluation; psychological testing and evaluation; individual, group, family/parent, couple counseling. Refers and provides consultation to other agencies for other counseling/social work services.
Educational: General academic; career education; ungraded

secondary for adult multiply disabled, deaf-blind and severely multiply disabled persons.
Professional Training: Low vision; orientation/mobility; social work; special education; field placement. Regular in-service training programs; short-term or summer training.
Reading: Talking book record player and cassette player; talking book records and cassettes; braille books; large-print books; braille magazines; recorded magazines; information and referral.
Residential: Cottages on 42-acre campus one mile from State Capitol Building. Emphasis on training in cooperation with school program.
Rehabilitation: Personal management; braille; handwriting; listening skills; Optacon; typing; electronic mobility aids; remedial education; sensory training.
Recreational: Leisure services; afterschool programs; arts and crafts; hobby groups; residential summer camp; bowling; swimming; skiing; ice skating; horseback riding.
Employment: Prevocational evaluation; career skill counseling; occupational skill development; training in massage therapy. Refers and provides consultation to other agencies for employment services.
Low Vision Follow-up: Y.

Call school office for program information.

INFANT AND PRESCHOOL

Alpena-Montmorency-Alcona Intermediate Schools
2118 U.S. 23 South
Alpena, MI 49707
(517) 354-3101
FAX: (517) 356-3385
Tom Miller, Director of Special Education

Type of Agency: Public school program.
County/District Where Located: Alpena County.
Funded by: P.L. 89-313 and 94-142 funds, private donations, state funds.
Budget: $3,000,000.
Staff: 28 full time (includes teachers of visually impaired children, psychologist, occupational/speech/physical therapist); 1 part time.
History/Date: Est. 1951.
Area Served: Alpena, Montmorency and Alcona Counties.
Transportation: Y.
Age Requirements: 0-26 years.

Health: Adaptive equipment; low vision exams.
Counseling/Social Work/Self-Help: Counseling for students.
Educational: Provides instruction in developmental areas. Orientation/mobility available on consultant or referral basis.

Home-based and center-based programs for visually impaired children, with or without other disabilities. Consultant services to other schools and programs.

STATEWIDE OUTREACH SERVICES

Michigan School for the Deaf and Blind
West Court and Miller Road
Flint, MI 48503
(810) 257-1400
FAX: (810) 238-1220
Alex Davlantes, Acting Superintendent

Funded by: State and local funds.
History/Date: Est. 1879.
Age Requirements: 0-25 years.

Assessment: Orientation and mobility; social evaluation; academic evaluation; psychological evaluation.
Consultation to Public Schools: Assist local school districts with transition plans to return students to home districts.
Direct Service: Residential placement for legally blind students.
Parent Assistance: Counseling, referral, and networking.
Materials Production: Large-print.
Professional Training: Low vision; orientation and mobility; social work; special education; field placement. Regular in-service training programs; short-term or summer training.

INSTRUCTIONAL MATERIALS CENTERS

PIA Media Center
1023 South U.S. 27
St. Johns, MI 48879
(517) 224-0330
FAX: (517) 224-0330
Thomas Blair, Director

Area Served: Statewide.

Types/Content: Textbooks.
Media Formats: Large print, braille.

UNIVERSITY TRAINING PROGRAMS

Eastern Michigan University
Department of Special Education
Ypsilanti, MI 48197
(313) 487-0028
Dr. George Barach, Contact Person, (313) 487-0028

County/District Where Located: Washtenaw County.

Programs Offered: Undergraduate and graduate (master's) program for teachers of visually impaired students.

Distance Education: Y.

Michigan State University
Department of Counseling, Educational Psychology
331 Erickson Hall
East Lansing, MI 48824
(517) 355-1871
FAX: (517) 353-6393
E-mail: alonsol@pilot.msu.edu
Lou Alonso, Contact Person

County/District Where Located: Ingham County.

Programs Offered: Bachelor's and master's programs for teachers of visually impaired students; program for dual competency teachers of visually impaired students, including deaf-blind, and orientation and mobility specialists. Ph.D. program in Special Education.

Wayne State University
Teacher Education Division
Detroit, MI 48202
(313) 577-0918
FAX: (313) 577-4091
Sharon Elliott, Visually Handicapped, (313) 577-0918
Dr. Marshal Zumberg, Multihandicapped Blind

County/District Where Located: Wayne County.

Programs Offered: Undergraduate and graduate (master's, doctoral) programs for teachers of visually impaired and multiply disabled persons.

Western Michigan University Department of Special Education
3506 Sangren Hall

Kalamazoo, MI 49008
(616) 387-5935
Elizabeth Whitten, Department of
Special Education
Dr. William Wiener, Orientation
and Mobility
Susan Ponchillia, Rehabilitation
Teaching

County/District Where Located:
Kalamazoo County.

Programs Offered: Undergraduate
program for teachers of visually
impaired and multiply disabled
students; master's program for
orientation and mobility
specialists, rehabilitation teachers
of blind students, and dual
competency teachers of visually
impaired students/orientation and
mobility.

♦ Information Services

LIBRARIES

Blue Water Library Foundation Blind and Physically Handicapped Library
210 McMorran Boulevard
Port Huron, MI 48060
(313) 982-3600
FAX: (313) 987-7327
Debra Oyler, Librarian

Subregional library.

Downtown Detroit Subregional Library for the Blind and Physically Handicapped
121 Gratiot Avenue
Detroit, MI 48226
(313) 224-0580 or TDD (313) 224-0584
FAX: (313) 965-1977
Joan Gartland, Librarian

Subregional library.

Grand Traverse Area Library for the Blind and Physically Handicapped
332 Sixth Street
Traverse City, MI 46984
(616) 922-4824 or TDD (616) 922-4843
FAX: (616) 922-4836
Carol Hubbell, Librarian

Subregional library.

Kent County Library for the Blind and Physically Handicapped
775 Ball Avenue, N.E.
Grand Rapids, MI 49503
(616) 774-3262
FAX: (616) 774-3256
Linda Hilton, Librarian

Subregional library.

Library of Michigan Services for the Blind and Physically Handicapped
717 West Allegheny Street
Lansing, MI 48913
(517) 373-5353 or (800) 992-9012
Maggie Bacon, Vision Coordinator

County/District Where Located:
Ingham County.
Funded by: Federal grant.
Hours of Operation: 8:00 AM-5:00 PM.
Staff: 11.
History/Date: Est. 1935.
Number of Clients Served: 5,700
locally.
Eligibility: Legally blind,
physically handicapped.
Area Served: Michigan. Will
exchange braille textbooks
nationally for brailon.
Age Requirements: None.

Offers/lends cassette tape players,
braille books. Also offers book
selection and information/referral
services.

Library of Michigan Services for the Blind and Physically Handicapped
P.O. Box 30007
Lansing, MI 48909
(517) 373-5614 or TDD (517) 373-1592
FAX: (517) 373-5865
Margaret Bacon, SBPH Supervisor
Cecelia Marlow, Regional
Coordinator

Type of Agency: State.
County/District Where Located:
Ingham County.
Mission: Provide recreational
reading materials to individuals
who are unable to read standard
printed material.
Funded by: Public funds.
Budget: $487,000.
Hours of Operation: Mon. - Fri.
8:00 AM - 6:00 PM.
Staff: 11.
History/Date: Est. 1928.
Number of Clients Served:
18,000.
Eligibility: For individuals unable
to read standard printed material
due to a physical or visual
disability.
Area Served: Michigan, excluding
Wayne County, with recorded
materials, talking book machines,
cassette machines and their
accessories. Serves entire state,
including Wayne County, with
braille.
Age Requirements: None.

Regional library supplying
recorded materials, talking book
machines, cassette machines.

Macomb Library for the Blind and Physically Handicapped
16480 Hall Road
Mount Clemens, MI 48044-3198
(313) 286-1580 or TDD (313) 286-9940
FAX: (313) 286-0634
Linda Champion, Librarian

Subregional library.

**Mideastern Michigan Library
Co-op
Library for the Blind and
Physically Handicapped**
G-4195 West Pasadena Avenue
Flint, MI 48504
(810) 230-3325
FAX: (810) 732-1715
Patricia Peterson, Librarian

Subregional library.

**Muskegon County Library for
the Blind and Physically
Handicapped**
635 Ottawa Street
Muskegon, MI 49442
(616) 724-6257
FAX: (616) 724-6675
Linda G. Glapp, Librarian

Subregional library.

Northland Library Cooperative
316 East Chisholm Street
Alpena, MI 49707
(517) 356-1622 or toll-free in
Michigan (800) 446-1580
FAX: (517) 354-3939
Catherine Glomski, Librarian

Subregional library.

**Oakland County Library for the
Blind and Physically
Handicapped**
Farmington Community Library
1200 North Telegraph
Pontiac, MI 48341
(810) 858-5050
Carole Hund, Librarian

Subregional library.

**Upper Peninsula Library for the
Blind and Physically
Handicapped**
1615 Presque Isle Avenue

Marquette, MI 49855
(906) 228-7697 or toll-free in
Michigan (800) 562-8985
FAX: (906) 228-5627
Suzanne Dees, Librarian

Subregional library.

**Washtenaw County Library for
the Blind and Physically
Handicapped**
P.O. Box 8645
Ann Arbor, MI 48107
(313) 971-6059
FAX: (313) 971-3892
Mary E. Udoji, Librarian

Subregional library.

**Wayne County Regional
Library for the Blind and
Physically Handicapped**
33030 Van Born Road
Wayne, MI 48184
(313) 274-2600 or TDD (313) 274-2600
FAX: (313) 326-3008
E-mail: wcrlbph@tln.lib.mi.us
URL: http://tln.lib.mi.us/~wcrlbph
Pat Klemans, Regional Librarian

County/District Where Located:
Wayne County.
Funded by: Public funds.
Hours of Operation: Mon.-Fri.
8:00AM-4:30PM.
History/Date: Est. 1931.
Area Served: Wayne County.

Regional library supplying talking
books, large type books, and
cassette and talking book
machines. Has volunteer taping
group.

MEDIA PRODUCTION SERVICES

**Library of Michigan
Services for the Blind and
Physically Handicapped**
717 West Allegan Street
P.O. Box 30007
Lansing, MI 48913
(517) 373-5353 or (800) 992-9012
FAX: (517) 373-5865
Maggie Bacon, Supervisor

County/District Where Located:
Ingham County.
Area Served: Primarily Michigan.
Will exchange braille textbooks
nationally for brailon exchange.
Groups Served: All ages.

Types/Content: Recreational
reading.
Media Formats: Braille books,
talking books/cassettes.
Title Listings: Available on
request.

**Michigan Association of
Transcribers for the Visually
Impaired**
1400 North Drake Road, #218
Kalamazoo, MI 49006
(616) 381-9566
Elizabeth M. Lennon, President

Area Served: Michigan.
Groups Served: K-12; college
students; other adults.

Types/Content: Textbooks;
career/vocational; menus;
directories.
Media Formats: Braille; cassettes;
large-print.
Title Listings: Prvided at no
charge.

**Recording for the Blind and
Dyslexic**
5600 Rochester Road

Troy, MI 48098
(810) 879-0101
FAX: (810) 879-9927
Margaret Sellgren, Executive
Director

County/District Where Located:
Oakland County.

See Recording for the Blind and
Dyslexic in U.S. national listings.

RADIO READING

**Detroit Radio Information
Service**
4600 Cass Avenue
Detroit, MI 48201
(313) 577-4146
Kim Walsh, Director

County/District Where Located:
Wayne County.
Hours of Operation: 24 hours a
day.
History/Date: Est. 1978.
Area Served: Southeast Michigan.

The Sight Seer
3333 East Beltine Avenue, N.E.
Grand Rapids, MI 49505
(616) 363-8838
FAX: (616) 363-2584
E-mail: seer@serv.net
URL: http://www.serv.net/
~seer/
Ken Van Prooyen, Sr., Director

County/District Where Located:
Kent County.
Hours of Operation: Mon.-Fri.
9:00 AM-9:00 PM.
Staff: All volunteer.
History/Date: Est. 1983.
Area Served: 35-mile radius from
Grand Rapids on local station,
100-mile radius from Grand
Rapids on regional station.
Age Requirements: Over 18.

WKAR Radio Talking Book
c/o WKAR Radio
Michigan State University
283 Communication Arts Building
East Lansing, MI 48824-1212
(517) 353-9124
E-mail: brigid@wkar.msu.edu
URL: http://www.wkar.msu.edu
Brigid King Jansen, Producer

County/District Where Located:
Ingham County.
Funded by: Gifts, grants,
donations, and in-kind services.
Hours of Operation: Mon.-Fri.
6:30 AM-11:00 PM; Sat.-Sun.
10:00 AM-12:00 PM (for local
programs). Mon.-Fri. 11:00PM-
9:00AM; Sat-Sun. 12:00 Midnight-
10:00AM (In Touch Network).
History/Date: Est. 1973.
Area Served: 60-mile radius from
East Lansing.
Age Requirements: None.

PHONE-IN NEWSPAPERS

Newspapers for the Blind
P.O. Box 441
Clio, MI 48420
(810) 762-3656
Jim Doherty, Director

County/District Where Located:
Genesee County.

Newspapers Read: *Detroit Free
Press, Flint Journal, Kalamazoo
Gazette* and *Detroit News.* Selections
of announcements, bulletins, and
magazines also read.

INFORMATION AND REFERRAL

**The Foundation Fighting
Blindness
Michigan Affiliate**
20202 Lennon
Harper Woods, MI 48225
(810) 574-0220
Debi Howells, Contact Person

See The Foundation Fighting
Blindness in U.S. national listings.

See also in national listings:

**4-Sights Network
Upshaw Institute for the Blind**

Blind Children's Fund

Braille Communication Services

**Michigan Braille Transcribing
Service**

**Seedlings: Braille Books for
Children**

Thorndike Press

Zondervan Publishing House

♦ *Rehabilitation Services*

STATE SERVICES

**Commission for the Blind
Family Independence Agency**
201 North Washington Square
P.O. Box 30652
Lansing, MI 48909
(517) 373-2062 or TDD (517) 373-
4026
FAX: (517) 335-5829
Philip E. Peterson, Director

Type of Agency: State.
Mission: Provides opportunities
for employment and independent
living to persons who are blind.
Funded by: Federal and state
funds.
Budget: 1992-93: $12,465,900.
Hours of Operation: Mon.-Fri.
8:00 AM-5:00 PM.
Program Accessibility: Itinerant
services and accessible offices;
TDD; adapted reading material;
interpreters as needed; braille and
voice-output computers; large-
print hardware or software.
Staff: 118 full time.

History/Date: Services for the Blind est. 1944. Commission for the Blind est. 1978.

Number of Clients Served: 4,000 annually.

Eligibility: Legally blind for vocational rehabilitation, independent living, business enterprise programs. Vision acuity of 20/70 or less for youth low vision program.

Age Requirements: Vocational rehabilitation: 16 years and older; youth low vision program: birth through high school; independent living: 55 years and older.

Health: Diagnostic, medical and surgical treatment; spectacles; low vision clinic.

Counseling/Social Work/Self-Help: Counseling, guidance, and referral.

Educational: Sponsors clients in college or technical programs.

Professional Training: Regular in-service training.

Reading: Information and referral regarding sources of braille, large-print and taped material.

Residential: Michigan Commission for the Blind Training Center is a short-term residential facility.

Rehabilitation: Personal management; orientation and mobility; braille reading/writing; home mechanics; adaptive kitchen skills; low vision; electronic and computerized communication devices; college preparatory; job-seeking skills.

Recreational: Orientation to adaptive leisure activities.

Employment: Evaluation; prevocational and vocational training; vocational placement; follow-up service.

Computer Training: Training sequence as needed by client and determined by job requirements. Further information: Robert

Tinney, (616) 385-1294; Roger Yake, (616) 385-1550.

Low Vision: Low vision evaluation and aids for children and adults.

Low Vision Aids: Prescriptive and nonprescriptive.

Low Vision Follow-up: Y.

Local Offices:

Detroit: Commission for the Blind, State of Michigan Plaza Building, North Tower, 15th Floor, 1200 Sixth Avenue, Detroit, MI 48226, (313) 256-1524.

Escanaba: Commission for the Blind, State Office Building, 305 Ludington Street, Escanaba, MI 49829, (906) 786-8602.

Flint: Commission for the Blind, Flint State Office Building, 125 East Union, 7th Floor, Flint, MI 48502, (313) 768-2030.

Gaylord: Commission for the Blind, 209 First Street, Gaylord, MI 49735, (517) 732-2448.

Grand Rapids: Commission for the Blind, State Office Building, 4th Floor, 350 Ottawa, N.W., Grand Rapids, MI 49503, (616) 451-8265.

Kalamazoo: Commission for the Blind, 1541 Oakland Drive, Kalamazoo, MI 49008, (616) 385-1294.

Lansing: Commission for the Blind, 201 North Washington Square, P.O. Box 30015, Lansing, MI 48909, (517) 373-6425 or (517) 373-2062.

Saginaw: Commission for the Blind, Saginaw State Office Building, 411-G East Genesee, Saginaw, MI 48607, (517) 771-1765.

REHABILITATION

Association for the Blind and Visually Impaired (formerly Vision Enrichment Services)
215 Sheldon, S.E.

Grand Rapids, MI 49503
(616) 458-1187 or (800) 458-7113
Beverly Geyer, Executive Director

Type of Agency: Private; non-profit.

Mission: Services for totally blind, legally blind, and visually impaired persons.

Funded by: United Way; fees, and donations.

Budget: 1996: $568,457.

Hours of Operation: Mon.-Fri. 8:30 AM - 4:30 PM. Examinations by appointment only.

Staff: 6 full time, 6 part time. Uses volunteers.

History/Date: Est. 1913.

Number of Clients Served: 1995: 706.

Eligibility: Any problem related to vision.

Area Served: 13 counties in western Michigan, surrounding the Grand Rapids area.

Health: Complete low vision service. Refers for other health services.

Counseling/Social Work/Self-Help: Social evaluation; individual, group, family/parent, couple counseling; referral to community services. Refers for other counseling/social work services.

Professional Training: Regular in-service training programs.

Reading: Information and referral; transcription to braille.

Rehabilitation: All rehabilitation services available in client's home and community, except low vision clinic; personal management; braille; handwriting; listening skills; typing; home management; orientation/mobility; remedial education.

Recreational: Arts and crafts. Provides consultation to other agencies on other recreational services.

Low Vision: Low vision examinations by certified low vision doctors.
Low Vision Aids: Prescription of aids.
Low Vision Follow-up: In-home low vision follow-up.

Goodwill Industries of Greater Detroit

3132 Trumbull
Detroit, MI 48216
(313) 964-3900
FAX: (313) 964-3909
Felicia R. Hunter, Chief Operating Officer

Type of Agency: Private; non-profit.
County/District Where Located: Wayne County.
Mission: To help people with disabilities achieve greater independence and self-esteem through training and work experience.
Funded by: United Way of Southeastern Michigan, Michigan Jobs Commission, Detroit-Wayne County Community Health, Oakland County Community Health, Oakland County Employment and Training, Fees-for-Service.
Budget: $17 million.
Hours of Operation: 8:30 AM-4:30 PM.
Staff: 256 full time; 25 part time.
History/Date: Est. 1921.
Number of Clients Served: 2,245.
Eligibility: Accepts deaf-blind persons or blind persons who are also emotionally disturbed, learning disabled, mentally retarded, or orthopedically disabled or who have other disabilities.
Area Served: Wayne, Oakland, Macomb, Washntnaw, and Livingston Counties.

Counseling/Social Work/Self-Help: Social evaluations; individual and group counseling.
Educational: Vocational/skill development.
Employment: Vocational evaluations; career and skill counseling; occupational skill development; job retention; job retraining; work adjustment; job placement; sheltered employment.
Low Vision Aids: Available at cost from our Handy Aids Department.

Local Offices:

Detroit: Salvage, 7940 Livernois, Detroit, MI 48210, (313) 898-2040.
Detroit: New Center Vocational Program, 1401 Ash Street, Detroit, MI 48208, (313) 964-3900.
Holly: Employment and Training, 115 Battle Alley, Holly, MI 48442, (313) 634-0250.
Mt. Clemens: Macomb, 195 Malow, Mt. Clemens, MI 48043, (313) 465-3707.
Oak Park: South Oakland Club House, 13200 Oak Park Boulevard, Oak Park, MI 48237, (313) 547-7712.
Taylor: South West Wayne Vocational Project, 15530 Racho Road, Taylor, MI 48180, (313) 287-9600.

Goodwill Industries of Mid-Michigan, Inc.

501 South Averill Avenue
Flint, MI 48506
(810) 762-9960
FAX: (810) 762-9957
Gary Smith, President

Type of Agency: Non-profit.
County/District Where Located: Genessee County.
Funded by: Workshop sales, sub-contracts, fees, contributions and United Way.
Budget: 1995: $6,000,000.

Hours of Operation: Mon. - Fri. 6:30 AM - 5:00 PM.
Staff: 8 full time, 1 part time.
History/Date: Est. 1931; inc. 1938.
Number of Clients Served: 1995: 250 plus.
Eligibility: Any person age 16 or older with a disabling or disadvantaging condition.
Area Served: Bay, Genesee, Lapeer, Midland, Saginaw, Shiawasee, Arenac, Iosco and Tuscola counties.
Age Requirements: 16 and older.

Counseling/Social Work/Self-Help: Consultation and referral services.
Educational: Job readiness and job-seeking skills.
Rehabilitation: Special program in vocational rehabilitiation for persons who are multiple disabled and blind. Includes work adjustment, daily living and orientation.
Employment: Evaluation; prevocational and vocational training; vocational placement; follow-up services; sheltered workshops.
Low Vision Aids: Y.

Michigan Commission for the Blind Training Center

1541 Oakland Drive
Kalamazoo, MI 49008
(616) 337-3848
FAX: (616) 337-3872
Paul Glatz, Superintendent

Type of Agency: State.
County/District Where Located: Kalamazoo County.
Mission: Services for totally blind, legally blind, visually impaired, and deaf-blind persons.
Funded by: State and federal funds.
Hours of Operation: 24 hours per day, 7 days per week.

Staff: 30 full time, 11 part time. Uses volunteers.
History/Date: Est. 1969.
Number of Clients Served: 300-400 annually.
Eligibility: Legally blind.
Area Served: Michigan.
Transportation: Y.
Age Requirements: 16 years or older.

Health: Provides occupational therapy. Contracts for other health services.
Counseling/Social Work/Self-Help: Social evaluations; individual, group, family/parent counseling. Refers for other counseling/social work services. Contracts for psychological services.
Professional Training: Internship/fieldwork placement in industrial arts, orientation/mobility, rehabilitation counseling, social work, vocational rehabilitation. Regular in-service training program. Modified short-term or summer training.
Reading: Talking book record player and cassette player; braille books; large print books; braille magazines; recorded magazines; Optacon.
Residential: Dormitories.
Rehabilitation: Personal management; braille; handwriting; listening skills; Optacon; typing; video magnifier; electronic mobility aids; home management; orientation/mobility; industrial arts; adaptive kitchen skills, etc.
Recreational: Arts and crafts; hobby groups; offers instruction and/or assistance for any student activity. Refers to community programs for other recreational services.
Employment: Prevocational evaluation; vending facility training.

Computer Training: For beginners.
Low Vision: Service provided through MSU Kalamazoo Center for Medical Studies.
Low Vision Aids: Prescribed by low vision specialist.
Low Vision Follow-up: Y.

Midwest Enterprises for the Blind

422 E. South Street
Kalamazoo, MI 49007
(616) 383-0713
FAX: (616) 349-6852
E. Ann Seaman, Executive Director

Type of Agency: Non-profit.
Mission: To create employment opportunities for legally blind and multidisabled persons, thus providing a means to economic independence.
Budget: $250,000.
Hours of Operation: Mon.-Fri. 8:30AM-5:00PM.
History/Date: Est. 1993.
Age Requirements: 16 years and older.

Penrickton Center for Blind Children

26530 Eureka Road
Taylor, MI 48180
(313) 946-7500
Kurt M. Sebaly, Executive Director

Type of Agency: Private; non-profit.
County/District Where Located: Wayne County.
Mission: Services for totally blind, legally blind, visually impaired, and children with additional disabilities, such as seizures, deafness, developmental delays, mental retardation, and orthopedic disabilties.
Funded by: Fund raising, donations.
Budget: $625,000.

Hours of Operation: Residential facility open weekdays.
Staff: 17 full time, 18 part time. Uses volunteers.
History/Date: Est. 1952.
Number of Clients Served: 21.
Eligibility: Blind or legally blind; at least one additional disability.
Area Served: Southeastern Michigan.
Age Requirements: 12 years and under.

Health: Occupational therapy; nursing.
Counseling/Social Work/Self-Help: Social evaluations; informal family counseling; referral to community services.
Educational: Children over 3 attend public school programs.
Professional Training: Internship/fieldwork placement in occupational therapy. Regular in-service training programs for staff.
Residential: Dormitories.
Rehabilitation: Activities of daily living; listening skills; sensory training; orientation/mobility, field trips.
Recreational: Arts and crafts; music therapy; field trips.

Upshaw Institute for the Blind

16625 Grand River
Detroit, MI 48227
(313) 272-3900
FAX: (313) 272-6893
E-mail: upshaw@wwnet.com
URL: http://www.wwnet:com/~upshaw
Carroll L. Jackson, Executive Director

Type of Agency: Private; non-profit.
County/District Where Located: Wayne County.
Mission: Prevention of blindness, reduction of the impact of blindness, and advocacy for those with severe vision loss.

Funded by: United Way; contributions; endowments; bequests, and sub-contracts from the state of Michigan.
Budget: $650,000.
Hours of Operation: Mon. - Fri. 8:30 AM - 4:30 PM.
Program Accessibility: Wheelchair accessible.
Staff: 15.
History/Date: Inc. 1961.
Number of Clients Served: 4,799.
Eligibility: Legally blind, blind, and visually impaired persons.
Area Served: Wayne, Macomb, Oakland, Livingston, St. Clair, Washtenaw, and Monroe Counties.
Age Requirements: Varies according to program funding source.

Health: Prevention of blindness and public education programs.
Counseling/Social Work/Self-Help: Psychosocial assessment; individual and group counseling; referral to community resources. Serves family members as well as clients. Specialized services for children include parent counseling, and school consultation.
Professional Training: Internships/fieldwork placements for rehabilitation teaching and social work. In-service workshops and training opportunities.
Rehabilitation: Individual and group rehabilitation teaching in client's home or the community. Personal adjustment training; communications systems and media; home management; follow-up training for low vision clinics; leisure activities; limited orientation/mobility. Refers for other rehabilitation services. Provides consultation to other agencies in cases where blindness is a secondary disability.
Recreational: Deaf-blind club for social interaction and ongoing case management services.

Employment: Consultation, specialized information services. Use of 4-Sights Network, a national computer system for vocational, educational, technological, and professional information for blind and visually impaired persons.

Visually Handicapped Services Detroit Receiving Hospital and University Health Center
4201 St. Antoine
Detroit, MI 48201
(313) 745-4510
Margaret M. Smith, Manager

Type of Agency: Private; non-profit.
Mission: Services for totally blind and legally blind persons.
Funded by: Contract with Michigan Commission for the Blind and private donations.
Hours of Operation: Mon.-Fri. 8:30 AM-5:00 PM.
Staff: 5 full time, 4 contingent.
History/Date: Est. 1964.
Number of Clients Served: 200 a year.
Eligibility: Legally blind.
Area Served: Wayne, Oakland, Macomb and Washtenaw Counties.
Age Requirements: 16 years and up.

Health: General medical services; emergency medical services; occupational therapy; speech therapy. Refers for other health services.
Counseling/Social Work/Self-Help: Social evaluations; individual, group counseling. Refers for and provides consultation to other agencies in other counseling/social work services.
Educational: College prep program.

Professional Training: Internship/fieldwork placement in rehabilitation counseling; vocational rehabilitation.
Reading: Talking book record players and cassette players; talking book records and cassettes; braille books; braille magazines; large print books; information and referral.
Rehabilitation: Personal management; braille; handwriting; typing; computerized speech synthesis; video magnifier; electronic mobility aids; home management; orientation/mobility; Kurzweil Personal Reader. Refers for other rehabilitation services. Distributes canes without charge to legally blind persons upon request. Provides commonly used aids and devices to students without charge.
Recreational: Makes arrangements for summer camp attendance.
Employment: Prevocational evaluation; career counseling.
Computer Training: Training on computer aids and devices.
Low Vision Aids: Wide variety of low vision aids.

Visually Impaired Center
725 Mason Street
Flint, MI 48503
(810) 235-2544
FAX: (810) 235-2597
Donald Stevens, Executive Director

Type of Agency: Private; non-profit.
County/District Where Located: Genesee County.
Mission: To share skills and resources for independent life with vision loss.
Funded by: United Way; endowments; fees, grants, contributions.

Budget: $365,000.
Hours of Operation: Mon.-Fri.,
8:00AM-4:00PM.
Program Accessibility: ADA
compliance.
Staff: 5 full time, 5 part time. Uses
volunteers.
History/Date: Est. 1970; as SCVI;
1986 as Visually Impaired Center.
Number of Clients Served: 240
blind and visually impaired
annually; 1500 education and
outreach consumers.
Eligibility: Totally blind, legally
blind, visually impaired.
Area Served: Genesee,
Shiawassee, and Lapeer Counties.
Transportation: Y.
Age Requirements: None.

Health: Requires eye and medical
reports prior to srvice delivery.
**Counseling/Social Work/Self-
Help:** Social work assessment and
referral for needed services
including: peer support group;
rehabilitation teaching orientation
and mobility; vocational
assessment.
Educational: Braille Classes:
Grade I and II; Blind Diabetics
Educational Program.
Professional Training:
Internships, Field placements for
social work (BA&MSW), and
O&M.
Reading: Information and referral;
transpcription to braille; tape
recording services; large print
resources.
Rehabilitation: Personal
management; braille; handwriting;
typing; video magnifier; home
management; orientation/
mobility; rehabilitation teaching in
client's home and community;
diabetes education; sensory
training. Refers for other services.
Recreational: Refers for
recreational services.
Employment: Prevocational
evaluation; occupational skill

development; job retention; job
retraining. Refers for other
employment-oriented services.
Computer Training: Computer
users selfhelp and exploration
group.
Low Vision: Refers for low vision
evaluations.
Low Vision Aids: Demonstrates
aids recommended by low vision
evaluation.
Low Vision Follow-up: Trains in
functional use of recommended
low vision devices.

Welcome Home for the Blind
1953 Monroe Street, N.W.
Grand Rapids, MI 49505
(616) 363-9088
Kathy Higgins, Administrator

Type of Agency: Non-profit.
County/District Where Located:
Kent County.
Funded by: Lions Club of
Michigan, private funds.
Hours of Operation: 7 days a
week, 24 hours a day.
Program Accessibility: Fully
accessible.
Staff: 12 full time, 18 part time.
History/Date: Est. 1952.
Number of Clients Served: 36.
Eligibility: Legally blind,
ambulatory, ability to dress and
care for normal personal needs.
Area Served: Michigan.
Transportation: Y.
Age Requirements: 60 years and
older; can obtain a waver for
younger persons.

Educational: Educational
programs provided.
Residential: Home for blind men
and women, including those with
hearing impairments.
Recreational: Opportunities
provided in and out of
home;lectures, physical activity,
crafts, church services.

Low Vision: Services provided.

COMPUTER TRAINING CENTERS

Association for the Blind and Visually Impaired (formerly Vision Enrichment Services)
215 Sheldon, S.E.
Grand Rapids, MI 49503
(616) 458-1187
URL: http://www.grcmc.org/
blindser
George Kremer, Teacher
Linda Haven, Teacher
Kathy Konow, Teacher

Computer Training: Speech
output systems; optical character
recognition systems; closed-circuit
television systems; word
processing; computer operating
systems.

Michigan Commission for the Blind Training Center
1541 Oakland Drive
Kalamazoo, MI 49008
(616) 337-3877
FAX: (616) 337-3872
Robert Tinney, Computer
Specialist

County/District Where Located:
Kalamazoo County.

Computer Training: Speech
output systems; screen
magnification systems; braille
access systems; optical character
recognition systems; closed-circuit
television systems; word
processing; database software;
computer operating systems.

Visually Handicapped Services Detroit Receiving Hospital and University Health Center
4201 St. Antoine
Detroit, MI 48201
(313) 745-4510
Carolee Moss, Communications
Technology Instructor

Computer Training: Speech output systems; screen magnification systems; closed-circuit television systems; word processing; adaptive technology.

Visually Impaired Center
725 Mason Street
Flint, MI 48503
(810) 235-2544
FAX: (810) 235-2597
Donald Stevens, Director
Laura Bates, Instructor
Michelle Wilson, Social Worker

County/District Where Located: Genesee County.
Mission: School-to-work transition.

Computer Training: Speech output systems; screen magnification systems; braille access systems; word processing; database software; computer operating systems.

DOG GUIDE SCHOOLS

Leader Dogs for the Blind
1039 South Rochester Road
Rochester, MI 48307
(810) 651-9011 or (810) 651-7115
FAX: (810) 651-5812
William Hansen, President/Executive Director

Type of Agency: Non-profit.
Mission: Trains dogs to serve as guides for blind persons. Conducts a supervised course of training to coordinate the work of blind persons with their dogs.
Funded by: Lions and Lioness Clubs, sororities, public-supported agencies, and individuals.
Hours of Operation: 7 days a week, 8:00AM- 4:00PM.
Staff: 72.
History/Date: Est. 1939.
Number of Clients Served: 10,000.

Eligibility: Legally blind, in good health, 18 years of age, out of high school, with basic orientation and mobility skills.
Area Served: Unlimited.
Transportation: Y.

♦ Low Vision Services

EYE CARE SOCIETIES

Michigan Ophthalmological Society
120 West Saginaw
East Lansing, MI 48823
(517) 333-8279
Andrew Lott, Executive Director

Michigan Optometric Association
530 West Ionia Street, Suite A
Lansing, MI 48933
(517) 482-0616
FAX: (517) 482-1611
William Dansby, C.A.E.

County/District Where Located: Ingham County.

LOW VISION CENTERS

Association for the Blind and Visually Impaired (formerly Vision Enrichment Services)
215 Sheldon, S.E.
Grand Rapids, MI 49503
(616) 458-1187 or (800) 466-8084
FAX: (616) 458-7113
Beverly Geyer, Executive Director
Bruce Dragoo, M.D., Consulting Ophthalmologist
George Kremer, Director of Vision Services

Type of Agency: Non-profit.
Mission: Provision of low vision devices to assist in meeting daily needs.
Funded by: District 11-C-1 Lions Clubs, Area Agency on Aging of

Western Michigan, United Way of Kent County, United Way of Muskegon County, client fees.
Budget: 1991: $512,032.
Hours of Operation: By appointment only, 8:30 AM-4:30 PM.
Staff: Ophthalmologist; optometrist; social worker; orientation/mobility instructor; rehabilitation teacher.
History/Date: Est. 1913.
Number of Clients Served: 1991: 568 regular service and 5,571 through glaucoma screening.
Eligibility: Referral by ophthalmologist or optometrist.
Area Served: 13 counties in western Michigan, surrounding the Grand Rapids area.

Low Vision Aids: Provided on loan for trial; no rental fee; on-site training provided.
Low Vision Follow-up: By return appointment and/or home visit in 1 month; after 1 month, as needed.

Burns Clinic Medical Center Low Vision Clinic
560 West Mitchell
Petoskey, MI 49770
(616) 347-7000
FAX: (616) 348-6166
John H. Tanton, M.D., Director

Type of Agency: Medical clinic.
Funded by: Client fees, foundation grants, state funds.
Hours of Operation: Tues. 9:00 AM-5:00 PM.
Staff: Ophthalmologist; low vision assistant; audiologist; psychologist.
History/Date: Est. 1982.
Number of Clients Served: More than 1,000.
Eligibility: Referral and current ophthalmological report.
Area Served: Primarily northern lower Michigan and eastern upper peninsula.

Age Requirements: None.

Health: Patient referrals.
Counseling/Social Work/Self-Help: Social worker on staff for immediate assistance. Various other programs.
Educational: Educational material available.
Rehabilitation: Orientation and mobility; life skills.
Recreational: Many physical activities; swimming pool.
Employment: Job placement.
Computer Training: 2-4 week program.
Low Vision: Evaluation interview to obtain visual history; examination; on and off site.
Low Vision Aids: Provided for loan/purchase; prescriptions and fittings.
Low Vision Follow-up: Return appointment; home visit; phone interview; referrals.

College of Optometry
Ferris State University
1310 Kramer Circle
Room 501
Big Rapids, MI 49307
(616) 592-3715
FAX: (616) 592-3991
Dr. Robert Foote, Chief, Low Vision Service

County/District Where Located: Mecosta County.
Mission: Educational clinic.
Funded by: Commission for the Blind, patient fees, Ferris State University.
Hours of Operation: Tues. 1:00-5:00 PM.
Staff: Optometrist.
Eligibility: None.
Area Served: Unlimited.

Low Vision: Complete low vision evaluations, including available electrodiagnostic testing.

Low Vision Aids: Rents or sells aids; closed circuit television will be recommended where it can be obtained.
Low Vision Follow-up: By return appointment.

Detroit Institute of Ophthalmology
Low Vision Program
Friends of Vision
15415 East Jefferson
Grosse Pointe Park, MI 48230
(313) 824-4710
Philip C. Hessburg, M.D., Medical Director

Type of Agency: Private; non-profit.
County/District Where Located: Wayne County.
Mission: Provides low vision and community services, including support groups at the Gorey Resource Center for the Visually Impaired.
Funded by: Contributions and annual fund raiser, "Eyes on the Classics".
Hours of Operation: Mon. - Fri. 9:00 AM-5:00 PM.
Staff: 3 full time.
History/Date: Est. 1972.
Area Served: Metropolitan Detroit and tricounty area.

Counseling/Social Work/Self-Help: Support groups/workshops on mobility and daily living skills for visually impaired persons.
Reading: Circulates cassette tape of local newspaper to members of support groups.
Low Vision: Assessments by appointment.
Low Vision Aids: Provided for purchase.

Kresge Eye Institute Low Vision Service
4717 St. Antoine

Detroit, MI 48201
(313) 577-1320 or (313) 577-1319
Shirley Sherrod, M.D., Director, Low Vision Services

Type of Agency: Non-profit.
County/District Where Located: Wayne County.
Funded by: Client fees.
Hours of Operation: Mon. - Fri. 9:00 AM - 5:00 PM.
Area Served: Unlimited.

Computer Training: Computer access available.
Low Vision: On-site training available.
Low Vision Aids: Loan/sell, prescribed/fitted.
Low Vision Follow-up: Return appointment.

Low Vision Consultants
2000 Green Road
Suite 200
Ann Arbor, MI 48105
(313) 930-2373
Steven I. Bennett, F.A.A.O., Certified Low Vision Consultant

Type of Agency: Non-profit.
Funded by: Client fees.
Hours of Operation: Mon., Thurs., Fri., 9:00 AM-8:30 PM; Sat. 9:00 AM-1:00 PM.
Staff: Ophthalmologist; optometrist.
Eligibility: Complete medical examination.
Area Served: Michigan, referrals from Ohio and Indiana.

Computer Training: Training on computer aids and devices.
Low Vision Aids: For sale.
Low Vision Follow-up: By return appointment.

Special Needs Vision Clinic
3660 Southfield Drive

Saginaw, MI 48601
(517) 777-1040
FAX: (517) 777-3509
E-mail: snvc@aol.com
Dr. Dolores Kowalski, Executive
Director

Type of Agency: Non-profit.
Mission: To provide optometric
vision care for developmentally
disabled persons and low vision
services for visually impaired
persons.
Funded by: Foundation grants;
private funds; and service
organizations.
Budget: $138,000.
Hours of Operation: Mon. - Thurs.
8:30 AM - 4:30 PM.
Staff: Low vision specialist.
History/Date: Founded in 1982.
Number of Clients Served: 1,200
persons per year (approximately).
Eligibility: Mentally, physically,
emotionally, visually, or otherwise
handicapped.
Area Served: State of Michigan.
Transportation: N.
Age Requirements: None.

Low Vision: Low vision services
provided by certified low vision
specialist.
Low Vision Aids: Available for
purchase through the clinic.
Low Vision Follow-up: As per the
doctors' recommendations.

Vision Rehabilitation Institute, Sinai Hospital

14800 West McNichols, Suite 310
Detroit, MI 48235
(313) 493-5514
Mary Jo Frence, O.D., Director
Elaine Roman, Vision Therapist

County/District Where Located:
Wayne County.
Funded by: Sinai Hospital of
Detroit, Detroit Medical Center.
Hours of Operation: Mon.-Fri.
8:30 AM - 5:00 PM.

Staff: Ophthalmologist;
ophthalmology resident;
optometrist; ophthalmic
assistant/technician; social
worker; optician; orientation/
mobility instructor; rehabilitation
teacher; special educator;
occupational therapist;
psychologist/counselor;
rehabilitation counselor;
audiologist.
Eligibility: Referral not necessary.
Area Served: Unlimited.

Low Vision: Testing, evaluation,
and training.
Low Vision Aids: Provided on
loan for trial; on-site training
provided.
Low Vision Follow-up: Based on
patient need and progress report.

Visual Rehabilitation and Research Center of Southeast Michigan

1501 East Jefferson Avenue
Grosse Point Park, MI 48230
(313) 824-2401
FAX: (313) 824-3850
Julian J. Nussbaum, M.D.,
Chairman
Lylas Mogk, Director

Type of Agency: Non-profit.
County/District Where Located:
Wayne County.
Funded by: Private funds and
foundation grants.
Hours of Operation: Mon.-Fri.
Staff: Ophthalmologists,
optometrists.
Eligibility: Referral.
Area Served: Metropolitan Detroit
area and surrounding
communities.

Low Vision: Examination and
evaluation.
Low Vision Aids: On-site or in-
home training.
Low Vision Follow-up: By return
appointment.

Western Michigan University Vision Rehabilitation Clinic

1000 Oakland Drive
KCMS Building, Third Floor
Kalamazoo, MI 49008
(616) 387-7000
Robert Unser, O.D.
Helen Lee, Coordinator

Type of Agency: Non-profit.
County/District Where Located:
Kalamazoo County.
Funded by: Client fees.
Hours of Operation: Wed.
9:30 AM-5:00 PM.
Staff: Optometrist; orientation/
mobility instructor;
ophthalmologist; rehabilitation
teacher; rehabilitation counselor;
audiologist.
Eligibility: Eye report; referral;
functional impairment due to poor
vision.
Area Served: Michigan.

Low Vision Aids: Provided on
loan for trial; no fee; on-site
training provided.

W.K. Kellogg Eye Center/Low Vision Services University of Michigan Medical Center

1000 Wall Street
Ann Arbor, MI 48105
(313) 764-5106
FAX: (313) 936-1991
Donna M. Wicker, O.D.
Mark Ventocilla, O.D.
Cheryl Caudill, O.T.R.

Type of Agency: Non-profit.
County/District Where Located:
Washtenaw County.
Mission: To help individuals
optimize use of remaining vision
for daily living, recreation, and
occupational goals.
Hours of Operation: Mon.-Fri.
8:00AM-5:00PM as needed.
Staff: Optometrists, social worker,
ophthalmologists, occupational
therapist.

Eligibility: Referral.
Area Served: Unlimited.

Counseling/Social Work/Self-Help: Available.
Rehabilitation: Occupational therapist is available for both clinic and home-based intervention.
Employment: Referrals for Michigan's vocational rehabilitation services as needed.
Low Vision Aids: Provided on loan for trial; on-site training provided.
Low Vision Follow-up: By return appointment.
Other services include Turner Geriatric Low Vision support group, occupational and physical therapy, and computer center support.

◆ *Aging Services*

STATE UNITS ON AGING

Office of Services to the Aging
P.O. Box 30026
Lansing, MI 48909
(517) 373-8230
FAX: (517) 373-4092
Carol Parr, Director

Provides referrals to Area Agencies on Aging and information on other local aging services.

INDEPENDENT LIVING PROGRAMS

**Commission for the Blind
Family Independence Agency**
201 North Washington Square
Lansing, MI 48909
(517) 373-2062 or (800) 292-4200
FAX: (517) 335-5140
Philip E. Peterson, Director

Provides independent living services for persons age 55 and over. For further information, contact the Project Director or general phone number listed.

MINNESOTA

♦ Educational Services

STATE SERVICES

Division of Special Education
Minnesota Department of
Children, Families and Learning
550 Cedar Street
811 Capitol Square Building
St. Paul, MN 55101
(612) 296-1793
FAX: (612) 297-7368
Wayne Erickson, Manager

Type of Agency: State.
County/District Where Located:
Ramsey County.
Mission: Administers
supplemental state funds for
visually impaired children
attending local schools.
Funded by: Public funds.
Area Served: Minnesota.

Counseling/Social Work/Self-
Help: Provides consultation on
educational services to local
schools and to the state residential
school.
Reading: Provides reader service
and special materials as needed.

For information about local
facilities, consult the
superintendent of schools or
director of special education in the
area.

EARLY INTERVENTION COORDINATION

Interagency Early Intervention
Planning Project
Minnesota Department of
Children, Families and Learning
550 Cedar Street
Capitol Square Building, Room 987
St. Paul, MN 55101
(612) 296-7032
FAX: (612) 297-5695
Jan Rubenstein, Part H Early
Childhood Coordinator

County/District Where Located:
Ramsey County.

SCHOOLS

Minnesota State Academy for
the Blind
Highway 298
P.O. Box 68
Faribault, MN 55021
(507) 332-3226
FAX: (507) 332-3631
Elaine Sveen, Superintendent
Wade Karli, Director of Education

Mission: Services for visually
impaired and deaf-blind persons.
Funded by: Public funds.
History/Date: Est. 1866.
Eligibility: Visually impaired.
Area Served: Minnesota.
Transportation: Y.
Age Requirements: 4-21 years.

Health: Occupational therapy;
physical therapy; contracts for
other health services.
Counseling/Social Work/Self-
Help: Career and guidance
counseling.
Educational: K through 12th
grade.
Residential: Dormitories.
Rehabilitation: Personal
management; orientation/
mobility; home mechanics; home
economics.
Recreational: Recreational
therapy.
Employment: Vocational training;
work adjustment program; refers
for other vocational services.
Computer Training: Speech,
screen magnification, braille
access. Word processing,
database, spreadsheet application.

INFANT AND PRESCHOOL

J.I.S.D. #287
1820 North Xenium Lane
Minneapolis, MN 55441
(612) 550-7147
FAX: (612) 550-7300
Ron Carter, Superintendent
Sande Scholzharson, Program
Supervisor

Type of Agency: Public school
program.
County/District Where Located:
Hennepin County.
Mission: To provide educational
support services for students with
low incidence impairments.
Funded by: State funds.
Staff: 22 full time for total vision
program (includes visually
handicapped and dually certified
teachers). Advisory board with
parent members for overall
program.
History/Date: Est. 1973.
Number of Clients Served: 350.
Area Served: Western
metropolitan area of the Twin
Cities of St. Paul and Minneapolis.
Age Requirements: 0-5 years.

Educational: Itinerant program
serves 13 school districts; braillers,
orientation and mobility teachers.
Reading: Adaptive materials
(braille, large print) available.
Recreational: Support clubs for all
ages.
Employment: Job coaching.
Computer Training: Technical
support; adaptive technology.

Provides instruction in
orientation/mobility, visual
development, use of special or
adaptive equipment. Consultant
services to other programs for
visually impaired children.

STATEWIDE OUTREACH SERVICES

Minnesota State Academy for the Blind

Highway 298
P.O. Box 68
Faribault, MN 55021
(507) 332-3226
FAX: (507) 332-3631
Elaine Sveen, Superintendent
Wade Karli, Principal

County/District Where Located:
Rice County.
Funded by: State funds.
History/Date: Est. 1866.
Age Requirements: 3-21 years.

Assessment: Available upon request in all areas relative to blindness and school functioning.
Consultation to Public Schools: On request.
Direct Service: Orientation and mobility services available on contractual basis.
Parent Assistance: Program to help the transition-aged student and family.
Materials Production: Braille and large print books.
Professional Training: As requested.

INSTRUCTIONAL MATERIALS CENTERS

Minnesota Resource Center Blind/Visually Impaired

P.O. Box 308
Faribault, MN 55021
(507) 332-5510
FAX: (507) 332-5494
E-mail: mnrcblnd@edu.gte.net
Jean Martin, Contact Person

Area Served: State of Minnesota.
Groups Served: K-12.

Performs computerized media searches but is not a statewide depository for materials.

UNIVERSITY TRAINING PROGRAMS

Mankato State University

Rehabilitation Counseling Department
MSU Box 52
P.O. Box 8400
Mankato, MN 56001-8400
(507) 389-1318
Dr. Donald Clark, (507) 389-5439

Programs Offered: Graduate (master's) program for rehabilitation counseling.

University of Minnesota Department of Educational Psychology

178 Pillsbury Drive, SE
233 Burton Hall
Minneapolis, MN 55455
(612) 624-1859
FAX: (612) 626-7496
E-mail: knowl001@maroon.tc.umn.edu
URL: http://www.coled.umn.edu/edpsy/speceduc/faculty/knowlton/knowltonhp.html
Dr. Marie Knowlton, (612) 624-1859

County/District Where Located:
Hennepin County.

Programs Offered: Graduate (master's, doctoral) programs for teachers of visually impaired students. Additional casework and related field emphasis available in early childhood, mental retardation, administration, and rehabilitation.
Distance Education: Y.

◆ Information Services

LIBRARIES

Minnesota Library for the Blind and Physically Handicapped

Highway 298
P.O. Box 68
Faribault, MN 55021
(507) 332-3279 or toll-free in Minnesota (800) 722-0550
FAX: (507) 332-3260
E-mail: 0999@mab.informns.k12.mn.us
Nancy Walton, Library Director

Type of Agency: Public.
County/District Where Located:
Rice County.
Mission: To provide reading materials in multiple formats for recreational and lifelong learning needs of visually and physically disabled.
Funded by: Public funds.
Budget: $483,000.
Hours of Operation: Mon.- Fri. 7:30 A.M.-5:00 P.M.
Staff: 10.
History/Date: Est. 1931.
Number of Clients Served: 11,000.
Eligibility: NLS requirements.
Area Served: Minnesota.

Regional library supplying talking books, braille and large-type books and cassettes.

Minnesota State Services for the Blind Communication Center

2200 University Avenue West
St. Paul, MN 55114
(612) 642-0500 or toll-free in Minnesota (800) 652-9000
FAX: (612) 649-5927
E-mail: dandrews@ssb.state.mn.us
David Andrews, Director, Communication Center

Type of Agency: Public.
County/District Where Located: Ramsey County.
Mission: Meet literacy needs of blind people.
Funded by: State, federal and private monies.
Budget: $2.1 million.
Hours of Operation: 8:00 AM - 4:30 PM.
Program Accessibility: Y.
Staff: 40.
History/Date: Est. 1954.
Number of Clients Served: 15,000.
Eligibility: Unable to read regular newsprint.
Area Served: Minnesota.

Radio talking books; tape and braille library; distributor of talking book machines; original transcriptions for educational materials in braille and tape forms.

TALKING BOOK MACHINE DISTRIBUTORS

Special Library and Transcription Services Minnesota State Services for the Blind Communication Center
2200 University Avenue West
Suite 240
St. Paul, MN 55114
(612) 642-0500 or toll-free in Minnesota (800) 652-9000
FAX: (612) 649-5927
David Andrews, Director, Communication Center

County/District Where Located: Ramsey County.

Machine-lending agency for the Library of Congress National Library Service for the Blind and Physically Handicapped. Other machines are distributed by the state regional libraries.

MEDIA PRODUCTION SERVICES

Minnesota Library for the Blind and Physically Handicapped
P.O. Box 68
Faribault, MN 55021
(507) 332-3279 or toll-free in Minnesota (800) 722-0550
FAX: (507) 332-3260
E-mail: 0999@mab.informns.k12.mn.us
Nancy Walton, Library Director

County/District Where Located: Rice County.
Area Served: Minnesota.
Groups Served: Blind, visually impaired, physically and reading disabled.

Types/Content: Recreational, lifelong learning.
Media Formats: Talking books/cassettes, Braille, large print.
Title Listings: None specified.

Minnesota State Services for the Blind
2200 University Avenue West, #240
St. Paul, MN 55114
(612) 642-0513 or toll-free in Minnesota (800) 652-9000
FAX: (612) 649-5927
E-mail: dandrews@ssb.state.mn.us
David Andrews, Director, Communication Center

County/District Where Located: Ramsey County.
Area Served: Minnesota.
Groups Served: K-12; college students; other adults.

Types/Content: Textbooks; recreational; career/vocational; religious.
Media Formats: Braille books; talking books/cassettes.
Title Listings: No title listings available.

RADIO READING

Radio Talking Book Network
Minnesota State Services for the Blind and Visually Handicapped Communication Center
2200 University Avenue West
St. Paul, MN 55114
(612) 642-0500
Stephen Rosenthal, Director

County/District Where Located: Ramsey County.
Hours of Operation: 24 hours daily.
History/Date: Est. 1969.
Area Served: State of Minnesota, portion of eastern South Dakota.

INFORMATION AND REFERRAL

The Foundation Fighting Blindness Minnesota Affiliate
4059 Yosemite Avenue, South
St. Louis Park, MN 55416
(612) 920-5651
Linda Frankenstein, President

See The Foundation Fighting Blindness in U.S. national listings.

Sight and Hearing Association Minnesota Society for the Prevention of Blindness and Preservation of Hearing
674 Transfer Road
St. Paul, MN 55114-1402
(800) 992-0424
FAX: (612) 645-2742
Vi Anne Traynor, CEO

Type of Agency: Non-profit.
County/District Where Located: Ramsey County.
Mission: To prevent loss of vision and hearing.
Funded by: Foundation grants; foundation and corporate donations.
Budget: $370,000.
Hours of Operation: Mon. - Fri. 9:00 AM - 5:00 PM.

Staff: 3 full time, 17 part time.
History/Date: Est. 1939.
Number of Clients Served: 10,000 per year.
Area Served: Minnesota.

Health: Free vision and hearing screenings.
Preschools: Vision and hearing screening.
Professional Training: Continuing education programs and seminars for medical and health professionals.

See also in national listings:

ELCA (Evangelical Lutheran Church in America) Braille and Tape Service

Joint Commission on Allied Health Personnel in Ophthalmology

Lutheran Braille Evangelism Association

Volunteer Braille Services

♦ *Rehabilitation Services*

STATE SERVICES

Minnesota State Services for the Blind and Visually Handicapped
2200 University Avenue West, Suite 240
St. Paul, MN 55114-1840
(612) 642-0500 or TDD (612) 642-0506
FAX: (612) 649-0506
Richard C. Davis, Assistant Commissioner

Type of Agency: State.
Mission: To facilitate the achievement of vocational and personal independence by children and adults who are blind or visually impaired.

Funded by: Public funds and private contributions.
Budget: $11 million.
Hours of Operation: 8:00 AM-4:30 PM.
Program Accessibility: Totally accessible.
Staff: 120 full time.
History/Date: Est. 1923.
Eligibility: Blind; visually impaired.
Area Served: State of Minnesota.

Health: Diagnostic services; low vision rehabilitation services; restoration services.
Counseling/Social Work/Self-Help: Rehabilitation counseling; consultation to parents and schools.
Professional Training: Internship in rehabilitation counseling.
Reading: Talking book record players and cassette players; talking book records and cassettes; braille books; large-print books; reader service; closed-frequency radio broadcasting; dial-in news.
Rehabilitation: Vocational and independent living rehabilitation services; home services.
Recreational: Provides consultation to other agencies.
Employment: Evaluation; vocational training; vocational placement; follow-up service; vending facility training; home employment programs.
Computer Training: Rehabilitation engineering and rehabilitation technology; training on computer aids and devices.
Low Vision: Preassessment.
Low Vision Aids: Provision of and training in use of low vision aids.
Low Vision Aids: Y.

Local Offices:

Brainerd: Services for the Blind, 1919 South Sixth Street, Brainerd, MN 56401, (218) 828-2490, FAX (218) 828-2262.
Duluth: Services for the Blind, 320 West Second Street, Room 111, Duluth, MN 55802, (218) 723-4600, FAX (218) 723-4712.
Hibbing: Services for the Blind, 750 East 34th Street, Hibbing, MN 55746, (218) 262-6754, FAX (218) 262-7315.
Mankato: Services for the Blind, 1650 Madison Avenue, Mankato, MN 56001, (507) 389-6324, FAX (507) 389-6070.
Marshall: Services for the Blind, 1424 East College Drive, Marshall, MN 56258, (507) 537-7114, FAX (507) 537-6061.
Moorhead: Services for the Blind, Townsite Centre, 715-11th Street North, Moorhead, MN 56560, (218) 236-2422, FAX (218) 299-5810.
Rochester: Services for the Blind, 300-11th Avenue N.W., Rochester, MN 55901, (507) 285-7282, FAX (507) 280-5592.
St. Cloud: Services for the Blind, 3333 West Division Street, St. Cloud, MN 56301, (612) 255-4800, FAX (612) 255-4801.

REHABILITATION

Blind, Inc.
100 East 22nd Street
Minneapolis, MN 55404
(612) 872-0100
Joyce Scanlan, Executive Director

Lighthouse for the Blind
4505 West Superior Street

Duluth, MN 55807-2728
(218) 624-4828
FAX: (218) 624-4479
E-mail: rehabsrv@cp.duluth.mn.
us
Paul Almirall, CEO
Georgia Guite, Director of
Rehabilitation Services

Type of Agency: Private; non-profit.
County/District Where Located: St. Louis County.
Mission: To foster the independence of blind and visually impaired persons, therby assisting them in the realization of their full potential as members of society.
Funded by: Workshop and sub-contract sales; fees; endowment and contributions.
Budget: 1996: $9,390.000.
Hours of Operation: 8:00 AM - 4:30 PM (rehabilitation facility); 6:30 AM - 2:30 AM (production operation).
Program Accessibility: All programs and facilities are fully accessible.
Staff: 10 full time.
History/Date: Est. 1919.
Number of Clients Served: 1996: 150.
Eligibility: Visually impaired, legally blind and deaf-blind.
Area Served: Duluth, northwest Wisconsin and all of Minnesota.
Transportation: Y.
Age Requirements: None.

Health: Diabetes information services.
Counseling/Social Work/Self-Help: Consultation and referral services; individual, group and family counseling.
Professional Training: Internships in orientation and mobility; in-service training when requested by schools or other facilities.

Residential: Housing provided for clients while in rehabilitation program.
Rehabilitation: Personal management; braille; handwriting; listening skills; typing; home management; orientation/mobility; talking calculators; communication skills; itinerant rehabilitation teaching in client's home and community. Outreach programs for low vision elderly and deaf-blind populations.
Recreational: Instruction in leisure skills.
Employment: Evaluation and training in industrial skills; work activity center.
Computer Training: Hands-on training in assistive technology lab. Speech output, magnification and braille access systems.
Low Vision: Evaluation and referral.
Low Vision Aids: Training on- or off-site.
Low Vision Follow-up: Yes.

Vision Loss Resources
1936 Lyndale Avenue South
Minneapolis, MN 55403
(612) 871-2222
FAX: (612) 872-0189
URL: http://
www.visionlossresources.com
Steven A. Fischer, Executive Director

Type of Agency: Private; non-profit.
County/District Where Located: Hennepin County.
Mission: Services for visually impaired persons.
Funded by: United Way; fees; Enterprise sales; capital funds; grants and contributions.
Budget: 1997: $8,000,000.
Hours of Operation: 8:00 AM-4:30 PM.
Program Accessibility: Fully accessible.

Staff: 17 full time, 7 part time. Uses volunteers.
History/Date: Est. 1917.
Eligibility: 20/60 vision or less or field restriction.
Area Served: Unlimited. Primarily 9-county metropolitan area and state of Minnesota.
Age Requirements: Preferably over 15 years.

Health: Diabetes information service; physical conditioning. Refers for other health services.
Counseling/Social Work/Self-Help: Group, individual and family. Refers for and provides consultation to other agencies in other counseling/social work services.
Educational: Diabetic education.
Professional Training: Internship/fieldwork placement in orientation/mobility; rehabilitation counseling; vocational rehabilitation; rehabilitation teaching; low vision internship.
Reading: Information and referral.
Residential: Non-residential facility. Uses community housing facilities.
Rehabilitation: Activities of daily living; braille and talking calculator; keyboarding; handwriting; adaptive computer technology; crafts and shop; orientation/mobility; rehabilitation teaching in client's home and other community settings. Contracts for rehabilitation services.
Recreational: Refers for recreation services.
Employment: Prevocational evaluation; career and skill counseling; job retention; follow-up services.
Computer Training: Training available on site and in community.

Low Vision Follow-up: Support group.

Services to seniors; provides an array of services including in-home assessment, in-home vision evaluation, independent living skills, and mutual help groups dealing with vision loss and concomitant needs of aging. Peer Counselors.

COMPUTER TRAINING CENTERS

FACES Access Services
1006 West Lake Street
Minneapolis, MN 55408
(612) 627-2925
FAX: (612) 627-3101
Deb Clark, Coordinator

County/District Where Located: Hennepin County.

Computer Training: Speech output systems; braille access systems; word processing; database software; computer operating systems.

Gillette Children's Hospital
550 West County Road D
New Brighton, MN 55112
(612) 636-9443
Patti Bahr, Rehabilitation Engineer

County/District Where Located: Ramsey County.

Computer Training: Screen magnification systems; word processing; computer operating systems.

Minnesota State Academy for the Blind
P.O. Box 68
Faribault, MN 55021
(507) 332-3226
FAX: (507) 332-3631
Steve Wasserman, Contact Person

County/District Where Located: Rice County.

Computer Training: Speech output systems; screen magnification systems; braille access systems; closed-circuit television systems; word processing.

Sister Kenny Institute
800 East 28th Street
Minneapolis, MN 55407
(612) 863-4400
FAX: (612) 863-1141
Becki Schwanke, Training Manager

Computer Training: Speech output systems; screen magnification systems; closed-circuit television systems; word processing; computer operating systems.

Vision Loss Resources
1936 Lyndale Avenue South
Minneapolis, MN 55403
(612) 871-2222
FAX: (612) 872-0189
Jean Christy, Sensory Aids Trainer

Computer Training: Speech output systems; screen magnification systems; braille access systems; closed-circuit television systems; word processing; access to internet.

♦ Low Vision Services

EYE CARE SOCIETIES

Minnesota Academy of Ophthalmology
676 Transfer Road
St. Paul, MN 55114
(612) 645-2452
FAX: (612) 645-2742
E-mail: kwmao@aol.com
Kristin M. H. Wallerich, Director
JoAnn R. Reed, M.D., President

Minnesota Optometric Association
2277 West Highway 36
Roseville, MN 55113
(612) 639-2555
FAX: (612) 639-2520
David N. Kunz, CEO

LOW VISION CENTERS

Mayo Clinic
Eye Department
Mayo West 7A
200 1st Street, S.W.
Rochester, MN 55905
(507) 284-2787
FAX: (507) 284-4612
E-mail: viggiano.suzanne@mayo.edu
Suzanne Viggiano, M.D.

Funded by: Client fees.
Hours of Operation: Mon.-Fri. by appointment.
Staff: Ophthalmologist; ophthalmology resident; ophthalmology technician.
Eligibility: None.
Area Served: Unlimited.

Low Vision: Examinations.
Low Vision Aids: Low vision aid prescriptions. Low vision optical aid rooms. Dispenses prescriptions. No loans.
Low Vision Follow-up: On regular basis.

Referrals to state department for rehabilitation.

St. Paul-Ramsey Medical Center Low Vision Clinic
640 Jackson Street
St. Paul, MN 55101
(612) 221-8782
Dianna Graves, M.D., C.O.M.T.

Type of Agency: Non-profit.
County/District Where Located: Ramsey County.
Mission: Optimization of residual vision.

Funded by: Client fees; county and state funds; medicare.
Hours of Operation: Thurs. 8:30 AM -12 noon, by appointment only.
Staff: Ophthalmic technician; ophthalmologist; social worker.
Number of Clients Served: 50 annually.
Eligibility: Referral; current ophthalmological report.
Area Served: Unlimited.
Age Requirements: None.

Low Vision: Residual vision and needs evaluated.
Low Vision Aids: Prescribed.
Low Vision Follow-up: Varies according to patient.

University of Minnesota Department of Ophthalmology

Box 493, UMHC
516 Delaware Street, S.E.
Minneapolis, MN 55455-0501
(612) 625-4400
Jay Krachmer, M.D., Chairman

County/District Where Located: Hennepin County.
Funded by: Client fees; private donors; Lions Club.
Hours of Operation: Mon.-Fri. 8:00 AM-4:30 PM.
Staff: Ophthalmologist; ophthalmology residents; ophthalmic assistant/technician; ophthalmic nurse.
Eligibility: None.
Area Served: Unlimited.

Low Vision Aids: Some provided on loan for trial; on-site training is provided.
Low Vision Follow-up: None.

Vision Loss Resources

1936 Lyndale Avenue South
Minneapolis, MN 55403
(612) 871-2222
FAX: (612) 872-0189
Steven A. Fischer, Executive Director

Type of Agency: Non-profit; private.
County/District Where Located: Hennepin County.
Mission: To assist people who are blind or visually impaird to achieve their full potential.
Funded by: Client fees; United Way.
Budget: $7 million.
Hours of Operation: Mon. - Fri. 7:00 AM - 4:30 PM.
Program Accessibility: Fully accessible.
Staff: Registered nurse, rehabilitation counselor, low vision instructors.
History/Date: Est. 1914.
Eligibility: Vision impairment.
Area Served: Unlimited.

Counseling/Social Work/Self-Help: Mutual help groups.
Low Vision: On-site/in-home training provided.
Low Vision Aids: Sell aids and appliances.
Low Vision Follow-up: Varies according to client.

Local Offices:

St. Paul: Vision Loss Resources, 216 South Wabash Street, St. Paul, MN 55107, (612) 224-7662.

♦ Aging Services

STATE UNITS ON AGING

Board on Aging
444 Lafayette Road
St. Paul, MN 55155-3843
(612) 296-2770 or Information and referral in-state (800) 652-9747 or (800) 882-6262
FAX: (612) 297-7855
Jim Varpness, Executive Director

Provides referrals to Area Agencies on Aging and information on other local aging services.

INDEPENDENT LIVING PROGRAMS

Minnesota Services for the Blind Career and Independent Living Services

2200 University Avenue West
St. Paul, MN 55114
(612) 642-0863 or (800) 652-9000
Lyle Lundquist, Supervisor

Provides independent living services for persons age 55 and over. For further information, contact the Project Director or general phone number listed.

MISSISSIPPI

♦ *Educational Services*

STATE SERVICES

Mississippi Department of Education

Sillers State Office Building
P.O. Box 771
Jackson, MS 39205
(601) 359-3513
Tom Burnham, Superintendent

County/District Where Located: Hinds County.
Mission: Serves as registration agency for blind and partially sighted students in public schools who are eligible for American Printing House for the Blind materials. Approves programs for visually handicapped in public schools.
Funded by: Public funds.
Area Served: Mississippi.

For information about local facilities, consult the superintendent of schools in the area.

EARLY INTERVENTION COORDINATION

Infant and Toddler Program Mississippi Department of Health

2423 North State Street
Room 107A
P.O. Box 1700
Jackson, MS 39215-1700
(601) 960-7427 or (800) 451-3903
FAX: (601) 354-6087
Roy Heart, Director, Infant and Toddler Program

County/District Where Located: Hinds County.

Information and referral services, technical assistance, central directory of early intervention services.

SCHOOLS

Mississippi School for the Blind

1252 Eastover Drive
Jackson, MS 39211
(601) 984-8200 or (601) 984-8203
FAX: (601) 984-8230
E-mail: jparmsb@misnet.com
Dr. John Parrish, Superintendent

Type of Agency: State.
County/District Where Located: Hinds County.
Mission: Services for totally blind; partially sighted; deaf-blind; multihandicapped.
Funded by: Public funds.
Hours of Operation: Mon.- Fri. 8:00A.M - 5:00P.M.
History/Date: Est. 1848.
Eligibility: 50 percent loss of vision; resident of Mississippi.
Area Served: Mississippi.
Age Requirements: 0-21 years.

Health: General medical services for students; refers for other health services.
Counseling/Social Work/Self-Help: Limited psychological testing and evaluation; individual, group, family/parent counseling; placement in school; referral to community services. Consultation provided to other schools and agencies upon request.
Educational: Grades K-12, deaf-blind-multihandicapped unit. Programs: general academic; vocational skill development; daily living. Ages 5-21, school program; 0-5 homebound program.
Preschools: Homebound program; developmental training and premobility.
Professional Training: Internship/fieldwork placement. In-service training programs.

Reading: Braille books and magazines; large print books.
Residential: Dormitories for residential students.
Rehabilitation: Personal management; orientation/mobility; home economics; refers for other rehabilitation services.
Recreational: Afterschool activities; swimming; track; wrestling; cheerleading.
Employment: Occupational skill development; work-study program.
Low Vision: Operates Low Vision Clinic. Provides exams, assists in ordering low vision aids, provides training and follow-up.
Low Vision Aids: Loan program.

Contact local school superintendent for program availability.

INFANT AND PRESCHOOL

Mississippi School for the Blind

1252 Eastover Drive
Jackson, MS 39211
(601) 984-8200 or (601) 984-8223
FAX: (601) 984-8230
Dr. John Parrish, Superintendent
Ted Dear, Director

Type of Agency: State residential school.
County/District Where Located: Hinds County.
Funded by: Title I, P.L. 89-313.
Staff: 2 full time (visually handicapped and early childhood teachers). Orientation/mobility specialist, other related services personnel available as consultants. Uses volunteers. Advisory board with parent members for overall program.
History/Date: Est. 1974.
Area Served: Mississippi.
Age Requirements: 0-5 years.

Counseling/Social Work/Self-Help: Parent and other counseling.

Educational: Adaptive equipment. Provides instruction in all developmental areas.

Low Vision: Exams available. Provides training and follow-up and assists in ordering low vision aids.

Home-based and consultant services to other programs for visually handicapped children, with or without other impairments.

UNIVERSITY TRAINING PROGRAMS

Jackson State University Department of Special Education and Rehabilitative Services
P.O. Box 17870
Jackson, MS 39217
(601) 968-2370
Dr. Celestine R. Jefferson, Chairman, Department of Special Education & Rehabilitative Services
Dr. Glenda Winfield, Assistant Professor, Department of Special Education

County/District Where Located: Hinds County.

Programs Offered: Undergraduate and graduate certification programs for teachers of visually impaired students (coursework offered only when there is sufficient demand).

Mississippi State University Rehabilitation Research and Training Center on Blindness and Low Vision
P.O. Drawer 6189

Mississippi State, MS 39762
(601) 325-2001
FAX: (601) 325-8989
E-mail: rrtc@ra.msstate.edu
URL: http://www.msstate.edu/dept/rrtc/blind.html
Dr. J. Elton Moore, Director

Programs Offered: In-service training and continuing education programs; graduate credit offered for vision specialists in vocational rehabilitation program.
Distance Education: Y.

♦ Information Services

LIBRARIES

Mississippi Library Commission Talking Book and Braille Services
5455 Executive Place
Jackson, MS 39206
(601) 354-7208 or TDD (601) 354-6411
FAX: (601) 354-6077
E-mail: tbbs@mlc.lib.ms.us
URL: http://www.mlc.lib.ms.us
Rahye Puckett, Manager
John Whitlock, Coordinator

County/District Where Located: Hinds County.
Mission: To provide library and information services to all Mississippi residents unable to read standard print due to a physical disability.
Funded by: Public funds and contributions.
Hours of Operation: Mon. - Fri. 8:00 AM - 5:00 PM.
Staff: 7 full time.
History/Date: Est. 1970.
Number of Clients Served: 3,000.
Eligibility: Unable to read standard print, by application.
Area Served: Mississippi.

Transportation: Y.

Regional library of the National Library Service, Library of Congress, providing talking books, audio cassettes, and braille books. Distributes talking book and audio cassette playback equipment. Renders repair service. Provides reference and information referral services by telephone, mail, fax, e-mail, and in person. Produces quarterly newsletter.

MEDIA PRODUCTION SERVICES

Mississippi Library Commission Talking Book and Braille Services
5455 Executive Place
Jackson, MS 39206
(601) 354-7208 or TDD (601) 354-6411
FAX: (601) 354-6077 (call before transmitting)
E-mail: tbbs@mlc.lib.ms.us
URL: http://www.mlc.lib.ms.us
Rahye L. Puckett, Coordinator

County/District Where Located: Hinds County.
Area Served: Mississippi.
Groups Served: K-12, college students, other adults.

Types/Content: Recreational.
Media Formats: Braille, cassettes, large-print.
Title Listings: No title listings available.

Mississippi School for the Blind
1252 Eastover Drive
Jackson, MS 39211
(601) 984-8200 or (601) 984-8221
FAX: (601) 984-8230
E-mail: msbkgc@misnet.com
Dr. John Parrish, Superintendent
Kevan Clinard, Coordinator

County/District Where Located: Hinds County.

Area Served: Statewide.
Groups Served: Public schools.

Types/Content: None specified.
Media Formats: Braille/large print books.
Title Listings: None specified.

RADIO READING

Radio Reading Service of Mississippi
3825 Ridgewood Road
Jackson, MS 39211
(601) 982-6301
Mike Duke, Manager

County/District Where Located: Hinds County.
Hours of Operation: Mon.-Sun. 24 hours.
History/Date: Est. 1986.
Area Served: Mississippi.

INFORMATION AND REFERRAL

Preserve Sight Mississippi
5455 Executive Place
Jackson, MS 39206-4104
(601) 362-6985
FAX: (601) 362-6987
Lois Russell, Executive Director

Type of Agency: Non profit.
County/District Where Located: Hinds County.
Mission: To preserve sight and prevent blindness.
Funded by: Contributions.
Budget: $80,000.
Hours of Operation: Mon.-Fri. 9:00AM-4:00PM.
Staff: 2.
History/Date: Est. 1967.
Area Served: Statewide.
Age Requirements: None.

Health: Glaucoma screening for adults.
Educational: Brochures, pamphlets.

Preschools: Visual acuity screening.

See Prevent Blindness America in U.S. national listings.

See also in national listings:

American Blind Lawyers Association

♦ *Rehabilitation Services*

STATE SERVICES

Office of Vocational Rehabilitation for the Blind Mississippi Department of Rehabilitation Services
P.O. Box 1698
Natchez, MS 39215-1698
(601) 853-5100
FAX: (601) 853-5205
E-mail: 102476.3621@compuserve.com
Dr. Michael J. Gandy, Director

Type of Agency: State.
Mission: Vocational rehabilitation and independent living services for the totally blind; legally blind; visually impaired; deaf-blind.
Funded by: State and federal funds; some donations.
Budget: $12.8 million.
Hours of Operation: Mon.-Fri. 8:00 AM-5:00 PM.
Program Accessibility: Fully accessible.
Staff: 90 full time.
History/Date: Est. 1928.
Number of Clients Served: 2,500.
Eligibility: Federal guidelines.
Area Served: Statewide.
Transportation: Y.
Age Requirements: 17 years of age and up.

Health: As needed to reach program goals.

Counseling/Social Work/Self-Help: Social evaluation; individual, group, family/parent, couple counseling; placement in training. Contracts and refers for other counseling/social work services.
Educational: Remedial, vocational, college and graduate.
Professional Training: Internship/fieldwork placement in orientation/mobility; rehabilitation counseling; vocational rehabilitation; regular in-service training programs, short-term or summer training.
Reading: Remedial as needed to reach program goals.
Residential: Dormitories available.
Rehabilitation: Personal management; braille; handwriting; listening skills; Optacon; Kurzweil Reading Machine; typing; video magnifier; home management; orientation/mobility. Provision of direct and purchased services for individuals not qualified for vocational rehabilitation but in need of intervention to pursue independent living goals.
Employment: Career and skill counseling; vocational placement; follow-up service; vending stand training. Contracts for other employment services.
Computer Training: Training on computer aids and devices.

Local Offices:

Columbus: 48 Datco Industrial Drive, P.O. Box 582, Columbus, MS 39703, (601) 328-8807.
Ellisville: Ellisville State School, Ellisville, MS 39437, (601) 477-9384.
Greenville: 1427 South Main Street, Suite 105, Greenville, MS 38702, (601) 335-1502.
Greenwood: 706 Highway 49-82 By-pass, P.O. Box 543, Greenwood, MS 38935, (601) 455-1432.

Gulfport: 625 Courthouse Road, Suite 113, Gulfport, MS 39506, (601) 897-7620.

Hattiesburg: 4015 Hardy Street, P.O. Box 17949, Hattiesburg, MS 39404, (601) 264-6210.

Jackson: Addie McBryde Rehabilitation Center for the Blind, 2550 Peachtree Street, P.O. Box 5314, Jackson, MS 39296-5314, (601) 364-2700.

Jackson: 300 Capers Avenue, Jackson, MS 39203, (601) 351-1527, (601) 351-1486.

McComb: 1400-A Harrison Drive, Box 1408, McComb, MS 39648-1408, (601) 684-3392.

Meridian: 1003 College Drive, P.O. Box 4317, Meridian, MS 39304, (601) 483-5391.

Natchez: 115 Jefferson Davis Boulevard, Natchez, MS 39120, (601) 442-7322.

Oxford: Nine Lafayette Park Drive, P.O. Box 1111, Oxford, MS 38655-1111, (601) 234-6092.

Tupelo: 615-A Pegram Drive, Tupelo, MS 38801-6321, (601) 844-5830.

Vicksburg: 1713 Clay Street, Vicksburg, MS 39180, (601) 638-1621.

REHABILITATION

Addie McBryde Rehabilitation Center for the Blind

2550 Peachtree Street
P.O. Box 5314
Jackson, MS 39296-5314
(601) 364-2700
Carrie Bahr, Director

Type of Agency: Personal adjustment center with evaluation and training in personal and vocational areas.
County/District Where Located: Hinds County.
Mission: To provide evaluation, training, and counseling services to persons who are blind/visually impaired.
Funded by: Mississippi Vocational Rehabilitation for the Blind, Independent Living Services and fees for out-of-state trainees.
Hours of Operation: 24 hours/day.
Program Accessibility: Accessible to wheelchair users and deaf persons.
Staff: Approximately 32.
History/Date: Est. 1972.
Number of Clients Served: 1991: 176.
Eligibility: Blind or visually impaired; deaf-blind or multihandicapped.
Area Served: Mississippi; accepts out-of-state referrals as space is available.
Age Requirements: 16 and older.

Health: General medical and ophthamological evaluations.
Counseling/Social Work/Self-Help: Comprehensive social and psychological evaluations; personal and group counseling provided.
Educational: Evaluations.
Reading: Library services; aids; computer literacy.
Residential: Dormitory space available for 34 trainees.
Rehabilitation: Home and personal management; braille; handwriting; typing; orientation/mobility.
Recreational: Training and activities for independent participation in community programs; physical conditioning.
Employment: Vocational evaluation; vocational information and job-seeking skills; vocational training in business enterprise program; clerical work and data entry.
Computer Training: Access and word-processing skills.
Low Vision: Evaluation and training; specialized evaluation/treatment available on site; treatment and services as needed.
Low Vision Aids: Recommended as needed.

Mississippi Industries for the Blind

P.O. Drawer 4417
Jackson, MS 38296
(601) 984-3200
FAX: (601) 987-3892
Jack Williams, Executive Director

County/District Where Located: Hinds County.
Mission: To provide blind persons with employment.
Hours of Operation: 7:30 AM-4:30 PM.
Staff: 20.
History/Date: Est. 1938.

Employment: Employment training.

Local Offices:

Meridian: Mississippi Industries for the Blind, 6603 Laurel Drive, Meridian, MS 39307, (601) 693-5525, FAX (601) 693-5569, Ronny Salter, Manager.

Signature Works, Inc.

P.O. Drawer 30
1 Signature Drive
Hazlehurst, MS 39083
(601) 894-1771 or (800) 647-2468
FAX: (601) 894-2993
E-mail: sigworks@techlink.net
URL: http://www.signatureworks.com
Howard Becker, President, C.E.O.

Type of Agency: Private; non-profit.
Mission: To provide competitive vocational training for persons who are totally blind, legally blind, deaf-blind, multiply disabled blind, learning disabled blind, mentally retarded blind,

emotionally disturbed blind, and clients with epilepsy and other disabilities if also blind.

Funded by: Workshop sales, service fees, and grants.

Hours of Operation: Mon.-Fri. 7:30 AM - 4:30 PM.

Program Accessibility: All locations meet accessibility guidelines.

Staff: 72 full time.

History/Date: Est. 1966.

Number of Clients Served: Approximately 450 annually.

Eligibility: Legally blind.

Area Served: Nationwide.

Transportation: Y.

Age Requirements: 16 years and over.

Health: Full time registered nurse; outsource for other medical services.

Counseling/Social Work/Self-Help: Individual counseling.

Educational: Vocational/skill development; GED classes.

Professional Training: Regular training programs; summer and short-term training.

Residential: Group homes for developmentally disabled blind adults. On-site residences for trainees; off-site apartments for employees.

Rehabilitation: Refers for rehabilitation services.

Recreational: Evening and weekend programs.

Employment: Career and skill counseling; occupational skill development; job retention; job retraining; competitive and transitional employment; post-retirement centers.

Computer Training: Beginner classes.

Local Offices:

Ellisville: Signature Works, Ellisville State School Division, P.O. Box 667, Ellisville, MS 39437, (601) 477-9384, ext. 252.

Gulfport: Signature Works, Gulf Coast Division, 424 34th Street, Gulfport, MS 39501, (601) 865-0324, FAX (601) 864-0605.

Jackson: Signature Works, Youth Program, 1252 Eastover Drive, Jackson, MS 39211, (601) 987-3952.

Jackson: Post-Retirement Center, 300 Capers Avenue, Jackson, MS 39203, (601) 969-3649.

Natchez: Signature Works Post-Retirement Center, 800 Washington Street, Natchez, MS 39120, (601) 442-2090.

Sanitorium: Signature Works, Boswell Division, P.O. Box 128, Sanitorium, MS 39112, (601) 849-3321.

Tupelo: Signature Works, Tupelo Division, 1151 South Veterans Boulevard, Tupelo, MS 38801, (601) 841-1640.

Whitfield: Signature Works, Hudspeth Center, Whitfield, MS 39193, (601) 939-8640.

COMPUTER TRAINING CENTERS

Addie McBryde Rehabilitation Center for the Blind
2550 Peachtree Street
P.O. Box 5314
Jackson, MS 39296-5314
(601) 364-2700
Carrie Bahr, Director

County/District Where Located: Hinds County.

Computer Training: Speech output systems; screen magnification systems; braille access systems; optical character recognition systems; closed-circuit television systems; word processing; database software; computer operating systems.

Mississippi School for the Blind
1252 Eastover Drive
Jackson, MS 39211
(601) 984-8200
FAX: (601) 984-8230
Ernestine Hubbard, Teacher

County/District Where Located: Hinds County.

Computer Training: Speech output systems; screen magnification systems; braille access systems; optical character recognition systems; closed-circuit television systems; word processing; computer operating systems.

◆ Low Vision Services

EYE CARE SOCIETIES

Mississippi Eye, Ear, Nose, and Throat Association
561 Medical Drive
Clarksdale, MS 38614
(601) 627-5256
Tom S. Cooper, M.D., President

County/District Where Located: Coahoma County.

Mississippi Optometric Association, Inc.
P. O. Box 16441
Jackson, MS 39236-0441
(601) 956-7412
Helen A. St. Clair, CAE, Executive Director

County/District Where Located: Hinds County.

LOW VISION CENTERS

University Medical Center, Department of Ophthalmology
2500 North State Street

Jackson, MS 39216-4505
(601) 984-5020
FAX: (601) 984-5031
Samuel B. Johnson, M.D.,
Chairman of Ophthalmology
Mark Cloer, Director, Low Vision

Funded by: Client fees and state
funds.
Hours of Operation: Mon., Tues.,
Thurs., Fri. 8:00 AM-4:30 PM.
Staff: Ophthalmologist;
ophthalmology resident;
ophthalmic assistant/technician;
low vision assistant; social worker;
orientation/mobility instructor;
rehabilitation teacher;
psychologist/counselor;
rehabilitation counselor; genetic
counselor; audiologist.
Area Served: Unlimited.

Low Vision Aids: Provided on
loan for trial; on-site training
provided.
Low Vision Follow-up: By return
appointment.

♦ *Aging Services*

STATE UNITS ON AGING

Council on Aging
Division of Aging and Adult
Services
750 North State Street
Jackson, MS 39202
(601) 359-4929 or Information and
referral in-state (800) 222-7622 or
(800) 948-3090
FAX: (601) 359-4370
Eddie Anderson, Director

Provides referrals to Area Agencies
on Aging and information on other
local aging services.

INDEPENDENT LIVING PROGRAMS

Office of Vocational
Rehabilitation for the Blind
Mississippi Department of
Rehabilitation Services
P.O. Box 1698
Jackson, MS 39215-1698
(601) 853-5100 or (800) 443-1000
Mike Gandy, Program Director

Provides independent living
services for persons age 55 and
over. For further information,
contact the Project Director or
general phone number listed.

MISSOURI

♦ *Educational Services*

STATE SERVICES

Missouri Department of Elementary and Secondary Education
P.O. Box 480
Jefferson City, MO 65102
(573) 751-4909
FAX: (573) 526-4404
Dr John Heskett, Commissioner of Division of Special Education
Melodie Friedebach, Coordinator of Special Education Programs

County/District Where Located: Cole County.
Mission: Administers supplementary state funds for visually impaired students attending local schools. Provides consultation on educational services.
Funded by: Public funds.
Area Served: Missouri.

For information about local facilities, consult the superintendent of schools in the area.

Specific questions regarding services should be directed to the local school district. All services are provided in compliance with IDEA, P.L. 94-142.

EARLY INTERVENTION COORDINATION

Section of Special Education Missouri Department of Elementary and Secondary Education
P.O. Box 480
Jefferson City, MO 65102
(573) 751-0185
FAX: (573) 526-4404
Melodie Friedebach, Assistant Director

Early intervention and special education services to children with disabilities, ages birth to five years.

SCHOOLS

Blue Springs Special Services Center
2103 West Vesper
Blue Springs, MO 64015
(816) 224-1360
Linda Nichols, Principal

Type of Agency: Public school program.
Funded by: P.L. 94-142 monies.
Staff: 46 full time (includes teachers, occupational and speech therapists, and aides), 1 part time; uses volunteers as classroom and occupational therapy aides.
History/Date: Est. 1976.
Number of Clients Served: 156.
Transportation: Y.

Educational: Instruction in all developmental areas; adaptive equipment. Center-based day program for severely disabled deaf-blind/multiply disabled students from 3 to 21 years of age.

Missouri School for the Blind
3815 Magnolia Avenue
St. Louis, MO 63110
(314) 776-4320 or toll-free in Missouri (800) 622-5672
FAX: (314) 776-1875
E-mail: yvonne.howze@together.org
Dr. Yvonne S. Howze, Superintendent

Type of Agency: Educational with residential component and outreach services.
County/District Where Located: St. Louis County.

Mission: To teach students to master basic academic, social, life, and work skills; to communicate effectively; to make responsible decisions, and to become life-long learners and productive citizens.
Funded by: State and federal funds; some private donations.
Budget: 1996: $6.0 million.
Hours of Operation: 24 hours; 7 days.
Staff: 182.
History/Date: Est. 1851.
Number of Clients Served: 1996: 120.
Eligibility: Legally blind; resident of Missouri.
Area Served: Missouri.
Transportation: Y.
Age Requirements: 0-5 (outreach); 5-21 (centerbased).

Health: On-site and in conjunction with local hospitals.
Counseling/Social Work/Self-Help: Available as needed.
Educational: Grades K-12. Educational and vocational preparation programs for children who are blind, multiply disabled or deaf-blind.
Preschools: Home-based services through Parent Involvement Network.
Professional Training: Weekends with the Experts training program for all professionals working with children, youths and adults who are blind/visually impaired; insite and VIISA training; teacher certification offerings in conjunction with the University of Missouri, St. Louis.
Reading: Print; braille; electronics.
Residential: Dormitories.
Rehabilitation: Offered in conjunction with adult-service providers.
Recreational: NCASVH conference participant for varsity sports; special olympics.

Employment: On- and off-campus jobs for students; supported work program.
Computer Training: Y.
Low Vision: Functional vision assessments on request.
Low Vision Aids: Issued by school optometrist.
Low Vision Follow-up: Conducted through Outreach Services Division.

INFANT AND PRESCHOOL

Children's Center for the Visually Impaired(CCVI)
400 West 57th Street
Kansas City, MO 64113
(816) 333-3166
FAX: (816) 333-3268
Mary Lynne Dolembo, Executive Director

Type of Agency: Private; non-profit.
Mission: To prepare young blind and visually impaired children, including those with multiple disabilities, to function at their highest potential in the sighted world.
Funded by: United Way; private donations; income from endowment, state and local funds, fund-raising events.
Budget: $780,000.
Hours of Operation: Mon.-Fri. 8:30 AM-5:00 PM; September-May; July summer session.
Program Accessibility: Y.
Staff: 31.
History/Date: Est. 1952.
Number of Clients Served: 110.
Eligibility: Any child with a visual impairment. Birth through school age.
Area Served: Serves 35-mile radius of Kansas City (consultation beyond in Kansas and Missouri).
Transportation: Y.
Age Requirements: Birth through school age.

Health: Hearing screening.
Counseling/Social Work/Self-Help: Parent counseling; other social and health services available on consultant or referral basis.
Preschools: For children aged 2 to kindergarten.
Professional Training: Sponsored workshops and seminars.
Reading: Braille and print.
Rehabilitation: Placement assistance, orientation/mobility, adaptive equipment, occupational therapy, speech pathology, physical therapy, braille.
Recreational: Summer school for children aged 3-7.
Low Vision: Examination and evaluation.
Low Vision Aids: Y.
Low Vision Follow-up: Y.

Center-based program with home component for visually impaired 0-3 year olds, with or without other impairments. Classes for visually impaired 3-5 year olds.

Consultant services to other programs available.

Delta Gamma Center for Children with Visual Impairments
5030 McRee
St. Louis, MO 63110
(314) 776-1300
FAX: (314) 776-7808
Debbie Naucke, Executive Director

Type of Agency: Private; non-profit.
Mission: Educational, developmental, and support services to visually impaired, deaf-blind, and multiply disabled children birth-3 and their families.
Funded by: Private donations; income from capital funds; local fund raising efforts; insurance; state/local contracts; special events.

Budget: 1992.: $380,000.
Hours of Operation: Mon. - Fri. 8:30 AM - 5:00 PM; some evenings/weekends.
Staff: 8 full time, 5 part time.
History/Date: Est. 1951.
Number of Clients Served: 90 annually.
Eligibility: Visually impaired.
Area Served: Serves 50-mile radius (includes city of St. Louis; St. Louis, St. Charles, Jefferson, Franklin, and Illinois Counties).
Transportation: Y.
Age Requirements: Birth - 3.

Health: Health and social services available on consultant or referral basis.
Counseling/Social Work/Self-Help: Parent support group; parent counseling; referrals to community programs; placement in school assistance; social evaluations.
Preschools: Developmental training; vision training; infant stimulation program. Provides instruction in most developmental areas. Speech therapy, state certified itinerant and center-based program. Orientation and mobility specialist on staff.
Reading: Library.
Rehabilitation: Toy-lending program.
Recreational: Parent activities.
Low Vision: Functional vision evaluation.
Low Vision Aids: Refers to other sources.
Low Vision Follow-up: On-going or consulting.

Home and center-based programs for visually impaired children, 0-3 years, with or without additional disabilities.

Consultant services to other programs.

STATEWIDE OUTREACH SERVICES

Missouri School for the Blind

3815 Magnolia Avenue
St. Louis, MO 63110
(314) 776-4320, ext. 250 or (in
Missouri only) (800) 622-5672
FAX: (314) 776-1875
Linda Van Eck-Niedringhaus,
Division Director, Outreach
Services
Jennie Mascheck, Vision
Supervisor

County/District Where Located:
St, Louis County.
Funded by: State and federal
funds.
History/Date: Est. 1851.
Age Requirements: 0-5 years for
preschool program; 3-21 years for
other services.

Assessment: Functional vision
assessment, orientation and
mobility assessment, and other
assessments available on a direct
service basis.
Consultation to Public Schools:
Consultation services available.
Direct Service: Outreach services
include indirect consultation,
assessment and training.
Parent Assistance: Direct in-home
services.
Materials Production:
Coordinates requests for service
with American Printing House for
the Blind Materials Center on
campus.
Professional Training: INSITE;
deafblind coursework in
collaboration with University of
Missouri, St. Louis.

INSTRUCTIONAL MATERIALS CENTERS

Missouri School for the Blind

3815 Magnolia Avenue
St. Louis, MO 63110
(314) 776-4320, ext. 256 or toll-free
in Missouri (800) 622-5672
FAX: (314) 776-1875
E-mail: bvz000@mail.connect.
more.net
Brian Forney, Librarian, APH
Materials Center

County/District Where Located:
St. Louis County.
Area Served: Entire state.
Groups Served: K-12.

Types/Content: Textbooks and
other educational aids.
Media Formats: Regular print;
braille; large-print.
Title Listings: No title listings
available.

◆ Information Services

LIBRARIES

Wolfner Library for the Blind and Physically Handicapped

600 West Main
P.O. Box 387
Jefferson City, MO 65102-0387
(573) 751-8720 or TDD (800) 347-
1379 or toll-free in Missouri
(800) 392-2614
FAX: (573) 526-2985
Elizabeth Eckles, Librarian

Type of Agency: Regional Library.
County/District Where Located:
Cole County.
Mission: To provide library and
information services to any
Missouri resident unable to read
standard print due to a physical
disability.
Funded by: State and federal.
Budget: $550,000.
Hours of Operation: Mon.-Fri.
8:00 AM-5:00 PM.
Program Accessibility: Fully
accessible.

Staff: 18.5 full-time equivalents.
History/Date: Est. 1924.
Number of Clients Served:
14,200.
Eligibility: Unable to use standard
print.
Area Served: Missouri.

Low Vision Aids: Low vision aids
for in-library and demonstration
purposes.

Regional library supplying talking
books, braille and large-type
magazines, tapes. Reader service
available.

MEDIA PRODUCTION SERVICES

Beth Shalom Braille Committee

12100 Wornall Road
Apt. 246
Kansas City, MO 64145
(816) 942-8334
Sylvia Katz, Secretary

County/District Where Located:
Jackson County.
Groups Served: K-12, college
students, other adults.

Types/Content: Recreational,
career/vocational, religious,
musical.
Media Formats: Braille.
Title Listings: No title listings
available.

Low Vision Library
Kansas City Association for the Blind

Kansas City Public Library
311 East 12th Street
Third Floor
Kansas City, MO 64106
(816) 842-7559
Jim Fettgather, System Librarian
for Low Vision Library

County/District Where Located:
Jackson County.
Groups Served: All groups;
individuals, schools, businesses.

Types/Content: Textbooks, business materials, items of personal interest.
Media Formats: Braille, cassette tape.

Midwestern Braille Volunteers

325 North Kirkwood Road
St. Louis, MO 63122
(314) 966-5828
FAX: (314) 966-0388
Sue Zahra, Office Manager

County/District Where Located: St. Louis County.
Groups Served: K-12, college students, other adults.
Types/Content: Textbooks, recreational, career/vocational, religious, miscellaneous.
Media Formats: Braille books.
Title Listings: Available on request.

Special School District, Saint Louis County

12110 Clayton Road
Town and Country, MO 63131
(314) 569-8251
FAX: (314) 569-8186
James Baker, Area Vision Coordinator

County/District Where Located: St. Louis County.
Groups Served: Age 3-21.
Types/Content: Textbooks, supplementary academic.
Media Formats: Braille books, talking books/cassettes, large-print books.
Title Listings: No title listings available.

Talking Tapes for the Blind

3015 South Brentwood Boulevard
St. Louis, MO 63144
(314) 968-2557
FAX: (314) 968-2557
Margaret A. Stroup, Executive Director

Area Served: Entire U.S.
Age Requirements: School-age and college students; adults.
Types/Content: Textbooks and leisure reading.
Media Formats: 2-track cassettes.
Title Listings: Catalog available on request.

Records textbooks and other printed material for blind, visually impaired, and learning disabled persons.

Circulating library of 5,250 books on tape.

INFORMATION AND REFERRAL

The Foundation Fighting Blindness
Greater Kansas City Affiliate

1000 S.W. Eight Court
Lees Summit, MO 64081
(816) 524-6443
Mary Lucas, President

See The Foundation Fighting Blindness in U.S. national listings.

The Foundation Fighting Blindness
Greater St. Louis Affiliate

8973 Lindenhurst Drive
St. Louis, MO 63126
(314) 843-1212
Pauline Krueger, Contact Person

See The Foundation Fighting Blindness in U.S. national listings.

See also in national listings:

American Optometric Association

Herald House

Lutheran Library for the Blind

Services to the Blind Reorganized Church of Jesus Christ of Latter-Day Saints

◆ Rehabilitation Services

STATE SERVICES

Missouri Rehabilitation Services for the Blind

3418 Knipp Drive
Jefferson City, MO 65109
(573) 751-4249
FAX: (573) 751-4984
Sally Howard, Deputy Director

Type of Agency: State.
County/District Where Located: Cole County.
Mission: To provide vocational and independent living rehabilitation services. To create opportunities for eligible blind and visually impaired persons so they may attain personal and vocational success.
Funded by: Public funds.
Budget: 1997: $9 million.
Hours of Operation: Mon. - Fri. 8:00 AM - 5:00 PM.
Program Accessibility: Fully accessible.
Staff: 100 full time.
History/Date: Est. 1915.
Number of Clients Served: 1996: 6,000.
Eligibility: Legal blindness; 20/70 or worse corrected acuity in the better eye, if individual has a progressive eye disease.
Area Served: Missouri.
Transportation: Y.
Health: Vision screening and glaucoma testing services. Additional eye care services to eligible persons include diagnosis and follow-up treatment that may include surgery, hospitalization, eyeglasses, medication, and prostheses.
Counseling/Social Work/Self-Help: Consultation and referral services; psychological testing;

counseling with parents of blind children.

Educational: Postsecondary for vocational rehabilitation clients, based on economic need.

Preschools: Instruction in preschool developmental activities.

Rehabilitation: Diagnosis and evaluation; counseling and guidance; referral; physical and mental restoration; instruction in personal management, communication techniques, homemaking activities, travel; home mechanics and economics; orientation/mobility.

Employment: Evaluation; vocational training; job development and placement; support services; post-employment services; services to family members; training and placement of blind persons in vending facilities and other small business enterprises; supervision and management services.

Computer Training: For vocational rehabilitation clients, based on economic needs.

Low Vision: Vision testing at designated site.

Low Vision Aids: Based on economic need.

Low Vision Follow-up: As needed.

Local Offices:

Jefferson City: 210C East High Street, Jefferson City, MO 65101, (573) 751-2714, FAX (573) 526-4526.
Kansas City: 615 East Thirteenth Street, Kansas City, MO 64106, (816) 889-2677, FAX (816) 889-2504.
St. Ann: 10449 St. Charles Rock Road, St. Ann, MO 63074-1827, (314) 426-4949, FAX (314) 426-3560.
St. Louis: Number Two Campbell Plaza, Suite 300, St. Louis, MO 63139, (314) 877-0151, FAX (314) 877-0168.

Sikeston: P.O Box 369, 808 Hunter, Sikeston, MO 63801, (573) 472-5240, FAX (573) 472-5393.
Springfield: 149 Park Central Square, Springfield, MO 65806, (417) 895-6386, FAX (417) 895-6392.

REHABILITATION

Alphapointe Association for the Blind
1844 Broadway
Kansas City, MO 64108
(816) 421-5848
FAX: (816) 421-6523
E-mail: richardk@alphapointe.org
Thomas Healy, President
Richard Knight, Executive Vice president

Type of Agency: Private; non-profit.
County/District Where Located: Jackson County.
Mission: To assist blind and visually impaired persons through rehabilitation and other social services.
Funded by: Workshop sales, donations, bequests.
Budget: $6 million.
Hours of Operation: Mon.-Fri. 8:00AM-4:30PM.
Program Accessibility: Fully accessible.
Staff: 12.
History/Date: Est. 1916.
Number of Clients Served: 700 annually.
Eligibility: Legally blind.
Area Served: Western Missouri, eastern Kansas.
Age Requirements: 16 years or older.

Counseling/Social Work/Self-Help: Counselor on staff.
Educational: Tuition assistance for blind work services clients.
Reading: Records and cassettes; braille transcription.

Rehabilitation: Employment and work training; in-home assistance for seniors.
Employment: Vocational training; sheltered workshop.
Computer Training: Adaptive technology.
Low Vision: Referrals.
Low Vision Aids: In-home demonstrations of aids.
Low Vision Follow-up: Yes.

Local Offices:

Kansas City: Low Vision Library, 311 East 12th, Kansas City, MO 64106, (816) 842-7559.

Center for Blindness and Low Vision
Rehabilitation Institute
2801 Wyandotte Street, Third Floor
Kansas City, MO 64108
(816) 753-6533
FAX: (816) 531-4570
Tory Brust, Supervisor

Type of Agency: Private; non-profit.
County/District Where Located: Jackson County.
Mission: Comprehensive rehabilitation as requested by referral.
Funded by: Client fees.
Budget: 1997: $1,400,000.
Hours of Operation: Mon.-Fri. 8:00 AM-4:30 PM.
Program Accessibility: Fully accessible.
Staff: 31.
History/Date: Est. 1974.
Number of Clients Served: 127.
Eligibility: Fee sponsorship.
Area Served: Primarily Missouri and Kansas; other states on request.
Transportation: Y.
Age Requirements: 14 years or over.

Health: Refers for eye health; provides occupational/physical/speech therapy.

Counseling/Social Work/Self-Help: Provides social and psychological evaluation/testing, counseling. Refers for community services, school placement.

Educational: College prep and general academics.

Professional Training: Provides internships in occupational therapy, social work, rehab counseling and orientation and mobility.

Reading: Talking book records/cassette players; braille/recorded magazines; transcription; closed-circuit television; information and referral services available.

Residential: 6 two-bedroom apartments.

Rehabilitation: Vocational/daily living/communication skills/orientation and mobility. Both on-site and in the community.

Recreational: Variety of recreational activities.

Employment: Vocational evaluation and counseling; placement; training; job coaching. Refers for job retraining.

Computer Training: Computers accessible to blind persons. Adaptive computer technology training.

Low Vision: Refers for low vision evaluations.

Low Vision Aids: Automated perimeter system, Dyna-vision 2000, CCTVs, magnifiers, large print computers.

Low Vision Follow-up: Prescribed therapy.

Lighthouse for the Blind

10440 Trenton Avenue
St. Louis, MO 63132-1223
(314) 423-4333
FAX: (314) 423-0139
Ed Lanser, President

Type of Agency: Blind Industries.

County/District Where Located: St. Louis County.

Mission: Provides training and employment for blind and legally blind men and women.

Funded by: Workshop sales; sub-contracts; endowment.

Budget: $5 million.

Hours of Operation: Mon. - Fri. 7:00 AM - 5:30 PM.

Staff: 40 full time and part-time.

History/Date: Est. 1933.

Number of Clients Served: 90.

Eligibility: 20/200 vision or worse in both eyes with best correction. Field restriction of 10 degrees.

Area Served: St. Louis metropolitan area.

Age Requirements: 18 years and older.

Counseling/Social Work/Self-Help: Consultation services.

Rehabilitation: Personal management, skill-training, work opportunity.

Employment: Evaluation and prevocational training.

Local Offices:

Berkeley: LHB Industries, 8833 Fleischer Place, Berkeley, MO 63134, (314) 522-3141, FAX (314) 522-8808, Steve Wenger, Plant Manager.

St. Louis: LHB Industries, 10616 Trenton, St. Louis, MO 63132, (314) 423-7955, FAX (314) 423-6918, Rex Osborn, Plant Manager.

The Mary Culver Home

221 West Washington Avenue
Kirkwood, MO 63122
(314) 966-6034
Colleen Hill, Administrator

Type of Agency: Non-profit: intermediate care home and licensed nursing facility.

County/District Where Located: St. Louis County.

Mission: To provide life care to blind or legally blind women.

Funded by: Contributions, endowment.

Budget: $850,000.

Hours of Operation: 24 hours a day.

Staff: 40.

History/Date: Est. 1866.

Number of Clients Served: 28.

Eligibility: Female; blind or legally blind; residents of Missouri; ambulatory.

Area Served: Missouri.

Transportation: Y.

Age Requirements: Over 21; average age 89.

Counseling/Social Work/Self-Help: Contracted as needed. In-house support group.

Reading: Braille material/library. Talking book program available.

Residential: Intermediate care home; private rooms.

Rehabilitation: Services contracted. Mobility training and orientation training provided.

Recreational: Daily activities provided.

Low Vision Aids: Quarterly eye exams provided.

St. Louis Society for the Blind and Visually Impaired

7954 Big Bend Boulevard
Webster Groves, MO 63119
(314) 968-9000
FAX: (314) 968-9003
David Ekin, Executive Director

Type of Agency: Private; non-profit.

County/District Where Located: St. Louis County.

Mission: To provide education and training to facilitate physical, psychological, and social rehabilitation and independence for blind and visually impaired adults; to promote prevention of blindness; to provide public information about visual impairment.

Funded by: Lions Clubs; capital income, community contributions and individual donations.

Budget: $680,000.

Hours of Operation: Mon.-Fri. 8:30 AM-4:00 PM.

Program Accessibility: Program accessible.

Staff: 11 full time, 5 part time. Uses and trains volunteers.

History/Date: Est. 1911.

Number of Clients Served: 600.

Eligibility: Visually impaired and multiply disabled.

Area Served: St. Louis.

Transportation: Y.

Age Requirements: Adult.

Health: Public education program; eye safety programs for school and industry; post-operative eye care; visual acuity and glaucoma screening. Provides eyeglasses/prostheses for medically indigent. Provides consulting services to low vision clinics and health care professionals.

Counseling/Social Work/Self-Help: Family, individual, counseling; information and referral. Group counseling on site and at senior living sites.

Professional Training: Low vision training. Provides in-service training for universities, schools and hospitals.

Rehabilitation: Rehabilitation teaching; orientation/mobility; sensory training. Refers for other rehabilitation services at nursing homes, hospitals, technical schools, schools and universities.

Recreational: Trips to symphony, Muni-opera. In-home and on-site recreation program for older adults. St. Louis teams of the U.S. Blind Bowlers Association. Community groups.

Employment: Refers for employment-oriented services.

Low Vision: Low vision clinic; has loan program.

Low Vision Aids: Provides low vision aids.

Low Vision Follow-up: Through clinic and home follow-up.

Service Club for the Blind

3719 Watson Road
St. Louis, MO 63109
(314) 674-3306
Fred Keller, President

Mission: Services for children and adults. Provides clothing, medicine, food vouchers, and shoes.

Funded by: Endowment and contributions.

Staff: 4 full-time, 1 volunteer.

History/Date: Est. 1934.

Eligibility: Blind or legally blind only.

Area Served: St. Louis and St. Louis County.

Health: Sells aids and appliances on order.

Counseling/Social Work/Self-Help: Consultation and referral services.

COMPUTER TRAINING CENTERS

Low Vision Library
Kansas City Association for the Blind

Kansas City Public Library
311 East 12th Street
Kansas City, MO 64106
(816) 842-7559
Kelly Guthrie

County/District Where Located: Jackson County.

Computer Training: Speech output systems; screen magnification systems; braille access systems; word processing; computer operating systems.

Missouri School for the Blind

3815 Magnolia Avenue
St. Louis, MO 63110
(314) 776-4320
FAX: (314) 776-1875
Doris Gros, Teacher

County/District Where Located: St. Louis County.

Computer Training: Speech output systems; screen magnification systems; braille access systems; optical character recognition systems; closed-circuit television systems; word processing; database software; training for instructors.

◆ Low Vision Services

EYE CARE SOCIETIES

Missouri Ophthalmological Society

Ten West Phillips Road
Metro Square One, Suite 120
Vernon Hills, IL 60061
(847) 680-1666
FAX: (573) 882-8474
E-mail: joseph_giangiacomo@missouri.edu
Richard H. Paul, Executive Director

County/District Where Located: Boone County.

Missouri Optometric Association, Inc.

112 East High Street
Jefferson City, MO 65101-3274
(573) 635-6151
Zoe Lyle

LOW VISION CENTERS

Barnes Eye Clinic
1 Barnes Hospital Plaza

St. Louis, MO 63110
(314) 362-5312
FAX: (314) 362-3725
Mary Dobbs, Supervisor

Type of Agency: Non-profit.
County/District Where Located:
Jefferson County.
Funded by: Client fees and
hospital.
Staff: Ophthalmology resident;
optometrist; social worker;
optician.
Number of Clients Served:
Referral.
Area Served: Unlimited.

Low Vision: Evaluation.
Low Vision Aids: Provided for
purchase. On-site training
provided.
Low Vision Follow-up: Varies
according to patient.

Eye Institute
St. Louis University
1755 South Grand
St. Louis, MO 63104
(314) 577-6038
John B. Selhorst, Interim

Type of Agency: Non-profit.
County/District Where Located:
St. Louis County.
Funded by: Client fees.
Hours of Operation: Wed.
9:00AM-4:00PM; Thurs. 1:00 PM -
5:00 PM.
Staff: Counselors;
ophthalmologist; optometrist;
optometry students;
ophthalmology resident.
History/Date: 1986.
Number of Clients Served:
500-600 annually.
Eligibility: Referral and current
ophthalmological report.
Area Served: Unlimited.

Professional Training: Clinical
training for ophthalmology
residents and optometry students.

Low Vision: Complete evaluation
and prescription service.
Low Vision Aids: Loaned at no
charge; prescribed/fitted.
Low Vision Follow-up: Return
appointment.

Kansas City Veterans Affairs
Medical Center
VICTORS Program
4801 Linwood Boulevard
Kansas City, MO 64128
(816) 861-4700, ext. 661, 662
FAX: (816) 922-3382
E-mail: maino@kansas_city.va.
gov
Dr. Joseph Maino, Chief

County/District Where Located:
Jackson County.
Mission: To assist in the low
vision rehabilitation of verterans.
Funded by: Federal funds.
Hours of Operation: Mon. - Fri.
8:00 AM - 4:30 PM.
Staff: 6.
History/Date: Est. 1979.
Eligibility: Visually impaired
veterans.
Area Served: Missouri, Kansas,
Iowa, Oklahoma, Arkansas,
Nebraska; referrals from other
areas considered.
Age Requirements: None.

Counseling/Social Work/Self-
Help: Individual and family
counseling available.
Professional Training: Optometry
residents and students on rotation.
Residential: In-patient and lodger
programs.
Rehabilitation: Intensive 5-day
inpatient rehabilitation program
for partially sighted veterans.
Low Vision: Evaluation and on-
site training provided.
Low Vision Aids: Provided on
loan for trial purpose at no charge.
Low Vision Follow-up: Return
appointment; home visits; phone
interviews; support groups.

Low Vision Rehabilitation
Program
University of Missouri - Kansas
City
Department of Ophthalmology
2300 Holmes Street
Kansas City, MO 64108
(816) 881-6157
FAX: (816) 881-6246
Camille Matta, M.D., Director

Type of Agency: Non-profit.
Mission: Provide low vision
rehabilitation services to all,
regardless of ability to pay.
Funded by: Client fees; insurance
payments.
Hours of Operation: Mon. - Fri.
9:00 AM - 4:00 PM.
Staff: Ophthalmologist;
occupational therapist; orientation
and mobility specialist.
Number of Clients Served:
Approximately 1,000 annually.
Eligibility: None.
Area Served: Metropolitan Kansas
City area.
Age Requirements: Adults age 18
and older.

Counseling/Social Work/Self-
Help: Support groups.
Rehabilitation: Outpatient
rehabilitation training for
independence in activities of daily
living.
Computer Training: Job-site
assessments for assistive
technology.
Low Vision: Training to maximize
usefulness of residual vision.
Low Vision Aids: Prescribed and
fitted for variable charge; on-site or
in-home training provided.
Low Vision Follow-up: Return
appointment; home visits.

Optometric Center of St. Louis
3940 Lindell Boulevard

St. Louis, MO 63108
(314) 535-5016
FAX: (314) 535-4747
Dr. Jane Shea, Coordinator

Type of Agency: Non-profit.
Owned by University of Missouri-
St. Louis School of Optometry.
County/District Where Located:
St. Louis County.
Funded by: Client fees; Lions
Club; state funds.
Hours of Operation: Mon.-Fri.
8:00 AM-4:30 PM.
Staff: Ophthalmic assistant;
ophthalmic technician;
optometrist; optometry students.
History/Date: Est. 1982.
Eligibility: Current
ophthalmologist report.
Area Served: Unlimited.

Professional Training: Training
for optometry students.
Low Vision: Optical rehabilitation
services.
Low Vision Aids: Provided for
purchase; sold at cost. Refers for
training.
Low Vision Follow-up: Varies
according to patient.

St. Louis Society for the Blind and Visually Impaired

7954 Big Bend Boulevard
Webster Groves, MO 63119
(314) 968-9000
FAX: (314) 968-9003
E-mail: slsbvi.org
Linda Barbier Bularzik, Low Vision
Clinic Coordinator

Type of Agency: Private; non-
profit.
County/District Where Located:
St. Louis County.
Mission: To provide education
and training.
Funded by: Capital income,
individual and community
donations.
Budget: $670,000.

Hours of Operation: Mon.-Fri.
9:00 AM-4:00 PM.
Program Accessibility: Yes.
Staff: Optometrist; low vision
specialist.
History/Date: Est. 1911.
Number of Clients Served: 300.
Transportation: Y.
Age Requirements: None.

Low Vision: Low vision exams;
instruction on use of aids; referrals
to related services.
Low Vision Aids: Prescription
and nonprescription devices for
sale and loan.
Low Vision Follow-up: After one
month, office or in-home.

Washington University Eye Center
Department of Ophthalmology and Visual Sciences
Low Vision Service

660 South Euclid Avenue
St. Louis, MO 63110
(800) 543-2733
Carrie S. Gaines, O.D., Director,
Low Vision Services

Type of Agency: Non-profit.
County/District Where Located:
St. Louis County.
Funded by: Client fees.
Hours of Operation: Variable.
Staff: Optometrist; ophthalmic
technician; social worker;
occupational therapist; physical
therapist; psychologist; diabetic
nurse specialist; audiologist;
optician; ophthalmologist.
Eligibility: Referral.
Area Served: Unlimited.

Low Vision Aids: Provided on
loan for trial purposes or purchase.
On-site or in-home or at-work
training provided.
Low Vision Follow-up: Varies
according to patient.

◆ Aging Services

STATE UNITS ON AGING

Division of Aging
**Missouri Department of Social
Services**
615 Howerton Court
P.O. Box 1337
Jefferson City, MO 65102-1337
Elderly Abuse and Neglect Hotline
(800) 392-0210 or (573) 751-3082
Gregg Vadner, Director

Provides referrals to Area Agencies
on Aging and information on other
local aging services.

MONTANA

◆ *Educational Services*

STATE SERVICES

Montana Department of Curriculum
Division of Special Education
Capitol Station
Helena, MT 59620
(406) 444-4429
FAX: (406) 444-3924
E-mail: brunkel@opi.mt.gov
Robert Runkel, State Director of Special Education
Marilyn Pearson, Education of the Handicapped Act/Part B
Francisco J. Roman, Deaf-Blind Specialist

Type of Agency: A unit of the Office of the Superintendent of Public Instruction.
Mission: Administers through affiliate, the Montana School for the Deaf and the Blind, the federal quota system for providing visually impaired children with materials from the American Printing House for the Blind. Through the same affiliate, it provides braille, large- type, and recorded material to the visually impaired students in local schools and has a repository of large-type textbooks. Also provides training on computer aids and devices.
Funded by: Public funds.
Budget: $163,000.
Hours of Operation: Mon.-Fri. 7:00 AM-4:00 PM.
Staff: One full time.
Number of Clients Served: 82.
Area Served: Montana.
Age Requirements: 0-21 years of age.

For information about local facilities, consult the Director of Special Education or Superintendent, Montana School for the Deaf and the Blind, Great Falls, Montana 59401.

EARLY INTERVENTION COORDINATION

Developmental Disabilities Program
Department of Public Health and Human Services
P.O. Box 4210
Helena, MT 59604
(406) 444-2995
FAX: (406) 444-0230
Jan Spiegle, Early Intervention Division

County/District Where Located: Lewis and Clark County.

Children in Montana who meet eligibility requirements and their families may receive a broad array of services based on individual need, including family training and support, assistive technology services, audiology services, family counseling, home visits, medical services for diagnostic purposes, nursing services, occupational therapy services, physical therapy services, psychological services, service coordination services, social work services, speech/ language services, transportation, and vision services.

SCHOOLS

Montana School for the Deaf and the Blind
3911 Central Avenue
Great Falls, MT 59405-1697
(406) 771-6000
FAX: (406) 771-6164
C. John Kinna, Superintendent
Bill Davis, Principal

Type of Agency: State residential school.

Mission: Services for totally blind, legally blind, visually impaired, and deaf-blind persons.
Funded by: State funds.
Budget: $3.2 million annually.
Hours of Operation: 24 hours/ day.
Staff: 13 full time. Shared speech and physical therapist.
History/Date: Est. 1893.
Number of Clients Served: 27 on campus; 160 in outreach program.
Eligibility: Auditory or visual impairment that is educationally significant.
Area Served: Montana.
Transportation: Y.

Health: Speech and physical therapy. Refers, contracts, and provides consultation to other agencies for other health services.
Counseling/Social Work/Self-Help: Psychological testing and evaluation; placement in school. Contracts and provides consultation to other agencies for other counseling/social work services.
Educational: Grades K through 12 and nongraded. General academic programs.
Preschools: Home-based parent-infant program for children birth-3 years. On-campus preschool program.
Professional Training: Internship/fieldwork/placement in orientation/mobility; special education.
Reading: Lends cassette players; braille books; large-print books. Information and referral; transcription to braille; tape recording services on demand.
Residential: Cottages.
Recreational: Arts and crafts; residential summer/camp. Provides for other recreational services.

Employment: Refers and provides consultation to other agencies for employment services.
Computer Training: Computer lab.
Low Vision: Low vision evaluation and low vision aids available through Montana low vision services.

Contact local school superintendent for program information.

STATEWIDE OUTREACH SERVICES

Montana School for the Deaf and the Blind
3911 Central Avenue
Great Falls, MT 59405-1697
(406) 771-6000
FAX: (406) 771-6164
Bill Davis, Principal

County/District Where Located: Cascade County.
Funded by: State funds.
Age Requirements: 0-21 years.

Assessment: Visual impairment assessment team performs assessments of visually impaired students at the request of parents or teachers.
Consultation to Public Schools: Three resource consultants provide services throughout the state.
Direct Service: Orientation and mobility; speech therapy; physical therapy.
Parent Assistance: Parent-teacher Houseparent Aide Program.
Materials Production: Braille.

INSTRUCTIONAL MATERIALS CENTERS

Montana School for the Deaf and the Blind
3911 Central Avenue
Great Falls, MT 59405
(406) 771-6000
Tee Holcomb, Contact Person

Area Served: Statewood.

Types/Content: Textbooks.
Media Formats: Computer materials; braille; large print.

♦ Information Services

LIBRARIES

Montana Talking Books Library
1515 East Sixth Avenue
Helena, MT 59620
(406) 444-2064 or (800) 332-3400
FAX: (406) 444-5612
Sandra Jarvie, Librarian
Alberta Blanton, Machine Lending Information

Hours of Operation: Mon.-Fri. 8:00 AM-5:00 PM.
Staff: 6.
Number of Clients Served: 2,600.
Eligibility: People who cannot read standard print because of a visual or physical disability.
Area Served: Statewide.

Regional library supplying recorded books on cassette. Distributes talking book machines. Braille readers served by Utah State Library.

RADIO READING

LIFTT Radio Reading Service
929 Broadwater Square
Billings, MT 59101
(406) 259-5181
FAX: (406) 259-5259
Dan Worneck, Director of Reading
Patricia Lockwood, Director

Hours of Operation: Mon.-Fri. 9:00 AM-5:00 PM.
History/Date: Est. 1988.
Area Served: Montana and northern Wyoming.

Western Montana Radio Reading Services
924 South Third West
Missoula, MT 59801
(406) 721-1998
Jan Bicha, Director
Evelyn Hawkins, Coordinator

Hours of Operation: Mon.-Fri. 9:00 AM-5:00 PM.
History/Date: Est. 1979.
Area Served: 150-mile radius from Missoula, covers 10 counties in western and central Montana.

♦ Rehabilitation Services

STATE SERVICES

Vocational Rehabilitation/Blind and Low Vision Services
Montana Department of Public Health and Human Services
111 Sanders
P.O. Box 4210
Helena, MT 59604-4210
(406) 444-2590
FAX: (406) 444-3632
E-mail: jmathews@mt.gov
Joe A. Mathews, Administrator

Type of Agency: Federal and state.
Mission: Services for totally blind, legally blind, visually impaired, and deaf-blind persons.
Funded by: Fees, government grants.
Hours of Operation: 8:00 AM - 5:00 PM.
Staff: 20 full time. Uses volunteers.
History/Date: Est. 1937.
Eligibility: Visual condition that is a vocational handicap.
Area Served: Statewide.
Age Requirements: Adults.

Health: Contracts and refers for health services.

Counseling/Social Work/Self-Help: Social evaluation; individual, group, family/parent, couple counseling. Refers for other counseling/social work services.

Professional Training: Internship/fieldwork placement in rehabilitation counseling; vocational rehabilitation. Regular in-service training programs. Short-term or summer training, open to enrollment from other agencies.

Rehabilitation: Personal management; braille; handwriting; listening skills; Optacon; typing; video magnifier; electronic mobility aids; home management; orientation/mobility; rehabilitation teaching in client's home and community; sensory training. Refers for other rehabilitation services.

Employment: Career and skill counseling; occupational skill development; job retention; job retraining; vocational placement; follow-up service; vending facility training. Contracts and refers for other employment-oriented services.

Computer Training: Training on computer aids and devices.

Local Offices:

Billings: 1211 Grand, Billings, MT 59102, (406) 252-5601.
Butte: Executive Village, 517 East Front, Butte, MT 59701, (406) 723-6537.
Great Falls: 1818 Tenth Avenue South, Great Falls, MT 59405, (406) 727-7740.
Missoula: 1018 Burlington, Room 101, Missoula, MT 59801, (406) 721-4910.

REHABILITATION

Rocky Mountain Development Council
201 South Main
P.O. Box 1717
Helena, MT 59624
(406) 447-1680 or Montana only
(800) 356-6544
FAX: (406) 447-1629
Cindy Baril, Program Manager

Type of Agency: Non-profit; Multi-county community action agency.
Funded by: Title VII, Chapter II.
Transportation: Y.

Recreational: Senior Companion Program, offering companion and chore services to elderly blind and sight impaired persons who are 55 years of age and older.

COMPUTER TRAINING CENTERS

Parents, Let's Unite for Kids (PLUK)
1500 North 30th Street
Billings, MT 59101-0298
(406) 657-2055
FAX: (406) 657-2061
Roger Holt, Database Technician

Computer Training: Speech output systems; screen magnification systems; word processing; computer operating systems.

♦ Low Vision Services

EYE CARE SOCIETIES

Montana Academy of Ophthalmology
1025 Strawberry
P.O. Box 803

Helena, MT 59624
(406) 449-2334
FAX: (406) 449-3156
Gloria Hermanson, Executive Director

Montana Optometric Association, Inc.
36 South Last Chance Gulch
Helena, MT 59601
(406) 443-1160
FAX: (406) 443-4614
Sue Weingartner, Executive Director

LOW VISION CENTERS

Montana Low Vision Service, Inc.
715 North Fee Street
Helena, MT 59601
(406) 442-0668 or toll-free in Montana and Idaho (800) 451-3226
FAX: (406) 443-5425
Christine Amundson, Manager

Type of Agency: Non-profit.
County/District Where Located: Lewis & Clark County.
Mission: Provide low vision evaluations and dispense optical/nonoptical aids to all who can benefit. Also act as a referral source to other helpful organizations.
Funded by: Client fees; foundation grants; Lions and Lioness Clubs of Montana.
Budget: $350,000.
Hours of Operation: Helena: Mon.-Fri. 9:00 AM - 12:00 PM; Billings: 10:00 AM - 2:00 PM.
Staff: Helena: 1. Billings: 2.
History/Date: Helena: est. 1977; Billings: 1986.
Number of Clients Served: Approximately 270 per year.
Eligibility: Referral.
Area Served: Unlimited, primarily Montana and northern Wyoming.
Age Requirements: None.

Computer Training: Access for demonstration; training for aids/devices.

Low Vision: On-site training provided.

Low Vision Aids: Loaned for trial (no charge); purchase; prescribed/fitted.

Low Vision Follow-up: Return appointment; phone interview.

Local Offices:

Billings: Low Vision Clinic, Securities Building, Room 510, 2708 First Avenue North, Billings, MT 59101, (406) 248-1941 (800) 228-1941 toll-free in Montana and Wyoming. Fax: (406) 248-1941.

◆ *Aging Services*

STATE UNITS ON AGING

Department of Public Health and Human Services Office on Aging

111 Sanders Street
Helena, MT 59604
(406) 444-4088 or Information & Referral (800) 332-2272
FAX: (406) 444-7743
Charles Rahbein, Aging Coordinator

Provides referrals to Area Agencies on Aging and information on other local aging services.

INDEPENDENT LIVING PROGRAMS

Department of Public Health and Human Services
Blind and Low Vision Services

111 Sanders Street
Helena, MT 59604
(406) 444-2590
FAX: (406) 444-3463
Joe A. Mathews, Administrator
Bob Maffit, Program Supervisor

Provides independent living services for persons age 55 and over. For further information, contact the Project Director or general phone number listed.

NEBRASKA

♦ *Educational Services*

STATE SERVICES

Nebraska Department of Education
301 Centennial Mall South
P.O. Box 94987
Lincoln, NE 68509
(402) 471-2471
FAX: (402) 471-0117
Gary Sherman, Director of Special Education
Don Anderson, Co-Director

Type of Agency: State.
County/District Where Located: Lancaster County.
Mission: Provides consultative services for the establishment and operation of educational programs for children with visual impairments.
Funded by: Public funds (state, local, and federal funds).
Area Served: Nebraska.
Age Requirements: Birth to 21 years.

Educational: Consultation with educators serving students with visual impairments, to assist with program planning, instructional and material modifications, and accessing resources.
Professional Training: Staff development for regular and special educators.

EARLY INTERVENTION COORDINATION

Special Education, Part H Program
Nebraska Department of Education
301 Centennial Mall South
P.O. Box 94987
Lincoln, NE 68509
(402) 471-2471
FAX: (402) 471-0117
Joan Luebber, Part H Coordinator

Special education services provided through local school districts for eligible children from birth or date of diagnosis.

SCHOOLS

Nebraska School for the Visually Handicapped
824 Tenth Avenue
P.O. Box 129
Nebraska City, NE 68410
(402) 873-5513
FAX: (402) 873-3463
William Mann, Superintendent

Type of Agency: State.
Mission: Services for totally blind, legally blind, visually impaired, learning disabled, mentally retarded, emotionally disturbed, and orthopedically disabled persons.
Funded by: State and federal funds, local schools through tuition, out-of-state contracts, and limited trust fund dollars.
Budget: 1996: $1,650,000.
Hours of Operation: Office hours: Mon. - Fri. 8:00 AM - 5:00 PM.
Staff: 33 full-time equivalents.
History/Date: Est. 1875.
Number of Clients Served: 1995-6: 19.
Eligibility: Visually impaired.
Area Served: State of Nebraska; will accept out-of-state contracts.
Transportation: Y.
Age Requirements: Kindergarten to age 21.

Health: Contracts and refers for health services.
Counseling/Social Work/Self-Help: Social evaluations; placement in school. Contracts for other counseling/social services.

Educational: Grades K through 12. Programs for college prep; general academic; vocational/skill development.
Preschools: Open during summer months for assessment purposes.
Professional Training: Pre-service and in-service training site for University of Nebraska-Lincoln vision teacher endorsement program.
Reading: Talking book record players and cassette players; talking book records and cassettes; braille books; large-print books; braille magazines; recorded magazines; information and referral; special collection; transcription to braille.
Residential: 5 days per week during regular school months.
Rehabilitation: Personal management; braille; handwriting; listening skills; typing; home management; orientation/mobility.
Recreational: Arts and crafts; hobby groups; bowling; swimming; track; wrestling; speech; music.
Employment: Job training opportunities available for some students.
Computer Training: Training on computer aids and devices. Word processing.
Low Vision: Assessments conducted and recommendations supplied to school.
Low Vision Aids: Assessments or referral available.

Contact local school superintendent for program information.

INFANT AND PRESCHOOL

Early Childhood Special Education Services
Omaha Public Schools
3215 Cuming Street

Omaha, NE 68131-2024
(402) 557-2420
FAX: (402) 557-2499
Gene Schwarting, Project Director,
(402) 557-2360
Donna Huttman, Visually
Impaired Program, (402) 557-2653

Type of Agency: Public school.
County/District Where Located:
Douglas County.
Funded by: P.L. 94-142 (incentive grants).
Hours of Operation: Mon.-Fri. 8:30AM-4:00PM.
Staff: 43 full time (includes early childhood/visually impaired teachers); orientation/mobility specialist available as consultant. 7 service coordinators.
History/Date: Est. 1979.
Area Served: Omaha area.
Transportation: Y.

Counseling/Social Work/Self-Help: Parent and other counseling; psychological evaluations; other social services.
Educational: Instruction in all developmental areas; auditory and sensory training; adaptive equipment. Home teaching for children with health restrictions; classrooms for visually impaired, multihandicapped, and noncategorical; and consultant services to other programs for visually impaired/multihandicapped children, with or without other disabilities, 3-5 years.
Preschools: Home-based program and consultation to primary caretaker for visually handicapped/multihandicapped infants, with or without other disabilities, 0-2 years.
Rehabilitation: Physical, occupational, and speech therapy.
Low Vision: Low vision exams.

Nebraska Department of Education
301 Centennial Mall South
P.O. Box 94987
Lincoln, NE 68509
(402) 471-2471
Gary Sherman, Director of Special Education

Type of Agency: State.
Funded by: State general funds and federal IDEA funds.
Staff: Outreach cadre teachers with certifications in visual impairment; services brokered by consultant.
Area Served: Nebraska.
Age Requirements: 0-5 years.

Counseling/Social Work/Self-Help: Parent counseling.
Educational: In-home and center-based assistance to meet needs of students with visual impairments in all developmental areas.

STATEWIDE OUTREACH SERVICES

Nebraska School for the Visually Handicapped
824 Tenth Avenue
P.O. Box 129
Nebraska City, NE 68410
(402) 873-5513
FAX: (402) 873-3463
William Mann, Superintendent

Funded by: State, federal, and local funds.
History/Date: Est. 1875.
Age Requirements: Birth through 21 years.

Assessment: Birth through 21 years.
Consultation to Public Schools: By request from school districts.
Direct Service: On campus.
Parent Assistance: On request.
Materials Production: Limited to serving Nebraska city public schools.

INSTRUCTIONAL MATERIALS CENTERS

Nebraska School for the Visually Handicapped
824 Tenth Avenue
Nebraska City, NE 68410
(402) 873-5513
FAX: (402) 873-3463
Jean Gotschall, Contact Person

Area Served: Statewide.

Types/Content: Textboosk, instructional materials.
Media Formats: Braille; large print; audio.

UNIVERSITY TRAINING PROGRAMS

University of Nebraska
Department of Special Education
250 Barkley Center
Lincoln, NE 68583-0732
(402) 472-7211
FAX: (402) 472-7697
E-mail: dalcorn@unlinfo.unl.edu
Dr. John Bernthal, (402) 472-3955

Programs Offered: Graduate (master's) program for teachers of visually impaired students (summer only).

◆ *Information Services*

LIBRARIES

Talking Book and Braille Service
The Atrium
1200 N Street, Suite 120

Lincoln, NE 68508-2023
(402) 471-2045 or toll-free in
Nebraska (800) 742-7691 or TDD
(402) 471-4038
FAX: (402) 471-2083
E-mail: jake@neon.ncl.state.ne.
us
URL: http://
www.nlc.state.ne.us/
Paul Jacobsen, Machine Lending
Information

Type of Agency: State library.
Mission: Free library service to
individuals unable to use regular
print because of visual or physical
impairment.
Funded by: Public funds.
Budget: $513,214.
Hours of Operation: Mon.- Fri.
8:00 AM - 5:00 PM.
Staff: 10.5 full-time equivalents.
History/Date: Est. 1952.
Number of Clients Served: 4,800.
Eligibility: Blind, visually
impaired, physically disabled, and
reading disabled persons.
Area Served: Nebraska.

Reading: Talking books,
magazines, playback equipment,
and braille.
Computer Training: Assistive
technology computer workstation
within facility for public access.

Regional library providing talking
books on disk or tape.

MEDIA PRODUCTION SERVICES

Special Education Media Center
3215 Cuming Street
Room 4029
Omaha, NE 68131-2024
(402) 554-6310
Donna Hultman

Area Served: Omaha public
schools.
Groups Served: K-12.

Types/Content: Textbooks.
Media Formats: Braille.
Title Listings: Registered with
American Printing House for the
Blind.

Talking Book and Braille Service
The Atrium
1200 N Street, Suite 120
Lincoln, NE 68508-2023
(402) 471-2045 or toll-free in
Nebraska (800) 742-7691 or TDD
(402) 471-4038
FAX: (402) 471-6244
E-mail: doertli@neon.nlc.state.
ne.us
URL: http://www.nlc.state.ne.us
David Oertli, Director

Area Served: Nebraska.
Groups Served: K-12, college
students, other adults.

Types/Content: Recreational,
newsletter information.
Media Formats: Braille books,
talking books/cassettes.
Title Listings: Provided at no
charge.

RADIO READING

Radio Talking Book Service
7101 Newport Avenue
Suite 205
Omaha, NE 68152
(402) 572-3003 or (800) 729-7826
FAX: (402) 572-3002
Richard Zlab, Station Manager
John Fullerton, Executive Director

Hours of Operation: Mon-Fri.
5:00 AM-Midnight; Sat.-Sun.
6:00 AM-6:30 PM.
History/Date: Est. 1974.
Area Served: All of Nebraska and
border areas of neighboring states.

INFORMATION AND REFERRAL

**The Foundation Fighting
Blindness
Nebraska/Iowa Affiliate**
P.O. Box 754
Omaha, NE 68101-0754
(402) 339-5604
Kay Konz, President

See The Foundation Fighting
Blindness in U.S. national listings.

Prevent Blindness Nebraska
7101 Newport Avenue
Suite 308
Omaha, NE 68152
(402) 572-3520
FAX: (402) 572-3522
E-mail: 104706.1123@compuserve.
com
Beverly J. Rudloff, Executive
Director

County/District Where Located:
Douglas County.

See Prevent Blindness America in
U.S. national listings.

See also in national listings:

Christian Record Services

**National Camps for Blind
Children**

Prose & Cons Braille Unit

♦ Rehabilitation Services

STATE SERVICES

**Nebraska Division of
Rehabilitation Services for the
Visually Impaired**
4600 Valley Road
Lincoln, NE 68510-4844
(402) 471-2891
FAX: (402) 483-4184
Dr. James S. Nyman, Director

Type of Agency: State.

Mission: Provide training and counseling to assist blind and visually impaired persons to overcome the difficulties of vision loss.

Funded by: Public funds.

Budget: $2.3 million.

Hours of Operation: Mon.-Fri. 8:00 AM-5:00 PM.

Staff: 46 full time equivalents.

History/Date: Est. 1943.

Number of Clients Served: 1,428.

Eligibility: All persons whose sight is so defective as to seriously limit ability to participate in the ordinary vocations and activities of life.

Area Served: Nebraska.

Counseling/Social Work/Self-Help: Individual, family counseling; consultation with schools, families of blind children; referral services.

Educational: Assistance with tuition, books, and other school supplies.

Residential: Apartment living for orientation and adjustment center students.

Rehabilitation: Braille, independent travel, homemaking skills; home teaching program; center training program; counseling/education on understanding of blindness, social attitudes.

Employment: Vocational counseling/career development; prevocational training; contracts for vocational training; placement and follow-up services; small business assistance; vending program.

Computer Training: Y.

Low Vision: Referral.

Low Vision Aids: Y.

Local Offices:

Kearney: Services for the Visually Impaired, 906 East 25th Street, Kearney, NE 68847-4603, (308) 865-5441.

Norfolk: Services for the Visually Impaired, 600 South 13th Street, Norfolk, NE 68701-4969, (402) 370-3436.

North Platte: Services for the Visually Impaired, North Platte State Office Building, 200 South Silber, North Platte, NE 69101-4298, (308) 535-8170.

Omaha: Services for the Visually Impaired, 1313 Farnam On the Mall, Omaha, NE 68102, (402) 595-2041.

Scottsbluff: Services for the Visually Impaired, 4500 Avenue I, Scottsbluff, NE 69361, (308) 632-1304.

COMPUTER TRAINING CENTERS

Nebraska Division of Rehabilitation Services for the Visually Impaired

600 South 13th Street
Norfolk, NE 68701-4969
(402) 370-3436
FAX: (402) 370-3508
Glenn Ervin, Counselor

Computer Training: Speech output systems; closed-circuit television systems; word processing; database software; computer operating systems; training for instructors.

Nebraska School for the Visually Handicapped

P.O. Box 129
Nebraska City, NE 68410
(402) 873-5513
FAX: (402) 873-3463
William Mann, Superintendent

Computer Training: Speech output systems; screen magnification systems; braille access systems; optical character recognition systems; word processing; training for instructors.

◆ Low Vision Services

EYE CARE SOCIETIES

Nebraska Academy of Ophthalmology

233 South 13th Street, Suite 1512
Lincoln, NE 68508
(402) 474-4472
Eric Carstenson, Executive Director

Nebraska Optometric Association, Inc.

P.O. Box 81706
Lincoln, NE 68501-1706
(402) 474-7716
FAX: (402) 476-6547
David S. McBride, Executive Director

LOW VISION CENTERS

Ophthalmology Department University of Nebraska Medical Center

3925 Dewey Avenue
Omaha, NE 68198
(402) 559-4170
FAX: (402) 559-5514
Howard Dinsdale, M.D., Director
Kathy Von Dollen, R.N., Coordinator

Type of Agency: Non-profit.

County/District Where Located: Douglas County.

Mission: Provide low vision services.

Funded by: Client fees; foundation grants.

Hours of Operation: Mon.-Fri. 9:00 AM-5:00 PM.

Staff: Ophthalmologist; R.N. low vision specialist.

Eligibility: None.
Area Served: Unlimited.

Low Vision Aids: Provided on loan for trial at no charge; on-site and in-home training.
Low Vision Follow-up: At regular intervals by appointment or by telephone.

◆ *Aging Services*

STATE UNITS ON AGING

Nebraska Department on Aging
301 Centennial Mall South
P.O. Box 95044
Lincoln, NE 68509
(402) 471-2306 or (800) 430-3244
FAX: (402) 471-4619
Dennis Loose, Director

Provides referrals to Area Agencies on Aging and information on other local aging services.

INDEPENDENT LIVING PROGRAMS

Rehabilitation Services for the Visually Impaired
Nebraska Department of Public Institutions
4600 Valley Road
Lincoln, NE 68510
(402) 471-2891
Dr. Pearl Van Zandt, Director

Provides independent living services for persons age 55 and over. For further information, contact the Project Director or general phone number listed.

NEVADA

♦ Educational Services

STATE SERVICES

Nevada Department of Education
700 East Fifth Street
Carson City, NV 89701
(702) 687-9171
FAX: (702) 687-9123
Gloria Dopf, Leader, Educational Equity

Type of Agency: State.
Mission: Provides training, technical assistance, consultation, information dissemination, funds administration, and planning for special education services in Nevada's 17 school districts and in other agencies which provide services to students with disabilities, ages 3 through 21. Conducts comprehensive monitoring to ensure compliance with state and federal statutes and regulations in programs which serve students with disabilities.
Funded by: Public funds.
Hours of Operation: Mon.-Fri. 8:00 AM - 5:00 PM.
Area Served: Nevada.

Contact local school superintendent for program information or Mike Becker, Area Supervisor, Services to the Blind, 308 North Curry, Carson City, NV 89710, (702) 687-4444.

EARLY INTERVENTION COORDINATION

Early Childhood Services Division of Child and Family Services Nevada Department of Human Resources
3987 South McCarran Boulevard
Reno, NV 89502
(702) 688-2284
FAX: (702) 688-2558
Marilyn K. Walter, Chief

Writes grants to fund outreach programs to rural areas; contracts with professionals specializing in visual impairment; operates home-based, statewide outreach program to serve young children and their families outside a 50-mile radius of Sparks.

♦ Information Services

LIBRARIES

Nevada State Library and Archives Regional Library for the Blind Talking Book Program
100 North Stewart Street
Carson City, NV 89701
(702) 687-5154 or toll-free in Nevada (800) 922-9334 or TDD (702) 687-5160
FAX: (702) 887-2630
Keri Putnam, Regional Librarian

Funded by: Public funds.
Hours of Operation: Mon.-Fri. 8:00 AM-5:00 PM.
Area Served: Nevada.

Regional library supplying talking books on disk and cassette.

Talking Book Program Las Vegas-Clark County Library Subregional Library for the Blind and Handicapped
1401 East Flamingo Road

Las Vegas, NV 89119
(702) 733-1925
FAX: (702) 733-1567
Doug Henderson, Librarian, (702) 687-5154

County/District Where Located: Clark County.
Funded by: Public funds.
Budget: $60,000.
Hours of Operation: Mon.-Fri. 9:00 AM-5:00 PM.
Staff: 2.
Number of Clients Served: 1,100.
Area Served: Southern Nevada.

Subregional library supplying talking books on disk and cassette.

MEDIA PRODUCTION SERVICES

Clark County School District
4101 West Bonanza Road
Las Vegas, NV 89107
(702) 799-4196
FAX: (702) 799-0389
Andrew Macklberg, Coordinating Teacher, Visually Impaired Program
Ronald Malcolm, Coordinator, Sensory Deficit Program, (702) 799-5266

County/District Where Located: Clark County.
Area Served: Clark County.
Groups Served: Preschool through 12th grade. Ages 3 to 22.

Types/Content: Textbooks, recreational, career/vocational.
Media Formats: Braille books, talking books/cassettes, large print books.
Title Listings: No title listings available.

Nevada Bureau of Services to the Blind
Kinkead Building
505 East King Street, Room 503

Carson City, NV 89710
(702) 687-4444
FAX: (702) 687-5980
Maynard Yasmer, Bureau Chief

Area Served: Statewide.
Groups Served: 164; college students; other adults.

Types/Content: Recreational; career/vocational.
Media Formats: Braille books; talking books/cassettes; large-print books.
Title Listings: Print and braille lists available at no charge.

Nevada State Library
Regional Library for the Blind

100 North Stewart Street
Carson City, NV 89701
(702) 887-2245
FAX: (702) 887-2630
Keri Putnam, Regional Librarian

Groups Served: K-12, college students, other adults.

Types/Content: Recreational.
Media Formats: None specified.
Title Listings: Printed at no charge.

Talking Book Program
Las Vegas–Clark County Library

1401 East Flamingo Road
Las Vegas, NV 89119
(702) 733-7810
Mary Anne Morton, Librarian

County/District Where Located: Clark County.
Area Served: Southern Nevada.
Groups Served: All ages.

Types/Content: Recreational, educational, informational.
Media Formats: Flexible disks and cassettes.
Title Listings: None specified.

RADIO READING

Nevada Public Radio Corporation
KNPR

5151 Boulder Highway
Las Vegas, NV 89122
(702) 456-6695
FAX: (702) 458-2787
URL: http://http.//
www.knpr.org
Lamar Marchese, General Manager
Jay Bartos, Radio Reading Services

Funded by: Listener contributions, grants and gifts.
Hours of Operation: 24 hours, 7 days.
History/Date: Est. 1980.
Area Served: Nevada.

See also in national listings:

Northern Nevada Braille Transcribers

◆ Rehabilitation Services

STATE SERVICES

Nevada Bureau of Services to the Blind

Kinkead Building
505 East King Street, Room 501
Carson City, NV 89710
(702) 687-4440
FAX: (702) 687-5980
Maynard Yasmer, Bureau Chief
Elizabeth Breshears, Administrator

Type of Agency: State.
Mission: Services for blind and visually impaired individuals.
Funded by: Public funds.
Budget: 1997.: $2,500,000.
Hours of Operation: Mon.-Fri. 8:00 AM-5:00 PM.
Program Accessibility: Fully accessible.

Staff: 31 full time.
History/Date: Est. 1965.
Number of Clients Served: 1,160.
Eligibility: Visual impairment that constitutes handicap to employment or independent living.
Area Served: Statewide.
Transportation: Y.
Age Requirements: Over 16 years old.

Health: Provides aids and appliances; low vision clinic; diagnostic and evaluation services.
Counseling/Social Work/Self-Help: Consultation and referral services; psychological testing; counseling and guidance; adaptive living skills.
Educational: Postsecondary, college, and special diabetic education.
Reading: Reader service available.
Rehabilitation: Personal management; orientation/mobility; home mechanics; home economics; communications.
Recreational: Summer and winter recreation and leisure time activities.
Employment: Evaluation, prevocational and vocational training; vocational placement; business enterprise program; follow-up service and post-employment services.
Computer Training: Access; training on computer aids and devices.
Low Vision: Evaluations.
Low Vision Aids: Magnafiers and other aids available.
Low Vision Follow-up: Therapy as prescribed.

Local Offices:

Fallon: 31 North Maine Street, Fallon, NV 89406, (702) 786-4444.
Las Vegas: 628 Belrose, Las Vegas, NV 89158, (702) 647-4111.

Reno: 1050 Matley Lane, Reno, NV 89502, (702) 789-0450.

REHABILITATION

Southern Nevada Sightless
1001 North Bruce Street
Las Vegas, NV 89101
(702) 642-6000
Catherine Law, Director

Type of Agency: Non-profit.
County/District Where Located: Clark County.
Funded by: Subcontracts, sale of products, individual and corporate contributions.
Hours of Operation: Mon.-Thurs. 8:30 AM-3:30 PM.
History/Date: Est. 1955.
Eligibility: Visually impaired or blind.
Area Served: Las Vegas.
Transportation: Y.

Counseling/Social Work/Self-Help: Instruction in independent living skills; recreation; children's program; work activities program.
Employment: Prevocational workshop and adjustment training.

◆ Low Vision Services

EYE CARE SOCIETIES

Nevada Ophthalmological Society
600 Whitney Ranch Road
Henderson, NV 89014
(702) 456-8389
Rudy R. Manthei, M.D., President

Nevada Optometric Association, Inc.
3311 South Rainbow Boulevard, Suite 132

Las Vegas, NV 89102
(702) 220-7444
Shanda Badger, Executive Director

LOW VISION CENTERS

Low Vision Clinic
Nevada Bureau of Services to the Blind
628 Belrose Street
Las Vegas, NV 89107
(702) 486-5333
Al Roybal, District Manager

County/District Where Located: Clark County.
Funded by: State and federal funds.
Hours of Operation: Mon.-Fri. 8:00 AM-5:00 PM.

Low Vision Aids: Provided on loan for trial; no rental fee; on-site training provided.
Low Vision Follow-up: By phone interview, visit to home, place of employment at 3 and 6 months.

◆ Aging Services

STATE UNITS ON AGING

Division for Aging Services
Nevada Department of Human Resources
340 North 11th Street
Suite 203
Las Vegas, NV 89101
(702) 486-3545 or in-state, referral only (800) 243-3638
Mary Liveratti, Acting Administrator

Provides referrals to Area Agencies on Aging and information on other local aging services.

INDEPENDENT LIVING PROGRAMS

Rehabilitation Division
Nevada Department of Human Resources
505 East King Street
Fifth Floor
Carson City, NV 89710
(702) 687-4440
FAX: (702) 687-5980
Elizabeth Breshears, Administrator
Maynard Yasmer, Chief, Bureau of Services for the Blind
Michael Becker, Project Director, (702) 687-4444

Provides independent living services for persons age 55 and over. For further information, contact the Project Director or general phone number listed.

NEW HAMPSHIRE

◆ *Educational Services*

STATE SERVICES

New Hampshire Department of Education
State Office Park South
101 Pleasant Street
Concord, NH 03301
(603) 271-6051
Robert T. Kennedy, Director,
Educational Improvement
Ruth Littlefield, Early Childhood
Consultant

Type of Agency: State.
County/District Where Located: Merrimack County.
Mission: Administers the federal quota system for providing visually handicapped children in local schools with materials from the American Printing House for the Blind. Provides information about local facilities.

EARLY INTERVENTION COORDINATION

New Hampshire's Early Support and Services
Division of Mental Health and Developmental Services
New Hampshire Department of Health and Human Services
105 Pleasant Street
Hospital Administration Building
Concord, NH 03301
(603) 271-5144
FAX: (603) 271-5166
Pam Miller Sallet, Part H Early Childhood Coordinator

County/District Where Located: Merrimack County.

Early intervention programs for children aged 0-5.

SCHOOLS

New Hampshire Educational Services for the Sensory Impaired
117 Pleasant Street
Dolloff Building
Concord, NH 03301
(603) 226-2900
FAX: (603) 226-2907
William Finn, Coordinator

Type of Agency: Special education project contracted by state to provide educational support services.
Mission: To provide educational support to local education agencies relative to low incidence populations.
Funded by: State and federal funds.
Staff: 13 staff provide consultation and materials support.
Number of Clients Served: 1,000 per year.
Eligibility: Determined by local education agency through special education placement and program process.
Area Served: Statewide.
Age Requirements: 3-21 years of age.

Educational: Services provided to schools and homes. Staff consults on educational needs.
Professional Training: Agency provides in-service and staff training.
Low Vision: Information, evaluation, referral.
Low Vision Aids: Available on case basis.
Low Vision Follow-up: Y.

INFANT AND PRESCHOOL

Multi-Sensory Intervention Through Consultation and Education (MICE)
Dolloff Building
117 Pleasant Street
Concord, NH 03301
(603) 226-2908
FAX: (603) 226-2907
Janet Halley, Contact Person

Type of Agency: Cooperative public-private agency.
Mission: To enhance quality services to families with infants who have sensory impairments, and provide technical assistance to community based agencies.
Funded by: State funds, federal funds; private donations; in-kind contributions.
Hours of Operation: Mon.-Fri. 8:30 AM - 4:30 PM.
Staff: 3 full time; 3 part time.
History/Date: Est. 1973.
Number of Clients Served: 150 annually.
Eligibility: Visually impaired children; deaf-blind children; with or without additional impairments, including those at risk.
Area Served: Entire state.
Age Requirements: 0-3 years.

Health: Provides direct visual and auditory training; consultative service; coordination with other involved agencies (health, early intervention, school districts, day care).
Educational: Instruction in all developmental areas; parent training; community and home-based services using itinerant model for visually impaired children.
Professional Training: In-service training regarding the developmental needs of sensory impaired infants for community-based professionals.

Reading: Parent/professional library.

INSTRUCTIONAL MATERIALS CENTERS

New Hampshire Educational Services for the Sensory Impaired

117 Pleasant Street
Dolloff Building
Concord, NH 03301
(603) 226-2900
FAX: (603) 226-2907
William Finn, Coordinator

Area Served: Statewide.
Groups Served: Students ages 3-21 with sensory impairments.

Types/Content: Educational.
Media Formats: Braille, large-print, electronic, audio visual.

◆ Information Services

LIBRARIES

New Hampshire State Library Library Services to the Handicapped Division

117 Pleasant Street
Concord, NH 03301
(603) 271-3429 or (800) 491-3429
E-mail: talking@lilac.nhsl.lib.nh.us
URL: http://www.state.nh.us
Eileen Keim, Librarian

Type of Agency: Regional library for visually and physically impaired people.
Funded by: Public funds.
Hours of Operation: Mon.- Fri. 8:00 AM - 4:30 PM.
Staff: 4.
History/Date: Est. 1970.
Number of Clients Served: More than 2,000.
Area Served: New Hampshire. Braille readers served by Braille

and Talking Book regional library in Massachusetts.
Age Requirements: Four years of age and older.

Regional library providing talking books, tapes, cassettes, and large type.

See also in national listings:

Chivers North America

◆ Rehabilitation Services

STATE SERVICES

Services for the Blind and Visually Impaired New Hampshire Division of Vocational Rehabilitation

78 Regional Drive
Building #2
Concord, NH 03301-8508
(603) 271-3537
FAX: (603) 271-3816
Colleen Ives, Supervisor
Paul Leather, Director

County/District Where Located: Merrimack County.
Mission: Administers the federal-state vocational rehabilitation program.
Funded by: Public funds.
Budget: $1,084,439.
Hours of Operation: Mon.-Fri. 8:30 AM-4:30 PM.
Staff: 15.
History/Date: Est. 1913.
Eligibility: Visually impaired.
Area Served: New Hampshire.

Counseling/Social Work/Self-Help: Consultation and referral; psychological testing.
Reading: Talking book record player and cassette player; talking book records and cassettes. Reader service available.

Rehabilitation: Personal management; home mechanics; home economics; communications; orientation/mobility.
Employment: Evaluation; prevocational and vocational training; vocational placement; follow-up service; vending facility program; postemployment programs.
Computer Training: Y.
Low Vision: Services available for a fee.

Local Offices:

Concord: Blind Services, Two Industrial Park Drive, Concord, NH 02301, (603) 271-2327.
Keene: Blind Services, 25 Roxbury Street, Keene, NH 03431, (603) 357-0266.
Manchester: Blind Services, 361 Lincoln Street, Manchester, NH 03103, (603) 669-8733.
Nashua: Blind Services, 547 Amherst Street, Nashua, NH 03060, (603) 889-6844.
Portsmouth: Blind Services, 30 Maplewood Avenue, Suite 201, Portsmouth, NH 03801, (603) 436-8884.

REHABILITATION

Camp Allen, Inc.

56 Camp Allen Road
Bedford, NH 03110-6606
(603) 622-8471
FAX: (603) 626-4295
Lori Stuntfol, Director

Type of Agency: Private; non-profit.
County/District Where Located: Hillsboro County.
Funded by: Maintained jointly by the Kiwanis Club of Boston and the Lions Club of Manchester, New Hampshire.
History/Date: Est. 1932.

Camp provides residential summer program for people with

developmental and/or physical disabilities.

New Hampshire Association for the Blind

25 Walker Street
Concord, NH 03301
(603) 224-4039 or toll-free in New Hampshire (800) 464-3075
FAX: (603) 224-4378
E-mail: gtnhab@aol.com
URL: http://
www.peekaboo.net/nhab
George F. Theriault, President
John Ferraro, Program Director

Type of Agency: Private; non-profit.
Mission: Provision of basic rehabilitation/independent living services, for all ages of blind and visually impaired persons statewide.
Funded by: Contributions, capital income, sales contracts for service; client fee (sliding scale).
Budget: $800,000.
Hours of Operation: Mon.-Fri. 8:00 AM-4:30 PM.
Program Accessibility: Fully accessible.
Staff: 15 full time, 2 part time. Uses volunteers.
History/Date: Est. 1912.
Number of Clients Served: 800-1,000 annually.
Eligibility: State resident with severe visual impairment.
Area Served: New Hampshire.

Counseling/Social Work/Self-Help: Social work evaluations; limited individual, counseling. Refers to and provides consultation to other agencies for other counseling/social work services.
Educational: Conducts extensive statewide public education program; speakers bureau; slides; films; displays; literature.

Professional Training: Provides consultation and training programs for staff and personnel of other organizations/agencies/institutions serving populations that include visually impaired persons.
Rehabilitation: Orientation/mobility and rehabilitation teaching programs. Provides instruction for independent, safe travel; personal and home management; communication skills in the home and community. Refers for other rehabilitation services as appropriate.
Low Vision: Low vision service; low vision eye exams.
Low Vision Aids: Low vision aid prescriptions; optical aids loan and training.
Low Vision Follow-up: Y.

COMPUTER TRAINING CENTERS

Services for the Blind and Visually Impaired
New Hampshire Division of Vocational Rehabilitation

78 Regional Drive
Building 2
Concord, NH 03301-8508
(603) 271-3537
FAX: (603) 271-3816
Colleen Ives, Contact Person

County/District Where Located: Merrimack County.

Computer Training: Speech output systems; screen magnification systems; braille access systems; optical character recognition systems; closed-circuit television systems; word processing; database software; computer operating systems.

◆ Low Vision Services

EYE CARE SOCIETIES

New Hampshire Society of Eye Physicians and Surgeons

Department of Ophthalmology
Lahey-Hitchcock Clinic
Lebanon, NH 03756
(603) 650-5123
Dr. Rosalind A. Stevens, Section Chief

County/District Where Located: Grafton County.

New Hampshire Optometric Association, Inc.

195 Hanover Street
Portsmouth, NH 03801
(603) 436-3717
Brian Klinger, O.D.

LOW VISION CENTERS

New Hampshire Association for the Blind
Low Vision Program

25 Walker Street
Concord, NH 03301
(603) 224-4039 or toll-free in New Hampshire (800) 464-3075
FAX: (603) 224-4378
E-mail: gtnhab@aol.com
URL: http://
www.peekaboo.net/nhab
George Theriault, President
Rene P. Paguin, Supervisor
John Ferraro, Program Director

Type of Agency: Private; non-profit.
Mission: Assists low vision persons to maximize use of remaining vision through prescription of optical aids and training in their use.
Funded by: Grants; purchase of service from third party funders; clients' fees; donations.

Budget: $850,000.
Hours of Operation: Mon.-Fri. 8:00 AM-4:00 PM.
Program Accessibility: Fully accessible.
Staff: Optometrists; rehabilitation teacher; orientation/mobility instructor; low/vision trainers, social worker.
History/Date: Est. 1979.
Number of Clients Served: 900 annually.
Eligibility: Current ophthalmological report.
Area Served: New Hampshire.

Counseling/Social Work/Self-Help: Social work intake; information referral services; limited counseling.
Rehabilitation: Low vision; orientation/mobility/rehabilitation teaching; short-term social work counseling.
Low Vision: Ophthalmological consultations; eye examinations; training; and instruction.
Low Vision Aids: Prescriptions; loans and training.
Low Vision Follow-up: By return appointment, phone interview or on-site at home, school or place of employment.

Mobile clinic scheduled at central locations statewide.

◆ *Aging Services*

STATE UNITS ON AGING

Division of Elderly and Adult Services
New Hampshire Department of Health and Human Services
115 Pleasant Street
State Office Park South, Annex Building #1

Concord, NH 03301-3843
(603) 271-4680 or Information & Referral In State (800) 351-1888
FAX: (603) 271-4643
Richard Crocker, Director

Provides referrals to Area Agencies on Aging and information on other local aging services.

INDEPENDENT LIVING PROGRAMS

Bureau of Vocational Rehabilitation
New Hampshire Department of Education
78 Regional Drive
Concord, NH 03301
(603) 271-3471 or (800) 299-1647
Paul Leather, Director

Provides independent living services for persons age 55 and over. For further information, contact the Project Director or general phone number listed.

NEW JERSEY

♦ *Educational Services*

STATE SERVICES

Office of Special Education Programs
New Jersey Department of Education
CN 500
Trenton, NJ 08625-0500
(609) 984-8422
Barbara Gantwerk, Director

Type of Agency: A division of the New Jersey Department of Education.
County/District Where Located: Mercer County.
Funded by: Public funds.
Area Served: New Jersey.

For information about local facilities, consult the New Jersey Commission for the Blind and Visually Impaired.

EARLY INTERVENTION COORDINATION

Office of Special Education Programs
New Jersey Department of Education
CN 500
Trenton, NJ 08625
(609) 633-6833
FAX: (609) 292-5558
E-mail: njse@ix.netcom.com
URL: http://www.state.nj.us/education/
Barbara Gantwerk, Director

County/District Where Located: Mercer County.

A free public awareness and referral service to assist parents, professionals, and the general public by identifying free available early intervention, preschool, or special education programs and services throughout New Jersey (Project Child Find, (800) 322-8174); and an initiative to provide technical assistance to parents and professionals regarding the education of children experiencing hearing and vision diffculties (NJ TAP, (609) 292-5894).

SCHOOLS

Matheny School and Hospital
Main Street
Peapack, NJ 07977
(908) 234-0011
FAX: (908) 719-2137
Robert Schonhorn, President
Doreen Glut, Admissions

Type of Agency: Private, non-profit agency.
County/District Where Located: Somerset County.
Mission: Services for physically disabled persons with additional learning, perceptual, and behavioral difficulties; persons who are learning disabled or mentally retarded; clients with cerebral palsy.
Staff: 296 full time.
Eligibility: Cerebral palsy or muscular distrophy or spina bifida.
Age Requirements: 5 to 25 years of age.

Health: Diagnosis and evaluation of eye health; treatment of eye condition; prescription of spectacles or aids; follow-up evaluation of eye treatment or prescription; general medical services.
Counseling/Social Work/Self-Help: Psychological testing and evaluation. Refers for social evaluation.
Educational: Grades K through 6 and non-graded; general academic study; life skills; occupational therapy; physical therapy; speech therapy; music therapy.
Professional Training: Internship/fieldwork placement in special education. Regular in-service training program.
Reading: Talking book record player and cassette player; talking book records and cassettes; recorded magazines.
Residential: Dormitories.
Rehabilitation: Personal management; handwriting; typing.
Recreational: Recreational therapy.
Computer Training: Access; training on computer aids and devices.

St. Joseph's School for the Blind
253 Baldwin Avenue
Jersey City, NJ 07306
(201) 653-0578
FAX: (201) 653-4087
Herbert Miller, Administrator
Gerald Kitzhoffer, Assistant Administrator

Type of Agency: Private, Catholic nondenominational, nonsectarian, nonprofit.
Mission: Services for blind, visually impaired, multiply disabled, or deaf-blind infants, children, and adults.
Funded by: Public donations, public funds, endowments, and contributions.
Hours of Operation: School: Mon. - Fri. 8:00 AM - 4:00 PM. School residence: Mon. - Thurs. 2:30 PM - 8:00 AM. Community residence: Sun. - Sat. 24 hours.
Staff: 95 full-time, 15 part-time. Uses volunteers.
History/Date: Est. 1891.
Number of Clients Served: 85.
Eligibility: Blindness plus other disabilities.

Area Served: New Jersey, especially the Northern New Jersey metropolitan area.

Age Requirements: Birth - 40 years.

Health: Physical therapy; speech therapy; occupational therapy; nursing; consulting physicians; music therapy. Refers for other health services.

Counseling/Social Work/Self-Help: Social evaluations; individual, family/parent, couple counseling; placement in training; referral to community services. Refers for other counseling/social work services.

Educational: Nongraded. Infant, preschool, school-age, young adult, educational programs; activities of daily living, vocational training, and special summer programs.

Preschools: Early Intervention Program.

Professional Training: Internship/fieldwork placement in special education, social work, speech, and language therapy. Regular in-service training programs.

Reading: Talking book record players and cassette players; computer reading; prebraille.

Residential: Dormitory for multiply disabled children. Five-day students return home on weekends. Community residence for adults 7 days a week.

Rehabilitation: Orientation/mobility; independent living.

Recreational: Afterschool programs; arts and crafts; swimming; community integration.

Employment: Occupational skill development; prevocational training. Vocational training.

Computer Training: Training on computers.

Low Vision: Consultants on an individual basis.

INSTRUCTIONAL MATERIALS CENTERS

George Meyer Instructional Resource Center
375 McCarter Highway
Newark, NJ 07114
(201) 648-2547
FAX: (201) 824-8926
Donald H. Potenski, Manager

Area Served: Primarily New Jersey; informational services to other states.

Groups Served: New Jersey Commission for the Blind clients. (aged birth-21).

Types/Content: Textbooks.
Media Formats: Large print, braille.
Title Listings: Available through APH (at the American Printing House for the Blind).

◆ *Information Services*

LIBRARIES

New Jersey Library for the Blind and Handicapped
2300 Stuyvesant Avenue, CN501
Trenton, NJ 08625-0501
(609) 292-6450 or toll-free in New Jersey (800) 792-8322 or TDD (609) 633-7250
Vianne Connor, Librarian
Christine Lisiecki, Machine Lending Information

Type of Agency: Library.
County/District Where Located: Mercer County.
Mission: To provide reading materials on tape, large print and disk.
Funded by: Public funds.

Budget: $1.5 million.
Hours of Operation: Mon. - Fri. 8:30 AM - 4:30 PM. and Sat. (except July and August) 9:00 AM - 3:00 PM.
Program Accessibility: Fully accessible.
History/Date: Est. 1967.
Number of Clients Served: 11,000.
Eligibility: New Jersey residents who are unable to use print as a result of a physical or visual impairment.
Area Served: New Jersey.
Age Requirements: 5 years and older.

Regional library providing talking books, braille, cassettes, large-print books, magazines, closed-circuit radio reading service, and video cassettes with discriptive narrative.

MEDIA PRODUCTION SERVICES

Madison-Chatham Braille Association
Box 541
Chatham, NJ 07928
(201) 377-4683
Helen Henshaw, President

County/District Where Located: Morris County.
Groups Served: K-12; college students; other adults.

Types/Content: Textbooks; including mathematics; recreational; career/vocational; religious.
Media Formats: Braille books.
Title Listings: None specified.

Recording for the Blind and Dyslexic
20 Roszel Road

Princeton, NJ 08540
(609) 452-0606
FAX: (609) 987-8116
E-mail: info@rfbd.org
URL: http://www.rfbd.org
Ritchie L. Geisel, President and
CEO

Groups Served: Individuals with visual impairments, learning disabilities, or other disabilities that prevent them from reading standard print.

Title Listings: Catalog of titles available.

See Recording for the Blind and Dyslexic in U.S. national listings.

Recording for the Blind and Dyslexic

36-A Hibben Road
Princeton, NJ 08540
(609) 921-6534
FAX: (609) 921-3916
Anne Young, Studio Director

County/District Where Located: Mercer County.

See Recording for the Blind and Dyslexic in U.S. national listings.

TFB Publications

238 75th Street
North Bergen, NJ 07047
(201) 662-0956

County/District Where Located: Hudson County.

Types/Content: Text materials other than music, including computer-related materials.
Media Formats: Braille, large print, and tape.

RADIO READING

Audiovision
New Jersey Library for the Blind and Handicapped

2300 Stuyvesant Avenue, CN 501

Trenton, NJ 08625
(609) 530-3260
FAX: (609) 530-6384
Christine Lisiecki, Director

County/District Where Located: Mercer County.
Funded by: Federal and state funds.
Hours of Operation: Mon.-Thurs. 8:00 AM-4:00 PM; Fri. 8:00 AM-4:00 PM; on air Mon.-Sun 1PM-12 midnight.
Staff: 2 full time.
History/Date: Est. 1984.
Area Served: 40-45 mile radius from Trenton and 40-45 mile radius from Waterford Works, NJ.
Age Requirements: None.

Electronic Information and Education Service

59 Scotland Road
P.O. Box 411
South Orange, NJ 07079
(201) 762-0552
John F. Mulvihill, General Manager

County/District Where Located: Essex County.
Hours of Operation: Mon.-Fri. 7:00 AM-11:00 PM; Sat.-Sun. 9:00 AM-12:00 midnight.
History/Date: Est. 1974.
Area Served: Nine counties in north New Jersey.

INFORMATION AND REFERRAL

The Foundation Fighting Blindness
New Jersey Affiliate

P.O. Box 449
Princeton, NJ 08542-0449
(609) 924-8034
FAX: (609) 921-7697
Llura Gund, President

County/District Where Located: Mercer County.

See The Foundation Fighting Blindness in U.S. national listings.

The Foundation Fighting Blindness
Northern New Jersey Affiliate

P.O. Box 38
Livingston, NJ 07039
(201) 994-1532
Edward Gollob, Contact Person

See The Foundation Fighting Blindness in U.S. national listings.

New Jersey College Resource Center for Adaptive Aids

CN 501
Trenton, NJ 08625
(609) 530-3259
Christine Lisiecki, Director
John Noecker, Technical Coordinator

Type of Agency: Non-profit resource center.
County/District Where Located: Mercer County.
Funded by: New Jersey State Commission on Higher Education.
Area Served: New Jersey colleges and universities.

Loans technical and nontechnical adaptive aids to New Jersey colleges and universities for use by students who are blind or visually impaired, learning disabled and deaf or hard of hearing. Provides resource information and basic technical assistance to New Jersey colleges. Conducts annual workshop.

Prevent Blindness New Jersey

2525 Route 130, Building D
Cranbury, NJ 08512
(609) 409-0770
FAX: (609) 409-0755
E-mail: 104706.1113@compuserve.com
Margo L. Asay, Director

County/District Where Located: Middlesex County.

See Prevent Blindness America in U.S. national listings.

See also in national listings:

Audio Optics, Inc.

Council of Schools for the Blind

G.K. Hall and Company
Simon and Schuster

Isis Large Print Books
Transaction Publishers

New Eyes for the Needy

Recording for the Blind and
Dyslexic

Simon & Schuster Publishing

◆ *Rehabilitation Services*

STATE SERVICES

New Jersey Commission for the Blind and Visually Impaired

153 Halsey Street
P.O. Box 47017
Newark, NJ 07101
(201) 648-2324 or (201) 648-2325
FAX: (201) 648-7364
Jamie Casabianca Hilton,
Executive Director

Type of Agency: State
government agency providing
various services to blind and
visually impaired residents of New
Jersey.
Mission: Administers the federal-
state vocational rehabilitation
program.
Funded by: State and federal
monies.
Budget: $18,734,000.
Hours of Operation: 9:00AM-
5:00PM.
Staff: 274 full time. Uses
volunteers.
History/Date: Est. 1910.
Number of Clients Served: 1995:
10,200 rehabilitation clients; 29,000
persons receiving eye exams.

Eligibility: 20/40 visual acuity or
field restriction to 20 degrees or
less.
Area Served: New Jersey.
Age Requirements: None.

Health: Eye health nursing;
diabetic retinopathy detection;
preschool vision screening;
glaucoma screening follow-up;
vision screening of children of
migratory workers and other at-
risk populations.
**Counseling/Social Work/Self-
Help:** Contracts with a
community organization to set up
self-help groups all over the state.
On-staff social workers and
counselors.
Educational: Itinerant services to
visually impaired children, ages
birth to 21; institutional and day
training center technical assistance;
deaf-blind program; summer
programs; residential/special
placement programs.
Reading: Textbook and materials
center; technical aids center.
Residential: Joseph Kohn
Rehabilitation Center, New
Brunswick, New Jersey.
Rehabilitation: Orientation/
mobility; home instruction
programs, vocational and
independent living skills.
Employment: Prevocational
evaluation; rehabilitation center;
vending facility program; college
unit; deaf-blind services;
vocational training and job
placement; follow-up services.
Computer Training: Technology
center.
Low Vision: Low vision services.
Low Vision Aids: Referrals.
Low Vision Follow-up: Y.

Statewide Services:

New Brunswick: Joseph Kohn
Residential Rehabilitation Center,
130 Livingston Avenue, New
Brunswick, NJ 08901, (908) 937-
6363, Ron Parent, Manager.
Trenton: Business Enterprise
Program, 222 South Warren Street,
Trenton, NJ 08625, (609) 777-2083,
John Klein, Manager.

Regional Offices:

Camden: Southern Regional
Office, 101 Haddon Avenue,
Camden, NJ 08103, (609) 757-2815,
Donald Potenski, Manager.
Egg Harbor: Township Office,
6712 Washington Avenue, Egg
Harbor, NJ 08232, (609) 645-6740.
Paterson: Northern Regional
Office, 100 Hamilton Plaza,
Paterson, NJ 07505, (201) 977-4200,
John Reiff, Manager.
Toms River: Central Regional
Office, 1510 Hooper Avenue, Suite
2400, Toms River, NJ 08753,
(908) 255-0723, Edward Gorczyca,
Manager.

REHABILITATION

Bestwork Industries for the Blind

209 Highland Avenue
Westmont, NJ 08108
(609) 854-3388
FAX: (609) 854-3565
Belinda S. Moore, Executive
Director

County/District Where Located:
Camden County.

Employment: Provides workshop
employment services.

Catholic Community Services

494 Broad Street
Newark, NJ 07102
(201) 242-1999
FAX: (201) 242-3789
George Piegaro, Program Director

Type of Agency: Private; non-profit.
County/District Where Located: Essex County.

Rehabilitation: Orientation/mobility; home mechanics; home economics; communications; clerical training.
Employment: Evaluation; prevocational and vocational training and placement; contract workshop.
Computer Training: Medical secretary course.

Family and Social Service Federation

44 Armory Street
Englewood, NJ 07631
(201) 568-0817
FAX: (201) 568-0913
Mitchell Schonfeld, Executive Director

Type of Agency: Private; non-profit.
County/District Where Located: Bergen County.
Funded by: United Way, Title XX, private donations.
Staff: 4 full time, 20 part time. Uses volunteers.
Eligibility: Mentally alert, visually impaired.
Transportation: Y.

Counseling/Social Work/Self-Help: Social evaluation. Refers for other counseling/social work services.
Professional Training: Regular in-service training; short-term or summer training; open to enrollment from other agencies.
Reading: Lends talking book record players and cassette player; talking book records and tapes; recorded magazines; information and referral; closed circuit television; machine which magnifies and then projects onto TV screen.

Rehabilitation: Personal management; braille; typing; home management; orientation/mobility; refers for and provides consultation to other agencies on other rehabilitation services.
Recreational: Arts and crafts; special programs for elderly; bowling; swimming; dancing. Refers for and provides consultation to other agencies on other recreational/leisure services.

New Jersey Foundation for the Blind

230 Diamond Spring Road
P.O. Box 929
Denville, NJ 07834
(201) 627-0055
FAX: (201) 627-1622
John Gromann, President
Terry Fioretto, Administrator

Type of Agency: Non-profit.
County/District Where Located: Morris County.
Mission: Training center for independent living skills.
Funded by: Private contributions.
Hours of Operation: 7 days, 24 hours.
History/Date: Est. 1942.
Eligibility: Legally or totally blind. Must be ambulatory.
Area Served: New Jersey.
Age Requirements: 18 years.

Counseling/Social Work/Self-Help: Referral services.
Rehabilitation: Activities of daily living.
Recreational: Arts and crafts.

St. Joseph's Home for the Blind

537 Pavonia Avenue
Jersey City, NJ 07306
(201) 653-8300
Sister Teresa Catherine, CSJP, Administrator

Type of Agency: Nursing home.

Mission: Services for aged and infirm blind and sighted persons.
Funded by: Medicaid and private fees.
Hours of Operation: 24 hours.
Program Accessibility: Accessible to wheelchair users.
History/Date: Est. 1899.
Number of Clients Served: 129 residents.
Transportation: Y.
Age Requirements: 65 years and older.

Health: Physical therapy, occupational therapy.
Counseling/Social Work/Self-Help: Services available.
Residential: Nursing home.
Rehabilitation: Orientation/mobility.

COMPUTER TRAINING CENTERS

National Institute for Rehabilitation Engineering

P.O. Box T
Hewitt, NJ 07421
(201) 853-6585 or toll-free (800) 736-2216
E-mail: dons@warwick.net
Donald Selwyn, Contact Person

Computer Training: Speech output systems; screen magnification systems; optical character recognition systems; braille access systems; word processing; database software; computer operating systems; training for instructors; on-site hardware, software and training services.

Closed-circuit TV reading systems: desktop and portable, black and white and color; integrated CCTV and computer systems with scanners and text (character) recognition; computer and technology aids training given on-site, in clients' homes, in schools and places of employment.

Technical Aids Center
New Jersey Commission for the
Blind and Visually Impaired
153 Halsey Street
P.O. Box 47017
Newark, NJ 07101
(201) 648-3330
FAX: (201) 648-7364
Joseph Tomasko, Coordinator

County/District Where Located:
Essex County.

Computer Training: Speech
output systems; screen
magnification systems; braille
access systems; optical character
recognition systems; closed-circuit
television systems; word
processing; database software;
computer operating systems;
evaluation and installation offered
as well.

DOG GUIDE SCHOOLS

Seeing Eye, Inc.
Washington Valley Road
Morristown, NJ 07960
(201) 539-4425
Judy Deuschle, Director of Student
Services

Mission: Trains dog guides and
instructs blind persons in their use.
Funded by: Endowment, bequests,
trusts and contributions.
Hours of Operation: Mon.-Fri.
8:30 AM -5:00 PM.
History/Date: Est. and Inc. 1929.
Area Served: United States, Puerto
Rico and Canada.
Transportation: Y.

Educational: Has public education
program, including films and
speakers by special request.

Provides follow-up services for
graduates.

◆ *Low Vision Services*

EYE CARE SOCIETIES

**New Jersey Academy of
Ophthalmology**
15 Brant Avenue
Unit #1
Clark, NJ 07066
(908) 388-7130
FAX: (908) 388-7138
Reni Erbos, Executive Director

County/District Where Located:
Union County.

**New Jersey Optometric
Association**
652 Whitehead Road
Trenton, NJ 08648
(609) 695-3456
David Grimm, Director

LOW VISION CENTERS

Camden Optometric Center
612 Benson Street
Camden, NJ 08103
(609) 365-1811
FAX: (609) 964-9054
Dr. Lawrence A. Ragone, Director
MaryAnn Ragone, Assistant
Director

Type of Agency: Non-profit.
County/District Where Located:
Camden County.
Mission: Eye care services for
poor, low income, uninsured
patients.
Funded by: United Way; Lions
Clubs; county funds.
Budget: $280,000.
Hours of Operation: Daily.
Program Accessibility: Three
outreach facilities, mobil vision
clinic.
Staff: Low vision assistants;
ophthalmologist; optometrist;
optometry students; optometry
residents.

History/Date: Est. 1961.
Number of Clients Served: 5,000
to 6,000 yearly.
Eligibility: None.
Area Served: Camden County and
South Jersey.
Age Requirements: None.

Low Vision: Assessments and
rehabilitation available.
Low Vision Aids: Available on
case basis.
Low Vision Follow-up: Yes.

Call for information on local
offices.

**Eye Institute of New Jersey
University of Medicine and
Dentistry**
Doctors Office Center
90 Bergen Street, Suite 6174
Newark, NJ 07103-2469
(201) 982-2054
FAX: (201) 982-2069
Mark Kirstein, O.D., Director
Maria Costa, Administrator

Type of Agency: Non-profit.
County/District Where Located:
Essex County.
Funded by: Client fees.
Hours of Operation: Tuesdays.
Staff: Ophthalmologist;
optometrist; ophthalmology
residents; optician; psychologist/
counselor; audiologist.
Eligibility: None, but referral
report requested.
Age Requirements: None.

Low Vision: Evaluations.
Low Vision Aids: Provided on
loan for trial; no rental fee; on-site
training provided.
Low Vision Follow-up: None.

**The Gerald E. Fonda, M.D., Low
Vision Center of Saint Barnabas**
101 Old Short Hills Road
Suite 102B

West Orange, NJ 07052
(201) 325-6720 or (201) 325-6721
FAX: (201) 325-6522
Marilyn Osman, Administrator

Type of Agency: Non-profit.
Mission: Clinical services, teaching, and research.
Funded by: Client fees and contributions.
Hours of Operation: Thurs.-Fri. 8:00 AM - 1:00 PM.
Staff: Optometrist; low vision assistant.
Eligibility: None.
Area Served: Unlimited.

Counseling/Social Work/Self-Help: Support groups and yearly seminar, "Coping with Macular Degeneration."
Low Vision Aids: Provided on loan for trial; no rental fee. Aids also available for sale.
Low Vision Follow-up: By return appointment in 1-3 months.

◆ *Aging Services*

STATE UNITS ON AGING

**Division on Aging
New Jersey Department of
Community Affairs**
CN807
South Broad and Front Streets
Trenton, NJ 08625-0807
(609) 292-3766 or Information & Referral In State (800) 792-8820
FAX: (609) 633-6609
Ruth Reader, Director

Provides referrals to Area Agencies on Aging and information on other local aging services.

INDEPENDENT LIVING PROGRAMS

New Jersey Commission for the Blind and Visually Impaired
153 Halsey Street, Sixth Floor
P.O. Box 47017

Newark, NJ 07101
(201) 648-2324
FAX: (201) 648-7364
Judith Liebman, Project Director,
(201) 648-4799

Provides independent living services for persons age 55 and over. For further information, contact the Project Director or general phone number listed.

NEW MEXICO

◆ *Educational Services*

STATE SERVICES

New Mexico State Department of Education
Special Education Office
300 Don Gaspar Street
Santa Fe, NM 87501-2786
(505) 827-6541
FAX: (505) 827-6791
Diego D. Gallegos, State Director of Special Education

Type of Agency: State.
Mission: To provide equal educational opportunities for all students; to guarantee that students reach their full potential by mastering learning skills and knowledge and by acquiring desirable personal qualities and values.
Funded by: Public funds.
Staff: 21 special education staff members.
Number of Clients Served: Approximately 35,000 children with disabilities.
Eligibility: In need of special education services as specified under the Individuals with Disabilities Education Act, New Mexico state statutes, and New Mexico Standards for Excellence.
Area Served: New Mexico.

Educational: Special education services are provided by local education agencies and assured by the New Mexico State Department of Education.

For information about local facilities, consult the local superintendent of schools.

EARLY INTERVENTION COORDINATION

Developmental Disabilities Division
New Mexico Department of Health
1190 St. Francis Drive
P.O. Box 26110
Santa Fe, NM 87502-6110
(505) 827-2575
FAX: (505) 827-2455
Marilyn Price, Early Childhood Coordinator

County/District Where Located: Santa Fe County.

SCHOOLS

New Mexico School for the Visually Handicapped
1900 North White Sands Boulevard
Alamogordo, NM 88310
(505) 437-3505
FAX: (505) 439-4411
Kirk Walter, Superintendent
Diane Baker, Principal

Type of Agency: State.
County/District Where Located: Otero County.
Mission: Services for totally blind, legally blind, and visually impaired students, including those with multiple disabilities.
Funded by: Public funds.
Budget: $7.7 million.
Staff: 148 full time. Uses volunteers.
History/Date: Est. 1903.
Eligibility: State resident, blind or visually impaired.
Area Served: New Mexico.
Transportation: Y.

Health: Prescription of spectacles or aids; follow-up evaluation of eye treatment or prescription; general medical services; physical therapy; speech therapy. Contracts for other health services.
Counseling/Social Work/Self-Help: Social evaluation; psychological testing and evaluation; individual, group, family/parent, couple counseling; referral to community services. Refers for other counseling/social work services.
Educational: Grades K through 12. Programs for play/nursery school; college prep; general academic; vocational/skill development. Compensatory skill, technology and transition planning.
Professional Training: Regular in-service training program, short-term or summer training, open to enrollment from other agencies.
Reading: Talking books record players and cassette players; talking book records and cassettes; braille books; large-print books; braille magazines; recorded magazines; information and referral; transcription to braille; translation into Spanish; tape recording services; Optacon; Kurzweil Reading Machine.
Residential: Dormitories.
Rehabilitation: Personal management; braille; handwriting; listening skills; Optacon; typing; home management; orientation/mobility; remedial education; sensory training. Refers and provides consultation to other agencies for other rehabilitation services.
Recreational: Afterschool programs; arts and crafts; hobby groups; swimming; track; wrestling; skiing; gymnastics. Refers for other recreational services.
Employment: Prevocational evaluations; career and skill counseling; occupational skill development; job retention; follow-up service. Refers and provides consultation to other agencies for other employment-oriented services.

Computer Training: Access; training on computer aids and devices.
Low Vision: Evaluations.
Low Vision Aids: Training in the use of prescribed devices.
Low Vision Follow-up: Yes.

Contact local school superintendent for program availability or Special Education Office, New Mexico State Department of Education, Santa Fe, NM 87501-2786, (505) 827-6541.

INFANT AND PRESCHOOL

New Mexico School for the Visually Handicapped Preschool
230 Truman, N.E.
Albuquerque, NM 87108
(505) 268-9506 or (800) 437-3505
FAX: (505) 265-4866
Patrika Griego, Site Facilitator

Type of Agency: State.
County/District Where Located: Bernalillo County.
Mission: To meet the educational needs of visually impaired infant and preschool students who are residents of the state.
Funded by: State.
Hours of Operation: Mon.-Fri. 8:30 AM-3:30 PM.
Program Accessibility: Completely accessible.
Staff: 12.
History/Date: Est. 1975.
Number of Clients Served: 50.
Eligibility: Visual impairment.
Area Served: Albuquerque and surrounding areas.
Age Requirements: 0-6 years.

Health: Functional vision evaluations and adaptive equipment.
Counseling/Social Work/Self-Help: Provides social evaluation; psychological testing/evaluation; counseling; parent counseling

through public school system via a joint powers agreement.
Educational: Instruction in all developmental areas. Consultant services to other programs.
Preschools: Center-based programs: parent, infant, and toddler program (birth through age 3); preschool program (age 3 through 6); home-based program for medically fragile children.
Reading: Talking book records/tapes; braille books; large-print books; magazines in braille/recorded format.
Low Vision: Functional vision evaluations.

STATEWIDE OUTREACH SERVICES

New Mexico School for the Visually Handicapped
1900 North White Sands Boulevard
Alamogordo, NM 88310
(505) 437-3505
FAX: (505) 439-4411
Eileen Kuhre, Director of Outreach Services

Funded by: New Mexico School for the Visually Impaired.
History/Date: Est. 1975.
Age Requirements: Birth to 21.

Assessment: Functional vision assessments, orientation and mobility evaluation, assistive technology assessment.
Consultation to Public Schools: Provides information and support to parents, teachers, therapists, and administrators.
Parent Assistance: Parent counseling.
Materials Production: Braille and recorded books.

INSTRUCTIONAL MATERIALS CENTERS

New Mexico School for the Visually Handicapped
1900 North White Sands Boulevard
Alamogordo, NM 88310
(505) 437-3505, ext. 193
FAX: (505) 439-4411
E-mail: snekuhre@arriba.nm.org
Eileen Kuhre, Director, Outreach/Media Services.

Groups Served: K-12.

Types/Content: Textbooks, recreational, professional.
Media Formats: Braille books, talking books/cassettes, large print books.
Title Listings: No title listings available.

◆ Information Services

LIBRARIES

New Mexico State Library for the Blind and Physically Handicapped
325 Don Gaspar Street
Santa Fe, NM 87501
(505) 827-3830 or toll-free in New Mexico (800) 456-5515
FAX: (505) 827-3888
John Brewster, Manager

Funded by: Public funds.
History/Date: Est. 1967.
Area Served: New Mexico.

Distributes talking books and play-back machines to blind and physically handicapped patrons in New Mexico.

PHONE-IN NEWSPAPERS

Newsline for the Blind
New Mexico Commission for the Blind
2200 Yale Boulevard, S.E.

Albuquerque, NM 87106
(505) 841-8844
Nancy J. Hendrickson, Contact
Person
Michael J. Santullo, Director

Newspapers Read: *Albuquerque Journal, Albuquerque Tribune, University of New Mexico Lobo, Wall Street Journal, Time Magazine, New Mexico Magazine, NM Business Journal, Santa Fean, Los Alamos Monitor (daily).*

♦ *Rehabilitation Services*

STATE SERVICES

New Mexico Commission for the Blind
PERA Building, Room 553
Santa Fe, NM 87503
(505) 827-4479
FAX: (505) 827-4475
Gary Haug, Director

Type of Agency: State.
Mission: Services for totally blind, legally blind, visually impaired, deaf-blind, and older blind persons.
Funded by: State funds.
Hours of Operation: Mon. - Fri. 7:30 AM - 5:00 PM.
Staff: 52 full time, 2 part time. Uses volunteers.
History/Date: Est. 1935.
Eligibility: Visual impairment or deteriorating eye condition.
Area Served: Statewide.
Transportation: Y.
Age Requirements: 18 years and older.

Health: Occupational therapy. Contracts, refers, and provides consultation to other agencies for other health services.
Counseling/Social Work/Self-Help: Psychological testing and evaluation; individual, group, family/parent, couple counseling. Contracts, refers for and provides consultation to other agencies on counseling/social work services.
Educational: Accepts deaf-blind, emotionally disturbed, mentally retarded, or orthopedically disabled persons. Programs for college prep; vocational/skill development.
Professional Training: Internship/fieldwork placement in industrial arts; low vision; orientation/mobility; vocational rehabilitation. Regular in-service training programs.
Residential: Dormitory for adults; elderly persons; multiply disabled persons.
Rehabilitation: Personal management; braille; handwriting; typing; video magnifier; Optacon; home management; orientation/mobility; rehabilitation teaching in client's home and community; remedial education; sensory training.
Recreational: Adult continuing education; arts and crafts; hobby groups; special programs for elderly; bowling; swimming. Contracts, refers, and provides consultation to other agencies for recreational services.
Employment: Prevocational evaluation; career and skill counseling; occupational skill development; job retention; job retraining; sheltered workshops; vocational placement; follow-up service; vending facility training and placement.
Computer Training: Training on computer aids and devices.
Low Vision: Low vision service/clinic.
Low Vision Aids: Prescription of spectacles and low vision aids and devices.
Low Vision Follow-up: Follow-up evaluation of eye treatment or prescriptions.

Local Offices:

Alamogordo: Field Office, Commission for the Blind, 408 North White Sands Boulevard, Alamogordo, NM 88310, (505) 437-8008, FAX (505) 434-3713.
Alamogordo: Rehabilitation-Orientation Center for the Blind, 408 North White Sands Boulevard, Alamogordo, NM 88310, (505) 437-0401, FAX (505) 434-3713.
Albuquerque: New Mexico Industries for the Blind, 2200 Yale Boulevard S.E., Albuquerque, NM 87106, (505) 841-8844, FAX (505) 841-8850.
Albuquerque: Field Office, Commission for the Blind, 2200 Yale Boulevard, S.E., Albuquerque, NM 87106, (505) 841-8844, FAX (505) 841-8854.
Albuquerque: Newsline for the Blind, 2200 Yale Boulevard, S.E., Albuquerque, NM 87106, (505) 841-8844, FAX (505) 841-8850.
Farmington: Field Office, Commission for the Blind, 800 East 30th Street, Suite E, Farmington, NM 87401, (505) 327-7789.
Las Cruces: Field Office, Commision for the Blind, 301 South Church, Suite C, Dona Ana Savings Office Plaza, Las Cruces, NM 88001, (505) 524-6450, FAX (505) 524-6455.
Las Vegas: Field Office, Commission for the Blind, 700 Friedman Avenue, Las Vegas, NM 87701, (505) 425-3546, FAX (505) 454-6120.
Roswell: Field Office, Commission for the Blind, 400 North Pennsylvania, Suite 1080, Roswell, NM 88201, (505) 624-6140, FAX (505) 624-6142.
Santa Fe: Field Office, Commission for the Blind, 1313 St. Francis Drive, Santa Fe, NM 87503, (505) 827-3768, FAX (505) 827-3759.

COMPUTER TRAINING CENTERS

New Mexico School for the Visually Handicapped
1900 North White Sands Boulevard
Alamogordo, NM 88310
(505) 437-3505
FAX: (505) 437-7851
Retha Coburn, Coordinator

County/District Where Located:
Otero County.

Computer Training: Speech output systems; screen magnification systems; braille access systems; optical character recognition systems; closed-circuit television systems; word processing; database software; training for instructors.

♦ Low Vision Services

EYE CARE SOCIETIES

New Mexico Ophthalmological Society
1100 Lead S.E.
Albuquerque, NM 87106
(505) 842-1844
FAX: (505) 768-1360
Richard A. Gray, MD, President

New Mexico Optometric Association, Inc.
10131 Coors Road, NW, #227
Albuquerque, NM 87114
(505) 898-6885
Richard Montoya, President

LOW VISION CENTERS

New Mexico Commission for the Blind
Low Vision Clinic
2200 Yale Boulevard, S.E.

Albuquerque, NM 87106
(505) 841-8844
FAX: (505) 841-8850
Adelmo Vigil, Deputy Director

County/District Where Located:
Bernalillo County.
Funded by: State.
Hours of Operation: 40 hours per week.
Staff: 3.
Number of Clients Served: 39 weekly.
Eligibility: Legally blind; ophthalmologist's report.
Area Served: New Mexico.

Counseling/Social Work/Self-Help: Self-help group.
Low Vision Aids: On-site or at home training provided.
Low Vision Follow-up: By return appointment.

♦ Aging Services

STATE UNITS ON AGING

State Agency on Aging
228 East Palace Avenue
La Villa Rivera Building,
Fourth Floor
Santa Fe, NM 87501
(505) 827-7640 or Information & Referral In State (800) 432-2080
FAX: (505) 827-7649
Michelle Lujan Grishan, Director

Provides referrals to Area Agencies on Aging and information on other local aging services.

INDEPENDENT LIVING PROGRAMS

New Mexico Commission for the Blind
PERA Building, Room 553
Santa Fe, NM 87503
(505) 827-4479
FAX: (505) 827-4475
Gary Haug, Director

Provides independent living services for persons age 55 and over. For further information, contact the Project Director or general phone number listed.

NEW YORK

◆ *Educational Services*

STATE SERVICES

New York State Education Department
Office for Special Education Services
One Commerce Plaza
Room 1624
Albany, NY 12234
(518) 486-9592
FAX: (518) 473-5387
Thomas B. Neveldine, Executive Coordinator

Type of Agency: State.
Mission: Provides in-service training for teachers of visually impaired children in local schools. Provides consultation on educational services for school-age legally blind and severely visually impaired students. Processes state appointments for legally blind children to the state-operated and state-supported schools for the blind. Administers the federal subsidy American Printing House for the Blind quota program for the purchase of reading material and educational aids for legally blind students in primary and secondary schools in New York State.
Funded by: Public funds.
Hours of Operation: 8:30 AM - 4:00 PM.
History/Date: Est. 1926.
Eligibility: Blind and visually impaired persons.
Area Served: New York State.
Age Requirements: Birth - 21 years.

Educational: Y.
Preschools: Consulting services available.

Contact regional Board of Cooperative Educational Services or local school superintendent for program availability.

EARLY INTERVENTION COORDINATION

Early Intervention Program
New York Department of Health
Empire State Plaza
Corning Tower, Room 208
Albany, NY 12237-0618
(518) 473-7016
FAX: (518) 473-8673
E-mail: dmn02@health.state.ny.us
Donna Noyes, Director

SCHOOLS

Lavelle School for the Blind
3830 Paulding Avenue
Bronx, NY 10469
(718) 882-1212
FAX: (718) 882-0005
Sister Louis Marie Baxter, O.P., Superintendent
Maria Galloway, Intake Coordinator
Sister Angelus Healy, O.P., Intake Coordinator

Type of Agency: Private; non-profit.
Mission: To provide an integrated education program for children with blindness and multiple handicaps who often need to interact socially and environmentally to facilitate learning.
Funded by: Private donations; and state funds.
Hours of Operation: 8:00 AM - 4:00 PM.
Staff: 70 full time.
History/Date: Est. 1904.
Number of Clients Served: 100.
Eligibility: Blind/visually impaired with multiple disabilities; ambulatory.

Area Served: The five boroughs of New York City, Nassau County and lower Westchester County.
Transportation: Y.
Age Requirements: 3 - 21 years.

Health: Full-time registered nurse. Contracted medical professionals to assess and monitor medical needs and concerns.
Counseling/Social Work/Self-Help: Career counseling; psychological testing and evaluation; individual, group, family/parent counseling; referral to community services.
Educational: New York State curriculum with adaptations to meet children's individual education programs; orientation/mobility; self-help; use of special equipment; auditory training; visual training; occupational education; daily living skills.
Preschools: Classroom for visually impaired, multiply disabled children.
Professional Training: Inservice and ongoing workshops.
Reading: Talking book record players and cassette players; talking book records and cassettes; braille books; large-print books; braille magazines; recorded magazines on disk.
Rehabilitation: Training in orientation and mobility; daily living skills; occupational education; use of adaptive equipment; speech therapy.
Employment: Experience-based career education.
Low Vision: Clinic with 2 low vision specialists.
Low Vision Aids: As prescribed.
Low Vision Follow-up: On-staff optomotrists.

New York Institute for Special Education
999 Pelham Parkway

Bronx, NY 10469
(718) 519-7000
FAX: (718) 231-9314
E-mail: nyise@ao.com
URL: http://www.nyise.org
Robert L. Guarino, Ph.D.,
Executive Director

Type of Agency: Educational.
County/District Where Located:
Bronx County, District 11.
Funded by: Public funds,
endowment and contributions.
Budget: 1996: $18,000,000.
Hours of Operation: 8:30 AM -
5:00 PM.
Staff: 250 full time.
History/Date: Est. 1831 as the
New York Institute for the
Education of the Blind.
Number of Clients Served: 1996:
300.
Eligibility: Legally blind,
emotionally disturbed and
learning disabled students, and
developmentally delayed
preschoolers.
Area Served: New York State.
Transportation: Y.
Age Requirements: 3 - 5 years:
developmentally delayed program;
5 - 21 years: visually impaired
program; 5 - 13 years: learning
disabled program.

Health: Diagnosis and evaluation
of eye, ear conditions; speech
therapy; adaptive program;
occupational and physical
therapies.
**Counseling/Social Work/Self-
Help:** Psychological testing and
evaluation; casework.
Educational: K through 12th
grade. Music and art education
and therapies.
Professional Training: Serves as
pre-service training site for many
universities and colleges.
Residential: 5 days a week.
Rehabilitation: Personal
management; orientation/

mobility; communications; skills
including adaptive technology.
Recreational: Evening program
for residential students; summer
day camp for visually impaired
children.
Employment: Evaluation,
prevocational and vocational
training.
Computer Training: Access;
training on computer aids and
devices.

New York State School for the Blind
Richmond Avenue
Batavia, NY 14020
(716) 343-5384
FAX: (716) 344-5557
Robert Seibold, Superintendent

Type of Agency: State.
County/District Where Located:
Genessee County.
Mission: Services for deaf-blind,
multiply handicapped blind.
Staff: 150 full time, 20 part time.
Uses volunteers.
History/Date: Est. 1868.
Eligibility: Legally blind.
Age Requirements: 5 to 21 years.

Health: General medical services;
physical, speech, occupational
therapies. Contracts and refers for
other health services.
**Counseling/Social Work/Self-
Help:** Social evaluation;
psychological testing and
evaluation; individual, group
counseling. Refers and provides
consultation to other agencies for
other counseling/social work
services.
Educational: Individualized
educational programs designed to
meet students' needs at varying
developmental levels. Includes
prevocational/skill training;
activities of daily living; leisure
time activities; orientation/
mobility; academics.

Professional Training:
Internship/fieldwork placement in
all program areas. Regular in-
service training programs.
Reading: Talking book record
player and cassette player; talking
book records and cassettes; braille
books; large print books; braille
magazines; recorded magazines;
information and referral; special
collection; transcription to braille;
tape recording services on
demand; Optacon and closed
circuit television.
Residential: Program will
accommodate those students
whose educational needs require
year-round, 7-day residential
status. Day programs and 5-day
residential capacity.
Rehabilitation: Personal
management; braille; gesticulation;
handwriting; listening skills;
Optacon; typing; video magnifier;
home management; orientation/
mobility; special education;
sensory training.
Recreational: Recreational
therapists develop individual/
group activities including
afterschool programs; bowling;
swimming; track; wrestling.
Low Vision: Low vision service;
low vision aids and devices.

INFANT AND PRESCHOOL
**Child Development Center
The Lighthouse Inc.**
111 East 59th Street
New York, NY 10022
(212) 821-9600
FAX: (212) 821-9656
Frank Simpson, Vice President for
Program Development
Catherine Kerins Wheeler,
Director, Early Childhood
Programs

Type of Agency: Private; non-
profit.
Mission: To enable the acquisition
of skills for functioning as

independently and interdependently as possible in school, at home and in the community. Integration of adaptive skills and adaptive equipment in everyday living and learning situations.

Funded by: Tuition; reimbursement from government agencies; private donations; fees for non-disabled students.

Program Accessibility: Handicaped accessible.

Staff: Specialists in early childhood education, special education, and education of students with visual impairments; staff in social work, occupational therapy, speech therapy, and physical therapy; other specialists are available to provide services in additional areas.

Number of Clients Served: FY '96: 104.

Transportation: Y.

Age Requirements: 0-6 years.

Health: Services available on consultant or referral basis.

Counseling/Social Work/Self-Help: Parent and family counseling; case management.

Educational: Instruction in all developmental areas.

Low Vision: Low vision exams, devices, and instruction available on premises.

Center-based programs and models (parent-infant training, early intervention, preschool, school-age program and an integrated classroom) for children with visual impairment and, often, other disabilities. Preschool children without disabilities are enrolled in the integrated classroom. A variety of specialists provide services. Programs are also located at The Lighthouse Inc., 65-05 Woodhaven Boulevard, Elmhurst, NY 11373, (718) 899-9100.

Helen Keller Services for the Blind

57 Willoughby Street
Brooklyn, NY 11201
(718) 522-2122
FAX: (718) 935-9463
URL: http://www.helenkeller.com
Fred W. McPhilliamy, President
John P. Lynch, Director
Garth White, Principal

Type of Agency: Private; non-profit.

Mission: To enable persons of all ages who are visually impaired, blind, or deaf-blind to lead as independent a life as possible.

Funded by: Income from capital funds; United Way, state, federal, and local government contracts and fees.

Hours of Operation: Mon.-Fri. 8:30 AM-4:30 PM.

Program Accessibility: Accessible.

Staff: 1 full-time principal; 4 full-time teachers; 6 full-time teaching assistants; 1 full-time social worker, part-time physical therapist, psychologist, physician, occupational therapist, and speech therapist.

History/Date: Est. 1950; founded 1892.

Number of Clients Served: 37.

Eligibility: Visually impaired children; legally blind.

Area Served: Kings and Queens Counties.

Transportation: Y.

Age Requirements: 0-5 years.

Health: Physical therapy, occupational therapy, and other health services available on consultant or referral basis.

Counseling/Social Work/Self-Help: Parent and family counseling.

Educational: Instruction in all developmental areas, home- and center-based with services for visually impaired multiply disabled infants, 0-5 years. Consultant services to other programs for children, 0-5 years, within itinerant model.

Preschools: Assists with placement in appropriate nursery schools, specialized programs, or public schools.

Low Vision: Low vision exams.

Local Offices:

Hempstead: Nassau Service Center, One Helen Keller Way, Hempstead, NY 11550, (516) 485-1234, Joanne Berger, Supervisor, Children's Services.

Huntington: Suffolk Service Center, Huntington, NY 11743, (516) 424-0022, Debbie Storace, Social Worker, Children's Services.

Jewish Guild for the Blind (The Guild)

15 West 65th Street
New York, NY 10023
(212) 769-6200
FAX: (212) 769-6266
Alan R. Morse, President and Chief Executive Officer
Ellen Trief, Ed.D., Director of Early Intervention Program

Type of Agency: Private; non-profit.

Mission: To simulate and enhance timely achievement of developmental milestones in early childhood; to help visually impaired children attain age-appropriate competencies and skills and become integrated into a preschool program; to lay the foundation for positive future educational experiences for visually impaired children.

Funded by: Private donations and other sources.

Hours of Operation: 8:00 AM-5:00 PM. Evening hours by appointment only.

Program Accessibility: Handicapped accessible.
Staff: Specialists in child development as well as social work and psychology.
Number of Clients Served: 60 infants and children.
Eligibility: Visual impairment.
Area Served: Metropolitan New York area.
Transportation: Y.
Age Requirements: 0-2 years.

Health: Low vision exams; immunizations and blood tests available on a consultant or referral basis.
Counseling/Social Work/Self-Help: Parent and other counseling.
Educational: Provides instruction in all developmental areas; orientation/mobility; bilingual. Community-based program for visually impaired multiply disabled infants. Preschool program for children ages 3 to 5.
Preschools: Preschool program for visually impaired children ages 3 to 5. Early Intervention Program for infants to age 3.
Low Vision: Low vision services on premises.
Low Vision Aids: Available.
Low Vision Follow-up: Y.

Staff provides instruction in areas of vision rehabilitation, sensory simulation, motor development, speech, music and art therapy, as well as physical and occupational therapy and socialization.

Lavelle School for the Blind
3830 Paulding Avenue

Bronx, NY 10469
(718) 882-1212
FAX: (718) 882-0005
Sister Louis Marie Baxter, O.P., Superintendent
Sister Angelus Healy, O.P., Principal
Maria Galloway, Intake Coordinator

Type of Agency: Private; non-profit.
Mission: To provide an integrated program for children with blindness and multiple handicaps who often need to interact socially and environmentally to facilitate learning.
Funded by: P.L. 914-142 monies, private donations and state funds.
Hours of Operation: 8:00 AM-4:00 PM.
Staff: 10 full time including related service providers.
History/Date: Est. 1988.
Number of Clients Served: 12.
Eligibility: Blind or visually impaired (with or without disabilities); ambulatory.
Area Served: The five boroughs of New York City; Nassau County; and lower Westchester County.
Transportation: Y.
Age Requirements: 3-5 years.

Health: Full-time registerd nurse, also contracted medical professionals assess and monitor medical needs and concerns.
Counseling/Social Work/Self-Help: Psychological testing and evaluation, family/parent counseling, referral to community services as appropriate. General social skills and counseling are provided and integrated into the education programs.
Educational: The modified, academic/funcitonal curriculum is tailored to meet the students' strengths and needs.
Preschools: Classrooms contain equipment adapted to meet the

needs of children who are blind/visually impaired and multiply-disabled.
Reading: Pre-readiness skills.
Rehabilitation: Orientation and mobility; sensory training (low vision, hearing services are provided as appropriate), self-help skills (including daily living skills).
Recreational: Field trips, adaptive physical education, weekly Achilles Club activities and special events.
Computer Training: Kindergarten only.
Low Vision: Clinic with two low vision specialists.
Low Vision Aids: As prescribed.
Low Vision Follow-up: On-staff optometrists.

The Lighthouse Inc.
Hudson Valley
44 Church Street
White Plains, NY 10601
(914) 761-3221
FAX: (914) 761-0484
Judith Millman, Vice President, Hudson Valley Region
Joanne Hallinan-Bases, Special Educator for Visually Impaired

Type of Agency: Private; non-profit.
Funded by: State, federal and local government contracts and fees; donations.
Staff: Teacher of early childhood/visually impaired; social worker; vision rehabilition therapists; low vision clinician.
Number of Clients Served: 31.
Age Requirements: 0-5.

Counseling/Social Work/Self-Help: Family counseling, self-help information/support groups.
Educational: Early intervention service. Evaluations of vision, gross and fine motor skills, language and social development. Instruction in all developmental

areas for visually impaired/ multiply disabled children; home or community-based individual sessions with children and parent/caregiver.

Consultation provided to center-based community programs, center-based agencies serving children with visual impairments. Low vision exams available with pediatric low vision specialist. Follow-up instruction in child's home or school.

STATEWIDE OUTREACH SERVICES

Resource Center for the Visually Impaired
New York State School for the Blind
Richmond Avenue
Batavia, NY 14020
(716) 343-5384 or (716) 343-8100
FAX: (716) 343-3711
E-mail: nysrescnter@aol.com
Emily Leyenberger, Ph.D.,
Coordinator

Funded by: Title VI B discretionary funds.
History/Date: Est. 1986.
Age Requirements: 0-21 years.

Assessment: Functional vision assessments provided when not available at local schools.
Consultation to Public Schools: Provides information and support to parents, teachers, administrators, and others concerning educational need of visually impaired students.
Parent Assistance: Library of resources for parents and professionals; facilitates communication and collaboration among parents and schools.
Professional Training: Specialized training and workshops according to need for teachers, aides, school nurses,

about the implications of visual impairments.

INSTRUCTIONAL MATERIALS CENTERS

Resource Center for the Visually Impaired
New York State School for the Blind
Richmond Avenue
Batavia, NY 14020
(716) 343-8100
FAX: (716) 343-3711
E-mail: nysrescntr@aol.com
Emily Leyenberger, Ph.D.,
Coordinator

Area Served: New York State.
Groups Served: 0-21 years of age.

Types/Content: Textbooks, recreational, career/vocational, professional topics.
Media Formats: Braille/large-print books, regular-print professional books, pamphlets.
Title Listings: Provides lists, at no charge, of assessments collection, curricula collection, large-print recreational reading, and Twin Vision books.

UNIVERSITY TRAINING PROGRAMS

Dominican College
10 Western Highway
Orangeburg, NY 10962
(914) 359-7800 or (914) 359-3577
FAX: (914) 359-2313
Dr. Rona Shaw, Visually
Handicapped Teaching

Programs Offered: Undergraduate programs for teachers of visually impaired.

D'Youville College
Division of Education
320 Porter Avenue

Buffalo, NY 14201
(716) 881-7629
Dr. Sheila Dunn, Director,
Education Department

County/District Where Located:
Erie County.

Programs Offered: Undergraduate program for teachers of the visually impaired.

Hunter College, City University of New York
Department of Special Education
695 Park Avenue
New York, NY 10021
(212) 772-4740
FAX: (212) 650-3542
E-mail: rsilberm@shiva.hunter.
cuny.edu
Dr. Rosanne K. Silberman

Programs Offered: Graduate (master's) programs for teachers of learners with blindness and visual impairments, severe/multiple impairments including deaf-blindness, rehabilitation teachers of individuals with blindness and visual impairments, and orientation and mobility instuctors.

New York University
School of Education
Rehabilitation Counseling Program
35 West Fourth Street, Suite 1200
Education Building
New York, NY 10012
(212) 998-5290
FAX: (212) 995-4192
Dr. Nancy Esibill, Director

County/District Where Located:
Manhattan County.

Programs Offered: Master's and doctoral degrees in rehabilitation counseling.

Teachers College, Columbia University
Department of Health and Behavioral Studies
525 West 120th Street
Box 223
New York, NY 10027
(212) 678-3814 or (212) 678-3878
E-mail: vss5@%columbia.edu
Virginia Stolarski, Coordinator

Programs Offered: Graduate (master's) programs for teachers of blind and visually impaired learners.

◆ Information Services

LIBRARIES

Andrew Heiskell Library for the Blind and Physically Handicapped
New York Public Library
40 West 20th Street
New York, NY 10011
(212) 206-5400 or (212) 206-5499
FAX: (212) 206-5418
Bonnie Birman, Regional Librarian

Regional library providing books and magazines in braille and on disk and cassette. Lends cassette players and special record players; provides reference, information, and referral services.

M.C. Migel Memorial Library/ Information Center
American Foundation for the Blind
11 Penn Plaza
Suite 300
New York, NY 10001
(212) 502-7660 or TDD (212) 502-7662 or (800) 232-5463
FAX: (212) 502-7771
E-mail: afbinfo@afb.org
URL: http://www.afb.org
Elga Joffee, Director

Type of Agency: Library and information center that houses one of the largest research collections of print materials related to all nonmedical aspects of blindness and low vision in the world.
Mission: Provides reference consultations and a wide range of information and referral services for the general public as well as for professionals in the blindness and low vision fields.
Program Accessibility: Wheelchair accessible; a wide range of adaptive equipment available, including Reading Edge, CCTV, and TDD equipment. Bibliographies on a wide range of subjects available in audio, braille, and disk formats.

Reading: Volunteer reading and taping.

Includes the Helen Keller Archives, photo collections of historic interest, and a rare book collection.

New York Public Library Project ACCESS
Mid-Manhattan Library
455 Fifth Avenue
New York, NY 10016
(212) 340-0843 or TDD (212) 340-0931

Type of Agency: Largest resource library in the New York Public Library's branch system.
County/District Where Located: Manhattan County.
Mission: Links patrons with visual, hearing, learning, and mobility impairments to the full range of the New York Public Library's materials and services.
Hours of Operation: All services by appointment so that individualized assistance may be provided.
Program Accessibility: Located on wheelchair-accessible second floor. Special equipment for blind and visually impaired persons: magnifiers; braille writer and audio playback equipment; Kurzweil Personal Reader with English, Spanish, and French language capabilities; Jaws for Windows, Open Book software, Large Print DOS; closed circuit televisions.

Reference collection of disability-related directories; pamphlets; newsletters; and publishers'/ vendors' catalogs.

New York State Talking Book and Braille Library
Cultural Education Center
Empire State Plaza
Albany, NY 12230
(518) 474-5935 or toll-free (800) 342-3688
FAX: (518) 474-5786
Jane Somers, Director

Type of Agency: State regional library for the Library of Congress National Library Service for the Blind and Physically Handicapped.
Hours of Operation: Mon.-Fri. 8:00 AM-4:30 PM.
Staff: 21.
History/Date: Est. 1896.
Number of Clients Served: 37,000.
Area Served: New York State (excluding New York City and Long Island).

Reading: Braille and recorded formats. Closed-circuit magnification devices available.

Provides books and magazines in braille and recorded on disks and cassettes. Lends cassette players and special record players for use with its recorded material. Reference, information, and referral services provided.

Queens Borough Public Library Special Services

89-11 Merrick Boulevard
Jamaica, NY 11432
(718) 990-0746 (voice) or TDD
(718) 990-0809
FAX: (718) 658-8312
URL: http://
www.queens.lib.ny.us
Nancy Titolo, Assistant Manager
Eileen Gellman, Community
Assistant

Type of Agency: Public.
Mission: Increases access to the materials and services of the Queens Borough Public Library for older adults and persons with disabilities.
Funded by: Public funds.
Hours of Operation: Mon.-Fri. 10:00 AM-5:00 PM.
History/Date: Est. 1981.
Area Served: Borough of Queens.

Low Vision Aids: Closed-circuit televisions; magnifiers.

Special equipment includes Kurzweil Personal Reader, VTEK, Perkins brailler, and telecommunication device for the deaf (TDD). Volunteer reading service provides recorded materials for visually impaired and learning disabled persons. Books in large print are available in all branch libraries. Mail-a-book service provides books in regular, large-print, and audio formats postage free to homebound users.

**Ruth M. Shellens Library
The Lighthouse Inc.**

111 East 59th Street
New York, NY 10022
(212) 821-9680 or TDD (212) 821-9713
FAX: (212) 821-9707
Andrew Stevenson, Director, Information Resources

Type of Agency: Library that houses a collection of Talking Books, commercial audio cassettes, large print books, and braille magazines and books, as well as collections in social work, education, psychology, sociology, and vision research.
Mission: Provides access to printed material for people who are blind or partially sighted.
Program Accessibility: Handicapped accessible; adaptive equipment and information systems available, including an accessible computerized library catalog; Kurzweil Reading Edge machines, CCTVs, and TDD.

Reading: Volunteer reading and recording service.

Stephanie Joyce Kahn Foundation (SJK)

2-12 West Park Avenue
Long Beach, NY 11561
(516) 889-5105
FAX: (516) 889-5201
Stephanie Joyce Kahn, Contact Person

County/District Where Located: Nassau County.
Area Served: Long Island, NY.

Mobile audio library that distributes audio cassette recordings of books and magazines to homebound individuals, hosptial patients, and nursing home residents.

**Talking Books
Nassau Library System**

900 Jerusalem Avenue
Uniondale, NY 11553
(516) 292-8920 or TDD (516) 579-8585
FAX: (516) 481-4777
Dorothy Puryear, Acting Librarian

Subregional library.

**Talking Books Plus
Outreach Services**

Suffolk Cooperative Library System
627 North Sunrise Service Road
Bellport, NY 11713
(516) 286-1600 or TDD (516) 286-4546
FAX: (516) 286-1647
Julie Klauber, Librarian

Subregional library.

MEDIA PRODUCTION SERVICES

Braille Transcribers of Central New York, Inc.

154 Homewood Drive
Clinton, NY 13323
(315) 853-2679
Catharine Hugo, Director of Reader Services

County/District Where Located: Oneida County.
Area Served: Central New York given priority; nationwide requests accepted.
Groups Served: K-12, college students, other adults.

Types/Content: Textbooks; recreational; career/vocational; religious.
Media Formats: Braille books, talking books/cassettes.
Title Listings: Not yet available.

**Educational Vision Services
New York City Public Schools, District 75**

22 East 28th Street
New York, NY 10016
(212) 481-5660
FAX: (212) 251-0602
Dr. Laurence R. Gardner, Interim Acting Director

County/District Where Located: Manhattan County.
Area Served: New York City.
Groups Served: K-12.

Types/Content: Textbooks, career/vocational.
Media Formats: Braille books, large print books, newspapers, magazines, books on cassette.

Helen Keller Services for the Blind/Braille Library

One Helen Keller Way
Hempstead, NY 11550
(516) 485-1234
FAX: (516) 538-6785
Geralyn Zuzze, Director

County/District Where Located: Nassau County.
Area Served: Nationwide.
Groups Served: K-12.

Types/Content: Textbooks.
Media Formats: Braille/large-print books.
Title Listings: No title listings available.

Jewish Heritage for the Blind

1655 East 24th Street
Brooklyn, NY 11229
(718) 338-4999
Rabbi David H. Toiv, Director

Nassau Community College Library

11530 Steward Avenue
Garden City, NY 11530
(516) 572-7883
FAX: (516) 572-7503
Arthur L. Friedman, Coordinator, "Round Pages" Program

County/District Where Located: Nassau County.
Groups Served: College students.

Types/Content: Textbooks.
Media Formats: Talking books/cassettes.

Onondaga Braillists

P.O. Box 326
Syracuse, NY 13215
(315) 475-6407
Jean Henderson, Director of Reading Services

County/District Where Located: Onondaga County.
Area Served: Canada and United States.
Groups Served: K-12, college students, other adults.

Types/Content: Textbooks, recreational, career/vocational, religious, general.
Media Formats: Braille books.
Title Listings: No title listings available.

Recording for the Blind and Dyslexic

545 Fifth Avenue
Suite 204
New York, NY 10017
(212) 557-5720
FAX: (212) 557-5789
E-mail: new_york@rfbd.org
Myra Shein, Studio Director

See Recording for the Blind and Dyslexic in U.S. national listings.

Sisterhood Braille Group of East Midwood Jewish Center

1625 Ocean Avenue
Brooklyn, NY 11230
(718) 338-3800 or (914) 235-4972
Sylvia Aig, Chairperson

County/District Where Located: Kings County.
Area Served: New York City metropolitan area.
Groups Served: None specified.

Types/Content: Textbooks, recreational, career/vocational, religious, foreign language.
Media Formats: Braille books.

Sisterhood of Temple Sinai

425 Roslyn Road
Roslyn Heights, NY 11577
(516) 621-6800
FAX: (516) 625-6020
Dr. Dorothy Axelroth, Chairperson

County/District Where Located: Nassau County.
Groups Served: Jewish Braille Institute of America; other requests considered whenever possible.

Types/Content: Recreational; religious.
Media Formats: Talking books.
Title Listings: None specified.

Sisterhood Temple Israel of Jamaica

188th Street and Grand Central Parkway
Holliswood, NY 11423
(718) 776-4400
FAX: (718) 740-8795
Gertrude Steinberg, Braille Chairperson

County/District Where Located: Queens County.
Groups Served: Jewish Braille Institute.

Media Formats: Braille books, talking books/cassettes, large-print books.
Title Listings: Braille lists supplied at no charge.

Spencerport Braille Association

43 Wainswright Circle
Rochester, NY 14626
(716) 227-1639
Beckie Cator, Work Chairperson

County/District Where Located: Monroe County.
Groups Served: K-12, college students, other adults.

Types/Content: Textbooks, recreational, career/vocational, religious, mathematics.
Media Formats: Braille books, computers.

Title Listings: No title listings available.

RADIO READING

IN TOUCH Networks
15 West 65th Street
New York, NY 10023
(212) 769-6270 or (800) 456-3166
FAX: (212) 769-6266
E-mail: bemass@aol.com
Bruce Massis, General Manager

Funded by: Donations.
Hours of Operation: 24 hours a day, 7 days a week.
Staff: 4.
History/Date: Est. 1978.
Area Served: New York metropolitan/tri-state area, closed circuit radio, cable service transmitted via satellite.

Niagara Frontier Radio Reading Service
P.O. Box 575
Buffalo, NY 14225
(716) 668-8888
Robert Sikorski, President

County/District Where Located:
Erie County.
Hours of Operation: 24 hours.
History/Date: Est. 1987.
Area Served: Western New York; Southern Ontario, Canada.

Northeast Radio Reading Service
159 Margaret Street
Suite 202
Plattsburgh, NY 12901
(518) 563-9058
FAX: (518) 563-0292
Andrew Pulrang, Director

County/District Where Located:
Clinton County.
Hours of Operation: Mon.-Fri 9:00 AM-5:00 PM.

Radio Vision-Ramapo Catskill Library System
619 North Street
Middletown, NY 10940
(914) 343-1131 or toll-free in New York State (800) 327-7343
FAX: (914) 343-1205
Dan Hulse, Director

County/District Where Located:
Orange County.
Hours of Operation: 24 hours a day, 7 days a week. Connects with In Touch Networks (NYC) Mon.-Fri. 9:00 PM-9:00 AM and on Saturday and Sunday all day.
Staff: 1.
History/Date: Est. 1979.
Area Served: Orange, Sullivan, Ulster, Dutchess, Putnam, parts of Columbia, Green, Rockland Counties.

RISE
c/o WMHT-FM
P.O. Box 17
Schenectady, NY 12301
(518) 357-1700
FAX: (518) 357-1709
Joyce M. Bach, Administrative Supervisor
Liz Hood, Radio Director

County/District Where Located:
Rotterdam County.
Hours of Operation: 24 hours a day, 7 days a week.
Staff: 3.
History/Date: Est. 1978.
Area Served: 13-county area surrounding Albany Capitol District of New York State.
Age Requirements: None.

UPDATE
Chautauqua-Cattaraugus Library System
106 West Fifth Street
P.O. Box 730

Jamestown, NY 14701-0730
(716) 484-7135
Helen K. Bolton, Outreach Librarian

County/District Where Located:
Chautauqua County.
Hours of Operation: Mon.-Fri. 8:00 AM- 5:00 PM.
History/Date: Est. 1996.
Area Served: Chautauqua and Cattaraugus Counties.

WCNY-READ-OUT Radio Reading Service
P.O. Box 2400
Syracuse, NY 13220-2400
(315) 453-2424
FAX: (315) 451-8824
E-mail: marian_carfagno@wcny. pbs.org
URL: http://www.wcny.org
Marian Carfagno, Reading Service Coordinator

Hours of Operation: 19 hours a day, 7 days a week.
History/Date: Est. 1982.
Area Served: Syracuse, Watertown, Utica, Ithaca and their environs.

WXXI Reachout Radio
280 State Street
Rochester, NY 14614
(716) 325-7500 or (716) 258-0333
FAX: (716) 258-0339
E-mail: ruth_phinney@wxxi.pbs. org
URL: http://www.wxxi.org
Ruth Phinney, Director

County/District Where Located:
Monroe County.
Funded by: WXXI Public Broadcasting Council, Inc. and Association for the Blind and Visually Impaired - Goodwill Industries of Greater Rochester, Inc.
Hours of Operation: Mon.-Fri. 9:00 AM-5:00 PM; Broadcast 24 hours a day.

Staff: 2 full-time, 1 part-time, 4 irregular.
History/Date: Est. 1984.
Eligibility: Visually or physically print handicapped.
Area Served: Rochester and 10 surrounding counties.
Age Requirements: None.

INFORMATION AND REFERRAL

American Foundation for the Blind

11 Penn Plaza, Suite 300
New York, NY 10001
(212) 502-7600 or (800) 232-5463 or
TDD (212) 502-7662
FAX: (212) 502-7777
E-mail: afbinfo@afb.org
URL: http://www.afb.org
Carl R. Augusto, President

See American Foundation for the Blind in U.S. national listings.

Cattaraugus County Association for the Blind and Visually Handicapped, Inc.

712 Wayne Street
Suite 1 West
Olean, NY 14760
(716) 373-2222
FAX: (716) 373-2222
Jacqueline Carroll, Administrator

Type of Agency: Private; non-profit.
County/District Where Located: Cattaraugus County.
Funded by: County funds.
Staff: 2 full time plus volunteers.
History/Date: Inc. 1957.
Number of Clients Served: 350.
Eligibility: Resident of Cattaraugus County.
Area Served: Cattaraugus County.

The Foundation Fighting Blindness Bronx-Westchester-Rockland Affiliate

7 Colvin Road
Scarsdale, NY 10583
(914) 472-6644
FAX: (914) 472-4470
Louise Boardman, President

See The Foundation Fighting Blindness in U.S. national listings.

The Foundation Fighting Blindness Brooklyn Affiliate

103 Ryerson Street
Brooklyn, NY 11205-2510
(718) 783-3942
Patsy Ross, President
Sara Kerber, Vice-President

See The Foundation Fighting Blindness in U.S. national listings.

The Foundation Fighting Blindness Long Island Affiliate

300 Garden City Plaza
Garden City, NY 11530
(516) 481-4287
Dr. Irving Barnett, Contact Person

See The Foundation Fighting Blindness in U.S. national listings.

The Foundation Fighting Blindness Manhattan Affiliate

Gracie Square Station
P.O. Box 229
New York, NY 10028
(212) 677-6711
Jackie Stein, President
Claire Feldman, Contact Person

See The Foundation Fighting Blindneses in U.S. national listings.

The Foundation Fighting Blindness Syracuse Affiliate

8752 Radburn Drive
Baldwinsville, NY 13027
(315) 638-2393
John Scala, President

See The Foundation Fighting Blindness in U.S. national listings.

The Lighthouse Inc.

111 East 59th Street
New York, NY 10022
TDD (212) 821-9713 or (800) 334-5497
FAX: (212) 821-9705
Barbara Silverstone, DSW, President and CEO

See The Lighthouse Inc. in U.S. national listings.

Prevent Blindness New York

160 East 56th Street
Eighth Floor
New York, NY 10022
(212) 980-2020
FAX: (212) 688-9641
Joseph Basile, President and CEO

See Prevent Blindness America in U.S. national listings.

See also in national listings:

American Bible Society

American Foundation for the Blind

Association for Macular Diseases

Association of Junior Leagues

AWARE (Associates for World Action in Rehabilitation and Education)

Bantam-Doubleday-Dell

Choice Magazine Listening

Eye Bank for Sight Restoration

Fight for Sight

The Glaucoma Foundation

HarperCollins Publishers

Helen Keller International

Helen Keller National Center for Deaf-Blind Youths and Adults

Helen Keller Services for the Blind/Braille Library

International Society on Metabolic Eye Disease

IN TOUCH Networks

Jewish Braille Institute of America

Jewish Guild for the Blind (The Guild)

John Milton Society for the Blind

The Lighthouse Inc.

March of Dimes Birth Defects Foundation

Matilda Ziegler Magazine for the Blind

Myopia International Research Foundation

National Accreditation Council for Agencies Serving the Blind and Visually Handicapped

National Association for Visually Handicapped

National Braille Association

National Marfan Foundation

National Multiple Sclerosis Society

National Self-Help Clearinghouse

Orbis International

Print Access Center
The Lighthouse Inc.

Random House Large Print

Research to Prevent Blindness

St. Martin's Press

Ulverscroft Large Print Books Limited

Xavier Society for the Blind

◆ *Rehabilitation Services*

STATE SERVICES

New York State Commission for the Blind and Visually Handicapped
40 North Pearl Street
Albany, NY 12243
(518) 473-1801
FAX: (518) 486-5819
Thomas A. Robertson, Acting Commissioner

Mission: Administration of services to legally blind residents of New York State for the purpose of ameliorating the disability imposed by visual impairments and to enhance individual employability. Through district offices across the state, provides and arranges for provision of vocational rehabilitation services and other services such as independent living skills and mobility training, business services and information and referral services.
Funded by: Public funds.
Budget: 1992: $29,000,000.
Staff: 168 full time.
History/Date: Est. 1913.
Number of Clients Served: 1992: 6,000.
Eligibility: Legally blind.
Area Served: New York State.

Health: Medical and specialist examinations.
Counseling/Social Work/Self-Help: Consultation and referral services; psychological testing and evaluations.
Educational: Post-secondary training programs.

Professional Training: Internships and practicums.
Reading: Readers services available to support program goals.
Rehabilitation: Training in activities of daily living, orientation and mobility, communications.
Employment: Vocational evaluation; career counseling; vocational training; vocational placement; follow-up services; vending facility training; self-employment program; homemaker training.
Computer Training: Available to support training and employment goals.
Low Vision: Available to support vocational rehabilitation goals.
Low Vision Aids: Available.

Local Offices:

Buffalo: Ellicott Square Building, 295 Main Street, Buffalo, NY 14203, (716) 847-3516.
Hempstead: 175 Fulton Avenue, Hempstead, NY 11550, (516) 564-4313.
New York: Commission for the Blind and Visually Handicapped (Brooklyn, Queens, and Staten Island), 270 Broadway, New York, NY 10007, (212) 417-5211.
New York: Commission for the Blind and Visually Handicapped (Manhattan and Bronx), Harlem State Office Building, 163 West 125th Street, New York, NY 10027, (212) 870-4440.
Rochester: 259 Monroe Avenue, Rochester, NY 14607, (716) 238-8110.
Syracuse: 333 East Washington Street, Syracuse, NY 13202, (315) 428-4147.
White Plains: 150 Grand Street, White Plains, NY 10601, (914) 993-5370.

REHABILITATION

Associated Blind

135 West 23rd Street
New York, NY 10011
(212) 255-1122
FAX: (212) 645-1638
Ruth Ellen Simmonds, Executive
Director

Type of Agency: Private; non-profit.
County/District Where Located: Manhattan County.
Funded by: Contributions, legacies, endowments and annuities.
Hours of Operation: Mon.-Fri. 8:30 AM-8:00 PM.
Staff: 12 full time, 3 part time.
History/Date: Est. 1938 and Inc. 1939.
Number of Clients Served: 1,200.
Eligibility: Adult, legally blind.
Area Served: New York City metropolitan area.
Age Requirements: Adult.

Counseling/Social Work/Self-Help: Individual counseling; support groups; referrals. Full social service agency.
Educational: Many programs in adult education, braille instruction.
Professional Training: Internships.
Reading: Volunteer readers available.
Rehabilitation: Personal management; home economics; communications; braille instruction; talking book machines; reader service.
Recreational: Life enrichment activities and programs, including social activities and physical fitness programs.
Employment: Career development programs.
Computer Training: Skills relevance programs, adaptive technology.

Association for the Advancement of Blind and Retarded, Inc.

123 - 14 14th Avenue
College Point, NY 11356
(718) 445-0752
FAX: (718) 739-4750
Chris Weldon, Executive Director

County/District Where Located: Kings County.
Mission: Services to persons with multiple disabilities.
Funded by: Medicaid, state grants, community groups and individuals interested in multiply disabled blind and severely retarded children and young adults.
Budget: $9 million.
Hours of Operation: Day treatment: Mon.-Fri. 8:30 AM-4:30 PM, Sat. 10:00 AM-4:00 PM; Residential facilities: 24-hour service.
Staff: 300.
History/Date: Est. 1956. Formerly (1974) Association for Advancement of Blind Children, Inc.
Number of Clients Served: 390.
Eligibility: Mild to profound retardation, blindness, multiple handicaps.
Area Served: New York City.
Transportation: Y.
Age Requirements: Over 18 years.

Counseling/Social Work/Self-Help: Available.
Residential: Eleven group residences providing intermediate care facilities for blind and retarded young adults.
Rehabilitation: Two six-day treatment centers for blind, multihandicapped and severely retarded young adults.
Recreational: All-year camp for blind and multihandicapped people.

Association for the Blind and Visually Impaired of Greater Rochester, Inc.

422 South Clinton Avenue
Rochester, NY 14620-1198
(716) 232-1111 or TDD (716) 232-1085
FAX: (716) 232-6707
A. Gidget Hopf, Executive Director
Dorothy H. Green, Director of Rehabilitation Services

Type of Agency: Non-profit.
Mission: To assist people who are blind and visually impaired to achieve their highest level of independence in their social and vocational lives; to provide comprehensive rehabilitation services and vocational training to people who are blind or visually impaired.
Funded by: Endowment, manufacturing and food service sales; New York State Commission for the Blind and Visually Handicapped; United Way; fundraising; sliding fee scale.
Budget: $10,000,000.
Hours of Operation: 8:00 AM-4:30 PM.
Program Accessibility: Totally accessible.
Staff: 120 direct-labor employees; 85 professional and non-exempt.
History/Date: Est. 1908; inc. 1913.
Number of Clients Served: 3,000 annually.
Eligibility: Blind or severely visually impaired.
Area Served: City of Rochester; Counties of Monroe, Ontario, Livingston, Orleans, Wayne, and Genesee.
Age Requirements: None.

Counseling/Social Work/Self-Help: Senior citizens; outreach and screening; support groups; individual counseling.
Educational: Summer children's program; computer assessment and training program for children,

adolescents, young adults and adults.

Preschools: Home training; early intervention services.

Reading: Volunteer readers available.

Rehabilitation: Full range of services including orientation and mobility, rehabilitation teaching, counseling, social work, and vocational preparation.

Recreational: Limited.

Employment: Supported employment, placement programs, and vocational preparation such as job skills club. Agency-based direct-labor employment available in such areas as manufacturing and food services.

Computer Training: Comprehensive evaluation and training.

Low Vision: On-site comprehensive low vision services.

Low Vision Aids: Consumer Resource Center on site.

Low Vision Follow-up: Y.

Association for the Visually Impaired

260 Old Nyack Turnpike
Spring Valley, NY 10977
(914) 574-4950
FAX: (914) 574-4944
Arlene Koeppel, CSW, President

Type of Agency: Private; non-profit.

County/District Where Located: Rockland, Orange Counties.

Mission: To help blind and visually impaired people retain or regain independence.

Funded by: County of Rockland; United Way; fees; contributions; N.Y. State Commission for the Blind and Visually Handicapped; and fundraising events.

Budget: $600,000.

Hours of Operation: Mon.-Fri. 9:00 AM-5:00 PM.

Staff: 14 full time, plus volunteers.

History/Date: Est. 1973.

Number of Clients Served: 1,500.

Eligibility: Visual impairment.

Area Served: Orange and Rockland counties.

Transportation: Y.

Counseling/Social Work/Self-Help: Social evaluation; crisis intervention; individual and group counseling; referral to community services.

Educational: In-service training programs to community agencies and public education to community members; internship/fieldwork placement in social work.

Reading: Large-print magazines; information and referral; instruction and use of video magnifier; volunteer reading service.

Rehabilitation: Personal and home management; braille; typing; writing and communication skills; orientation/mobility; daily living skills; instruction in client's home and community; skills instruction; low vision aids instruction.

Recreational: Educational social support groups.

Low Vision: Low vision aids referral.

Low Vision Follow-up: Y.

Aurora of Central New York

518 James Street Street
Syracuse, NY 13203
(315) 422-7263
FAX: (315) 422-4792
Donald Buodov, Executive Director

Type of Agency: Private; non-profit.

Mission: Services for totally blind, legally blind, visually impaired, and deaf-blind persons.

Funded by: Fees, United Way, capital income, government agency, contributions, sales.

Budget: 1997: $1,700,000.

Hours of Operation: Mon.-Fri. 8:30 AM-4:30 PM.

Staff: 35 full time, 8 part time. Uses volunteers.

History/Date: Est. 1917.

Number of Clients Served: 1,302.

Eligibility: Visual/hearing impairment.

Area Served: Central and northern counties.

Age Requirements: None.

Health: Refers for health services.

Counseling/Social Work/Self-Help: Social evaluation; individual, family, couple counseling. Refers for and provides consultation to other agencies on other counseling/social work services.

Professional Training: Internship/fieldwork placement in orientation/mobility; social work. Regular in-service training programs, open to enrollment from other agencies.

Reading: Lends talking book record players and cassette players; recorded magazines. Information and referral; tape recording services on demand.

Rehabilitation: Personal management; braille; gesticulation; handwriting; listening skills; typing; Optacon adapted computer equipment; video magnifier; electronic mobility aids; home management; orientation/mobility; rehabilitation teaching in client's home and community; remedial education; sensory training.

Recreational: Refers for recreation services.

Computer Training: On-site computer access technology center.

Low Vision: Evaluations.
Low Vision Aids: Available for sale.
Low Vision Follow-up: Y.

Blind Association of Western New York

1170 Main Street
Buffalo, NY 14209
(716) 882-1025
FAX: (716) 882-5577
Ronald S. Maier, Ph.D., Executive Director

Type of Agency: Private, non-profit, citizen-directed rehabilitation agency.
County/District Where Located: Erie County.
Mission: Services for totally blind, legally blind, visually impaired, deaf-blind, and multiply disabled blind or visually impaired persons.
Funded by: United Way, state funds, private donations.
Budget: Approximately $4 million.
Hours of Operation: Mon.-Fri. 8:30 AM-5:00 PM.
Program Accessibility: Fully accessible.
Staff: 40 full time. Uses volunteers.
History/Date: Est. 1907 and Inc. 1908.
Number of Clients Served: Over 10,000 through all services.
Eligibility: Blind or visually impaired.
Area Served: Eight counties of western New York.
Age Requirements: None.

Counseling/Social Work/Self-Help: Casefinding; assessment; social casework; information and referral; adjustment counseling; group, individual and family counseling.
Educational: Public information and education programs to schools, civic groups, professionals and the media.
Preschools: For visually impaired children, birth-5 years.
Professional Training: Fieldwork supervision and conferences for professionals and consumers.
Reading: Resource center dispenses talking books; adaptive and high-tech devices and assistance on usage.
Residential: 24 unit subsidized housing designed for physically disabled yet functionally independent individuals, particularly those who are blind and visually impaired.
Rehabilitation: Personal management; braille; handwriting; listening skills; Optacon; typing; video magnifier; home management: orientation/mobility; rehabilitation teaching; non-visual skills training; children's programs; services to children. Home, school, or agency-based.
Recreational: Services related to recreation groups meeting in the agency and integrated in the community.
Employment: Prevocational evaluation; career and skill development; job retention; vocational placement; employment services; sheltered workshop; work activities center; follow-up services.
Computer Training: Y.
Low Vision: Low vision clinic services available.
Low Vision Aids: Located in low vision clinic and resource center.
Low Vision Follow-up: Y.

Blind Work Association

55 Washington Street
Binghamton, NY 13901
(607) 724-2428
FAX: (607) 771-8045
M. Conrad Range, Jr., Executive Director

Type of Agency: Private; non-profit.
County/District Where Located: Broome County.
Mission: Services for totally blind, legally blind, and deaf-blind persons.
Funded by: Workshop sales, capital funds, contributions.
Hours of Operation: Mon.-Fri. 9:00 AM-5:00 PM.
Staff: 8 full time. Uses volunteers.
History/Date: Est. 1926.
Area Served: Broome, Chenango, Cortland, Delaware, Otsego, Tioga, and Tompkins Counties.

Counseling/Social Work/Self-Help: Individual, family/parent counseling; placement and training; referral to community services. Refers for other social work services.
Professional Training: In-service training when requested by schools, nursing homes, hospitals, and others. Trains volunteers for vision screening.
Reading: Information and referral; transcription to braille; tape recording services and large print on request.
Rehabilitation: Personal management; braille; typing; home management; orientation/mobility; rehabilitation teaching in client's home.
Recreational: Special programs for elderly. Refers for bowling.
Employment: Sheltered workshop.

Brooklyn Bureau of Community Service

285 Schermerhorn Street

Brooklyn, NY 11217
(718) 875-0710
FAX: (718) 855-1517
Donna A. Santarsiero, Executive
Director
Leslie Klein, Director, Adult
Rehabiliatiion Services

Type of Agency: Multi-service.
County/District Where Located:
Kings County.
Mission: Services to visually
impaired and other disabled
persons.
Funded by: Workshop sales and
sub-contracts, endowment, public
funds, contributions, Greater New
York Fund, and New York Times
Neediest.
Budget: $15 Million.
Staff: 49 full time (rehab services
only).
History/Date: Est. 1866.
Number of Clients Served: 600
(rehab services only).
Eligibility: Disabled adults.
Area Served: Kings County.
Transportation: Y.
Age Requirements: 17 years and
over.

Health: Psychological testing.
**Counseling/Social Work/Self-
Help:** Individual, family, and
group counseling. Psychological
counseling.
Rehabilitation: Personal
management; communication
skills; prevocational group work.
Employment: Sheltered
workshop; work training; job
placement services; diagnostic
vocational evaluation.

Catholic Charities
Office for Disabled Persons

191 Joralemon Street
Brooklyn, NY 11201
(718) 722-6000
FAX: (718) 722-6096
Thomas Destefano, Executive
Director

County/District Where Located:
Kings County.
Funded by: Contributions and
membership fees.
Staff: 1 full time.
History/Date: Est. 1945.
Eligibility: Visually impaired.
Area Served: Brooklyn and
Queens.
Transportation: Y.

**Counseling/Social Work/Self-
Help:** Religious counseling and
services. Mass for blind clients;
special events and services.
Advocacy and assistance with
housing.
Recreational: Monthly social
activities.

Catholic Charities Services for
Visually Impaired Persons

143 Schleigel Boulevard
Amityville, NY 11701
(516) 789-5213
FAX: (516) 789-9542
Paul Sauerland, Administrator

Type of Agency: Private, non-
profit. Catholic sponsored, non-
sectarian in service.
County/District Where Located:
Nassau County.
Mission: Provides services for
totally blind; legally blind; visually
impaired persons.
Funded by: Service fees from New
York State Commission for the
Blind and Visually Handicapped
and Catholic Charities.
Budget: $270,000.
Hours of Operation: Mon.-Fri.
9:00 AM-5:00 PM.
Program Accessibility:
Rehabilitation services are
provided in clients' homes.
History/Date: Est. 1957.
Number of Clients Served: 209.
Eligibility: Visually impaired,
except for contracted services that
are for those legally blind.

Area Served: Nassau and Suffolk
Counties.
Transportation: Y.

Health: Refers for health services.
**Counseling/Social Work/Self-
Help:** Social evaluations;
individual, group, family/parent,
couple counseling; referral to
community services. Refers for
other counseling/social work
services.
Rehabilitation: Personal
management; braille; handwriting;
mobility skills; typing; home
management; rehabilitation;
teaching in client's home and
community; remedial education;
sensory training. Refers for other
rehabilitation services.
Recreational: Special programs
for elderly.
Employment: Refers for
employment-oriented services.

Catholic Guild for the Blind

525 Washington Street
Buffalo, NY 14203
(716) 856-4494
Sister Rose Mary Cauley, Director.

Type of Agency: Private.
County/District Where Located:
Erie County.
Mission: To promote and enhance
spiritual and social interests of the
blind and visually impaired
population in the Diocese of
Buffalo.
Funded by: Catholic Charities
appeal.
Budget: $10,000.
Hours of Operation: Mon.-Fri.
9:00 AM - 5:00 PM.
Program Accessibility: Facilities
are fully accessible. Referrals from
other agencies and self referrals.
Staff: 1 full time. Uses volunteers.
History/Date: Est. 1939.
Number of Clients Served:
Approximately 300 in community
and nursing homes.

Eligibility: Legally blind.
Area Served: Buffalo diocese (8 western New York counties).
Transportation: Y.

Counseling/Social Work/Self-Help: Referral services; short-term counseling; spiritual counseling. Emergency financial aid. Sponsors social and religious programs.
Professional Training: Conducts training seminars for volunteers.
Rehabilitation: Social and spiritual programs.
Recreational: Sponsors picnics.

Catholic Guild for the Blind

1011 First Avenue
New York, NY 10022
(212) 371-1000, ext. 2017
FAX: (212) 826-8377
A. Therese Snyder, Director

Type of Agency: Private; non-profit.
County/District Where Located: Manhattan County.
Mission: Rehabilitation of legally blind persons.
Funded by: Catholic Charities and New York State Commission for the Blind and Physically Handicapped.
Budget: $300,000.
Hours of Operation: Mon.-Fri. 9:00 AM-5:00 PM.
Program Accessibility: Fully handicapped accessibility.
Staff: 5 full time; 5 part time.
History/Date: Est. 1953.
Number of Clients Served: Approximately 250 annually.
Eligibility: Legal blindness.
Area Served: New York City area.

Counseling/Social Work/Self-Help: Social work and counseling available when needed.
Educational: English as a second language; and remedial instruction.

Professional Training: Internships for rehabilitation teaching and mobility.
Rehabilitation: Personal management; orientation/mobility; adaptive communication skills training; homemaking; communications and casework services; consultation to other agencies.
Low Vision: Referrals.
Low Vision Follow-up: Y.

Central Association for the Blind and Visually Impaired

507 Kent Street
Utica, NY 13501
(315) 797-2233
FAX: (315) 797-4763
Donald D. LoGuidice, President

Type of Agency: Private; not-for-profit.
County/District Where Located: Oneida County.
Mission: To assist people who are blind or visually impaired to achieve their highest level of independence.
Funded by: Contributions, fees, grants, workshop/industries sales, investment income.
Budget: 1997: $8,550,789.
Hours of Operation: 8:30 AM-4:30 PM.
Staff: 38 full time, 14 part time. Uses volunteers.
History/Date: Inc. 1929.
Number of Clients Served: 2,439.
Eligibility: Legally blind, severely visually impaired, deaf and blind, multiply disabled blind persons.
Area Served: 6 counties in central New York: Oneida, Madison, Merrimac, Lewis, Montgomery, Fultch plus 5 additional counties for technology and other services.
Transportation: Y.
Age Requirements: No age restrictions.

Health: Glaucoma screening, preschool screening, and distance acuity vision screenings. Refers for health services.
Counseling/Social Work/Self-Help: Individual, group, family, crisis intervention counseling; referral to community services. Provides consultation to other agencies on counseling/social work services, adult support group meetings. Children's services; resource advocacy and training activities for visually impaired children.
Educational: Public education and in-service training programs provided upon request. Prevention, careers, and other educational material information available.
Preschools: Preschool Vision Training Program. Serves blind and visually impaired children, many with other disabling conditions. Individual training provided in visual and compensatory skills. Works in cooperation with all other area preschool programs.
Professional Training: Internship/fieldwork placement in orientation/mobility; social work; rehabilitation teaching. Regular in-service training program open to other agencies.
Reading: Braille transcribing services; braille books; large-print books; tape recording; information and referral.
Rehabilitation: Independent living skills, personal and home management, orientation and mobility, concept development, community and facility-based programs.
Recreational: Refers and provides consultation to other agencies for some recreational services.
Employment: Job evaluation and training, community placement,

supported employment, center industries, work activity center.
Computer Training: Regional technology center for visually impaired persons serving 10 counties. Assessment, training, and job/education site services on personal computers based adaptive equipment.
Low Vision: Low vision center. Adaptive equipment and low vision aids.
Low Vision Aids: Available through low vision center.
Low Vision Follow-up: Provided as necessary through low vision center.

Volunteer services: transportation, friendly visiting, grocery shopping, recreational activities, tutoring, clerical help, and assistance with vision screenings.

Chautauqua Blind Association, Inc.

406 East Fourth Street
Jamestown, NY 14701
(716) 664-6660 or (716) 487-7561
Joanne E. Nelson, Executive Director

Type of Agency: Private; non-profit.
County/District Where Located: Chautauqua County.
Mission: Services for visually impaired persons and blindness prevention programs.
Funded by: County; United Way; sub-contracts; donations; New York State Commission for the Blind; memberships; fund raising; grants.
Budget: 1996: $137,938.
Hours of Operation: Mon.-Fri. 8:00 AM-4:00 PM.
Staff: 3 full time, 4 part time. Uses volunteers.
History/Date: Est. 1921.
Number of Clients Served: 1991: 650.

Eligibility: Visually impaired.
Area Served: Chautauqua County, all programs. Cattaraugus County, one contracted program for legally blind persons.
Age Requirements: Must be old enough to understand instructions.

Health: Preschool vision screening; glaucoma screening.
Counseling/Social Work/Self-Help: Assistance in meeting medical, housing, financial, recreational and/or legal needs; referral to other service providers when appropriate.
Preschools: Vision screening offered to preschoolers aged 3-6.
Professional Training: In-service workshops available to other agencies and nursing homes.
Reading: Delivery of talking books and Radio Reading Service receivers; transcription to braille; referrals for large-print books and magazines. Aids and appliances available.
Rehabilitation: Orientation/mobility; home management; personal management; rehabilitation teaching in the client's home; communication skills.
Recreational: Large-print/braille recreational aids available.
Employment: Referral to appropriate agencies for training and placement, when applicable.
Low Vision: Low vision services available through subcontractors.
Low Vision Aids: Available through subcontractors.
Low Vision Follow-up: Available through subcontractor and agency staff.

Consolidated Industries of Greater Syracuse, Inc.

100 West Courts Street
Syracuse, NY 13204
(315) 476-4021
FAX: (315) 425-0461
George A. Manyo, Executive Director

Type of Agency: Private; non-profit.
Mission: Services for totally blind; legally blind; visually impaired; deaf-blind; learning disabled; mentally retarded; emotionally handicapped.
Funded by: Sub-contracts, capital income, fees and grants.
Staff: 65 full time, 8 part time. Uses volunteers.
History/Date: Est. 1964.
Eligibility: Emotionally, mentally, physically and socially disabled, unable to be assisted through ordinary vocational counseling and placement programs. Must be able to travel unescorted.
Transportation: Y.
Age Requirements: At least 17 years.

Health: Refers for health services.
Counseling/Social Work/Self-Help: Individual, group counseling; placement in training. Refers for other counseling/social work services.
Professional Training: Internship/fieldwork placement in rehabilitation counseling; social work; vocational rehabilitation. Regular in-service training program.
Reading: Large print books.
Rehabilitation: Remedial education. Refers for other rehabilitation services.
Recreational: Provides consultation to other agencies on recreational services.
Employment: Prevocational evaluation; career and skill counseling; work adjustment and work evaluation; occupational skill development; job retention; job retraining; skill training; sheltered

workshops; vocational placement; follow-up services. Refers for vending stand training.

Local Offices:

Syracuse: Consolidated Industries of Greater Syracuse, Inc., 100 West Court Street, Syracuse, NY 13203, (315) 476-4021.

Glens Falls Association for the Blind

144 Ridge Street
Glens Falls, NY 12801
(518) 792-3421
FAX: (518) 792-3430
Philip R. Jessen, Executive Director

Type of Agency: Private; non-profit.
Mission: Services for totally blind; legally blind; visually impaired.
Funded by: Capital funds, United Way, gifts, bequests, county allotment, contracts, Lions Club.
Budget: 1996: $308,174.
Hours of Operation: Mon.-Fri. 9:00 AM-5:00 PM.
Program Accessibility: Completely accessible.
Staff: 7 full-time.
History/Date: Est. 1937; inc. 1965.
Number of Clients Served: 1996: 2,200.
Eligibility: Legal blindness or severe visual impairment.
Area Served: Warren, Washington, north Saratoga, Hamilton Counties.
Transportation: Y.
Age Requirements: None.

Health: Preschool and elderly vision screening; in-service education programs. Refers for other health services.
Counseling/Social Work/Self-Help: Counseling/social work services; social casework; advocacy; outreach; visitation.
Reading: Information and referral.

Rehabilitation: Personal management; orientation/mobility training; social casework.
Recreational: Community-based programs for elderly.
Employment: Refers for employment services.
Low Vision: Monthly low vision clinic.
Low Vision Aids: Y.
Low Vision Follow-up: Y.

Helen Keller National Center for Deaf-Blind Youths and Adults Mid-Atlantic Region Office

111 Middle Neck Road
Sands Point, NY 11050
(516) 944-8900 (voice/TDD)
FAX: (516) 944-7302
Barbara Martin, Regional Representative
Susan Ruzenski, Assistant Director

Type of Agency: Vocational rehabilitation training.
Mission: To facilitate a national, coordinated effort to meet the social, rehabilitative and independent living needs of the deaf blind population.
Budget: $5 million.
Hours of Operation: Mon.-Fri. 8:45AM-4:30PM.
Program Accessibility: Fully accessible.
History/Date: Est. 1969.
Number of Clients Served: 1,700 annually, nationwide.

See Helen Keller National Center for Deaf-Blind Youths and Adults in U.S. national listings.

Helen Keller Services for the Blind

57 Willoughby Street

Brooklyn, NY 11201
(718) 522-2122
FAX: (718) 935-9463
URL: http://www.helenkeller.org
Fred W. McPhilliamy, President
John P. Lynch, Director
Frank Romano, Associate Director

Type of Agency: Private; non-profit.
Mission: To enable persons of all ages who are visually impaired, blind, or deaf-blind to lead as independent a life as possible.
Funded by: New York State Commission for the Blind and Visually Handicapped, New York State Office of Vocational and Educational Services for Individuals with Disabilities, New York State Office of Mental Retardation and Developmental Disabilities, capital income, public support, Medicaid, grants, and legacies.
Hours of Operation: Mon.-Fri. 8:30 AM-4:30 PM.
Program Accessibility: Accessible.
Staff: 141 full time, 31 part time.
History/Date: Est. 1893.
Number of Clients Served: 3,000-4,000 blind and visually impaired people annually. Plus 30,000 preschool children in a vision screening program on Long Island.
Eligibility: Visually impaired children or adults; legally blind.
Area Served: New York City metropolitan area and Long Island.
Transportation: Y.
Age Requirements: All ages accepted.

Health: Comprehensive low vision services; audiology; and vision screening services.
Counseling/Social Work/Self-Help: Social evaluation; psychological testing and evaluation; individual, group, family counseling; placement in

school, training; referral to community services.

Educational: Supplemental educational services to school-age visually impaired children. Summer career development seminars and mobility clinics for school-age children.

Preschools: Center-based services for visually impaired preschoolers. Vision screening services for preschool children.

Preschools: Center-based services for visually impaired preschoolers. Vision screening services for preschool children.

Professional Training: Internship/field work placement in low vision; rehabilitation counseling; social work, orientation and mobility; and education.

Reading: Produces and lends braille and large-print textbooks; information and referral; transcription to braille/large print.

Rehabilitation: Diagnostic and prevocational evaluation; vocational placement services; supported employment; psychological testing; social work services; rehabilitation counseling; communication skills; orientation/mobility; adaptive technology training; transcription/typing; audiology and rehabilitation teaching. Day treatment program provides diagnostic treatment and rehabilitative services to multiply disabled blind and deaf-blind adults. Operates the Helen Keller National Center for Deaf-Blind Youths and Adults.

Recreational: Senior citizens service centers in 4 locations; summer camp for children up to age 14; fishing; bowling. Refers for other recreation services. Co-op scouting program.

Employment: Career and skill counseling; occupational skill development; job retention; job retraining; vocational placement; follow-up service; and supported employment.

Computer Training: Comprehensive adaptive technology and computer training services for educational and vocational purposes.

Low Vision: Comprehensive low vision services.

Low Vision Aids: Low Vision Center prescribes aids and other low vision devices.

Low Vision Follow-up: Y.

Local Offices:

Hempstead: Helen Keller Services for the Blind, Nassau Service Center and Rehabilitation Center, One Helen Keller Way, Hempstead, NY 11550, (516) 485-1234, FAX (516) 538-6785.

Huntington: Helen Keller Services for the Blind, Suffolk Service Center, 40 New York Avenue, Huntington, NY 11743, (516) 424-0022, FAX (516) 424-0301.

Industries for the Blind of New York State

230 Washington Avenue Extension
Suite 106
Albany, NY 12203
(518) 456-8671
FAX: (518) 456-3587
Steven M. Ennis, President-Executive Director

Type of Agency: Sales.
County/District Where Located: Albany County.
Funded by: Fees for service.
Budget: $740,000.
Hours of Operation: Mon.-Fri. 8:00 AM-4:30 PM.
Staff: 10.
History/Date: Inc. 1946.
Area Served: New York State.

Sales organization actively markets blind-made products to state agencies, political subdivisions, and public benefit corporations under provisions of the New York State finance law, working with eight qualified, nonprofit workshops for blind persons.

Jefferson County Association for the Blind

321 Prospect Street
Watertown, NY 13601
(315) 782-2451
Shirley Cooper, Executive Director

Type of Agency: Private; non-profit.
County/District Where Located: Jefferson County.
Mission: Services for totally blind, legally blind, and visually impaired persons of all ages.
Funded by: United Way; capital funds; contributions.
Hours of Operation: Mon.-Fri. 9:00 AM-4:00 PM.
Staff: 2 full time, 2 part-time, uses volunteers.
History/Date: Est. 1919.
Number of Clients Served: 480.
Eligibility: Blind or visually impaired.
Area Served: Jefferson County.
Transportation: Y.

Counseling/Social Work/Self-Help: Home visits to individuals in Jefferson County; counseling. Referrals to community services.
Reading: Talking book machines. Placement of special radio receivers.
Low Vision: Low vision aids.

Jewish Guild for the Blind (The Guild)

15 West 65th Street
New York, NY 10023
(212) 769-6200
FAX: (212) 769-6266
Alan R. Morse, President and CEO

Type of Agency: Private; nonprofit; nonsectarian.

Mission: Services for totally blind; legally blind; deaf-blind; learning disabled; mentally retarded; emotionally disturbed; orthopedically disabled; multiply disabled.

Funded by: Fees, Medicaid, United Way, contributions.

Budget: $40,000,000.

Hours of Operation: 8:30 AM-5:00 PM. Evenings by appointment only.

Program Accessibility: Handicapped accessible.

Staff: 475 full time. Uses volunteers, in addition.

History/Date: Est. 1914.

Number of Clients Served: 1991: 4,800.

Eligibility: Visual impairment.

Area Served: No geographic limitations.

Transportation: Y.

Age Requirements: Serves all visually impaired/blind persons from infancy through extreme old age.

Health: Comprehensive Outpatient Rehabilitation Facility (CORF). Diagnostic and treatment center. Short-term medical rehabilitation. GuildCare: Adult Day Health Program provides comprehensive health care, case management, vision rehabilitation, and recreational services for visually impaired/blind adults with medical needs who can benefit from day services. Medicaid reimbursable program includes transportation. Available in Manhattan, the Bronx and Yonkers campuses, as well as in Albany, Buffalo and Niagara Falls.

Counseling/Social Work/Self-Help: Psychiatric clinic; continuing day treatment program; individual, group, family/parent, couple, crisis, substance abuse counseling; referral to community services. Case management services for visually impaired persons with HIV/AIDS. Provides consultation to other agencies for other counseling/social work services.

Educational: The Guild School accepts deaf-blind; emotionally disturbed; learning disabled; mentally retarded; developmentally disabled; orthopedically disabled; neurologically impaired or brain damage. Programs for adult continuing education; vocational/skill development; high school equivalency.

Preschools: Early Intervention Program for infants through age 3. Preschool for 3 to 5 year olds.

Professional Training: Internship/fieldwork placement in orientation/mobility; rehabilitation; social work; special education and other related disciplines. Regular in-service training programs.

Reading: Talking book records and cassettes; transcription to braille; tape recording services, upon request; volunteer reading service. Information and referral.

Residential: The Home for Aged Blind is a 219-bed skilled nursing facility in Yonkers, New York; includes a special 26-bed Alzheimer's unit and a 20-bed unit for visually impaired persons with AIDS.

Rehabilitation: Personal management; braille; handwriting; Optacon, typing; electronic mobility aids; home management; orientation/mobility; rehabilitation teaching; remedial education; communication skills; work adjustment training; adapted physical education; sensory training; physical therapy; occupational therapy; psychiatric evaluation and treatment. Provides consultation to other agencies for rehabilitation services.

Employment: Prevocational evaluation; career and skill counseling; occupational skill development; job retention; job retraining; vocational placement; word processing; supported employment, customer service representative training. Consultation to employers.

Computer Training: Includes adaptive devices, i.e., synthetic speech, large-print and braille.

Low Vision: Low vision services available.

Low Vision Aids: Available.

Low Vision Follow-up: Y.

Local Offices:

Yonkers: The Home for Aged Blind, 75 Stratton Street South, Yonkers, NY 10701, (914) 963-4662, (212) 365-3700.

Yonkers: Kramer Vision Rehabilitation Center, 75 Stratton Street South, Yonkers, NY 10701, (914) 963-4661, (212) 365-3700.

The Lighthouse Inc.

111 East 59th Street
New York, NY 10022-1202
(212) 821-9200 or (800) 334-5497 or TDD (212) 821-9713
FAX: (212) 821-9705
E-mail: info@lighthouse.org
URL: http://www.lighthouse.org
Barbara Silverstone, DSW, President and CEO

Type of Agency: Private; non-profit.

Mission: Vision rehabilitation services for all ages; research, education and advocacy programs.

Funded by: Fees; government grants; product sales; investment income; contributions.

Budget: $27,200,000 (excluding Lighthouse Enterprises).

Hours of Operation: Mon.-Fri. 9:00 AM-9:00 PM; Sat. 9:00 AM-5:00 PM.

Program Accessibility: Fully accessible.

Staff: 311 full time, 69 part time. Uses volunteers.

History/Date: Est. 1906 (as the New York Association for the Blind).

Number of Clients Served: FY '96: 4,606 received direct services.

Eligibility: Functional vision impairment.

Area Served: Greater New York.

Age Requirements: None.

Health: Diabetic education, insulin device training, health counseling, sex education.

Counseling/Social Work/Self-Help: Social evaluation; crisis intervention; psychological testing and evaluation; individual, group, family counseling; placement in school, training; referral to community services.

Educational: Afterschool programs for children and teenagers; leisure education; music; arts; high school equivalency.

Preschools: Center-based programs and consultation services to other programs for visually impaired multiply disabled children.

Professional Training: Internship/fieldwork placement in low vision; orientation/mobility; social work; special education; therapeutic recreation; rehabilitation counseling. Professional training programs and seminars for professionals in allied fields.

Reading: Full-service library including braille, cassettes, Kurzweil Reader and print enlarger; information and referral; transcription to braille; tape recording services; volunteer reading service.

Rehabilitation: Independent living skills; braille; handwriting; reading machines; typing; home management; orientation/mobility. Community and facility-based programs.

Employment: Prevocational evaluation; career and skill development; occupational skill development; clerical skills training; job retention; job retraining; vocational placement; follow-up service and job coaching; work activity program for individuals with multiple impairments.

Computer Training: Training on computer aids and devices; assessment, training, speech, braille and large print systems.

Low Vision: Evaluation and services.

Low Vision Aids: Prescriptions and training.

Local Offices:

Bronx: 350 East Gunhill Road, Bronx, NY 10467, (718) 920-0730.

Elmhurst: 60-05 Woodhaven Boulevard, Elmhurst, NY 11373, (718) 899-9100.

Medford: 1731 North Ocean Avenue, Medford, NY 11763, (516) 654-3522.

Poughkeepsie: 110 Main Street, Poughkeepsie, NY 12601, (914) 473-7350.

Staten Island: One Edgewater Plaza, Suite 316, Staten Island, NY 10305, (718) 816-9777.

White Plains: 44 Church Street, White Plains, NY 10601, (914) 761-3221.

New York City Industries for the Blind

2701 Queens Plaza North
Long Island City, NY 11101-4015
(718) 786-9300
FAX: (718) 786-9377
Richard C. Bland, President

County/District Where Located: Queens County.

Mission: To provide employment opportunities for people in the New York area who are blind or partially sighted.

Budget: $7.5 million.

Hours of Operation: Mon.-Fri. 8:30AM-5:00PM.

Staff: 13.

History/Date: Est. 1995.

Number of Clients Served: 60.

Area Served: Metropolitan New York.

Age Requirements: 18 years and older.

Employment: Manufacturing, office, and service positions.

North Country Association for the Visually Impaired

301 Main Street
Third floor
Lake Placid, NY 12946
(518) 523-1950
Karen Mergenthaler, Executive Director

Type of Agency: Private; non-profit.

Mission: To offer free professional assistance and support, as well as promote the physical and mental well-being of the legally blind and visually impaired.

Funded by: Gifts, donations, contracts, and Lions Clubs.

Budget: $200,000.

Hours of Operation: Mon.-Fri. 8:00 AM - 4:00 PM.

Staff: 7 full time; 1 part time.

History/Date: Est. 1989.

Number of Clients Served: 2,000.

Eligibility: Legally blind.

Area Served: Clinton, Franklin, Essex, and St. Lawrence Counties.

Age Requirements: None.

Counseling/Social Work/Self-Help: Home visits and counseling by the agency or by referral to another organization.

Educational: Braille classes available.

Preschools: Rehabilitation teaching and social casework for infants to school-age children.

Rehabilitation: Services for older persons; home-based and community-based training; homemaking skills, kitchen management; activities of daily living.

Employment: Vocational training.

Low Vision: Services and referrals.

Low Vision Aids: Low vision aids can be ordered through the agency.

Low Vision Follow-up: After two months.

Northeastern Association of the Blind

301 Washington Avenue
Albany, NY 12206
(518) 463-1211
FAX: (518) 436-4194
Carolyn Gebhardt, Executive Director

Type of Agency: Private; non-profit.

Mission: Services for totally blind; legally blind; severely visually impaired.

Funded by: Fees, workshop sales, sub-contracts, capital funds, fund raising, grants.

Budget: $2.5 million.

Hours of Operation: Mon.-Fri. 8:00 AM-4:00 PM.

Staff: 36 full time, 4 part time. Uses volunteers.

History/Date: Est. 1908.

Number of Clients Served: 650.

Eligibility: Legally blind, severely visually impaired.

Transportation: Y.

Health: Low vision service. Refers for other health services.

Counseling/Social Work/Self-Help: Case management; social evaluation; psychological testing and evaluation; referral to community services.

Professional Training: Internship/fieldwork placement; low vision; orientation/mobility; rehabilitation counseling; rehabilitation teaching; social work. In-service training programs.

Reading: Talking book referral and follow-up services; braille; large print; information and referral.

Rehabilitation: Independent living evaluation; personal management; braille; handwriting; listening skills; typing; home management; orientation/mobility; rehabilitation teaching and mobility training in client's home and community; remedial education; sensory training.

Employment: Vocational evaluation; career and skill counseling; occupational skill development; job retention; job retraining; sheltered workshop; vocational placement; follow-up service.

Computer Training: Access; training on computer aids and devices; vocational preparation in word and data processing.

Low Vision: In house clinic; home evaluations available.

Low Vision Aids: Evaluation and prescription of low vision aids.

Low Vision Follow-up: Y.

St. John's Episcopal Home for the Aged and Blind

452 Herkimer Street
Brooklyn, NY 11213
(718) 467-1885
Janet McNemar, Administrator

County/District Where Located: Kings County.

Funded by: Public funds, endowment, Greater New York Fund, and contributions.

History/Date: Est. 1851.

Area Served: Queens, Nassau and Suffolk counties, Brooklyn.

Health: Diagnostic, medical and surgical treatment. Eyeglasses available.

Residential: Facilities for adults.

Rehabilitation: Orientation/mobility training.

Southern Tier Association for the Visually Impaired

719 Lake Street
Elmira, NY 14901
(607) 734-1554
FAX: (607) 734-9467
Stephan Connors, Executive Director

Type of Agency: Private; non-profit.

County/District Where Located: Chemung County.

Mission: Provides services for legally blind and visually impaired individuals.

Funded by: Contributions; workshop sales; endowment; fees.

Budget: 1996: $607,000.

Hours of Operation: Mon.-Fri. 8:00 AM-4:00 PM.

Staff: 14 full time, 2 part time.

History/Date: Est. 1930.

Number of Clients Served: 250 annually.

Eligibility: Persons who are legally blind; visually impaired; able to benefit from service.

Area Served: Chemung, Schuyler, Steuben, Southern Seneca and Yates Counties.

Age Requirements: None.

Health: Glaucoma screening program/education outreach.

Counseling/Social Work/Self-Help: Counseling and referral services, public education and in-service training, peer support groups.
Educational: Public education and in-service training.
Rehabilitation: Personal management; orientation/mobility; home management; communication; low vision service.
Employment: On-the-job training; sheltered workshop.
Low Vision: Arthur P. Darling Low Vision Center, Corning, NY—functional assessments; adaptive equipment; low vision aides.
Low Vision Aids: Use of R.T. and R.T. aids for in-home training.
Low Vision Follow-up: Y.

VISIONS/Services for the Blind and Visually Impaired
120 Wall Street, 16th Floor
New York, NY 10005
(212) 425-2255
FAX: (212) 425-7114
E-mail: alwidman@aol.com
Nancy D. Miller, Executive Director

Type of Agency: Private; non-profit.
County/District Where Located: Manhattan County.
Mission: Community and rehabilitation services for adults and elders who are blind and visually impaired. Year-round residential camp services for visually impaired/blind and multiply disabled adults, elders and families. CIL Publications offering professional textbooks and audiobooks for newly blind individuals.
Funded by: Contributions; United Way; grants; legacies; fees; government contracts.

Budget: $2 million.
Hours of Operation: Mon.-Fri. 9:00 AM-5:00 PM.
Program Accessibility: Rehabilitation in home; camp fully accessible.
Staff: 24 full time. Uses volunteers.
History/Date: Est. 1926. Formerly called Vacations and Community Services for the Blind incorporating the Center for Independent Living.
Number of Clients Served: 1,500.
Eligibility: Blind or visually impaired adults and elders; multiply disabled persons; family members.
Area Served: New York City and metropolitan area.
Transportation: Y.
Age Requirements: Over 55 years; multiply disabled 18 and over.

Counseling/Social Work/Self-Help: General social services—short-term counseling, information, referral and concrete services. Group programs and social services in 31 neighborhood senior centers (Brooklyn, Queens, Bronx, Manhattan, Westchester) promote integration of elders who are visually impaired into community life. Self-study audiobooks for learning skills for independence.
Educational: Public education boroughwide forums; group education; and vision screening. Textbooks for instructors in mobility, housekeeping, personal management, and sensory development.
Professional Training: Internship/fieldwork placement in social work; orientation/mobility; rehabilitation teaching; occupational therapy. In-service program for professionals in allied fields.

Residential: Overnight respite care in the camp facility during weekends/summer sessions for blind multiply disabled adults living with a caregiver.
Rehabilitation: Rehabilitation teaching (personal management, communications, housekeeping); orientation/mobility; occupational therapy. Training provided in the client's home and community. Consultations to other agencies for rehabilitation services.
Recreational: Vacation Camp for the Blind near Spring Valley, New York in Rockland County. 5 summer sessions and special winter weekends. Full range of recreational and social activities with adapted facilities. Social work supervision.
Employment: Counselor in training; pre-employment mentoring project; summer employment for blind, visually impaired, or disabled persons.
Low Vision: Referral as part of a rehabilitation program.
Publications: Self-help audiobooks and in print for visually impaired adults and professionals. Publications teach sensory development, housekeeping skills, basic indoor mobility, and personal management. Instructional textbooks with structured tasks and behavioral objectives.

Westchester Independent Living Center, Inc.
297 Knollwood Road
White Plains, NY 10607
(914) 682-3926
FAX: (914) 682-8518
Joseph R. Bravo, Executive Director

Type of Agency: Private; non-profit.
County/District Where Located: Westchester County.

Mission: Direct services to disabled population.
Funded by: State Education Department.
Staff: On-site 15, off-site 35.
History/Date: Est. 1983.
Eligibility: Disability.
Area Served: Westchester and Rockland Counties.

Counseling/Social Work/Self-Help: Provides social evaluation, community services. Information, referral and advocacy for people with disabilities.
Professional Training: Social integration program for seniors who prc-legally blind.

COMPUTER TRAINING CENTERS

Aurora of Central New York

518 James Street
Syracuse, NY 13203
(315) 422-7263
FAX: (315) 422-4792
Director, Computer Access Technology Program

County/District Where Located: Onondaga County.

Computer Training: Speech output systems; screen magnification systems; braille access systems; closed-circuit television systems; word processing; database software; computer operating systems.

Baruch College Computer Center for Visually Impaired People

17 Lexington Avenue
P.O. Box H648
New York, NY 10010
(212) 802-2140
FAX: (212) 802-2103
Dr. Karen Luxton Gourgey, Director
Judith Gerber, Manager

Computer Training: Speech output systems; screen magnification systems; braille access systems; closed-circuit television systems; word processing; database software; computer operating systems; training for instructors.

ENABLE

1603 Court Street
Syracuse, NY 13208
(315) 455-7591
Carol Tytler, Director, Assistive Technology

County/District Where Located: Onondaga County.

Computer Training: Speech output systems; screen magnification systems; optical character recognition systems; word processing; database software; computer operating systems; assistive technology.

Finger Lakes Independent Center

609 West Clinton Street
Suite 112
Ithaca, NY 14850
(607) 272-2433
Richard Farruggio, Coordinator

County/District Where Located: Thompkins County.

Computer Training: Speech output systems; screen magnification systems; optical character recognition systems; closed-circuit television systems; word processing; database software; computer operating systems.

Helen Keller National Center for Deaf-Blind Youths and Adults

111 Middle Neck Road
Sands Point, NY 11050
(516) 944-8900 or TDD (516) 944-8637
FAX: (516) 944-7302
E-mail: 76215.1062@compuserve.com
Jim Belanich, Adaptive Technology Coordinator

Computer Training: Screen magnification systems; braille access systems; closed-circuit television systems; word processing; database software; computer operating systems; training for instructors.

Helen Keller Services for the Blind

57 Willoughby Street
Brooklyn, NY 11201
(718) 522-2122
FAX: (718) 935-9463
Frank Romano, Associate Director

Computer Training: Speech output systems; screen magnification systems; braille access systems; optical character recognition systems; closed-circuit television systems; word processing; database software; computer operating systems; training for instructors.

Lavelle School for the Blind

East 221th Street and Paulding Avenue
Bronx, NY 10469
(718) 882-1212
FAX: (718) 882-0005
Ronald D. Fedele, Computer Specialist

Computer Training: Speech output systems; screen magnification systems, braille access systems; OSCAR scanning systems, closed-circuit television systems; word processing.

LIFT

P.O. Box 1072

Mountainside, NY 07092
(908) 789-2443
FAX: (908) 903-0933
E-mail: liftinc@aol.com
Donna Walters Kozberg, President
Barbara Lee, Assessment
Counselor

Computer Training: Speech
output systems; screen
magnification systems; braille
access systems; optical character
recognition systems; closed-circuit
television systems; word
processing; database software;
computer operating system.

The Lighthouse Inc.

111 East 59th Street
New York, NY 10022
(212) 821-9681
Martin S. Yablonski, Vice
President, Manhattan, Bronx,
Brooklyn

Computer Training: Speech
output systems; screen
magnification systems; braille
access systems; closed-circuit
television systems, word
processing; database software;
computer operating systems.

The Lighthouse Inc.
Hudson Valley

44 Church Street
White Plains, NY 10601
(914) 761-3221
Judith Millman, Vice President,
Hudson Valley Region

Computer Training: Speech
output systems;
screenmagnification systems;
braille access systems; closed-
circuit television systems, word
processing; database software;
computer operating systems.

New York Institute for Special Education

999 Pelham Parkway

Bronx, NY 10469
(718) 519-7000
John Hernandez, Teacher

Computer Training: Speech
output systems; braille access
systems; optical character
recognition systems; closed-circuit
television systems; training for
instructors.

Northeastern Association of the Blind

301 Washington Avenue
Albany, NY 12206
(518) 463-1211
FAX: (518) 436-4194
Art Rizzino, Director

County/District Where Located:
Albany County.

Computer Training: Speech
output systems; screen
magnification systems; braille
access systems; optical character
recognition systems; closed-circuit
television systems; word
processing; database software;
computer operating systems.

Techspress/RCIL

409 Columbia Street
Utica, NY 13502
(315) 797-4642
FAX: (315) 797-4747
E-mail: txprsny@aol.com
Lana Grossin, Director

County/District Where Located:
Oneida County.

Computer Training: Speech
output systems; screen
magnification systems; word
processing; computer operating
systems.

DOG GUIDE SCHOOLS

Guide Dog Foundation for the Blind, Inc.

371 East Jericho Turnpike

Smithtown, NY 11787
(516) 265-2121 or (800) 548-4337
FAX: (516) 361-5192
E-mail: wjones@guidedog.org
Wells B. Jones, CAE, CFRE

Type of Agency: Non-profit.
Mission: Offers professional
training of blind persons with dog
guides, without fee. Maintains
breeding and puppy-raising
program.
Funded by: Contributions and
endowments.
Budget: $3 million.
Hours of Operation: Mon.-Fri.
8:00 AM-5:00 PM.
Staff: 49 full and part-time.
History/Date: Est. 1946 and Inc.
1949.
Number of Clients Served: 80-90
annually.
Eligibility: Legally blind.
Area Served: International in
scope.
Transportation: Y.
Age Requirements: 16 years and
older.

Guiding Eyes for the Blind, Inc.

611 Granite Springs Road
Yorktown Heights, NY 10598
(914) 245-4024
FAX: (914) 245-1609
William Badger, President

Mission: Breeds, raises, and trains
dog guides and instructs blind
individuals in their use. Trains
own instructors, maintains
follow-up service for graduates.
Funded by: Corporate,
foundation, and individual gifts.
Budget: 1996.: $6,699,769.
Hours of Operation: Mon.-Fri.
8:00 AM-6:00 PM.
Staff: 60 full time; 20 part time; 95
volunteers.
History/Date: Est. and Inc. 1954.
Number of Clients Served:
Approximately 160 annually.

Area Served: Unlimited.
Age Requirements: 16 years and older.

Educational: Has public education program, including speakers bureau.
Computer Training: Adaptive equipment available.

♦ Low Vision Services

EYE CARE SOCIETIES

New York State Ophthalmological Society
10 Colvin Avenue
Albany, NY 12206-1920
(518) 438-2020
Robin Pellegrino, Executive Director

New York State Optometric Association, Inc.
90 South Swan Street
Albany, NY 12210
(518) 449-7300 or (800) 342-9836
Jan Dorman

LOW VISION CENTERS

Association for the Blind and Visually Impaired of Greater Rochester, Inc.
Low Vision Clinic
422 South Clinton Avenue
Rochester, NY 14620-1198
(716) 232-1111
FAX: (716) 232-6707
Marilyn Kuchmek, Low Vision Coordinator

Type of Agency: Non-profit.
Mission: To maximize residual vision.
Funded by: Client fees (sliding scale); United Way; state funds.
Hours of Operation: Mon., Tues., Wed., Fri. mornings. Occasional Thurs.

Program Accessibility: Totally accessible.
Staff: 1 ophthalmologist; 3 optometrists; 1 optician.
History/Date: Est. 1976.
Number of Clients Served: 800 annually.
Eligibility: Current ophthalmological report.
Area Served: Unlimited.
Age Requirements: None.

Counseling/Social Work/Self-Help: Individual counseling, support groups, outreach and screening.
Educational: Children's program in partnership with public education, computer assessment and training.
Preschools: Home training; early intervention.
Reading: Volunteer readers available.
Rehabilitation: Full range of services including orientation and mobility, rehabiliation teaching, counseling, social work and vocational training.
Employment: Placement, supported employment, vocational preparations, agency based direct laboratories, food service, and manufacturing.
Computer Training: Comprehensive assessment and training.
Low Vision: On site comprehensive low vision service.
Low Vision Aids: For sale and loan only with doctor's prescription.
Low Vision Follow-up: After 2 months or 6 months, according to doctor's directions.

Blind Association of Western New York
1170 Main Street

Buffalo, NY 14209
(716) 882-1025
Sara A. Law MS, V.P.
Rehabilitation Services
Beverly Stana, Coordinator, Vision Rehabilitation Center

Type of Agency: Private, non-profit.
Mission: Services for persons of all ages who are visually impaired or legally blind.
Funded by: Client fees, third party payments, New York State Commission for the Blind and Visually Handicapped, Medicare, VESID.
Budget: $130,000.
Hours of Operation: By appointment only.
Program Accessibility: Fully accessible.
Staff: Certified low vision optometrists; low vision coordinator; orientation/mobility instructor; rehabilitation counselor; social caseworker; vocational evaluator; communication instructor.
History/Date: Est. 1907, Inc. 1908.
Number of Clients Served: 350 annually.
Eligibility: Recent eye report or ophthalmological exam at clinic.
Area Served: Western New York.
Transportation: Y.
Age Requirements: All ages.

Low Vision Aids: Provided on recommendation.
Low Vision Follow-up: Provided.

Buffalo General Hospital
Wettlaufer Eye Clinic
100 High Street

Buffalo, NY 14203
(716) 859-2533
Joseph F. Monte, M.D., Chief
Geraldine Schneider, Clinic
Supervisor
Paula A. Gowin, Administrative
Assistant, Department of
Ophthalmology

Type of Agency: Non-profit.
County/District Where Located:
Erie County.
Funded by: Client fees.
Hours of Operation: Mon.-Fri.
9:00 AM-4:30 PM.
Staff: Ophthalmologist;
ophthalmology resident; social
worker.
Eligibility: None.
Area Served: Unlimited.

Low Vision Aids: Not provided
on loan; on-site training provided.
Low Vision Follow-up: Variable
according to problem.

Eleanor E. Faye Low Vision Service
The Lighthouse Inc.

111 East 59th Street
New York, NY 10022-1202
(212) 821-9626
FAX: (212) 821-9710
E-mail: mfischer@lighthouse.org
URL: http://www.lighthouse.org
Martin S. Yablonski, Vice
President, Regional Director
Michael Fischer, O.D., Director

Type of Agency: Non-profit.
Mission: Provide low vision
evaluations and instruction as part
of comprehensive vision
rehabilitation services.
Funded by: Consumer/patient
fees; third-party payers; referral
sources and The Lighthouse, Inc.
Hours of Operation: By
appointment: Mon.-Fri. 9:00 AM-
5:00 PM; Thurs. till 7:00 PM.
Program Accessibility:
Handicapped accessible.

Staff: Low vision clinicians (MDs,
ODs); low vision instructors;
optician; social workers; vision
rehabilitation therapists in
orientation and mobility and/or
rehabilitation teaching;
employment and placement
specialists.
Number of Clients Served: FY
'96: 2,355.
Eligibility: Functional vision
impairment, proof of primary eye
care, diagnostic eye report
requested and required for certain
conditions.
Area Served: Unlimited.
Age Requirements: None.

Rehabilitation: Comprehensive
vision rehabilitation therapy
(orientation/mobility and/or
rehabilitation teaching); counseling
and employment services.
Low Vision Aids: Provided on
loan for trial. Dispensed by
optician or low vision clinician.
Instruction provided.
Low Vision Follow-up: Provided
as needed in accordance with
prescribed treatment plan.

Local Offices:

Bronx: Outreach Office, 350 East
Gunhill Road, Bronx, NY 10467,
(718) 920-0730.
New York: Mt. Sinai Hospital,
Five East 98th Street, Faculty
Practice Building, Seventh Floor,
New York, NY 10029, (212) 821-
9632, (212) 241-0939.

Erie County Medical Center

462 Grider Street
Buffalo, NY 14215
(716) 898-3716
FAX: (716) 898-3343
Norman Weiss, O.D.

County/District Where Located:
Erie County.
Funded by: County.

Hours of Operation: Second and
fourth Wednesday of each month
at 1:00 PM.
Staff: Ophthalmologist;
opthalmology residents; optician.
Eligibility: None.
Area Served: Unlimited.

Low Vision: Evaulation.
Low Vision Aids: Not provided
for trial on loan; on-site training
provided.
Low Vision Follow-up: By return
appointment at 3 and 6 months, as
indicated.

Jewish Guild for the Blind/Home for Aged Blind
Kramer Vision Rehabilitation Center

75 Stratton Street South
Yonkers, NY 10701
(212) 365-3700, ext. 544 or
(914) 963-4661, ext. 544
Bruce Mastalinski, Vice President
and Director
Laura Sperazza, Director, Low
Vision Services

Type of Agency: Non-profit.
County/District Where Located:
Westchester County.
Mission: Serving visually
impaired/blind persons.
Staff: Optometrist; social worker;
orientation/mobility instructor;
rehabilitation counselor;
communication skills instructor;
rehabilitation teacher.
Ophthalmologists available off
site.
Eligibility: By referral, with
diagnosis.
Area Served: Unlimited.

Low Vision: Evaluation, referral,
rehabilitation.
Low Vision Aids: On-site training
provided.
Low Vision Follow-up: By return
appointment.

Long Island Jewish Medical Center
Eye Care Center

600 Northern Boulevard, Room 214
Great Neck, NY 11021
(516) 470-2000
Ira Udell, M.D., Chairman,
Department of Ophthalmology
Joel Scheckner, O.D., Attending
Optometrist

County/District Where Located:
Nassau County.
Funded by: Insurance, fee for
service.
Hours of Operation: Fri. 9:00 AM -
4:00 PM.
Staff: Low vision specialist
(optometrist).
Eligibility: None.
Area Served: Nassau and Queens
Counties.

Low Vision Aids: Provided on
loan for trial, if necessary.
Low Vision Follow-up: By return
appointment and telephone.

Low Vision Clinic
Helen Keller Services for the Blind (HKSB)

57 Willoughby Street
Brooklyn, NY 11201
(718) 522-2122
FAX: (718) 935-9463
William Dale, Clinic Administrator

Type of Agency: Private; non-
profit.
Mission: To enable persons of all
ages who are visually impaired,
blind, or deaf-blind to lead as
independent a life as possible.
Funded by: Medicaid, Medicare,
client fees, New York State
Commission for the Blind and
Visually Handicapped.
Budget: $90,000.
Hours of Operation: Mon.-Fri.
9:00 AM-4:00 PM; by appointment.
Staff: Ophthamalogist;
optometrists; social worker;

rehabilitation teachers; orientation
and mobility instructors.
History/Date: Est. 1952.
Number of Clients Served: More
than 1,200 annually.
Eligibility: Recent eye report.
Area Served: New York City
metropolitan area and Long Island.

Low Vision: Comprehensive eye
care services.
Low Vision Aids: Available for
purchase with on-site training.
Low Vision Follow-up: Varies
according to patient needs.

Local Offices:

Hempstead: Helen Keller Services
for the Blind, Nassau Service
Center and Rehabilitation Center,
320 Fulton Avenue, Hempstead,
NY 11550, (516) 485-1234, FAX
(516) 538-6785.

Low Vision Service
The Lighthouse Inc.

60-05 Woodhaven Boulevard
Elmhurst, NY 11373
(718) 899-9100
FAX: (718) 899-9506
E-mail: mfischer@lighthouse.org
URL: http://www.lighthouse.org
Frank Simpson, Vice President,
Regional Director
Michael Fischer, O.D.

Type of Agency: Non-profit.
County/District Where Located:
Queens County.
Mission: Provide low vision
evaluations and instruction as part
of comprehensive vision
rehabilitation services.
Funded by: Client fees; approved
third party payers, referral sources
and The Lighthouse, Inc.
Hours of Operation: By
appointment: three days a week,
9:00 AM-5:00 PM.
Program Accessibility:
Handicapped accessible.

Staff: Low vision clinicians (MDs,
ODs); low vision instructors;
optician; social workers; vision
rehabilitation therapists in
orientation/mobility and/or
rehabilitation teaching;
employment and placement
specialists.
Number of Clients Served: 412.
Eligibility: Functional vision
impairment, proof of primary eye
care, diagnostic eye report
requested and required for certain
conditions.
Area Served: Unlimited, primarily
Queens County.
Age Requirements: None.

Rehabilitation: Comprehensive
vision rehabilitation therapy
(orientation/mobility and/or
rehabilitation teaching); counseling
and employment services.
Low Vision Aids: Provided on
loan for trial. Dispensed by
optician or low vision clinician.
Instruction provided.
Low Vision Follow-up: Provided
as needed in accordance with
prescribed treatment plan.

Low Vision Service
The Lighthouse Inc.

1731 North Ocean Avenue
Medford, NY 11763
(516) 654-3525
FAX: (516) 654-3280
E-mail: rfarand@lighthouse.org
URL: http://www.lighthouse.org
Frank Simpson, Vice President,
Regional Director
Teresa Halliwell, OD, Director

Type of Agency: Non-profit.
County/District Where Located:
Suffolk County.
Mission: Provide low vision
evaluations and instruction as part
of comprehensive vision
rehabilitation services.
Funded by: Consumer/patient
fees; third-party payers; referral
sources and The Lighthouse, Inc.

Hours of Operation: By appointment: Wed. 9:00AM-1:00PM; Fri: 9:30AM-12:30PM.
Program Accessibility: Handicapped accessible.
Staff: Low vision clinicians (ODs); low vision instructors; social workers; vision rehabilitation therapists in orientation/mobility and/or rehabilitation teaching.
Number of Clients Served: FY '96: 263.
Eligibility: Functional vision impairment, proof of primary eye care, diagnostic eye report requested and required for certain conditions.
Area Served: Unlimited, primarily Suffolk and Nassau Counties.
Age Requirements: None.

Rehabilitation: Comprehensive vision rehabilitation therapy (orientation/mobility and/or rehabilitation teaching); counseling and referral to employment services.
Low Vision Aids: Provided on loan for trial. Dispensed by low vision clinician. Instruction provided.
Low Vision Follow-up: Provided as needed in accordance with prescribed treatment plan.

Low Vision Service
State University of New York
College of Optometry
100 East 24th Street
New York, NY 10010
(212) 780-5013
FAX: (212) 420-5094
Roy Gordon Cole, O.D., Director

Type of Agency: University low vision service.
Mission: Provides low vision services and training for clinical internships and residencies in low vision.
Funded by: State funds, patient fees, Medicaid, Medicare.

Hours of Operation: Mon. - Fri. 9:00 AM-12:00 noon; 1:00-5:00 PM. Evenings by appointment.
Staff: Ophthalmologist; optometry interns; externs; residents; optician; social worker; pediatrician; internist; neurologist. Staff available through associated agencies in New York City include psychologist; rehabilitation teacher; orientation/mobility instructor; special educator; technology center.
Number of Clients Served: Low vision service: approximately 2,000.
Eligibility: None.
Area Served: Unlimited.

Computer Training: Access.
Low Vision: Complete evaluations and special testing including VEP's, ERG's, ultra sound, and color vision analysis.
Low Vision Aids: Provided on loan for trial; on-site training provided.
Low Vision Follow-up: Two weeks after initial visit, or as needed.

Low Vision Services
The Lighthouse Inc.
44 Church Street
White Plains, NY 10601
(914) 761-3221
FAX: (914) 761-0484
E-mail: woconnell@lighthouse.org
URL: http://www.lighthouse.org
Judith Millman, Vice President, Regional Director
William F. O'Connell, O.D., Director

Type of Agency: Non-profit.
County/District Where Located: Westchester County.
Mission: Provide low vision evaluations and instruction as part of comprehensive vision rehabilitation services.

Funded by: Consumer/patient fees, approved third party payers, referral sources and The Lighthouse, Inc.
Hours of Operation: By appointment: Mon.-Fri. 8:00 AM-5:00 PM; evening appointments also available.
Program Accessibility: Handicapped accessible.
Staff: Low vision clinicians (ODs); low vision instructors; social workers; vision rehabilitation therapists in orientation/mobility and/or rehabilitation teaching; employment and placement specialists.
Number of Clients Served: FY'96: 585.
Eligibility: Functional vision impairment, proof of primary eye care, diagnostic eye report requested and required for certain conditions.
Area Served: Unlimited, primarily the Hudson Valley Region.
Age Requirements: None.

Rehabilitation: Comprehensive vision rehabilitation therapy (orientation/mobility and/or rehabilitation teaching); counseling and employment services.
Low Vision Aids: Provided on loan for trial. Dispensed by low vision clinician. Instruction provided.
Low Vision Follow-up: Provided as needed in accordance with prescribed treatment plan.

Montefiore Hospital
Medical Center
Low Vision Service
3332 Rochambeau Avenue
Bronx, NY 10467
(718) 920-6244
FAX: (718) 655-3985
Lanny Binstock O.D. F.A.A.O., Director, Low Vision Service

Type of Agency: Non-profit.

Funded by: Client fees; third-party payments; New York State Commission for the Blind and Visually Handicapped.
Hours of Operation: Mon.-Fri. 9:30 AM-4:30 PM. By appointment only.
Staff: Ophthalmologist; ophthalmology resident; optometrist; social worker; optician.
Area Served: Unlimited.

Low Vision: Evaluation and referral.
Low Vision Aids: Provided on loan; on-site training provided.
Low Vision Follow-up: By return appointment.

New York Eye and Ear Infirmary

310 East 14th Street
New York, NY 10003
(212) 979-4375
Judith Gurland, M.D., Ophthalmologist, Director
Suzanne Schudel, Low Vision Assistant/Ophthalmic Technologist

Type of Agency: Non-profit.
Funded by: Client fees.
Hours of Operation: By appointment.
Staff: Ophthalmologist; ophthalmology residents; ophthalmic technologist; low vision assistant; optometrist; social worker; audiologist.
Eligibility: Poor visual acuity; clinic and private patients not in need of mobility training.
Area Served: Unlimited.

Low Vision Aids: Can be purchased directly; provided for trial; rental fee; on-site training.
Low Vision Follow-up: By return appointment and/or phone interview at 1 month.

Northeastern Association of the Blind

301 Washington Avenue
Albany, NY 12206
(518) 463-1211
FAX: (518) 463-3585
Albert M. Morier, O.D.
Susan Ebert, Clinic Coordinator

Type of Agency: Non-profit.
County/District Where Located: Albany County.
Hours of Operation: Tues. 8:00 AM-Noon.
Staff: Optometrist-low vision specialist; social worker; orientation/mobility instructor; rehabilitation teacher; psychologist; rehabilitation counselor; job placement specialists.
Eligibility: Ophthalmologic report.
Area Served: Central New York State.
Age Requirements: None.

Computer Training: Two full-time instructors, training 3-12 months; contact: Andy Davidson.
Low Vision Aids: On-site and community training provided.
Low Vision Follow-up: By return appointment with rehabilitation teacher.

Northport Veterans Affairs Medical Center
Low Vision Clinic and VICTORS Program

79 Middleville Road
Northport, NY 11768-2290
(516) 261-4400
Richard Soden, O.D., Supervisor, Low Vision Clinic
Allen H. Cohen, O.D., F.A.A.O., Chief, Eye/Vision Program
Brendal Waiss, O.D., F.A.A.O., Coordinator, VICTORS Program

County/District Where Located: Suffolk County.

Funded by: Federal government.
Hours of Operation: Tues., Wed., Thurs. 9:00 AM-11:00 AM.
Staff: Ophthalmologists; optometrists; audiologist; low vision assistant; occupational therapist; psychiatrist; psychologist; rehabilitation counselor; social worker; speech therapist; vocational counselor, diabetic nurse.
Eligibility: Visually impaired veterans with Honorable Discharge.
Area Served: Eastern Seaboard.

Counseling/Social Work/Self-Help: Visual impairment service team counselor available.
Rehabilitation: VICTORS Program, intensive 5-day inpatient rehabilitation program for partially sighted veterans.
Low Vision: On-site evaluations and training provided.
Low Vision Aids: Supplied free to eligible veterans (service-connected disability).
Low Vision Follow-up: By recall system.

North Shore University Hospital Low Vision Services

300 Community Drive
Manhasset, NY 11030
(516) 562-4530
Marc C. Epstein, O.D., Director

Type of Agency: Non-profit.
Mission: To serve the low vision needs of patients referred by physicians and optometrists.
Funded by: Client fees.
Hours of Operation: Alternate Fri., 9:00 AM-12:00 noon.
Staff: Ophthalmology resident; optometrist; social worker; occupational therapist; rehabilitation counselor; orthoptist; rehabilitation teacher; psychologist/counselor; audiologist.

Eligibility: Referral.
Area Served: Unlimited.
Age Requirements: None.

Low Vision Aids: Not provided on loan; on-site training provided.
Low Vision Follow-up: By return appointment.

University Eye Institute
SUNY Health Science Center at Syracuse

Vision Rehabilitation Center
550 Harrison Center #340
Syracuse, NY 13202
(315) 422-4412
FAX: (315) 422-4690
Mary M. Jackowski, Ph.D., O.D., Director

Type of Agency: Private.
County/District Where Located: Onondaga County.
Mission: Serving clients with visual dysfunction due to ocular disease, trauma, stroke and neurological deficit.
Funded by: Federal and state funds, private insurance, client fees.
Hours of Operation: Mon.-Sat.; evening hours available.
Staff: Optometrist, low vision coordinator, nurse-educator.
Area Served: Unlimited.
Age Requirements: All ages.

Computer Training: Assessment for assistance technology.
Low Vision Aids: Provided for purchase and rental.
Low Vision Follow-up: Return appointment.

Local Offices:

Fulton: 201 South Second Street, Fulton, NY 13069.
Syracuse: 1101 Erie Boulevard East, Syracuse, NY 13210.

◆ Aging Services

STATE UNITS ON AGING

Office for the Aging
New York State Plaza
Agency Building Two
Albany, NY 12223
(518) 474-4425 or Information & Referral In State, Senior Citizens Hotline (800) 342-9871
FAX: (518) 474-1398
Walter Hoefer, Director

Provides referrals to Area Agencies on Aging and information on other local aging services.

INDEPENDENT LIVING PROGRAMS

Department of Social Services New York State Commission for the Blind and Visually Handicapped
10 Eyck Office Building
40 North Pearl Street
Albany, NY 12243
(518) 473-1801
FAX: (518) 486-5819
Thomas Robertson, Assistant Commissioner
Neil Springfield, Project Director, (518) 474-2209

Provides independent living services for persons age 55 and over. For further information, contact the Project Director or general phone number listed.

NORTH CAROLINA

◆ *Educational Services*

STATE SERVICES

**North Carolina Department of Public Instruction
Exceptional Children Division**
Education Building
301 North Wilmington Street
Raleigh, NC 27601-2825
(919) 715-1565
FAX: (919) 715-1569
E. Lowell Harris, Director, Exceptional Children Division
Ed Stone, Textbook Consultant
Kathy Nisbet, Early Childhood Consultant
David Mills, Section Chief, Areas of Exceptionality

Type of Agency: State.
County/District Where Located: Wake County.
Mission: Provides braille, cassette tape and large-type textbooks for Grades 1-12. Offers consultation on education programs.
Funded by: Public funds.
Hours of Operation: Mon.-Fri. 7:30AM-5:30PM.
Staff: 20.
History/Date: Est. 1949.
Number of Clients Served: 687.
Eligibility: Must meet State Board of Education criteria.
Area Served: North Carolina.
Transportation: Y.
Age Requirements: Ages 3-21.

Low Vision: Evaluations, referrals, training.
Low Vision Aids: Yes.
Low Vision Follow-up: Yes.

For information about local facilities, consult the superintendent of schools in the area.

EARLY INTERVENTION COORDINATION

**Developmental Disabilities Section
Division of Mental Health, Mental Retardation and Substance Abuse Services
North Carolina Department of Human Services**
325 North Salisbury Street
Raleigh, NC 27603
(919) 733-3654
FAX: (919) 733-9455
Duncan Munn, Chief of Day Services

County/District Where Located: Wake County.

SCHOOLS

Governor Morehead School
301 Ashe Avenue
Raleigh, NC 27606
(919) 733-6381
FAX: (919) 733-1855
George Lee, Director of Students

Type of Agency: State.
Mission: Services for totally blind; legally blind.
Funded by: State and federal funds.
Budget: $7.7 million.
Hours of Operation: 8:00 AM - 5:00 PM, (office hours).
Staff: 260 full time. Uses volunteers.
History/Date: Est. 1845.
Number of Clients Served: 1997: 90 residential, 300 preschool at 12 sites and 30 more through outreach.
Eligibility: Legally blind and multiply disabled.
Area Served: North Carolina.
Transportation: Y.
Age Requirements: 0-5 years: preschool day program; 5-21 years: residential program.

Health: Treatment of minor eye conditions; follow-up evaluation of eye treatment or prescription; general medical services; speech, hearing, occupational and physical therapy; low vision. Refers for other health services.
Counseling/Social Work/Self-Help: Social evaluations; psychological testing and evaluations; individual counseling; transition services; placement in school, training. Refers for other counseling/social work services; access to Lions Clinic Assessment Center.
Educational: Preschool through 12. Programs for general academic studies; vocational/skill development; special programs for multiply disabled blind persons.
Preschools: 8 sites: Greensboro, Chapel Hill, Charlotte, Morganton, Fayetteville, Greenville, and Wilmington.
Professional Training: Internship/fieldwork placement in vocational areas; orientation/mobility; rehabilitation counseling; special education. Regular in-service training programs. Masters program with NC Central University.
Reading: Talking book record players and cassette players; talking book records and cassettes; braille books; large print books; braille and recorded magazines; Kurzweil Reader; computers; radio reader service.
Residential: Cottages for children.
Rehabilitation: Personal management; braille; handwriting; listening skills; keyboard; typing; home management; orientation/mobility; remedial education; sensory motor training; prevocational and vocational workcenters. Refers for

rehabilitation teaching in client's home and community.

Recreational: After-school programs; arts and crafts; hobby groups; leisure activities; fitness activities; residential summer camp; swimming; track; wrestling; cheerleading; goalball.

Employment: Career and skill counseling transition services; refers for some other employment services.

Computer Training: Y.

Contact local school superintendent for program availability or Visually Impaired Programs, Division for Exceptional Children, North Carolina Department of Public Instruction, Raleigh, NC 27603-1712, (919) 733-3004.

INFANT AND PRESCHOOL

North Carolina Department of Human Resources
Division of Services for the Blind
309 Ashe Avenue
Raleigh, NC 27606
(919) 733-9822
John B. DeLuca, Director

Type of Agency: State.
County/District Where Located: Wake County.
Funded by: State and Title XX funds and county funds.
Staff: 500 full time.
History/Date: Est. 1935.
Transportation: Y.
Age Requirements: For certain programs.

Health: Genetic and other counseling; adaptive equipment.
Educational: Instruction in all developmental areas.
Low Vision: Complete eye exams and follow-up including eyeglasses, surgery, treatment;

medical workshops for eligible clients.

Home-based program and consultant services to other programs for visually impaired multiply disabled children.

♦ Information Services

LIBRARIES

North Carolina Library for the Blind and Physically Handicapped
North Carolina State Library
1811 Capital Boulevard
Raleigh, NC 27635
(919) 733-4376 or (800) 662-7726 or TDD (919) 733-1462
FAX: (919) 733-6910
E-mail: nclbph@ncsl.dcr.state.nc.us
Francine Martin, Librarian

Type of Agency: Library.
Mission: To administer the National Library Service for the Blind and Physically Handicapped program in North Carolina.
Funded by: Public funds.
Staff: 33.
History/Date: Est. 1958.
Number of Clients Served: 9,555.
Eligibility: Inability to read standard print due to visual or physical disability as certified by competent authority.
Area Served: North Carolina. Also serves South Carolina with braille.

Regional library providing talking books on disk and on cassette, braille and large-type books, talking book machines, and accessories.

MEDIA PRODUCTION SERVICES

Blue Ridge Braillers
175 Bingham Road
Asheville, NC 28806-3800
(704) 255-5921
Helen Hicking, Assignment Chairman.

Area Served: Buncombe County, western North Carolina.
Groups Served: K-12; college students; other adults.

Types/Content: Textbooks; career/vocational.
Media Formats: Braille books.
Title Listings: Braille lists supplied at no charge.

North Carolina Department of Human Resources
Division of Services for the Blind
309 Ashe Avenue
Raleigh, NC 27606
(919) 733-9700
FAX: (919) 715-8871
E-mail: jdeluca@dhr.state.nc.us
URL: http://www.dhr.state.nc.us/dhr/dsb
John B. DeLuca, Director

Area Served: Statewide.
Groups Served: All ages.

Types/Content: Textbooks, career/vocational.
Media Formats: Braille books, cassettes, large-print books.
Title Listings: No title listings available.

RADIO READING

Central Piedmont Community College Radio Reading Service
P.O. Box 35009
Charlotte, NC 28235
(704) 330-6994
FAX: (704) 330-6597
Jim Bailey, Program Director

County/District Where Located:
Mecklenburg County.
Hours of Operation: 24 hours a day, seven days a week.
History/Date: Est. 1977.
Area Served: Mecklenburg (Charlotte), Gaston, Iredell, Lincoln, Rowan, Stanly, Union Counties.

Neighborhood News for the Blind
P.O. Box 7405
Winston-Salem, NC 27109
(910) 761-5257
T. Cleve Callison, Station Manager

Hours of Operation: Sat. 8:00 AM-9:00 PM.
History/Date: Est. 1976.
Area Served: 35-mile radius from Winston-Salem.

Radio Reading Services, Inc.
211 E. Six Forks Road
Suite 103
Raleigh, NC 27609-7743
(919) 832-5138
FAX: (919) 832-5138
E-mail: ah_trrs@juno.com
Annette Henry, Director

County/District Where Located:
Wake County.
Funded by: United Way; local groups, and individuals.
Hours of Operation: 24 hours a day, 7 days a week.
Staff: 2.
History/Date: Est. 1983.
Area Served: Metropolitan Raleigh, Wake County, and 16 counties in north central North Carolina.
Age Requirements: None.

Regional Audio Information Service Enterprise (RAISE)
75 Haywood Street, G-5

Asheville, NC 28801
(704) 251-2166
Robert Brummond, President

County/District Where Located:
Boncomb County.

Southeastern North Carolina Radio Reading Service
1200 Murchison Road
Fayetteville, NC 28301
(910) 486-7007
Thomas N. White, Executive Director

County/District Where Located:
Cumberland County.
Area Served: Southeastern North Carolina, thirteen counties.

INFORMATION AND REFERRAL

The Foundation Fighting Blindness
North Carolina Affiliate
1822 Cavendish Court
Charlotte, NC 28211
(704) 362-2611
Pam Allen, President

See The Foundation Fighting Blindness in U.S. national listings.

The Foundation Fighting Blindness
Piedmont Affiliate
44 Kemp Road East
Greensboro, NC 27410-6016
(910) 292-8124
Marilyn Green, President

See The Foundation Fighting Blindness in U.S. national listings.

The Foundation Fighting Blindness
Raleigh Affiliate
5321 Barclay Drive
Raleigh, NC 27606
(919) 851-2856
Rebekah Royster, Contact Person

See The Foundation Fighting Blindness in U.S. national listings.

Prevent Blindness North Carolina
3801 Lake Boone Trail
Suite 410
Raleigh, NC 27607
(919) 571-1014
FAX: (919) 571-1502
E-mail: 104706.1114@compuserve.com
Jennifer Green, Executive Director

See Prevent Blindness America in U.S. national listings.

See also in national listings:

Metrolina Association for the Blind

National Early Childhood Technical Assistance System (NEC*TAS)

◆ *Rehabilitation Services*

STATE SERVICES

North Carolina Department of Human Resources
Division of Services for the Blind
309 Ashe Avenue
Raleigh, NC 27606
(919) 733-9822
FAX: (919) 733-9769
E-mail: jdeluca@dhr.state.nc.us
URL: http://www.dhr.state.nc.us/dhr/dsb
John B. DeLuca, Director

Type of Agency: State.
Mission: Services for totally blind, legally blind, visually impaired, and deaf-blind persons.
Funded by: State, federal, and county funds.

Budget: $35 million.
Hours of Operation: Mon.-Fri. 8:00 AM - 5:00 PM.
Staff: 500 full time.
History/Date: Est. 1935.
Number of Clients Served: 57,886.
Eligibility: Legally blind or visually impaired.
Area Served: Statewide.
Age Requirements: For certain programs.

Health: Complete eye examinations and follow-up including eyeglasses, surgery and treatment; medical work-ups for eligible clients.
Counseling/Social Work/Self-Help: Social evaluation; psychological testing and evaluation; individual, group, family/parent, couple counseling; placement in training. Refers and provides consultation to other agencies for other counseling/social work services.
Educational: The Governor Morehead School includes a preschool, K-12, and outreach program.
Preschools: Morehead School for the Blind serves approximately 275 children in the 0-4 years age group from 10 sites covering approximately one half of state.
Professional Training: Regular in-service training programs; contracts with university system.
Reading: Reader services.
Residential: Rehabilitation center, Morehead School.
Rehabilitation: Personal management; braille; handwriting; listening skills; assistive technology; electronic mobility aids; home management; orientation/mobility; rehabilitation teaching in client's home and community; remedial education; sensory training.

Employment: Prevocational evaluation; career and skill counseling; occupational skill development; job retention; job retraining; sheltered workshops; vocational placement; follow-up service; Business Enterprises training.
Computer Training: Yes.
Low Vision: Low vision aids.
Low Vision Follow-up: Yes.

Local Offices:

Asheville: District Office, 50 South French Broad Avenue, Asheville, NC 28801, (704) 251-6732.
Charlotte: District Office, 500 W. Trade Street, Suite 347, Charlotte, NC 28202, (704) 342-6185.
Fayetteville: District Office, 225 Green Street, Fayetteville, NC 28301, (910) 486-1582.
Greenville: District Office, 404 St. Andrews Drive, Greenville, NC 27834, (919) 355-9016.
Raleigh: Evaluation Unit, Raleigh Lions Clinic, 315 Hubert Street, Raleigh, NC 27603, (919) 733-4281.
Raleigh: District Office, 309 Ashe Avenue, Raleigh, NC 27606, (919) 733-4234.
Raleigh: Rehabilitation Center for the Blind, 305 Ashe Avenue, Raleigh, NC 27606, (919) 733-5897.
Wilmington: District Office, 14 South 16th Street, Wilmington, NC 28401, (910) 251-5743.
Winston-Salem: District Office, 200 Miller Street, Winston-Salem, NC 27103, (910) 761-2345.

REHABILITATION

Industries of the Blind
920 West Lee Street
P.O. Box 3544
Greensboro, NC 27402
(910) 274-1591 or (910) 272-0927
FAX: (910) 274-9207
Derek M. Davis, Executive Director

Type of Agency: Sheltered workshop; vocational training agency.
County/District Where Located: Guilford County.
Mission: To assist visually impaired persons to develop their capabilities to the fullest and offer employment opportunities to those who wish to work.
Funded by: Workshop sales and sub-contracts.
Budget: $14.5 million.
Hours of Operation: 7:30 AM-4:00 PM.
Staff: 14.
History/Date: Est. 1933.
Number of Clients Served: 103.
Eligibility: Blind or visually impaired; referred from North Carolina Services for the Blind.
Area Served: North Carolina and parts of South Carolina and Virginia.
Transportation: Y.

Counseling/Social Work/Self-Help: Provided by Services for the Blind of North Carolina.
Rehabilitation: Vocational evaluations, vocational training, training in independent living skills.
Employment: Sheltered workshops; vocational training.
Low Vision Aids: Recommendations and referrals.

Lions Club Industries for the Blind, Inc.
1810 East Main Street
P.O. Box 11305
Durham, NC 27703
(919) 596-8277
FAX: (919) 598-1179
William L. Hudson, Executive Director

Type of Agency: Private; non-profit.
County/District Where Located: Durham County.

Mission: Services for totally blind; legally blind.
Funded by: Workshop sales.
Staff: 6 full time.
History/Date: Est. 1936.
Eligibility: Legally blind.

Counseling/Social Work/Self-Help: Individual counseling; placement in training.
Employment: Prevocational evaluation; sheltered workshops.

Lions Industries for the Blind

P.O. Box 2001
Kingston, NC 28502
(919) 523-1019
FAX: (919) 523-7090
Robert W. Smith, Executive Director

Mission: To provide employment and training for the blind and visually impaired.

Lions Services

4600 A North Tryon
Charlotte, NC 28213
(704) 921-1527
FAX: (704) 921-1577
David Marotta, Executive Director

County/District Where Located: Mecklenburg County.
Funded by: Workshop sales.
History/Date: Est. 1934.

Employment: Job training; job retention; sheltered workshops; vocational placement; supported employment; computer training.

Metrolina Association for the Blind

704 Louise Avenue
Charlotte, NC 28204
(704) 372-3870
FAX: (704) 372-3871
Robert Scheffel, Executive Director

Type of Agency: Private; non-profit.

County/District Where Located: Mecklenburg County.
Mission: Services for totally blind, legally blind, and visually impaired persons.
Funded by: Fees; United Way; endowment.
Budget: $850,000.
Hours of Operation: Mon. - Fri. 8:30 AM - 5:00 PM.
Staff: 20 full time. Uses volunteers.
History/Date: Est. 1934.
Number of Clients Served: 600 annually.
Eligibility: Visually impaired.
Area Served: Greater Charlotte area.
Transportation: Y.

Health: Refers for health services.
Counseling/Social Work/Self-Help: Individual, group, family/parent, couple counseling; referral to community services. Refers for other counseling/social work services.
Reading: Transcription to braille, large print, and tape. Computer braille and large print.
Rehabilitation: Personal management; orientation/mobility; braille; handwriting; typing; home management. Refers for other rehabilitation services. Electronic travel aids; audio devices.
Recreational: Arts and crafts; hobby groups; special programs for elderly; bowling. Refers for and provides consultation to other agencies for other recreational services.
Employment: Refers for and provides consultation to other agencies for employment-oriented services.
Low Vision: Spectacles or aids; resale of aids and appliances; follow-up evaluation of eye treatment or prescription.

Low Vision Aids: Lends and resells low vision aids.
Low Vision Follow-up: Y.

North Carolina Lions Foundation

P.O. Box 39
Sherrills Ford, NC 28673-0039
(704) 478-2135
FAX: (704) 478-4419
Steve W. Walker, Executive Director

Type of Agency: Private; non-profit.
Mission: To serve the needs of visually impaired and hearing impaired persons.
Funded by: Contributions and Lions Clubs of North Carolina.
Budget: $1,250,000.
Hours of Operation: 8:30 AM - 5:00 PM.
Staff: Uses volunteers.
History/Date: Est. 1934.
Number of Clients Served: 3,000.
Eligibility: Visually impaired and hearing impaired.
Area Served: North Carolina.
Age Requirements: All ages.

Health: Supports eye and human tissue bank. Supplementary medical help.
Counseling/Social Work/Self-Help: Consultation and referral service.
Recreational: Operates Camp Dogwood.

Raleigh Lions Clinic for the Blind

315 Hubert Street
Raleigh, NC 27603
(919) 833-8611
FAX: (919) 833-5664
James W. Wells, President

Type of Agency: Private non-profit rehabilitation facility.
County/District Where Located: Wake County.

Mission: To vocationally rehabilitate visually impaired persons by successfully placing them in competitive employment.
Funded by: Income from manufactured items for federal government under the Javits-Wagner-O'Day Program and subcontracting for private industry.
Budget: $2,826,000.
Hours of Operation: Clinic: Mon. 8:00 AM-4:00 PM, Tues.-Fri. 8:00 AM-4:30 PM. Administrative offices: 8:00 AM-5:00 PM daily.
Staff: 28.
History/Date: Est. 1966.
Number of Clients Served: 1996: 39 blind transitional employees and 184 clients.
Eligibility: Determined by the NC Division of Services for the Blind.
Area Served: Provides services for blind and visually impaired persons statewide through evaluation and work adjustment training. Provides employment for blind persons at local level.
Age Requirements: 18 and older.

Counseling/Social Work/Self-Help: Vocational counseling services provided through the NC Division of Services for the Blind. Human services personnel, available to assist in areas affecting employees outside of employment.
Educational: Vocationally related classes provided, as necessary, for clients in training.
Residential: No residential housing on site; residential arrangements for clients are made through the NC Division of Services for the Blind.
Rehabilitation: Provides for vocational evaluation, work adjustment training, limited sheltered employment, supported employment, medical services, and job placement services in competitive employment.

Employment: Provides limited sheltered employment.
Low Vision: Low vision screening provided for clients.
Low Vision Aids: Low vision clinic on site carries extensive array of low vision aids for clients being served.

Winston-Salem Industries for the Blind

7730 North Point Drive
Winston-Salem, NC 27106
(910) 759-0551
FAX: (910) 759-0990
Dan Boucher, President

Type of Agency: Private; non-profit.
County/District Where Located: Forsyth County.
Mission: Services for totally blind, legally blind, and deaf-blind persons.
Funded by: Workshop sales, sub-contracts, capital income.
Budget: $10,500,000.
Hours of Operation: Mon. - Fri. 7:30 AM - 4:00 PM.
Staff: 18.
History/Date: Est. 1936.
Number of Clients Served: 110.
Eligibility: Legally blind.
Area Served: Lexington, Thomasville, High Point, Kemersville, Yadkinville, Elkin, King, Rural Hall, North Wilkesboro.
Transportation: Y.
Age Requirements: 18 years of age.

Professional Training: Evaluations and training.
Employment: Evaluations; vocational training; job retention; job retraining; sheltered workshops; vocational placement.
Low Vision Aids: Vision technology.

Winston-Salem Industries for the Blind
Ashville Division

45 South French Broad Avenue
Asheville, NC 28801
(704) 258-2332
FAX: (704) 258-9814
Randy Buckner, Plant Manager

Type of Agency: Non-profit.
County/District Where Located: Buncombe County.
Funded by: Workshop sales and sub-contracts.
Staff: 5 full time.
History/Date: Est. 1938.
Eligibility: Blind or legally blind.
Transportation: Y.

Employment: Vocational training; sheltered workshops.

COMPUTER TRAINING CENTERS

North Carolina Rehabilitation Center for the Blind
305 Ashe Avenue
Raleigh, NC 27606
(919) 733-5897
FAX: (919) 715-0471
Pattie Barker, Teacher

County/District Where Located: Wake County.

Computer Training: Speech output systems; screen magnification systems; braille access systems; optical character recognition systems; closed-circuit television systems; word processing; database software; computer operating systems.

◆ Low Vision Services

EYE CARE SOCIETIES

North Carolina Society of Eye Physicians and Surgeons
222 North Person Street

Raleigh, NC 27611
(919) 833-3836
Alan Skipper, Executive Director

North Carolina State Optometric Society, Inc.

Box 1206
Wilson, NC 27894-1206
(919) 237-6197
Sue Gardner, Contact Person

LOW VISION CENTERS

Asheville Lions Club Eye Clinic

45-A South French Broad Avenue
Asheville, NC 28801
(704) 252-5706
Guy Penland, Chairman, Board of
Directors
Ann Rice, LPN

Type of Agency: Non-profit.
County/District Where Located:
Buncombe County.
Mission: To provide eye care
assistance for low-income visually
impaired individuals. To eliminate
the potential for blindness among
the citizens of Buncombe County.
Funded by: United Way; Asheville
Lions Club; Buncombe County
government.
Budget: $81,702.
Hours of Operation: Mon.-Thurs.
8:30AM-5:00PM; Fri. 8:00AM-
1:30PM.
Staff: Volunteer director, nurse,
office secretary, screening
technician.
Number of Clients Served: 150
for Low Vision Services; 16,156 for
other services.
Eligibility: Referral; current
ophthalmological report.
Area Served: Asheville and
Buncombe Counties.

Health: Public glaucoma and
diabetes screenings; individuals
may come to office by
appointment for eye pressure,
blood sugar or blood pressure

check. Hearing screening in office.
No charge for any services.
Preschools: Vision screenings
provided to private and public
schools; referrals to eye care
specialists for elevated readings.
Low Vision Aids: Provided on
loan for trial purpose at no charge;
sold at cost; on-site or in-home
training provided. No charge to
individual other than actual cost of
low vision aids. Assistance in
finding several aids to purchase if
needed.
Low Vision Follow-up: Return
appointment; home visit and/or
phone interview; varies according
to patient. As many visits as
necessary to satisfy needs.

Duke University Eye Center
Duke University Medical Center

Box 3802
Durham, NC 27710
(919) 684-6749
FAX: (919) 681-6474
Monica De La Paz, M.D., Medical
Director
Deborah Lapolice, Evaluator

Type of Agency: Non-profit.
Mission: To provide low vision
aids and training in their use for
patients with low vision.
Funded by: Client fees.
Hours of Operation: Low vision
service by appointment only.
Staff: Ophthalmologist; optician;
rehabilitation counselor, low
vision evaluator.
Eligibility: None.
Area Served: Unlimited.

**Counseling/Social Work/Self-
Help:** Available by social worker
on staff.
Low Vision: Examination and
rehabilitation referral by
ophthalmologists; low vision
evaluation, including prescriptions
for optical aids, spectacles,
magnifiers, and telescopes.

Low Vision Aids: Available for
purchase and on-site use.
Low Vision Follow-up: By return
appointment as needed.

North Carolina Memorial Hospital
Low Vision Clinic

CB7040
617 Clinical Sciences Building
Chapel Hill, NC 27599
(919) 966-2061 or (919) 966-5509
FAX: (919) 966-7908
Henry A. Greene, O.D., Director,
Low Vision Service

Type of Agency: Non-profit.
County/District Where Located:
Orange County.
Funded by: Client fees.
Hours of Operation: Fri.
9:00 AM-1:00 PM.
Staff: Genetic counselor;
ophthalmologist; optometrist.
Eligibility: None.
Area Served: Unlimited.

**Counseling/Social Work/Self-
Help:** By referral within medical
center.
Rehabilitation: By referral within
medical center.
Low Vision Aids: Refundable
return deposit for trial period;
provided for purchase; prescribed
and fitted for variable fee. On-site
training provided.
Low Vision Follow-up: Return
appointment.

Raleigh Lions Clinic for the Blind
Evaluation Unit
North Carolina Division of Services for the Blind

315 Hubert Street
Raleigh, NC 27603
(919) 833-8611
FAX: (919) 833-5664
W. A. Shearin, M.D.,
Ophthalmologist
Jerry Paul, Supervisor

Type of Agency: State.
County/District Where Located: Wake County.
Mission: Rehabilitation of blind, visually impaired and multiply disabled individuals.
Funded by: North Carolina Division of Services for the Blind.
Hours of Operation: Mon.-Fri. (Low vision clinic on Wednesday only).
Program Accessibility: Meets ADA standards.
Staff: Ophthalmologist; ophthalmic assistant / nurse; psychologist / counselor; rehabilitation counselor; audiologist; orientation / mobility instructor; rehabilitation teacher.
Eligibility: Ophthalmologist's report or referral by North Carolina Division of Services for the Blind Rehabilitation Program. Resident of North Carolina.
Area Served: North Carolina.
Transportation: Y.
Age Requirements: High school and above.

Low Vision Aids: Provided to eligible rehabilitation clients.
Low Vision Follow-up: By rehabilitation counselor.

◆ *Aging Services*

STATE UNITS ON AGING

Division of Aging
CB 29531
693 Palmer Drive
Raleigh, NC 27626-0531
(919) 733-3983 or Information & Referral In State (800) 662-7030
FAX: (919) 733-0443
Bonnie Cramer, Director

Provides referrals to Area Agencies on Aging and information on other local aging services.

INDEPENDENT LIVING PROGRAMS

Department of Human Resources
Division of Services for the Blind
309 Ashe Avenue
Raleigh, NC 27606
(919) 733-9700
Sally Syria, Director

Provides independent living services for persons age 55 and over. For further information, contact the Project Director or general phone number listed.

NORTH DAKOTA

◆ *Educational Services*

STATE SERVICES

North Dakota Department of Public Instruction
600 East Boulevard Avenue
State Capitol
Bismarck, ND 58505-0440
(701) 328-2277
Robert Rutten, Special Education Regional Coordinator

Type of Agency: State.
County/District Where Located: Burleigh County.
Mission: Administers supplemental state funds for visually impaired children attending local schools. Provides consultation on educational programs.
Funded by: Public funds.
Area Served: North Dakota.

For further information, consult the Division of Special Education.

EARLY INTERVENTION COORDINATION

Developmental Disabilities Division
North Dakota Department of Human Services
600 South Second Street, Suite 1-A
State Capitol
Bismarck, ND 58504-5729
(701) 328-8929
FAX: (701) 328-8969
Robert Graham, Part H Coordinator

SCHOOLS

North Dakota Vision Services/ School for the Blind
500 Stanford Road
Grand Forks, ND 58203-2799
(701) 795-2700
FAX: (701) 795-2727
E-mail: suminski@sendit.sendit.nodak.edu
Carmen Suminski, Superintendent and Administrator of Vision Services

Type of Agency: State residential school.
Mission: Services for totally blind; legally blind; visually impaired; deaf-blind; learning disabled; mentally retarded.
Funded by: State funds.
Budget: $3.1 million.
Staff: 28 full time, including 12 full-time visually handicapped and dually certified teachers, 1 speech pathologist, 1 occupational therapist, 1 half-time physical therapist, and 17 part-time staff. Various specialists are available as consultants. Uses volunteers.
History/Date: Est. 1908.
Number of Clients Served: 250.
Eligibility: Visual impairment that impedes school progress.
Area Served: Statewide.
Age Requirements: 3-26 years.

Health: Low vision exams, immunizations, blood tests, and other health services available on consultant or referral basis.
Counseling/Social Work/Self-Help: Family, parent, couple counseling; placement in school; genetic counseling. Refers for and contracts for other counseling/ social work services.
Educational: Grades preschool through 12. Accepts deaf-blind; emotionally disturbed; learning disabled; mentally retarded; orthopedically handicapped; speech impaired; autistic.

Programs for general academic; prevocational and vocational.
Reading: Talking book record player and cassette player; talking book records and cassettes; braille books; large print books; braille magazines; recorded magazines; Optacon and Kurzweil Reading Machine.
Residential: Independent living units.
Rehabilitation: Adaptive leisure activities.
Recreational: Afterschool programs; arts and crafts; swimming; track.
Employment: Occupational skill development. Contracts and refers for other employment-oriented services.
Computer Training: Access; training on computer aids and devices.
Low Vision: Aids or devices; functional vision evaluations.
Low Vision Aids: Available on loan and for purchase.
Low Vision Follow-up: Y.
Professional Training: Inservice training and staff development.

Consultant services to other programs for visually impaired, multiply disabled children.

Contact local school superintendent for program information and availability.

INSTRUCTIONAL MATERIALS CENTERS

North Dakota Vision Services/ School for the Blind
500 Stanford Road, Suite A
Grand Forks, ND 58203-2799
(701) 795-2700
FAX: (701) 795-2727
E-mail: suminski@sendit.sendit.nodak.edu
Betty Bender, Media Specialist
Carmen Suminski, Superintendent

County/District Where Located: Grand Forks County.
Area Served: Statewide.
Groups Served: K-12.

Types/Content: Instructional materials.
Media Formats: Braille available on a limited basis.
Title Listings: No title listings available.

Acts as a depository for large-print and braille materials.

UNIVERSITY TRAINING PROGRAMS

University of North Dakota
Department of Special Education
Grand Forks, ND 58202
(701) 777-3188
FAX: (701) 777-4393
E-mail: mrolson@badlands.nodak.edu
Dr. Myrna Olson, Visually Impaired Program

County/District Where Located: Grand Forks County.

Programs Offered: Graduate programs for teachers of visually impaired students.
Distance Education: N.

◆ Information Services

LIBRARIES

North Dakota State Library Services for the Disabled
604 East Boulevard
Bismarck, ND 58505-0800
(701) 328-1477
FAX: (701) 328-2040
E-mail: msmail.scone@ranch.state.nd.us
Stella Cone, Head of Services

Regional library lending talking books; cassettes, and braille books.

TALKING BOOK MACHINE DISTRIBUTORS

North Dakota Vision Services/ School for the Blind
500 Stanford Road, Suite A
Grand Forks, ND 58203
(701) 795-2700
FAX: (701) 795-2727
Colleen Sanford, Outreach Coordinator
Betty Bender, Contact Person

Mission: To provide a full range of services to the blind and visually impaired.
Funded by: State funds.
Budget: $3 million.
Hours of Operation: Mon.-Fri. 8:00 AM-5:00 PM.
Staff: 28.
History/Date: Est. 1908.
Number of Clients Served: 180.
Eligibility: Visually impaired.
Area Served: Statewide.
Age Requirements: None.

Distributor of talking machines.

RADIO READING

North Dakota State Library Services for the Disabled
604 East Boulevard
Bismarck, ND 58505-0800
(701) 328-1477
FAX: (701) 328-2040
E-mail: msmail.scone@ranch.state.nd.us
Stella Cone, Head of Services

Hours of Operation: Mon.-Fri. 8:00 AM-5:00 PM.
Staff: 5.
History/Date: Est. 1986.
Area Served: North Dakota.
Age Requirements: None.

◆ Rehabilitation Services

STATE SERVICES

Vocational Rehabilitation North Dakota Department of Human Services
600 South Second Street
Dacotah Foundation Building
Bismarck, ND 58504
(701) 328-8950 or (800) 472-2622 or TDD (701) 328-8968
FAX: (701) 328-8969
Mike Beck, Program Administrator, Vision Services
Gene Hysjulien, Director of Vocational Rehabilitation

Type of Agency: State.
Mission: To provide the opportunity for individuals with disabilities to achieve productive employment and increased independence.
Funded by: State and federal funds.
History/Date: Est. 1921.
Area Served: Statewide.

Counseling/Social Work/Self-Help: Individual, group.
Professional Training: In-service training programs.
Rehabilitation: Braille; home management; orientation/ mobility.
Employment: Career and skill counseling; vocational placement follow-up service. Contracts for and refers for other employment-oriented services.
Low Vision: Evaluation and referral.
Low Vision Follow-up: Yes.

Regional Offices:

Bismarck: Vocational Rehabilitation, West Central Human Service Center, 600 South Second Street, Bismarck, ND 58504, (701) 328-8800, FAX (701) 328-8803.

Devils Lake: Vocational Rehabilitation, Lake Region Human Service Center, Highway Two West, Devils Lake, ND 58301, (701) 662-7581 or TDD (701) 662-3404, FAX (701) 662-2830.

Dickinson: Vocational Rehabilitation, Badlands Human Service Center, Pulver Hall, Dickinson, ND 58601-4857, (701) 227-7500, FAX (701) 227-7575.

Fargo: Vocational Rehabilitation, Southeast Human Service Center, 2624 Ninth Avenue S.W., Fargo, ND 58102, (701) 298-4459 or TDD (701) 298-4450, FAX (701) 298-4400.

Grand Forks: Vocational Rehabilitation, Northeast Human Service Center, 1407 24th Avenue South, Grand Forks, ND 58201, (701) 795-3100 or TDD (701) 795-3060, FAX (701) 795-3050.

Jamestown: Vocational Rehabilitation, South Central Human Service Center, 520 Third Street N.W., P.O. Box 2055, Jamestown, ND 58402-2055, (701) 252-2641, FAX (701) 253-3033.

Minot: Vocational Rehabilitation, North Central Human Service Center, 400 22nd Avenue N.W., Minot, ND 58701-1080, (701) 857-8643, FAX (701) 857-8555.

Williston: Vocational Rehabilitation, Northwest Human Service Center, 316 Second Avenue West, P.O. Box 1266, Williston, ND 58802-1266, (701) 774-4600, FAX (701) 774-4620.

REHABILITATION

North Dakota Vision Services/ School for the Blind
500 Stanford Road
Grand Forks, ND 58203-2799
(701) 795-2700
Carmen Suminski, Superintendent

Type of Agency: Outreach and resource center.
County/District Where Located: Grand Forks County.

Mission: To provide a full range of services to persons who are blind and visually impaired, including multiple disabilities.
Funded by: State funds.
Budget: $3.1 million per biennium.
Program Accessibility: Fully accessible.
Staff: 28.
History/Date: Est. 1908.
Number of Clients Served: 250.
Eligibility: Visually impaired.

Rehabilitation: Daily living skills; orientation/mobility.
Employment: Comprehensive vocational evaluation services and training.
Low Vision: Functional evaluations.
Low Vision Follow-up: Y.

COMPUTER TRAINING CENTERS

Technology Center
North Dakota School for the Blind
500 Stanford Road
Grand Forks, ND 58203-2799
(701) 795-2700
FAX: (701) 795-2727
E-mail: sowokino@sendit.sendit.nodak.edu
Janice Sowokinos, Computer Specialist

Computer Training: Speech output systems; screen magnification systems; braille access systems; optical character recognition systems; word processing; computer operating systems; database software; closed-circuit television systems.

◆ Low Vision Services

EYE CARE SOCIETIES

North Dakota Society of Ophthalmology and Otolaryngology
Williston Basin Eye Clinic
1213 15th Avenue West
Williston, ND 58801
(701) 572-7641
John R. Herr, Jr., M.D., President

North Dakota Optometric Association, Inc.
204 W. Thayer Avenue
Bismarck, ND 58501
(701) 258-6766
FAX: (701) 258-9005
Virginia Corwin, Director

County/District Where Located: Burleigh County.

◆ Aging Services

STATE UNITS ON AGING

Aging Services Division
North Dakota Department of Human Services
600 South Second Street
Suite 1C
Bismarck, ND 58504
(701) 328-8909 or Information & Referral (800) 472-2622 or Aging Services (800) 642-6042
FAX: (701) 328-8969
Linda Wright, Director

Provides referrals to Area Agencies on Aging and information on other local aging services.

INDEPENDENT LIVING PROGRAMS

North Dakota Department of Human Services

Dacotah Foundation Building
600 South Second Street
Bismarck, ND 58504
(701) 328-8954 or (800) 755-2745
Mike Beck, Director

Provides independent living services for persons age 55 and over. For further information, contact the Project Director or general phone number listed.

OHIO

◆ Educational Services

STATE SERVICES

Ohio Department of Education Division of Special Education
933 High Street
Worthington, OH 43085-4087
(614) 466-2650
FAX: (614) 728-1097
E-mail: se-herner@a1.ode.ohio.
gov
John Herner, Director

Type of Agency: State.
County/District Where Located: Franklin County.
Mission: Administers state funds for visually handicapped children in local public schools. Provides consultation on educational services.
Funded by: Public funds.
Hours of Operation: Mon.-Fri. 8:00 AM-4:45 PM.
Area Served: Ohio.

EARLY INTERVENTION COORDINATION

Ohio Department of Health Bureau of Early Intervention Services
246 North High Street
Fifth Floor
P.O. Box 118
Columbus, OH 43266-0118
(614) 644-8389
FAX: (614) 728-9163
Cindy Oser, Early Intervention Chief

Coordination of early intervention services in Ohio for disabled infants and young children birth-3 years.

SCHOOLS

Ohio State School for the Blind
5220 North High Street
Columbus, OH 43214
(614) 888-1325
FAX: (614) 888-2158
Raymond A. Horn, Acting Superintendent

Type of Agency: State.
County/District Where Located: Franklin County.
Mission: Services for totally blind, legally blind and deaf-blind persons.
Funded by: State and federal funds.
Hours of Operation: Mon.-Fri. 8:00 AM-4:45 PM.
Staff: 127 full time. Uses volunteers.
History/Date: Est. 1837.
Number of Clients Served: Approximately 130 annually.
Eligibility: Resident of Ohio; legal school age for visually impaired children. Recommendation for placement by school district of residence.
Area Served: Statewide.
Age Requirements: 3-22 years.

Health: Speech and hearing therapy; occupational therapy; physical therapy; orientation/mobility training; adaptive physical education.
Educational: Grades K through 12. Programs for general academic studies; vocational/skill development; deaf-blind programming. Education Assessment Clinic schedules and provides free multifactored assessments of visually impaired and deaf-blind children, when requested by residence school district.
Professional Training: Internship/fieldwork placement in low vision; orientation/mobility; special education.
Residential: Cottages.
Recreational: Afterschool programs; arts and crafts; hobby groups; bowling; swimming; scouting; camping; wrestling; extracurricular cheerleading; boys' and girls' track; swimming; forensics; field trips. Refers for day residential summer camp.
Computer Training: Training on computer aids and devices.
Low Vision: Assessments for enrolled students.
Low Vision Aids: For enrolled students.
Low Vision Follow-up: For enrolled students.

Contact local school superintendent for program availability or John Saylor, Education Consultant, Ohio Department of Education, Division of Special Education, 933 High Street, Worthington, OH 43085, (614) 466-1470.

INFANT AND PRESCHOOL

Cincinnati Association for the Blind
2045 Gilbert Avenue
Cincinnati, OH 45202-1490
(513) 221-8558
FAX: (513) 221-2995
Gina Carroll, M.S.W., Program Supervisor

Type of Agency: Private; non-profit.
County/District Where Located: Hamilton County.
Mission: To provide services for families of young children who are visually impaired.
Funded by: United Way; client fees; contributions, state contract.
Budget: $7 million.
Hours of Operation: Mon.-Fri. 8:30AM-4:30PM.
Program Accessibility: Fully accessible.

Staff: Two early intervention vision specialists, social worker, orientation and mobility specialist, rehabilitation teacher available as consultants.
History/Date: Est. 1988.
Number of Clients Served: 125.
Eligibility: Visually impaired.
Area Served: Greater Cincinnati and northern Kentucky.

Cleveland Sight Center of the Cleveland Society for the Blind

1909 East 101st Street
Cleveland, OH 44106
(216) 791-8118
FAX: (216) 791-1101
Michael E. Grady, Executive Director
Janet Stone Bard, Manager, Children and Youth Services

Type of Agency: Private; non-profit.
County/District Where Located: Cuyahoga County.
Mission: Services to visually impaired persons.
Staff: 5 full time, 4 part time. Uses volunteers.
Transportation: Y.
Age Requirements: 0-5 years.

Health: Adaptive equipment; low vision evaluation with full agency services available; occupational, speech, and language therapy; other health services available on referral basis; other specialists available as consultants.
Counseling/Social Work/Self-Help: Family counseling; workshop for professionals and parents; parent support groups.
Educational: Provides consultation, training, and referral.
Low Vision: Evaluation, recommendation trial, and sale of vision aids.

Home- and center-based programs for children 0-5 years, with or without other disabilities.

Consultant service to other schools and programs.

Vision Rehabilitation Inc.

220 Oberlin Road
Elyria, OH 44035
(216) 322-1122 or toll-free
(800) 233-6777
FAX: (216) 322-2111
Kevin E. Walter, LPC

Type of Agency: Private; non-profit.
County/District Where Located: Lorain County.
Mission: Education and counseling services for parents, family members, and other caregivers. Developmental assessments, training, and referral services.
Funded by: Client fees, government agencies' fees, contributions, United Way.
Budget: $450,000.
Hours of Operation: Mon.-Fri. 8:30 AM-4:30 PM.
Program Accessibility: Fully accessible.
Staff: Rehabilitation teachers and counselors; orientation/mobility specialist; other specialists available for consultation.
History/Date: Est. 1941.
Eligibility: Visually impaired able to benefit from services.
Area Served: Northern central Ohio.

Counseling/Social Work/Self-Help: Counseling and education for parents, family, and providers; referral and advocacy.
Educational: Remedial and developmental services.
Low Vision: Clinic.
Low Vision Follow-up: Y.

Home-based services and consultation with other programs for visually impaired and multiply disabled infants and children.

Wood County Office of Education

1 Courthouse Square
Bowling Green, OH 43402
(419) 352-3933
Judy Cernkovich, Teacher/ Consultant, Preschool, Visually Impaired and Blind

Type of Agency: Public school.
Funded by: State funds.
Staff: 1 home-based preschool teacher also consults with preschool children attending existing programs.
History/Date: Est. 1975-76.
Number of Clients Served: 18.
Area Served: Serves children within a 60-mile radius of Bowling Green, Ohio.
Age Requirements: Birth through 5 or until child enters school.

Educational: Provides instruction, adaptions, and materials.

Home-based programs and consultation with other programs for visually impaired/multiply disabled children, 0-5 years.

STATEWIDE OUTREACH SERVICES

Ohio State School for the Blind

5220 North High Street
Columbus, OH 43214
(614) 888-1325
FAX: (614) 888-2158
Raymond A. Horn, Acting Superintendent

County/District Where Located: Franklin County.
Funded by: State funds.
Age Requirements: 0-22 years.

Assessment: Y.
Consultation to Public Schools: Y.
Parent Assistance: Y.
Materials Production: Y.

INSTRUCTIONAL MATERIALS CENTERS

ORCLISH (Ohio Resource Center for Low Incidence and Severely Handicapped)

470 Glenmont Avenue
Columbus, OH 43214
(614) 262-6131 or (800) 672-5474
FAX: (614) 262-1070
E-mail: mary_binion@coserrc.esu.k12.oh.us
URL: http://www.schoolimprovement.ode.ohio.gov/ordish/home.html
Mary Binion, Coordinator

County/District Where Located: Franklin County.
Area Served: Ohio.
Groups Served: K-12.

Types/Content: Textbooks; educational aids; resource information.
Media Formats: Braille/large print books.
Title Listings: No title listings available.

UNIVERSITY TRAINING PROGRAMS

Ohio State University School of Teaching and Learning

333 Arps Hall
1945 North High Street
Columbus, OH 43210
(614) 292-2437
FAX: (614) 292-7695
Dr. Marjorie E. Ward, Visually Handicapped Program

County/District Where Located: Franklin County.

Programs Offered: Graduate (master's, doctoral) programs for teachers of children with visual impairments.

University of Toledo Department of Special Education Services

2801 West Bancroft Street
Toledo, OH 43606
(419) 530-7733
Dr. Sakvi Malakpa, Professor of Visually Impaired

County/District Where Located: Lucas County.

Programs Offered: Undergraduate and graduate (master's, doctoral) program for teachers of the visually handicapped.

♦ Information Services

LIBRARIES

Cleveland Public Library Library for the Blind and Physically Handicapped

17121 Lake Shore Boulevard
Cleveland, OH 44110-4006
(216) 623-2911 or toll-free in Ohio (800) 362-1262 or TDD (216) 623-7116
FAX: (216) 623-7036
E-mail: info@library.cpl.org
Barbara T. Mates, Librarian

County/District Where Located: Cuyahoga County.
Funded by: Public funds; endowment; and contributions.
Hours of Operation: Mon.-Fri. 9:00AM-5:00PM.
Staff: 17 full time.
History/Date: Est. 1931.
Eligibility: Service is available to anyone who cannot use regular print materials because of a visual or physical handicap.
Area Served: Northern Ohio, including Columbus.
Age Requirements: None.

Regional library lending talking books, cassettes, and braille books. Provides reference and information referral services by telephone, mail, and in person using CD-ROM and OCR technology. Cooperates with the State Library of Ohio and other agencies to have talking book and cassette machines distributed.

Public Library of Cincinnati and Hamilton County Library for the Blind and Physically Handicapped

800 Vine Street
Library Square
Cincinnati, OH 45202-2071
(513) 369-6999 or toll-free in Ohio (800) 582-0335
Donna Foust, Librarian

Type of Agency: Library.
County/District Where Located: Hamilton County.
Mission: Provide talking books, cassettes and braille books to readers.
Funded by: Public funds.
Staff: 6 full time; 6 full-time equivalent.
History/Date: Est. 1903.
Number of Clients Served: 5,500.
Eligibility: Print disabled.
Area Served: Southern Ohio.

Regional library supplying talking books, braille books, cassette books, and tapes.

TALKING BOOK MACHINE DISTRIBUTORS

Talking Book Program State Library of Ohio

65 South Front Street
Columbus, OH 43215
(614) 644-6897 or toll-free in Ohio (800) 686-1531
FAX: (614) 466-3584
E-mail: jbow@winslo.state.oh.us
URL: http://winslo.state.oh.us
Judith Bow, Machine Lending Information

Type of Agency: State library.
Mission: To bring library service
to all residents of Ohio.
Funded by: State of Ohio and
federal funds.
Budget: $223,425.
Hours of Operation: Mon.-Fri.
8:00 AM-5:00 PM.
Staff: 5 full time.
History/Date: Est. 1981.
Number of Clients Served:
Approximately 27,000.
Eligibility: Print handicapped, by
application.
Area Served: State of Ohio.

Distributor of talking book
machines and accessories.

63 machine sublending agencies
throughout Ohio.

MEDIA PRODUCTION SERVICES

Aid to Visually Handicapped
6200 Montgomery Road
Cincinnati, OH 45213
(513) 631-2537
Phyllis Ringel, Coordinator

Area Served: Nationwide.
Groups Served: K-12, college
students, adults.

Types/Content: Textbooks,
general books (as time allows).
Media Formats: Braille books,
talking books/cassettes, large-
print books.
Title Listings: None specified.

Canton Program for the Visually Handicapped
Canton City Schools
617 McKinley, S.W.
Canton, OH 44707
(330) 438-2551 or (330) 455-1010
FAX: (330) 455-0682
Tamara Kelley, Director of Special
Education

County/District Where Located:
Stark County.

Area Served: Stark, Wayne, and
Tuscaraway counties.
Groups Served: Preschool-grade
12.

Types/Content: Textbooks.
Media Formats: Braille books,
talking books/cassettes, large-
print books.
Title Listings: No title listings
available.

Dayton Public Schools
Service Building
4280 North James H. McGee
Boulevard
Dayton, OH 45427
(513) 276-2141
Gerry Schooler, Librarian

County/District Where Located:
Montgomery County.
Groups Served: K-12.

Types/Content: Textbooks.
Media Formats: Braille books.
Title Listings: No title listings
available.

The Sight Center of the Toledo Society for the Blind
1819 Canton Avenue
Toledo, OH 43624-1380
(419) 241-1183
FAX: (419) 241-4510
John Davies Jr., Director

Area Served: 21 counties in
northwestern Ohio; 2 counties in
southeastern Michigan.
Groups Served: Preschool; K-12;
college students; other adults.

Types/Content: Textbooks;
recreational; career/vocational;
religious; individual requests; local
newspapers.
Media Formats: Talking books/
cassettes; large-print books; braille.
Title Listings: No title listings
available.

Temple Sisterhood Braille Group
6453 Sylvania Avenue
Toledo, OH 43560
(419) 885-3341
FAX: (419) 882-2778
Elaine Hershman, Chairperson,
Braille Group

County/District Where Located:
Lucas County.
Groups Served: K-12.

Types/Content: Literary,
textbooks, personal requests.
Media Formats: Braille.
Title Listings: None specified.

Vision Center of Central Ohio
1393 North High Street
Columbus, OH 43201
(614) 294-5571
FAX: (614) 294-5576
E-mail: 72630.2230@compuserve.
com
Joanna River, Executive Director

Area Served: Central Ohio.
Groups Served: K-12, college
students, other adults.

Types/Content: Textbooks,
recreational, career/vocational,
religious.
Media Formats: Braille books,
talking books/cassettes, large-
print books.
Title Listings: No title listings
available.

Visually Handicapped Materials Center
Cincinnati Public Schools
2355 Iowa Street
Cincinnati, OH 45206
(513) 369-4617
Elizabeth R. Collins, Materials
Coordinator for the Visually
Impaired

Groups Served: K-12, college
students, other adults.

Types/Content: Textbooks, recreational, career/vocational, academic.
Media Formats: Braille books, talking books/cassettes, large-print books.
Title Listings: No title listings available.

Youngstown Braille Service

100 Wadsworth Street
Canfield, OH 44406
(216) 533-5989
Al Henderson, Director

Groups Served: K-12, college students, other adults.

Types/Content: Textbooks.
Media Formats: Braille books.
Title Listings: No title listings available.

RADIO READING

Central Ohio Radio Reading Service

2955 West Broad Street
Columbus, OH 43204
(614) 464-2614
FAX: (614) 464-2302
Sandy Turner, Executive Director

County/District Where Located: Franklin County.
Hours of Operation: 24 hours a day, seven days a week.
History/Date: Est. 1975.
Area Served: Southeastern Ohio.

Cleveland Radio Reading Service

1909 East 101th Street
Cleveleand, OH 44106
(216) 791-8800
FAX: (216) 791-1101
Lynn Brewer, Supervisor, Communication Services

County/District Where Located: Cuyahoga County.
Funded by: Cleveland Sight Center.

Hours of Operation: Mon.-Fri. 10:00 AM-12:00 PM; Sat.-Sun. 10:00 AM-10:00 PM.
Staff: 6.
History/Date: Est. 1976.
Area Served: Greater Cleveland area, 50 miles radius.

Ohio Educational Telecommunications Network Commission

2470 North Star Road
Columbus, OH 43221
(614) 644-1714
FAX: (614) 644-3112
Dave L. Fornshell, Executive Director
Elmer E. Fischer, Coordinator

Type of Agency: State.
County/District Where Located: Franklin County.
Hours of Operation: 7:30 AM-12:00 midnight, 7 days a week.
History/Date: Est. 1961.

Radio Reading Services of Greater Cincinnati, Inc.

317 East Fifth Street
Cincinnati, OH 45202
(513) 621-4545
FAX: (513) 763-7763
Hank Baud, Interim Director

County/District Where Located: Hamilton County.
Funded by: Ohio Educational Telecommunications, private foundations, businesses, and individuals.
Hours of Operation: 6:00 AM - 12:00 midnight daily.
History/Date: Incorporated 1977.
Area Served: Greater Cincinnati area, including southwestern Ohio, northern Kentucky, and southeastern Indiana.

Sight Center Audio Network

1819 Canton Avenue

Toledo, OH 43624-1380
(419) 241-1183
FAX: (419) 241-4510
E-mail: sightctr@primenet.com
Gary P. Hoffman, Directort

Hours of Operation: Seven days 8:00 AM-11:00 PM.
History/Date: Est. 1819.
Area Served: Northwest Ohio and southwest Michigan.

Written Communications Radio Service (WCRS) for the Print Handicapped

1615 East Market Street
Akron, OH 44305
(330) 784-3393
FAX: (330) 784-3698
Marcia Jonke, Executive Director

County/District Where Located: Summit County.
Funded by: Fund raising and minimal state aid.
Hours of Operation: Office hours: Mon.-Fri. 9:00 AM-5:00 PM; broadcast hours: Mon.-Fri. 8:00 AM-10:00 PM; no Saturday broadcast; Sun. 10:00 AM-5:00 PM.
History/Date: Est. 1976.
Area Served: Summit, Stark, Portage, Medina, parts of Wayne, Ashland, Holmes, Tuscarawas, and Caroll Counties.
Age Requirements: None.

Youngstown Radio Reading Service

2747 Belmont Avenue
Youngstown, OH 44505-1819
(330) 759-0100
FAX: (330) 759-0678
E-mail: name@yrrs.oet.state.oh.us
Mike Bosela, Program Director

County/District Where Located: Mahoning County.
Funded by: State of Ohio, United Way, Lions Club, donations.

Hours of Operation: Mon.-Sun. 12:00 noon-12:00 midnight.
Staff: 2 full-time, 2 part-time, 1 intern.
History/Date: Est. 1976.
Area Served: Mahoning, Trumbull and Columbiana Counties in Ohio; Mercer and Lawrence Counties in Pennsylvania.
Age Requirements: None.

INFORMATION AND REFERRAL

The Foundation Fighting Blindness
Eastern Ohio Affiliate
644 University Avenue
Elyria, OH 44035
(216) 284-1487 or (800) 968-8242
Richard Walker, President

See The Foundation Fighting Blindness in U.S. national listings.

The Foundation Fighting Blindness
Toledo Affiliate
719 Sandralee Drive
Toledo, OH 43612
(419) 478-0652
Anne DeLong, President

See The Foundation Fighting Blindness in U.S. national listings.

Prevent Blindness Ohio
1500 West Third Avenue
Suite 200
Columbus, OH 43212-2874
(614) 464-2020
FAX: (614) 486-9670
E-mail: 75300.647@compuserve.com
Sherill K. Williams, President

County/District Where Located: Franklin County.

Local Offices:

Cincinnati: Southwest Ohio Chapter, 2652 Erie Avenue, Cincinnati, OH 45208, (513) 871-8373.
Cleveland: Northwest Ohio Chapter, 19929 Center Ridge Road, Cleveland, OH 44116, (216) 356-6914.

See Prevent Blindness America in U.S. national listings.

See also in national listings:

Association on Higher Education and Disability (AHEAD)

Cleveland Sight Center of the Cleveland Society for the Blind

The Clovernook Center Opportunities for the Blind

Delta Gamma Foundation

United States Braille Chess Foundation

◆ Rehabilitation Services

STATE SERVICES

Ohio Rehabilitation Services Commission
Bureau of Services for the Visually Impaired
400 East Campus View Boulevard
Columbus, OH 43235-4604
(614) 438-1255
FAX: (614) 438-1257
William A. Castro, III, Director
Robert L. Rabe, Administrator

Type of Agency: State.
Mission: To work in partnership with people with disabilities to assist them to achieve full community participation through employment and independent living opportunities.

Funded by: Public funds.
Budget: $19.7 million.
Hours of Operation: 8:00 AM-4:45 PM.
Program Accessibility: Fully accessible.
Staff: 150 (includes vocational rehabilitation counselors, rehabilitation teachers, vocational development specialists, and business enterprise specialists.
History/Date: Est. 1908.
Number of Clients Served: October 1992: 5,122.
Eligibility: A physical or mental disability that results in a substantial handicap to employment and a reasonable expectation that vocational rehabilitation may benefit the person in terms of employability. Prioroty is given to persons who are legally blind.
Area Served: Ohio.

Health: Medical and eye health services.
Counseling/Social Work/Self-Help: Counseling service.
Educational: Financial support for clients to attend technical or vocational college or a public university. Emphasis is on training to help clients become gainfully employed.
Rehabilitation: Contract for services.
Employment: Evaluation and vocational training; business enterprise programs.
Computer Training: Y.
Low Vision: Services available.
Low Vision Aids: Available for loan.
Low Vision Follow-up: Y.

Local Offices:

Cincinnati: 617 Vine Street, Suite 905, Cincinnati, OH 45202-2423, (513) 852-3223.

Cleveland: 310 Lakeside Avenue West, Second Floor, Cleveland, OH 44113-1000, (216) 787-3375.

Columbus: 3333 Indianola Avenue, Suite 402, Columbus, OH 43214-4192, (614) 466-7730.

Toledo: 5533 Southwyck Boulevard, Suite 101, Toledo, OH 43614-1592, (419) 866-5811.

REHABILITATION

Akron Blind Center and Workshop

325 East Market Street
Akron, OH 44304
(330) 253-2555
FAX: (330) 762-1313
Cindy Darin, Executive Director
Joseph Giovanni, Workshop Director

Type of Agency: Rehabilitation services and workshop.
County/District Where Located: Summit County.
Mission: To ensure a better quality of life for blind and visually impaired persons.
Funded by: Private grants and donations.
Budget: $375,000.
Hours of Operation: Rehabilitation services and activities: Mon.-Thurs. 9:00AM-3:00PM. Workshop: Mon.-Fri. 7:30AM-3:30PM.
Staff: School: 17 part-time teachers; 3 part-time non-teaching staff. Workshop: 4 full time.
Number of Clients Served: 1,400, talking book program. 120, rehabilitation services. 125, workers at the workshop.
Eligibility: Talking book program, visually impaired or physically disabled. Rehabilitation services, legally blind. Workshop, legally blind.
Area Served: Summit County.
Transportation: Y.

Age Requirements: None.
Educational: Braille, basic computer training, independent living skills.
Reading: Audio library and books recorded upon request.
Rehabilitation: Workshop and classes.
Recreational: Field trips, volunteer opportunities, supervised and unsupervised games and activities.
Employment: Workshop and training.
Computer Training: Basic.
Low Vision Aids: Magnifiers, talking calculators.

Local Offices:

Akron: Workshop, 25 North Fir Street, Akron, OH 44304, (303) 762-1313.

Cincinnati Association for the Blind

2045 Gilbert Avenue
Cincinnati, OH 45202-1490
(513) 221-8558
FAX: (513) 221-2995
Hank E. Baud, Ed.D., Executive Director

Type of Agency: Private, non-profit.
County/District Where Located: Hamilton County.
Mission: To provide services for blind and visually impaired persons to develop skills for independent living.
Funded by: Fees, United Way, capital income, contributions, fees from government agencies.
Budget: $7 million.
Hours of Operation: Mon.-Fri. 8:30 AM-4:30 PM.
Program Accessibility: Building is fully accessible.
Staff: 39 full time, 1 part time. Uses volunteers.

History/Date: Est. 1910.
Number of Clients Served: 3,800 annually.
Eligibility: Vision loss that interferes with normal functioning.
Area Served: Greater Cincinnati and northern Kentucky.
Age Requirements: None.

Health: Low vision services. Refers for other health services.
Counseling/Social Work/Self-Help: Individualized assessment; individual, group, family/parent, couple counseling. Refers and provides consultation to other agencies. Information and referral.
Preschools: Early childhood intervention service (community based).
Professional Training: Internships and field work placements in orientation and mobility, rehabilitation teaching, social work.
Reading: Lends talking book record player and cassette player.
Rehabilitation: Community-based instruction in personal and home management; braille and other communication skills; orientation/mobility.
Recreational: Arts and crafts as part of rehabilitation teaching. Refers and provides consultation to other agencies for other recreation services.
Employment: Sheltered workshop.
Computer Training: Training on applications and computer access technology; job site modulations.
Low Vision: Prescription and instruction in use of low vision aids and devices.
Low Vision Aids: Provided on trial basis; available for purchase after evaluation; instruction provided.
Low Vision Follow-up: As indicated.

Cleveland Sight Center of the Cleveland Society for the Blind

1909 East 101st Street
Cleveland, OH 44106
(216) 791-8118
FAX: (216) 791-1101
Michael E. Grady, Executive Director

Type of Agency: Private, non-profit.
County/District Where Located: Cuyahoga Conty.
Mission: Services for totally blind; legally blind; visually impaired; deaf-blind.
Funded by: Fees; United Way; capital income; contributions.
Hours of Operation: Mon.-Fri. 8:30 AM-5:00 PM.
Staff: 88 full time. Uses volunteers.
History/Date: Est. 1906.
Number of Clients Served: 1,200 new and reopened cases each year; 13,000 preschool children screened yearly.
Eligibility: Visually impaired.
Area Served: Primarily Cuyahoga, Lake, Geauga and parts of Medina and Summit Counties; other parts of Ohio and neighboring states for some programs.
Transportation: Y.

Health: Glaucoma and amblyopia screening and referral; audiology testing; diabetic education and counseling; refers for other health services.
Counseling/Social Work/Self-Help: Social evaluation; psychological testing and evaluation; individual, group, family, parent, and couple counseling; and referral to other community services; consultation. Senior to senior peer support program.
Educational: Educational consultation, orientation/mobility in schools. Summer pre-college and vocational training program, including assessment, counseling and remedial classes for high school juniors and seniors.
Preschools: Home- and center-based early intervention program for infants, toddlers, and preschoolers.
Professional Training: Internship/fieldwork placement in low vision; orientation/mobility; rehabilitation counseling; social work; vocational rehabilitation teaching; regular in-service training programs; open to enrollment from other agencies.
Reading: Lends talking book record and cassette players. Information and referral; transcription to braille; translation to other languages; tape recording services on demand; radio reading services; lending library.
Residential: On-site apartments for in-training students.
Rehabilitation: Counseling; activities of daily living; orientation/mobility; adaptive communications; college prep and vocational readiness program; STORER Computer Access Center and closed circuit televisions; aids and appliances shop. Services for school-age children and early intervention preschool program. Community rehabilitation for seniors. Deaf-blind services. Diabetes education/counseling for individuals with both diabetes and vision loss; office skills training program.
Recreational: Residential summer camp; full recreational therapy program.
Employment: Food service training and snack bar employment. Vocational counseling and consultation. Refers to other employment services.
Computer Training: Introduction to a variety of access software and hardware through STORER Computer Access Center.
Low Vision: Low vision clinic services.
Low Vision Aids: Recommendation and sale of aids.
Low Vision Follow-up: 3 months after visit.

Outreach offices in five suburbs.

Cleveland Skilled Industries

2239 East 55th Street
Cleveland, OH 44103
(216) 431-8085 or (216) 431-8234
FAX: (216) 431-5123
Brad E. Sommerfelt, Executive Director

Type of Agency: Non-profit vocational rehabilitation agency.
Mission: To provide training and work opportunities for visually impaired persons in the Cleveland area.
Funded by: Self-supporting.
Budget: $1,500,000.
Hours of Operation: 6:45 AM-4:30 PM.
Staff: 6.
History/Date: Inc. 1980.
Number of Clients Served: More than 100.
Eligibility: Visually impaired, 16 years of age and older.
Area Served: Greater Cleveland.
Transportation: Y.
Age Requirements: 16 and older.

Counseling/Social Work/Self-Help: Counselors on staff make referrals to outside direct sources.
Rehabilitation: Vocational.
Employment: In-house workshop provides full-time employment opportunities.
Low Vision: Evaluation, referrals.
Low Vision Aids: Adaptive aids available.
Low Vision Follow-up: Y.

The Clovernook Center Opportunities for the Blind

7000 Hamilton Avenue
Cincinnati, OH 45231
(513) 522-3860
FAX: (513) 728-3946
E-mail: clovernook@aol.com
URL: http://www.clovernook.org
Marvin Kramer, Executive Director

Type of Agency: Private, non-profit.
County/District Where Located: Hamilton County.
Mission: Provide visually impaired persons, particularly those with multiple handicaps, with services and training necessary for the attainment and maintenance of each individual's optimal level of independence.
Funded by: Workshop sales, capital income, contributions, fees.
Budget: $7 million.
Hours of Operation: Mon.-Fri. 8:00 AM-4:30 PM.
Staff: 32 full time, 12 part time. Uses volunteers.
History/Date: Est. 1903.
Eligibility: Visually impaired, legally blind.
Area Served: Services provided locally. Referrals accepted from the United States and other countries.
Transportation: Y.

Health: Some health services. Refers to community for primary care.
Counseling/Social Work/Self-Help: Individual, group counseling; case management; referral to community services.
Preschools: Cooperative venture with local school district provides preschool services to disabled and non-disabled students; Head Start Program.
Professional Training: Internship/fieldwork placement in orientation/mobility; rehabilitation counseling; social work; rehabilitation teaching.

Residential: Provide supported living program, training, and maintenance services for community living. Assessment center for supported living program.
Rehabilitation: Programs include: training and counseling; supported living program; vocational services program; summer program for youth; community-based instruction. Services offered: personal management (i.e. self-care, eating skills, telling time); communication skills (i.e. braille, typing, handwriting, listening skills, CCTV and computer assistance); homemaking/management; orientation and mobility; remedial education; sensory training.
Recreational: Individualized leisure programming with emphasis on community participation.
Employment: Vocational counseling; transitional work services; job coaching; job development; work adjustment sheltered workshop.
Low Vision: Referral to community low vision clinic with follow-up by Clovernook staff.

Fairfield Regional Vision Rehabilitation Center

784 East Main Street
Lancaster, OH 43130
(614) 687-4785
FAX: (614) 687-4541
Kathy Moos, Director

Type of Agency: Private; non-profit.
County/District Where Located: Fairfield County.
Mission: To promote independence for individuals with visual impairments.
Funded by: United Way; Lions Clubs; client fees; donations; Title XX; endowment funds; grants;

Passport; Rehabilitation Services Commission.
Budget: $157,000.
Hours of Operation: Mon.-Fri. 9:00 AM-4:00 PM and by appointment.
Program Accessibility: Handicapped accessible.
Staff: 3 full time, 4 part time. Uses volunteers.
History/Date: Est. 1970.
Number of Clients Served: 300 annually.
Eligibility: Visual impairment that interferes with independent functioning.
Area Served: Southeastern Ohio.
Transportation: Y.
Age Requirements: All ages served.

Health: Adult and preschool vision screenings; literature and guest speakers; referrals for financial assistance with cost of medical care.
Counseling/Social Work/Self-Help: Support groups and referral.
Preschools: Vision screenings.
Reading: Talking book cassette and record players; radio reading service; closed circuit televisions.
Rehabilitation: Rehabilitation teaching in clients' homes.
Recreational: Therapeutic activities for socialization.
Employment: Job development and placement; job coaching.
Low Vision: Functional low vision evaluations; electronic magnification evaluations.
Low Vision Aids: Assessment and provision of low vision aids.
Low Vision Follow-up: As needed.
Professional Training: Provide staff in-services.

Goodwill Industries of Dayton
1511 Kuntz Road

Dayton, OH 45404
(937) 461-4800
FAX: (937) 461-2112
William Jessee, President
Jerome Motter, President

Type of Agency: Non-profit.
County/District Where Located: Montgomery County.
Mission: To expand quality services for people with barriers to independence.
Funded by: Workshop sales and sub-contracts, United Way, contributions, and fees.
Budget: $3 million.
Hours of Operation: Mon.-Fri. 8:00 AM-4:45 PM.
Program Accessibility: Fully accessible.
Staff: 50 full time, 15 part time.
History/Date: Est. 1934.
Number of Clients Served: 1,100 annually.
Eligibility: Visually, physically, mentally, or emotionally disadvantaged.
Area Served: Montgomery, Greene, Logan, Miami, Shelby, Darke, and Preble counties.

Counseling/Social Work/Self-Help: Consultation and referral service; group work; psychological testing.
Educational: Literacy and GED program.
Reading: Talking book record players and cassette players; talking book records and cassettes.
Rehabilitation: Personal management; work adjustment; orientation/mobility training; rehabilitation teaching.
Employment: Evaluation; prevocational and vocational training; vocational placement; follow-up service; sheltered workshop; work activities center.
Computer Training: Business skills with current software applications.

Low Vision Aids: Sells aids and appliances.

Ohio Valley Goodwill Industries Rehabilitation Center

10600 Springfield Pike
Cincinnati, OH 45215
(513) 771-4800
FAX: (513) 771-4959
Joseph S. Byrum, Executive Director

Type of Agency: Non-profit.
County/District Where Located: Hamilton County.
Funded by: Workshop sales, sub-contracts, and United Way.
Staff: 60 full time.
History/Date: Est. 1916.
Eligibility: Any handicap.
Area Served: Indiana, Kentucky, Ohio.
Transportation: Y.
Age Requirements: Over 16 years.

Counseling/Social Work/Self-Help: Consultation and referral service; group work; psychological testing.
Residential: Facilities for adults.
Rehabilitation: Personal management.
Recreational: Social activities.
Employment: Evaluation; prevocational and vocational training; vocational placement; follow-up service; sheltered workshop; watch school; clerical and janitorial training.
Computer Training: Access; training on computer aids and office technology.

Philomatheon Society of the Blind, Inc.

2810 Tuscarawas Street West
Canton, OH 44708
(330) 453-9157
Gerald Dessecker, President

Type of Agency: Private.

County/District Where Located: Stark County.
Funded by: Private contributions.
Staff: 2 full time, 3 part time.
History/Date: Est. 1924.
Eligibility: Totally and legally blind only. Cannot accept diabetics or epilepsy patients. Clients in residential facilities must be able to navigate stairs.

Reading: Lends talking book record players and cassette players.
Residential: Boarding home for adults.

Samuel W. Bell Home for Sightless, Inc.

1507 Elm Street
Cincinnati, OH 45210
(513) 241-0720
FAX: (513) 241-2560
Louis A. Hoff, Director

Type of Agency: Non-profit.
County/District Where Located: Hamilton County.
Mission: Services for legally blind persons.
Funded by: Endowments and contributions.
Hours of Operation: 9:00 AM-5:00 PM.
Staff: 8.
History/Date: Est. 1925.
Number of Clients Served: 22.
Eligibility: Legally blind; must be able to care for themselves.
Age Requirements: Over 18.

Residential facilities for legally blind men, women, and couples.

The Sight Center of the Toledo Society for the Blind

1819 Canton Avenue
Toledo, OH 43624-1380
(419) 241-1183
FAX: (419) 241-4510
John Davies, Jr., Director

Type of Agency: Private; non-profit.

Mission: To provide services that maximize the independence of individuals who are visually impaired and blind and minimize the incidence of visual impairment.

Funded by: United Way, fees, donations, endowment, and Lions Clubs.

Budget: $750,000.

Hours of Operation: Mon.-Fri. 8:00 AM-4:30 PM.

Program Accessibility: Fully accessible.

Staff: 14 full time, 10 part time; more than 650 volunteers.

History/Date: Est. 1923.

Number of Clients Served: More than 30,000.

Eligibility: Legally blind; visually impaired. Prevention of blindness services available to general public.

Area Served: 21 counties of northwestern Ohio, 2 counties of southeastern Michigan.

Health: Vision screening (preschool; school age; adult glaucoma); industrial eye safety, prevention of blindness programs, low income eye clinics.

Counseling/Social Work/Self-Help: Individual, family, peer, and group counseling; information and referral.

Educational: Children's services.

Preschools: Children's services, vision stimulation.

Professional Training: Regular in-service training program for universities, hospitals, interns, nursing homes, and related institutions.

Reading: Talking book distribution and repair center; reading services including radio reading service; braille and large-print transcription and duplication; closed-circuit televisions; Optacon and Kurzweil Reading Machine.

Rehabilitation: Rehabilitation teaching; orientation/mobility; children's educational specialist.

Computer Training: Computer evaluation and training.

Low Vision: Vision rehabilitation services, low vision clinic.

Low Vision Aids: Prescribes spectacles; provides low vision aids training; sells aids and appliances.

Low Vision Follow-up: Performed by medical, rehabilitation, and technology staff.

Sight Society of Ohio, Inc.

3603 Washington Avenue
Cincinnati, OH 45229
(513) 221-2775
William Poole, Board Member

Funded by: Contributions and earnings.

History/Date: Est. 1929.

Area Served: Greater Cincinnati.

Vision Center of Central Ohio

1393 North High Street
Columbus, OH 43201
(614) 294-5571
FAX: (614) 294-5576
E-mail: 72630.2230@compuserve.com
Joanna River, Executive Director

Type of Agency: Private, non-profit.

Mission: Services for totally blind, legally blind, visually impaired, deaf-blind, learning disabled, and mentally retarded persons.

Funded by: Fees, sub-contracts, United Way.

Budget: $2.5 million.

Hours of Operation: 24 hours a day.

Staff: 40 full time. Uses volunteers.

History/Date: Est. 1927.

Number of Clients Served: 1,500 per year.

Eligibility: Visual impairment that constitutes a handicap to employment.

Area Served: State of Ohio.

Transportation: Y.

Health: Refers for some eye health services.

Counseling/Social Work/Self-Help: Social evaluations; psychological testing and evaluation; individual, group, family/parent, couple counseling; placement in institution. Refers and provides consultation to other agencies for other counseling/social work services.

Professional Training: Internship/fieldwork placement in social work; psychological evaluation. Short-term or summer training.

Reading: Lends talking book record player and cassette player. Information and referral.

Residential: Dormitory for adults.

Rehabilitation: Personal management; braille; gesticulation; handwriting; listening skills; Optacon; typing; video magnifier; home management; orientation/mobility; rehabilitation teaching in client's home and community; sensory perception; homebound teaching service.

Employment: Prevocational and vocational evaluation; career and skill counseling; sheltered workshops; work adjustment. Refers for and provides consultation to other agencies on other employment-oriented services. Job-seeking skills training; clerical training.

Low Vision: Low vision clinic serving all age groups.

Low Vision Aids: Y.

Low Vision Follow-up: Y.

Local Offices:

Columbus: Vision Center Industries, 3232 Cleveland Avenue, Columbus, OH 43211, (614) 261-9816.

Vision Rehabilitation Inc.

220 Oberlin Road
Elyria, OH 44035
(216) 322-1122 or (800) 233-6777
FAX: (216) 322-2111
Kevin E. Walter, Executive Director

Type of Agency: Private; non-profit.
County/District Where Located: Lorain County.
Mission: Services for totally blind; legally blind; visually impaired; deaf-blind; and multiply disabled persons.
Funded by: Fees, United Way, endowment funds, gifts, and contracted fees.
Budget: $450,000.
Hours of Operation: Mon.-Fri. 8:30 AM-4:30 PM.
Program Accessibility: Fully accessible.
Staff: 9 full time, and contract rehabilitation professionals. Uses volunteers.
History/Date: Est. 1941.
Eligibility: Visually impaired of all ages able to benefit from services.
Area Served: Northern Ohio.

Health: Vision screenings for preschool and adult populations; glaucoma testing. Provides educational seminars on a variety of topics including diseases of the eye and aids and appliances for individuals with diabetes.
Counseling/Social Work/Self-Help: Case management; advocacy; referral to community services; referral for other counseling/social work services;

job placement and employer consultation services.
Educational: In-school consultation and rehabilitation training.
Preschools: Early intervention services.
Professional Training: Internship and fieldwork placements in orientation/mobility, rehabilitation teaching, and social work.
Reading: Lends talking book machines and cassette players as a sublending agency. Information and referral.
Rehabilitation: Rehabilitation teaching; orientation/mobility; functional assessment and training. Low vision services; electronic applications assessment and training; occupational services at the job site; job placement.
Recreational: Tandem bicycling.
Employment: Job placement and training services.
Computer Training: Adaptive systems for IBM-compatible computers.
Low Vision: Full clinic and community-based services.
Low Vision Aids: Comprehensive lending library and catalog sales.
Low Vision Follow-up: Yes.

Vocational Guidance Services

2239 East 55th Street
Cleveland, OH 44103
(216) 431-7800 or (800) 227-6625
FAX: (216) 431-5123
Edward J. Jeschelnig, Case Services Coordinator

Type of Agency: Private; non-profit.
Mission: To furnish all visually impaired people with tools needed to participate in competitive employment.
Budget: $11,000,000.
Hours of Operation: 7:00 AM-4:30 PM.

Staff: 98.
History/Date: Est. 1890.
Number of Clients Served: 100 per year.
Eligibility: Documented disability.
Area Served: Northeastern Ohio.
Transportation: Y.
Age Requirements: 17 and over.

Counseling/Social Work/Self-Help: All services available.
Rehabilitation: Y.
Employment: Clerical and other employment training.
Computer Training: Y.
Low Vision: Y.
Low Vision Aids: Y.

COMPUTER TRAINING CENTERS

Cincinnati Association for the Blind

2045 Gilbert Avenue
Cincinnati, OH 45202-1490
(513) 221-8558
FAX: (513) 221-2995
Mark Foersterling, Coordinator

Computer Training: Speech output systems; screen magnification systems; braille access systems; optical character recognition systems; closed-circuit television systems; word processing; database software; computer operating systems; training for instructors.

Ohio State School for the Blind

5220 North High Street
Columbus, OH 43214
(614) 888-1325
E-mail: wbolsen@ossb.odc.ohio. gov
William Bolsen, Contact Person

Computer Training: Speech output systems; screen magnification systems; braille access systems; optical character recognition systems; word processing; training for instructors.

STORER Computer Access Center
Cleveland Sight Center of the Cleveland Society of the Blind
1909 East 101th Street
Cleveland, OH 44106
(216) 791-8118
FAX: (216) 791-1101
Michael Grady, Director

Computer Training: Speech output systems; screen magnification systems; braille access systems; optical character recognition systems; closed-circuit television systems; word processing; database software; computer operating systems; training for instructors.

Vision Center of Central Ohio
1393 North High Street
Columbus, OH 43201
(614) 294-5571
FAX: (614) 294-5576
E-mail: 72630.2230@compuserve.com
Jo Ann Slagle, Teacher

Computer Training: Speech output systems; screen magnification systems; optical character recognition systems; closed-circuit television systems; word processing; computer operating systems.

DOG GUIDE SCHOOLS

Pilot Dogs, Inc.
625 West Town Street
Columbus, OH 43215-4496
(614) 221-6367
J. Jay Gray, Executive Director

Type of Agency: Non-profit.
Mission: Provides guide dogs to blind persons and renders training in the satisfactory use of such guide dogs.

Funded by: Lions Club, Pilot Guide Dog Foundation, general public.
Budget: $890,000.
Hours of Operation: 8:00 AM-5:00 PM.
Staff: 28.
History/Date: Est. 1948; inc. 1950.
Number of Clients Served: 155 per year.
Eligibility: Legally blind; physically and mentally capable.
Area Served: United States, Canada, Mexico, and other countries.
Transportation: Y.
Age Requirements: High school.

Trains and supplies dog guides for blind persons. Provides consultation and referral services. Has public education program.

◆ Low Vision Services

EYE CARE SOCIETIES

Ohio Ophthalmological Society
1500 Lake Shore Drive
Columbus, OH 43204-3891
(614) 486-2401
FAX: (614) 486-3130
Todd Baker, Executive Director

County/District Where Located: Franklin County.

Ohio Optometric Association, Inc.
169 East Livingston Avenue
Columbus, OH 43215
(614) 224-2600 or (800) 874-9111
Earl K. Green

LOW VISION CENTERS

Cincinnati Association for the Blind
2045 Gilbert Avenue

Cincinnati, OH 45202-1490
(513) 221-8558
FAX: (513) 221-2995
Susan Kimbrough, Low Vision Supervisor

Type of Agency: Private, non-profit.
Mission: Services for blind and visually impaired persons.
Funded by: Client fees, contributions, United Way, fees from government agencies.
Budget: $7 million.
Hours of Operation: Mon.-Fri. 8:30 AM-4:30 PM.
Program Accessibility: Building is fully accessible.
Staff: Optometrists; low vision specialists; social worker; orientation/mobility specialists; rehabilitation teacher; computer specialist.
History/Date: Est. 1910.
Number of Clients Served: 3,000 annually.
Eligibility: Vision loss that interferes with normal functioning.
Area Served: Greater Cincinnati and northern Kentucky.

Health: Glaucoma screenings; refers for other health services.
Low Vision: Prescription and instruction in use of low vision aids and devices.
Low Vision Aids: Provided on trial; available for purchase after evaluation; instruction provided.
Low Vision Follow-up: As indicated.

Cleveland Sight Center of the Cleveland Society for the Blind
1909 East 101st Street
Cleveland, OH 44106
(216) 791-8118
FAX: (216) 791-1101
Barbara Tomko, Director, Community and Social Services
Robert V. Spurney, M.D., Medical Director

Type of Agency: Non-profit.
County/District Where Located: Cuyahoga County.
Funded by: Client fees on a sliding scale; contributions; Medicare; Medicaid; state fees; public school systems.
Hours of Operation: Mon.-Fri., by appointment.
Staff: 2 optometrists; 1 low vision specialist.
Number of Clients Served: 600 annually.
Eligibility: Vision loss.
Area Served: Unlimited.

Educational: Provides consultation, training, and referral.
Low Vision: Evaluation, recommendation, and trial, sale of vision aids.
Low Vision Aids: Provided for trial; on-site training provided; follow-up.
Low Vision Follow-up: 3 months.

Greater Akron Low Vision Clinic

33 North Union Street
Akron, OH 44304-1318
(330) 996-4080
FAX: (330) 996-4181
Dr. Cheryl J. Reed, Director

Type of Agency: Private; non-profit.
County/District Where Located: Summit County.
Mission: Provides assessment, training, and adaptive aids to assist visually impaired individuals of all ages to function in home, work, and school environments.
Funded by: Fees for service.
Hours of Operation: Tues.-Thurs. 9:00AM-5:00PM.
Program Accessibility: Handicapped accessible.
Staff: 4.
History/Date: Est. 1994.
Number of Clients Served: 250.

Area Served: Northeastern Ohio.
Low Vision: Evaluation, referral, rehabilitation.
Low Vision Aids: Available for loan or purchase; traiing in use of aids.
Low Vision Follow-up: Y.

Ohio State University College of Optometry
Low Vision Clinic

320 West Tenth Avenue
Columbus, OH 43210
(614) 292-1222
FAX: (614) 688-5603
Greg Good, O.D., Ph.D., Director

County/District Where Located: Franklin County.
Funded by: State funds.
Hours of Operation: Mon.-Fri. 8:30 AM - 5:00 PM.
Staff: Optometrist; residents; ophthalmologists.
Eligibility: Referrals from previous doctor.
Area Served: Unlimited.

Low Vision Follow-up: Return appointment in 6 months as necessary.

Vision Rehabilitation Inc.

220 Oberlin Road
Elyria, OH 44035
(216) 322-1122 or toll-free
(800) 233-6777
FAX: (216) 322-2111
Kevin E. Walter, LPC

Type of Agency: Private; non-profit.
County/District Where Located: Lorain County.
Mission: Personal adjustment and occupational rehabilitation services for blind and visually impaired persons of all ages.
Funded by: Client fees, government agencies' fees, contributions, United Way.

Budget: $450,000.
Hours of Operation: By appointment.
Program Accessibility: Fully accessible.
Staff: Optometrist; rehabilitation social worker; rehabilitation teacher; orientation/mobility instructor; employment consultant.
History/Date: Est. 1941.
Eligibility: Visually impaired able to benefit from services.
Area Served: North central Ohio.

Counseling/Social Work/Self-Help: Referral services.
Preschools: Early intervention program.
Employment: Placement and on-the-job support services.
Computer Training: Speech, large print and braille systems; skills assessment and training.
Low Vision: Clinic.
Low Vision Aids: Provided for trial period; available for purchase; community-based training and follow-up procedure.
Low Vision Follow-up: Y.

◆ Aging Services

STATE UNITS ON AGING

Ohio Department of Aging

50 West Broad Street
Ninth Floor
Columbus, OH 43266-0501
(614) 466-5500 or Golden Buck-eye Card, discount program (800) 422-1976
FAX: (614) 466-5741
Judith Brachman, Director

Provides referrals to Area Agencies on Aging and information on other local aging services.

INDEPENDENT LIVING PROGRAMS

Rehabilitation Services Commission
Bureau of Services for the Visually Impaired
400 East Campus View Boulevard
Columbus, OH 43235
(614) 438-1255
William A. Castro, Director

Provides independent living services for persons age 55 and over. For further information, contact the Project Director or general phone number listed.

OKLAHOMA

♦ *Educational Services*

STATE SERVICES

Oklahoma State Department of Education
Special Education Services
Oliver Hodge Memorial Education Building
2500 North Lincoln Boulevard
Oklahoma City, OK 73105-4599
(405) 521-3351
FAX: (405) 522-3503
Darla Griffin, Special Education Section Director
Rex S. Howard, State Coordinator
Dr. Jill Burroughs, Coordinator of Preschool Handicapped,
(405) 521-3351

Type of Agency: State.
County/District Where Located: Oklahoma County.
Mission: Administers supplemental state funds for visually handicapped children attending public schools. Provides consultation and in-service training for public schools. Distributes large type books through Library for the Blind and Physically Handicapped. Provides resource and program information through state coordinator.
Funded by: Public funds.
Hours of Operation: Mon.-Fri. 8:00 AM-4:30 PM.
Area Served: Oklahoma.

For information about local facilities, consult the superintendent of schools in the area or contact State office.

EARLY INTERVENTION COORDINATION

Interagency Coordinating Council for Early Childhood Intervention
Oklahoma Commission on Children and Youth
4545 North Lincoln Boulevard
Suite 114
Oklahoma City, OK 73105
(405) 521-4016, ext. 111
FAX: (405) 524-0417
E-mail: pdunkelgod@oklasof. state.ok.us
Patrice Dunkelgod, ICC Coordinator

County/District Where Located: Oklahoma County.

Provides planning and coordination for the implementation of early childhood intervention services for Oklahoma infants, toddlers, and preschoolers with developmental delays and disabilities. Does not provide direct services.

Oklahoma State Department of Education
Special Education Services/ Sooner Start Program
Oliver Hodge Memorial Education Building
2500 North Lincoln Boulevard
Oklahoma City, OK 73105-4599
(405) 521-4880
FAX: (405) 522-3503
Cathy Perri, Early Intervention Administrator

County/District Where Located: Oklahoma County.

Early intervention services for infants and toddlers with disabilities, birth to 3 years. Home-based programs. To be eligible, a child must have one of the following: 50 percent delay in one area, 25 percent delay in two or more areas, or diagnosed syndrome that may result in delay.

SCHOOLS

Parkview School (Oklahoma School for the Blind)
3300 Gibson Street
Muskogee, OK 74403
(918) 682-6641
FAX: (918) 682-1651
E-mail: osb@ok.azalea.net
Garold Conn, Superintendent

Type of Agency: State.
County/District Where Located: Muskogee County.
Mission: Services for totally blind, legally blind, visually impaired, learning disabled, mentally retarded, emotionally disturbed, orthopedically disabled, and multiply disabled persons.
Funded by: State funds.
Budget: $4,000,000.
Hours of Operation: 24 hours a day.
Program Accessibility: Fully accessible.
Staff: 133 full time. Uses volunteers.
History/Date: Est. 1897.
Number of Clients Served: 410.
Eligibility: Educable; resident of the state with a visual impairment not adequately served in school district.
Area Served: Statewide.
Transportation: Y.
Age Requirements: 0-21 years.

Health: Audiology services; speech therapy. On-campus dental, pediatric, ophthalmological and physical therapy. Referrals for other services.
Counseling/Social Work/Self-Help: Social evaluations; psychological testing and evaluation; individual, group, family/parent, couple counseling; placement in school.
Educational: Preschool through grade 12. Programs for college prep; general academic studies; vocational/skill development.

Preschools: Located at Oklahoma School for the Blind.

Professional Training: Internship/fieldwork placement in special education. Regular in-service training programs, short-term or summer training.

Reading: Talking book record players and cassette players; talking book records and cassettes; braille books; large-print books; braille magazines; recorded magazines; information and referral.

Residential: Dormitories, on-site apartments.

Rehabilitation: Personal management; braille; gesticulation; handwriting; listening skills; Optacon; typing; video magnifier; home management; orientation/mobility; remedial education; sensory training; computer training.

Recreational: After-school programs; hobby groups; bowling; swimming; track; wrestling; modified games; archery; weight lifting; goal ball.

Employment: Prevocational evaluation; career and skill counseling; occupational skill development; vending facility training; work-study. Refers for vocational placement.

Computer Training: Access. At all levels, literacy training for all students.

Low Vision: Low vision service. Sells or lends low vision aids.

Low Vision Aids: Some provided.

Low Vision Follow-up: Low vision clinic once a week.

Contact local school superintendent for information or Rex S. Howard, State Coordinator, Special Education Services, 2500 North Lincoln, Oklahoma City, OK 73105, (405) 521-3351.

INFANT AND PRESCHOOL

Little Light House, Inc.

5120 East 36th Street
Tulsa, OK 74135-5228
(918) 664-6746
FAX: (918) 664-2293
Marcia Mitchell, Executive Director

Type of Agency: Private; non-profit.

County/District Where Located: Tulsa County.

Funded by: Private donations.

Budget: 1992-93: $720,000.

Hours of Operation: Mon.-Fri. 8:00 AM-4:00 PM.

Staff: 30 full time (occupational/speech therapists, special educators).

History/Date: Est. 1972.

Eligibility: Physical or mental disability.

Area Served: Tulsa and surrounding areas.

Age Requirements: 0-6 years.

Preschools: Serving deaf, blind, learning disabled, and mentally retarded persons.

Professional Training: Vocational special education.

Reading: Braille and large-print books.

Developmental center for disabled children. Nonresidential day program.

Parkview School (Oklahoma School for the Blind)

3300 Gibson Street
Muskogee, OK 74403
(918) 682-6641
FAX: (918) 682-1651
E-mail: osb@ok.azalea.net
Garold Conn, Superintendent

Type of Agency: State residential school.

County/District Where Located: Muskogee County.

Mission: Services for totally blind, visually impaired, and multiply disabled students.

Funded by: P.L. 89-313 monies; private donations; income from capital funds; state funds.

Budget: $3,900,000.

Hours of Operation: Mon.-Fri., 24 hours; closed weekends.

Program Accessibility: Fully accessible.

Staff: Includes teachers of visually impaired students, early childhood specialists, orientation/mobility specialists, social workers, physical therapists, and psychologist.

History/Date: Est. 1907.

Number of Clients Served: 105.

Eligibility: Residents of Oklahoma.

Area Served: Oklahoma.

Transportation: Y.

Age Requirements: 3-21 years.

Health: Low vision exams; immunizations; adaptive equipment.

Counseling/Social Work/Self-Help: Parent and other counseling. Other consultants' services to parents.

Educational: Provides instruction in all developmental areas. Self-contained classes for visually impaired and for multiply impaired children, aged 3-5.

Professional Training: In-service training provided during school year.

Reading: Reading specialist.

Residential: Y.

Rehabilitation: Visual services and vocational counseling.

Recreational: Y.

Employment: Prevocational training and work experience.

Computer Training: Computer lab.

Low Vision: Low vision clinic held once per week.

Low Vision Follow-up: Provided by staff and low vision clinic.

Consultant services to other programs on request for visually impaired infants, 0-2 years, with or without other disabilities.

STATEWIDE OUTREACH SERVICES

Parkview School (Oklahoma School for the Blind)
3300 Gibson Street
Muskogee, OK 74403
(918) 682-6641
FAX: (918) 682-1651
E-mail: osb@ok.azalea.net
Mary Sue Oxtoby, Outreach Coordinator

County/District Where Located: Muskogee County.
Funded by: State funds.
History/Date: Est. 1984 (Outreach Program)/School 1897.
Age Requirements: Infancy to 21 years.

Assessment: Provided on campus at no charge. Low vision, psychoeducational; orientation and mobility; physical therapy; speech and language; audiological; academic; daily living skills; developmental.
Consultation to Public Schools: On request. Professionals come to Parkview for observation and training. Outreach Coordinator will go to schools on request.
Direct Service: Resources and consultation on-site; observation; functional vision assessment.
Parent Assistance: Provides information by telephone and mail. Workshops and conferences on campus for training purposes; observation of classrooms; demonstration of equipment and techniques.
Materials Production: Limited braille materials.
Professional Training: Conferences and in-service training in teaching braille;

orientation and mobility; early childhood intervention; daily living skills; low vision adaptation; computer technology.

♦ Information Services

LIBRARIES

Oklahoma Library for the Blind and Physically Handicapped
300 N.E. 18th Street
Oklahoma City, OK 73105
(405) 521-3514 or (405) 521-3833
FAX: (405) 521-4582
Geraldine Adams, Director
Paul Adams, Machine Lending Information

Type of Agency: State.
Funded by: Public funds administered under the Oklahoma Department of Rehabilitation Services.
Hours of Operation: Mon.-Fri. 8:00 AM-5:00 PM.
Staff: 25.
History/Date: Est. 1933.
Area Served: Oklahoma.

Regional library supplying talking books, braille, cassette tapes, talking book machines and repair service.

Special Services
Tulsa City-County Library System
1520 North Hartford
Tulsa, OK 74106
(918) 596-7920 or (918) 596-7922 or TDD (918) 596-7922
FAX: (918) 596-7283
Amy Stephens, Librarian

Subregional library.

MEDIA PRODUCTION SERVICES

Oklahoma Library for the Blind and Physically Handicapped
300 N.E. 18th Street
Oklahoma City, OK 73105
(405) 521-3514
FAX: (405) 521-4582
Geraldine Adams, Director

County/District Where Located: Oklahoma County.
Groups Served: K-12; college students; other adults.

Types/Content: Textbooks; recreational; career/vocational; religious; any requests.
Media Formats: Braille books; talking books/cassettes; Large Print textbooks.
Title Listings: No title listings available.

INFORMATION AND REFERRAL

Prevent Blindness Oklahoma
6 N.E. 63rd Street, #150
Oklahoma City, OK 73105
(405) 848-7123
FAX: (405) 848-6935

See Prevent Blindness America in U.S. national listings.

See also in national listings:

Narrative Television Network

♦ Rehabilitation Services

STATE SERVICES

Visual Services Division
Oklahoma Department of Rehabilitation Services
3535 N.W. 58th Street
Suite 500

Oklahoma City, OK 73112
(405) 951-3494
FAX: (405) 951-3529
Raymond Hopkins, Visual Services
Director

Type of Agency: State.
Mission: Services for totally blind, legally blind, visually impaired, and deaf-blind persons.
Funded by: Public funds.
Hours of Operation: 8:00 AM-5:00 PM.
History/Date: Est. 1920.
Eligibility: Visual impairment.

Health: Contracts for health services.
Professional Training: Internship/fieldwork placement in rehabilitation counseling; vocational rehabilitation; rehabilitation teaching; orientation and mobility training.
Reading: Lends talking book record players and cassette players; talking book records and cassettes; braille books; large-print books; braille magazines; recorded magazines. Transcription to braille; tape recording services on demand.
Rehabilitation: Personal management; braille; handwriting; listening skills; Optacon; typing; video magnifier; home management; orientation/mobility; rehabilitation teaching in client's home and community.
Employment: Career and skill counseling; vocational placement; vending facility training. Contracts for other employment-oriented services.
Low Vision Aids: Has low vision aids or devices.

Local Offices:

Ada: 1628 East Beverly, Ada, OK 74820, (405) 436-2430.

Chickasha: 1000 Choctaw, Suite 2, Plaza North Shopping Center, Chickasha, OK 73018, (405) 222-0685.
Enid: 528 North Van Buren, Enid, OK 73702, (405) 233-6514.
Idabel: 513 E. Washington, Idabel, OK 74745, (405) 286-3789.
Lawton: 1332 N.W. 53rd Street, Lawton, OK 73505, (405) 355-0127.
McAlester: 321 South Third, Suite 7B, McAlester, OK 74501, (918) 423-1296.
Muskogee: 727 South 32nd, Muskogee, OK 74402, (918) 686-0488.
Oklahoma City: 300 N.E. 18th, Oklahoma City, OK 73105, (405) 521-3873 (Library for the Blind).
Oklahoma City: 608 Stanton L. Young Drive, Oklahoma City, OK 73104, (405) 271-6632.
Oklahoma City: Evaluation Center, 5813 South Robinson, Oklahoma City, OK 73109, (405) 636-0140.
Oklahoma City: Vending Facility Warehouse, 300 N.E. 18th, Oklahoma City, OK 73105, (405) 521-3723.
Oklahoma City: 5813 South Robinson, Oklahoma City, OK 73109, (405) 636-0140.
Stillwater: 522 South Ramsey, Stillwater, OK 74076, (405) 372-2017.
Tulsa: 444 South Houston, Suite 200, Tulsa, OK 74127-8990, (918) 581-2352.
Tulsa: 130 North Greenwood, Suite T-8, Tulsa, OK 74120, (918) 587-3453.
Vinita: Eastern State Hospital, Building 8 East, Vinita, OK 74301, (918) 256-5509.
Weatherford: 1401 Lera Drive, Suite 204, Weatherford, OK 73096, (405) 772-5805.
Woodward: 1611 Main, Suite 204, Woodward, OK 73801, (405) 256-2565.

REHABILITATION

Oklahoma League for the Blind
P.O. Box 24020
Oklahoma City, OK 73124
(405) 232-4644
FAX: (405) 236-5438
Nasir Ahmed, Executive Director

Type of Agency: Private; non-profit.
Mission: Services for totally blind; legally blind; visually impaired; deaf-blind.
Funded by: Fees, workshop sales, sub-contracts, miscellaneous.
Hours of Operation: Mon.-Fri. 7:15 AM-3:45 PM.
Staff: 12 full time.
History/Date: Est. 1949.
Number of Clients Served: 60.
Eligibility: Visual impairment; 18 years or older.
Area Served: Oklahoma.
Age Requirements: 18 years or older.

Employment: Vocational evaluation; occupational skill development; job retention; job retraining; sheltered workshops; job placement within the agency. Provides consultation to other agencies for some employment services.
Computer Training: Some on-the-job training.

COMPUTER TRAINING CENTERS

Parkview School (Oklahoma School for the Blind)
3300 Gibson Street
Muskogee, OK 74403
(918) 682-6641
FAX: (918) 682-1651
E-mail: osb@ok.azalea.net
Jeanne Meyer, Teacher

County/District Where Located: Muskogee County.

Computer Training: Speech output systems; screen

magnification systems; braille access systems; word processing; database software.

◆ Low Vision Services

EYE CARE SOCIETIES

Oklahoma State Society of Eye Physicians and Surgeons
The Enid Eye, Inc.
615 East Oklahoma, Suite 101
Enid, OK 73701
(405) 233-4711
FAX: (405) 233-1532
Charles A. Lawrence, M.D.,
President

County/District Where Located: Garfield County.

Oklahoma Optometric Association
4545 North Lincoln Boulevard
Suite 105
Oklahoma City, OK 73105
(405) 524-1075
FAX: (405) 524-1077
Saundra Gragg, Executive Director

LOW VISION CENTERS

College of Optometry Northeastern State University
Tahlequah, OK 74464
(918) 456-5511, ext. 4014 or
(918) 458-3160 clinic
FAX: (918) 458-2104
E-mail:
edmondso@cherokee.nsuok.
edu
Linda Edmondson, A.M., O.D.,
Director of Low Vision Services

Type of Agency: Non-profit.
County/District Where Located: Cherokee County.
Funded by: Client fees; state funds.

Hours of Operation: Mon.-Fri. 8:00 AM-5:00 PM.
Staff: Optician; optometrist; optometry student; psychologist; social worker.
Eligibility: No restrictions (priority given to Indian Health Service eligible patients).
Area Served: Northeastern Oklahoma, Arkansas, Missouri.

Low Vision Aids: Sold at cost; prescribed and fitted for variable charge; on-site or in-home training provided.
Low Vision Follow-up: Varies according to patient.

Dean A. McGee Eye Institute
608 Stanton L. Young Boulevard
Oklahoma City, OK 73104
(405) 271-6060
FAX: (405) 271-4442
Gary W. Harris, M.D., Director,
Low Vision Services

Type of Agency: Non-profit.
Funded by: Client fees; county, state, federal funds; foundation grants; personal donations.
Hours of Operation: Mon.-Fri. 8:00 AM to 4:30 PM.
Staff: Ophthalmologist; ophthalmic assistant; ophthalmic technician. Through ancillary staff of McGee Eye Institute and Oklahoma Department of Human Services: optician; orientation/ mobility instructor; rehabilitation teacher; rehabilitation counselor.
Area Served: Unlimited.

Low Vision Aids: Provided for purchase; on-site training provided.
Low Vision Follow-up: By return appointment.

◆ Aging Services

STATE UNITS ON AGING

Aging Services Division Oklahoma Department of Human Services
312 N.E. 28th Street
Oklahoma City, OK 73105
(405) 521-2327 or (800) 211-2116
FAX: (405) 521-2086
Roy Keen, Division Administrator

Provides referrals to Area Agencies on Aging and information on other local aging services.

INDEPENDENT LIVING PROGRAMS

State Department of Rehabilitation Visual Services Division
3535 Northwest 58 Street
Suite 500
Oklahoma City, OK 73112-4812
(405) 951-3400 or (800) 845-8476
FAX: (405) 951-3529
Linda Parker, Director
Ray Hopkins, Administrator

Provides independent living services for persons age 55 and over. For further information, contact the Project Director or general phone number listed.

OREGON

♦ Educational Services

STATE SERVICES

Oregon Department of Education
255 Capitol Street, N.E.
Salem, OR 97310
(503) 378-3598
FAX: (503) 373-7968
E-mail: jane.mulholland@state.
or.us
Jane Mulholland, Assistant
Superintendent, Special Schools/
Regional Programs
Marilyn Gense, Program Specialist

Mission: Through eight regional
programs, provides supplemental
state funds for the education of
children who are visually
impaired, hearing impaired, deaf-
blind, orthopedically impaired, or
have autism or severe health
impairments. Offers consultation
to local school districts and
specialized instruction and related
services to children. Lends special
education material, including
braille and large type books, tape,
tape recorders, talking books, and
talking book machines, needed for
the education of visually impaired
children. Offers reading service.
Funded by: Public funds.
Staff: Teachers of visually
impaired students, orientation and
mobility teachers.
History/Date: Est. 1951.
Number of Clients Served: 800.
Eligibility: Meet Oregon
eligibility criteria for visual
impairment.
Area Served: Oregon.
Age Requirements: 0-21.

**Counseling/Social Work/Self-
Help:** Self-help groups.

For information about local
facilities, consult the Department
of Education at the above address.

EARLY INTERVENTION COORDINATION

**Early Intervention and Early
Childhood Special Education
Programs
Oregon Department of
Education**
Public Service Building
255 Capitol Street, N.E.
Salem, OR 97310
(503) 378-3598
FAX: (503) 373-7968
Jane Mulholland, Early Childhood
Coordinator
Valerie Miller-Case, Early
Intervention/Early Childhood
Specialist

County/District Where Located:
Marion County.

Provides early intervention
programs for children 0-5 years of
age.

SCHOOLS

**Oregon Office of Special
Education
Services to Children and Youth
with Deafblindness**
255 Capitol Street, N.E.
Salem, OR 97310
(503) 378-3598
FAX: (503) 373-7968
E-mail: jay.gense@state.or.us
D. Jay Gense, State Coordinator/
Specialist for Deaf-Blind

Type of Agency: State.
Mission: To provide technical
assistance and support to
educational programs serving
children who are deaf-blind.
Funded by: Title VI-C.
Staff: 9 part time.
Number of Clients Served:
approximately 90.

Eligibility: Eligible as both
visually and hearing impaired
acccording to Oregon
Administrative Rule eligibility
criteria.
Area Served: Oregon.
Age Requirements: 0-21 years.

Consultant services to programs
for deaf-blind children, 0-22 years;
services provided from program to
local education agency/state
schools and other agencies serving
deaf-blind persons.

Oregon School for the Blind
700 Church Street, S.E.
Salem, OR 97301
(503) 378-3820
FAX: (503) 373-7537
Ann Hicks, Director

Type of Agency: State.
County/District Where Located:
Marion County.
Mission: Services for totally blind;
legally blind; deaf-blind; learning
disabled; mentally retarded;
emotionally disturbed;
orthopedically handicapped.
Funded by: State funds.
Budget: 1992-93 school year:
$2,589,991.
Hours of Operation: 7 days a
week, 24 hours a day. School closes
one weekend per month.
Staff: 55 full time, 15 part time.
Uses volunteers.
History/Date: Est. 1873.
Number of Clients Served: 52
residential, 345 outreach.
Eligibility: Visually impaired;
resident of Oregon where no local
educational/training program is
appropriate.
Area Served: State of Oregon.
Transportation: Y.
Age Requirements: 3-21 years.

Health: Low vision service;
physical therapy; general health
services; refers for specific health
problems; vision stimulation.

Counseling/Social Work/Self-Help: Individual, group, family/parent counseling. Consultation for behavioral programs.

Educational: Preschool through grade 6 for general academic studies. Transition program for high school through age 21.

Preschools: Provided through regional programs.

Professional Training: In-service training for staff; internships and practice in cooperation with universities.

Reading: Y.

Residential: Dormitories.

Rehabilitation: Personal management; braille; handwriting; typing; closed circuit television; orientation/mobility; sensory training; remedial work skills; prevocational education.

Recreational: Services include swimming; bowling; social situations; community resources. Summer programs and student assessment for public school youngsters.

Employment: Work experience on and off campus provided.

Computer Training: Y.

Low Vision: Y.

Low Vision Aids: Y.

Low Vision Follow-up: Y.

INFANT AND PRESCHOOL

Oregon Department of Education

255 Capitol Street, N.E.
Salem, OR 97310
(503) 378-3598
FAX: (503) 373-7968
E-mail: jane.molholland@state.or.us
Jane Molholland, Assistant Superintendent, Special Schools/Regional Programs
Marilyn Gense, Program Specialist

Type of Agency: State.

Mission: Home-based programs and consultant services for preschool visually impaired/multiply impaired persons.

Funded by: Various federal funds and state general fund.

Staff: Certified teachers of visually impaired students plus orientation/mobility specialists.

History/Date: Est. 1951.

Area Served: Oregon.

Transportation: Y.

Health: Low vision exams; adaptive equipment; various health services.

Counseling/Social Work/Self-Help: Parent counseling and workshops; genetic counseling; other social services.

Educational: Provides direct instruction or consultation/referral in all developmental areas; scholarships for regular preschool attendance. Itinerant model for consultative and direct instruction to children.

Regional Offices:

Region I: Eastern Oregon Regional Program, 10100 North McAllister Road, Island City, OR 97850-2193, (541) 963-4106, Lenny Williams, Coordinator.

Region II: Central Oregon Regional Program, 520 N.W. Wall Street, Bend, OR 97701, (541) 383-6845, Kathy Emerson, Coordinator.

Region III: Southern Oregon Regional Program, 101 North Grape Street, Medford, OR 97501, (503) 776-8556, Paul Rickerson, Coordinator.

Region IV: Cascade Regional Program, 905 Fourth Avenue, S.E., Albany, OR 97321, (503) 967-8822, Lila Kuykendall, Coordinator.

Region V: Mid-Oregon Regional Program, 3400 Portland Road, N.E., Salem, OR 97303, (503) 588-6677, Maureen Casey, Coordinator.

Region VI: Columbia Regional Program, 531 S.E. 14th Street, Portland, OR 97214, (503) 916-5840, Bob Crebo, Coordinator.

Region VII: Lane Regional Program, 1200 Highway 99 North, Eugene, OR 97402, (541) 461-8264, Carol Knobbe, Coordinator.

Region VIII: Northwest Regional ESD, 5825 Northeast Ray Circle, Hillsboro, OR 97124, (503) 690-5428, Bud Moore, Coordinator.

Preschool services provided through regional programs. For information, contact: Assistant Superintendent, Special Schools/Regional Programs, Oregon Department of Education, Salem, OR 97310, (503) 378-3598.

Oregon School for the Blind

700 Church Street, S.E.
Salem, OR 97301
(503) 378-3820
FAX: (503) 373-7537
Ann Hicks, Director

Type of Agency: State.

County/District Where Located: Marion County.

Mission: Programs for children who are visually impaired or multiply disabled.

Funded by: Private donations and state funds.

Staff: 49 full time; 25 part time.

History/Date: Est. 1873.

Number of Clients Served: 50.

Eligibility: Visually impaired, ages 0-5.

Area Served: Oregon.

Transportation: Y.

Age Requirements: 0-5.

Health: Low vision exams; auditory training, immunizations, and blood tests available on consultant or referral basis; adaptive equipment.

Counseling/Social Work/Self-Help: Genetic counseling; parent

and other counseling; financial assistance.
Educational: Provides instruction in all developmental areas. Noncategorical classrooms for visually impaired/multiply disabled children.
Preschools: None on campus. Provides funds for preschool attendance in local district.
Reading: Y.
Low Vision: Y.
Low Vision Aids: Y.
Low Vision Follow-up: Y.

Services provided through 6 regional program offices of the Oregon Department of Education and through the School for the Blind.

STATEWIDE OUTREACH SERVICES

Oregon School for the Blind
700 Church Street, S.E.
Salem, OR 97301
(503) 378-3820
FAX: (503) 373-7537
Ann Hicks, Director

County/District Where Located: Marion County.
Funded by: State funds; private donations.
History/Date: Est. 1873.
Age Requirements: 0-21.

Assessment: Technology; day/living skills; orientation and mobility; functional vision; Low Vision clinic.
Consultation to Public Schools: Referrals.
Direct Service: On-campus services.
Parent Assistance: Parent workshops (both in-house and traveling); provide parent training materials.
Materials Production: On a limited basis.

Professional Training: In-service workshops held at school.

INSTRUCTIONAL MATERIALS CENTERS

Independent Living Resources
4506 S. E. Belmont
Suite 100
Portland, OR 97215
(503) 232-7411 or TDD (503) 232-8408
FAX: (503) 232-7480
Thomas Ciesielski, Executive Director

County/District Where Located: Multnomah County.
Groups Served: K-12, college students, other adults.

Types/Content: Textbooks, recreational, career/vocational, religious, any requests.
Media Formats: Braille books, cassettes, large print.
Title Listings: No title listings available.

Oregon Text and Media Center for the Visually Handicapped
531 S.E. 14th Street
Portland, OR 97214
(503) 916-5840, ext. 421
FAX: (503) 916-6224
E-mail: larrybrown@aol.com
Larry Brown, Director

County/District Where Located: Multnomah County.
Area Served: Statewide.
Groups Served: Birth-K; K-12; postgraduate school-aged students.

Types/Content: Textbooks; recreational.
Media Formats: Braille books; talking books/cassettes; large-print books; educational aids.
Title Listings: None specified.

UNIVERSITY TRAINING PROGRAMS

Portland State University Department of Special Education
P.O. Box 751
Portland, OR 97207
(503) 725-4686
FAX: (503) 725-5599
E-mail: shelly@ed.pdx.edu
Dr. Joel Arick

County/District Where Located: Multnomah County.

Programs Offered: Graduate (master's) programs for teachers of visually impaired and deaf-blind students.
Distance Education: Y.

◆ *Information Services*

LIBRARIES

Oregon State Library Talking Book and Braille Services
250 Winter Street, N.E.
Salem, OR 97310
(503) 378-3849 or toll-free in Oregon (800) 452-0292
FAX: (503) 588-7119
Mary Mohr, Operations Coordinator
Nanc Ripperda, Machine Lending Agent

Funded by: Public funds.
Hours of Operation: Mon.-Fri. 8:00 AM-5:00 PM.
History/Date: Est. 1933.
Number of Clients Served: 7,000 individuals, 500 institutions.
Area Served: Oregon.
Age Requirements: 4 years and older.

Regional library providing talking books, braille, tape, and large-print children's books.

MEDIA PRODUCTION SERVICES

Oregon State Library Talking Book and Braille Services
250 Winter Street, N.E.
Salem, OR 97310
(503) 378-3849
FAX: (503) 588-7119
E-mail: mary.c.mohr@state.or.us
URL: http://www.osl.state.or.us/tbabs/tbabs.html
Mary Mohr, Operations Coordinator, Librarian
Nanc Ripperda, Machine Lending Agent

County/District Where Located: Marion County.
Area Served: Oregon.
Groups Served: Pre-school to adults.

Types/Content: Recreational, career/vocational, religious. Oregon author collection.
Media Formats: Braille books, talking books/cassettes (large-print books for children).
Title Listings: No title listings available.

RADIO READING

Golden Hours, Inc.
7140 S.W. Macadam Drive
Portland, OR 97219-3013
(503) 293-1902
FAX: (503) 777-8469
Jerry Delaunay, Executive Director

Hours of Operation: 24 hours a day.
History/Date: Est. 1970.
Area Served: State of Oregon and southwestern Washington.

KBPS Seeing Sound
515 N.E. 15th Street
Portland, OR 97232
(503) 916-5828
FAX: (503) 916-2642
Tania Thompson

County/District Where Located: Multnomah County.
Hours of Operation: 24 hours, 7 days.
History/Date: Est. 1973.
Area Served: Portland metropolitan area.

See also in national listings:

Blindskills, Inc.

DB-LINK: The National Information Clearinghouse on Children Who Are Deaf-Blind

NTAC (National Technical Assistance Consortium for Children and Young Adults who are Deaf-Blind)
Teaching Research Division

♦ Rehabilitation Services

STATE SERVICES

Oregon Commission for the Blind
535 S.E. 12th Avenue
Portland, OR 97214
(503) 731-3221
FAX: (503) 731-3230
Charles E. Young, Administrator

Type of Agency: State.
Mission: Services for legally blind; totally blind. Independent living services for persons over 55 years of age with visual impairment.
Funded by: Federal and state appropriations; federal grants; donations.
Hours of Operation: Mon.-Fri. 8:00 AM-5:00 PM.
Program Accessibility: All facilities and programs are accessible to persons with disabilities, according to ADA specifications.
Staff: 47 full time, 5 part time.
Number of Clients Served: 1,500 per year.
Eligibility: Meets definition of legal blindness.
Area Served: Statewide.
Age Requirements: Over 17 years.

Health: Refers for medical services.
Counseling/Social Work/Self-Help: Vocational and personal counseling and guidance. Referral to community services. Refers for other counseling/social work services.
Educational: College prep; remedial education. Accepts legally blind persons and multiply disabled persons.
Professional Training: Regular in-service training programs; open to enrollment from other agencies.
Reading: Refers for reading services.
Residential: Dormitory for adults.
Rehabilitation: Personal management; braille; handwriting; Optacon; typing; video magnifier; electronic mobility aids; home management; orientation/mobility; rehabilitation teaching in client's home and community; remedial education.
Recreational: Challenge course; refers for other recreational/leisure services.
Employment: Prevocational evaluation; career and skill counseling; job retention; vocational placement; follow-up service; vending facility training. Refers for other employment-oriented services.
Computer Training: Speech output systems; screen magnification systems; braille access systems; word processing; computer operating systems. One

full-time instructor. Contact: Pat Macdonnell, Director of Orientation & Career Center for the Blind, (503) 731-3221.

Low Vision: Low vision assessments, sale or loan of low vision aids; instruction in techniques of daily living and vision therapy.

Low Vision Aids: Sells, lends, or rents low vision aids, including magnifiers, signature guides, cane tips, phone dials, braille paper, labelling tape, slate and stylus, Hi-marks.

Low Vision Follow-up: Recommends low vision devices/aids to clients and either loans aids to clients or orders devices for them. Follow-up assessment with decrease in vision.

Local Offices:

Eugene: 541 Willamette, Room 408, Eugene, OR 97401, (503) 686-7990.

Medford: 228 North Holly, Medford, OR 97501, (503) 776-6047.

Newport: Oregon State Commission for the Blind, P.O. Box 2053, Newport, OR 97365, (503) 563-5231.

Salem: 670 Church Street, S.E., Salem, OR 97301, (503) 378-8479.

REHABILITATION

Blind Enterprises of Oregon
1101 SE 12th Avenue
Portland, OR 97214-3602
(503) 233-8141
FAX: (503) 233-8536
Tami Foss, Executive Director

Type of Agency: Private.
County/District Where Located: Multnomah County.

Employment: Offers workshop employment for blind and visually impaired persons in manufacturing products.

Independent Living Resources
4506 S.E. Belmont
Suite 100
Portland, OR 97215
(503) 232-7411 or TDD (503) 232-8408
Thomas Ciesielski, Executive Director

Type of Agency: Private; non-profit.
County/District Where Located: Multnomah County.
Mission: Independent living services.
Funded by: Federal grants, donations.
Budget: $580,000.
Hours of Operation: Mon.-Fri. 8:30 AM-5:00 PM.
Staff: 17.
History/Date: Est. 1957 and Inc. 1980.
Number of Clients Served: 700 per year.
Eligibility: Severe vision loss, deaf-blindness, or multiple disabilities.
Age Requirements: None.

Counseling/Social Work/Self-Help: Individual/group/family counseling; community services. Refers for social/psychological testing and evaluation.
Educational: Refers for school/training placement.
Rehabilitation: Daily living/communication skills both on/off premises.
Recreational: Continuing education; arts/crafts; special programs for the elderly.
Low Vision: Referrals to eye care professionals.
Low Vision Aids: Magnification devices on loan and for sale.

Vision Northwest
621 S.W. Alder Street
Suite 500

Portland, OR 97205-3620
(503) 221-0705
FAX: (503) 243-2537
Gloria Patrick, Office Manager

Type of Agency: Non-profit.
County/District Where Located: Multnomah County.
Mission: Help reintegrate newly visually impaired persons into community.
Funded by: Foundation grants, private donations, charities.
Staff: 4. Uses volunteers.
History/Date: Est. 1983.
Eligibility: Newly blind, severe visual impairment.
Area Served: Oregon; Washington.

Counseling/Social Work/Self-Help: Counseling for adjustment to severe vision loss. Psychological services available.
Rehabilitation: Peer support groups; information and referral services.

COMPUTER TRAINING CENTERS

Oregon Commission for the Blind
535 S.E. 12th Avenue
Portland, OR 97214
(503) 731-3221
FAX: (503) 731-3230
Winslow Parker, Technology Specialist

Computer Training: Speech output systems; screen magnification systems; braille access systems; word processing; computer operating systems.

Oregon School for the Blind
700 Church Street, S.E.
Salem, OR 97301
(503) 378-8025
Margie Jordan, Media Specialist

County/District Where Located: Marion Country.

Computer Training: Screen magnification systems; braille access systems.

DOG GUIDE SCHOOLS

Guide Dogs for the Blind
32901 S.E. Kelso Road
Boring, OR 97009
(503) 668-2100
Steve Strand, Executive Director

For referral, contact Sue Sullivan, (415) 499-4000 or (800) 295-4050.

◆ Low Vision Services

EYE CARE SOCIETIES

Oregon Academy of Ophthalmology
208 S.W. Stark, #205
Portland, OR 97204
(503) 222-3937
FAX: (503) 243-6755
Nan Heim, Executive Director

Oregon Optometric Association
6901 S. E. Lake Road
Suite 26
Milwaukie, OR 97267
(503) 654-5036
Wayne Schumacher, Executive Director

LOW VISION CENTERS

Devers Eye Institute
1040 N.W. 22nd Avenue
Portland, OR 97210
(503) 413-8499
FAX: (503) 413-7006
Shari Katz, M.A., Vision Rehabilitation Specialist
Vasiliki D. Stoumbos, M.D.

Type of Agency: Outpatient clinic.
County/District Where Located: Multnomah County.

Funded by: Patient fees and donations.
Hours of Operation: Mon.-Thurs., by appointment.
Staff: Ophthalmologist; vision rehabilitation specialist.
Eligibility: None.
Area Served: Unlimited.

Low Vision Aids: Provided on loan for trial use and to purchase; on-site instruction provided; home visits as needed.
Low Vision Follow-up: As needed.

Oregon Health Sciences University
Department of Ophthalmology
Low Vision Aid Clinic
3375 S.W. Terwilliger Boulevard
Portland, OR 97201-4197
(503) 494-7672
FAX: (503) 494-2282
Nancy Harlburt, Coordinator

County/District Where Located: Multnomah County.
Funded by: Client fees; state funds.
Hours of Operation: By appointment only.
Staff: Ophthalmologist; optician; social worker; genetic counselor; audiologist; social worker; orientation/mobility instructor; rehabilitation teacher; special educator; occupational therapist; psychologist/counselor.
Eligibility: Referral by Oregon Commission for the Blind or by ophthalmologist with ophthalmology report.
Area Served: Oregon and southern Washington.

Low Vision Aids: Provided on loan for trial; no rental fee; on-site training provided.
Low Vision Follow-up: As needed.

Pacific University
College of Optometry
2043 College Way
Forest Grove, OR 97116
(503) 357-5800
John A. Smith, O.D., Coordinator, Low Vision Services

Type of Agency: Non-profit.
Funded by: Client fees.
Hours of Operation: Tues.-Fri. 9:00 AM-5:00 PM.
Staff: Optometrist; optician.
Eligibility: None.
Area Served: Unlimited.

Low Vision: Complete diagnostic evaluations and dispensation of low vision devices.
Low Vision Aids: Provided on loan for trial; on-site training provided.
Low Vision Follow-up: By return appointment.

Portland Family Vision Center
511 S.W. Tenth Street
Portland Medical Center Building, Suite 500
Portland, OR 97205
(503) 224-2323 or TDD (503) 241-0222
FAX: (503) 241-0222
Linda Fields, Director

Type of Agency: Non-profit.
County/District Where Located: Multnomah County.
Funded by: Client fees.
Hours of Operation: Low vision services: Tues., Wed., Thurs. 9:00 AM-5:00 PM. All other services: Mon.-Fri. 9:00 AM-5:00 PM.
Staff: Optometrist; optometry student/resident; orientation/mobility specialist; social worker; consulting ophthalmologist; optician; rehabilitation teacher; special educator; occupational therapist; psychologist/counselor; rehabilitation counselor; genetic counselor; audiologist.

Eligibility: None.
Area Served: Unlimited.

Low Vision Aids: Provided on loan for trial; on-site training provided.
Low Vision Follow-up: By return appointment.

♦ Aging Services

STATE UNITS ON AGING

Senior and Disabled Services Division
500 Summer Street N.E.
Second Floor
Salem, OR 97310-1015
(503) 945-5811 or (800) 232-3020 or (800) 282-8096
FAX: (503) 373-7823
Roger Auerbach, Administrator

Provides referrals to Area Agencies on Aging and information on other local aging services.

INDEPENDENT LIVING PROGRAMS

Oregon Commission for the Blind
535 Southeast 12th Avenue
Portland, OR 97214
(503) 731-3221
Pat Macdonnell, Director

Provides independent living services for persons age 55 and over. For further information, contact the Project Director or general phone number listed.

PENN-SYLVANIA

♦ *Educational Services*

STATE SERVICES

Pennsylvania Department of Education
Bureau of Special Education
333 Market Street
Seventh Floor
Harrisburg, PA 17126-0333
(717) 783-2311
FAX: (717) 783-6139
Dr. William Penn, Director of
Special Education

Type of Agency: State.
Mission: Administers state funds for education of visually handicapped children including deaf-blind enrolled in public schools and in approved private schools for the blind. Provides funds to local school districts for reader service, aids and appliances, materials, and other services for children attending local schools. Subsidizes statewide materials center for visually handicapped children. Provides consultation for local schools and agencies on education services. Administers small-grant program to assist blind college students.
Funded by: Public funds.
Area Served: Pennsylvania.

For information about local programs, consult the superintendent of schools in the area.

EARLY INTERVENTION COORDINATION

Division of Community Program Development
Office of Mental Retardation
Pennsylvania Department of Public Welfare
P.O. Box 2675
Harrisburg, PA 17105-8302
(717) 783-8302 or (717) 783-5661
FAX: (717) 772-0012
Jackie Epstein, Director
Norma Shoppel, Chief, Children's Services Unit

SCHOOLS

Capital Area Intermediate Unit
55 Miller Street
P.O. Box 489
Summerdale, PA 17093-0489
(717) 732-8400 or TDD (717) 732-8422
FAX: (717) 732-8414
Patricia Querry, Director of Special Education
Kathy Scott, Supervisor, Visually Impaired Program

Type of Agency: Intermediate education program.
Funded by: P.L. 89-313 and 94-142 monies.
Hours of Operation: 7:30 AM-4:15 PM.
Staff: Visually handicapped and dually certified teachers; various therapists available as consultants. Advisory board, including parent members, for overall preschool program.
History/Date: Est. 1975.
Number of Clients Served: 130.
Eligibility: Determined through multidisciplinary team assessment, as prescribed in the Pennsylvania Department of Education Regulations and Standards for the Operation of Special Education Programs.

Area Served: Cumberland, Dauphin, Perry, northern York Counties.
Transportation: Y.
Age Requirements: 0-21 years.

Counseling/Social Work/Self-Help: Various social and health services available on consultant or referral basis.
Educational: Provides instruction in all developmental areas.

Home-based, center-based, and consultant services using itinerant model for visually impaired students, 0-21 years, with or without other disabilities.

Overbrook School for the Blind
6333 Malvern Avenue
Philadelphia, PA 19151-2597
(215) 877-0313
FAX: (215) 877-2466
E-mail: bmk@obs.org
Bernadette M. Kappen, Director

Type of Agency: Residential school.
Mission: To enable each student to acquire the fund of knowledge and living skills that is required of the well-integrated adult.
Funded by: State and school district funds.
Hours of Operation: Office: 8:00 AM-4:30 PM. School: 8:15 AM-3:15 PM. Currently the majority of students attend school on a day basis.
Program Accessibility: Several buildings are accessible.
Staff: More than 200.
History/Date: Est. 1832.
Number of Clients Served: 199 (school aged); 93 (birth-three years).
Eligibility: Legally blind.
Area Served: Eastern Pennsylvania.
Transportation: Y.

Age Requirements: Early intervention: birth to 3 years. School age programs: 3 to 21 years.

Health: Adaptive equipment; medical services.

Counseling/Social Work/Self-Help: Family seminars; summer week for familes with blind infants and toddlers. Family weekends, transition services, career education, and counseling for students.

Educational: Life Elementary and Secondary Programs; Early Childhood Program; International program.

Preschools: Preschool program; Early Childhood Program 3 to 5, TEAMS (Early Intervention Program for 0-3 year olds in their homes).

Professional Training: On-going staff development. Teacher Trainee Program for teachers from foreign countries.

Reading: Braille, large print, tapes, computer access.

Residential: 5-day residential placement available.

Rehabilitation: Work Experience Program: prevocational training, on-campus job placement, supported employment, sheltered workshop, career education on campus and community opportunities.

Computer Training: All classrooms have computers and assistive technology. Computers are networked and staff and students have acceses to the Internet.

Royer-Greaves School for Blind
118 South Valley Road
Paoli, PA 19301-1444
(610) 644-1810
FAX: (610) 644-8164
E-mail: rgschool@aol.com
Carol T. Dale, Executive Director

Type of Agency: Private; non-profit.

County/District Where Located: Chester County.

Mission: To provide a supportive home education and training environment for individuals who are visually impaired and profoundly developmentally disabled. Residents learn to function to their full potential and thus enjoy an enhanced quality of life.

Funded by: Fees; capital income; grants; subscriptions; donations.

Hours of Operation: 24 hours, 7 days.

Program Accessibility: Wheelchair accessible.

Staff: 33 full time, 2 part time. Uses volunteers.

History/Date: Est. 1921.

Number of Clients Served: 33 residents; also day students.

Eligibility: Visual impairment and retardation; referral.

Area Served: Unlimited.

Age Requirements: 4 to 21 years: education program. Beyond age 21: licensed community home for individuals with mental retardation.

Health: Speech therapy; physical therapy; nursing services. Contracts and refers for other health services.

Counseling/Social Work/Self-Help: Social evaluation; psychological testing and evaluation; individual, family/parent, couple counseling.

Educational: Non-graded. Instruction of multiply disabled blind pupils includes orientation and mobility, occupational therapy, life skills, and adaptive physical education.

Preschools: Programs for play/nursery school run by Chester County Intermediate Unit.

Professional Training: Periodic in-service training programs. Attendance at seminars and conferences.

Reading: Talking book records and cassettes; braille books and magazines; large print-books; recorded magazines; radio link for newspaper and magazine readings.

Residential: Dormitories.

Rehabilitation: Daily living skills; personal management; braille; handwriting; listening skills; orientation/mobility (pre-cane); remedial education; sensory training.

Recreational: Arts and crafts; swimming; scouting; music; horticulture.

Employment: Prevocational evaluation and training. Contracts with sheltered workshops.

Computer Training: Low vision adaptations available for computer skill training.

Low Vision: Black light room; large-print.

Low Vision Aids: Large print books; CCTV; light tables.

Low Vision Follow-up: Yes.

St. Lucy Day School for Children with Visual Impairments
130 Hampden Road
Upper Darby, PA 19082
(610) 352-4550
FAX: (610) 352-4582
E-mail: 102142.3102@compuserve.com
Sister M. Margaret Fleming, Principal

Type of Agency: Private, non-profit day school.

Funded by: Catholic Charities.

Staff: 10 full-time, 3 part-time. Uses volunteers for supervision and as teachers' aides.

History/Date: Est. 1955.

Number of Clients Served: 30.

Eligibility: Visual acuity of 20/70 or less with best correction, 20 degrees field restriction; must be ambulatory and without mental handicaps.
Transportation: Y.
Age Requirements: 0-14 years.

Educational: K through eighth grade.
Preschools: Early intervention: birth-6 years. Preschool: 2½-5 years.
Professional Training: In-service training programs, summer and short term.
Reading: Talking books/cassettes; braille/large-print books; magazines; book selection services; information/referral; transcription; Optacon; closed circuit television; VersaBraille.
Rehabilitation: Daily living; communication skills; orientation/mobility; remedial education.
Recreational: Arts and crafts, summer day camps available.
Computer Training: On-site training provided.

Western Pennsylvania School for Blind Children
201 North Bellefield Avenue
Pittsburgh, PA 15213-1499
(412) 621-0100
FAX: (412) 621-4067
E-mail: jsimon@wpsbc.org
Janet Simon, Ph.D., Executive Director

Type of Agency: Non-profit and state supported.
County/District Where Located: Allegheny County.
Mission: To provide superior opportunities for training and education to students who in addition to visual impairment are disabled by other severe conditions.

Funded by: State allocation, contributions, endowment income.
Budget: $11 million.
Hours of Operation: Residential, 5 days a week.
Program Accessibility: Fully accessible.
Staff: 253 full time. Uses volunteers.
History/Date: Est. 1887.
Number of Clients Served: 195 full time.
Eligibility: Legally blind, resident of western Pennsylvania.
Area Served: Western Pennsylvania.
Age Requirements: 3-21 years.

Health: 24 hour health center staffed by licensed nurses.
Counseling/Social Work/Self-Help: Individual counseling; referal to community agencies.
Educational: Preschool through 12th grade; functional, community-referenced curriculum for blind students with moderate to severe disabilities.
Preschools: Ages 3 to 6.
Professional Training: Student teaching in special education; internship/fieldwork placement in orientation/mobility. Regular in-service training.
Reading: Talking book record players and cassette players; talking book records and cassettes; braille books and magazines; large print books; recorded magazines; closed-circuit television; information and referral; special collection; transcription to braille.
Residential: Dormitories.
Rehabilitation: Personal management; braille; handwriting; listening skills; typing; video magnifier; electronic mobility aids; orientation/mobility; sensory training.
Recreational: Afterschool programs; expressive arts; leisure time; bowling; dance; radio;

swimming; extended school year program.
Employment: Career and skill counseling; occupational skill development; sheltered workshops; follow-up service.
Computer Training: Augmentative communication.
Low Vision: Optometric consultation.

INFANT AND PRESCHOOL

Allegheny Intermediate Unit Project Dart
#4 Station Square
Floor #2
Pittsburgh, PA 15219-1178
(412) 394-5736
Mary McCormick, Program Administrator

Type of Agency: Intermediate education program.
County/District Where Located: Allegheny County.
Funded by: P.L. 94-142 monies.
History/Date: Est. 1975.
Area Served: Allegheny County and 42 school districts.

Counseling/Social Work/Self-Help: Parent counseling.
Educational: Provides instruction in most developmental areas.

Home-based, center-based, and consultant programs on itinerant model for children with visual and other disabilities, 0-3 years and 3-5 years.

Overbrook School for the Blind
6333 Malvern Avenue
Philadelphia, PA 19151-2597
(215) 877-0313
FAX: (215) 877-2709
Cassandra Giardina, Early Intervention Coordinator
Lynne Williams, Preschool Coordinator

Type of Agency: Day and residential school.

Mission: To help the families and caregivers of very young children who have impaired vision and who may have impaired hearing as well to learn special techniques to help stimulate maximum learning.
Funded by: State funds; county and school district funds.
Staff: 25.
Number of Clients Served: 60.
Eligibility: Legally blind.
Age Requirements: Birth to 3 years.

Preschools: Preschool program and home-based program for children 0-3 years.

Home-based early intervention program for children, birth to 3, and their families. Center-based summer seminar program with follow-up consultation for parents of visually impaired infants, 0-2 years, with or without other disabilities.

INSTRUCTIONAL MATERIALS CENTERS

Central Instructional Support Center
6340 Flank Drive, Suite 600
Harrisburg, PA 17112
(717) 541-4960
FAX: (717) 541-4968
Daniel Ficca, Production Services Coordinator

Area Served: Statewide.

Types/Content: Textbooks, novels.
Media Formats: Braille.

UNIVERSITY TRAINING PROGRAMS

Kutztown University Department of Special Education
Kemp 15

Kutztown, PA 19530
(610) 683-4651 or (610) 683-4290
FAX: (610) 683-1516
E-mail: dross@kutztown.edu
Dr. David B. Ross

County/District Where Located: Berks County.

Programs Offered: Undergraduate program for teachers of visually impaired students.

Pennsylvania College of Optometry Institute for the Visually Impaired
Department of Graduate Studies in Vision Impairment
1200 West Godfrey Avenue
Philadelphia, PA 19141
(215) 276-6093
FAX: (215) 276-6292
E-mail: kathyh@pco.edu
Dr. Audrey J. Smith, Orientation and Mobility
Dr. Kathleen M. Huebner, Visual and Multiple Impairments
Maureen Duffy, Rehabilitation Teaching
Dr. Laura Edwards, Vision Rehabilitation

Programs Offered: Master's programs in orientation and mobility, rehabilitation teaching, vision rehabilitation, and education of the visually impaired. Certificate programs in vision rehabilitation, orientation and mobility, and education of the visually impaired. Continuing education programs are also offered.
Distance Education: Y.

University of Pittsburgh School of Education Department of Instruction and Learning
4H01 Forbes Quadrangle

Pittsburgh, PA 15260
(412) 624-7254
FAX: (412) 648-7081
URL: http://www.pitt.edu/
~soeforum/sped_vis.html
Dr. George Zimmerman, Program Coordinator, (412) 624-7247
Dr. Christine Roman, (412) 648-7308

County/District Where Located: Allegheny County.

Programs Offered: Graduate (master's, doctoral) programs for teachers of visually impaired students, orientation and mobility specialists, and dual competency teachers of visually impaired students/orientation and mobility specialists. Additional coursework available in the area of early intervention.

♦ *Information Services*

LIBRARIES

Carnegie Library of Pittsburgh Library for the Blind and Physically Handicapped
The Leonard C. Staisey Building
4724 Baum Boulevard
Pittsburgh, PA 15213
(412) 687-2440 or toll-free in Pennsylvania (800) 242-0586
FAX: (412) 687-2442
E-mail: clbph@clpgh.org
URL: http://www.clpgh.org/
clp/lbph/intro.html
Sue Murdock, Librarian
Henry Picciafoco, Machine Lending Information

Type of Agency: Network library of the National Library Service for the Blind and Physically Handicapped (NLS/BPH).
Mission: To be a force for education, information, recreation, and inspiration in the communities it serves.

Funded by: Public funds.
Hours of Operation: Mon.-Fri.
9:00 AM-5:00 PM.
History/Date: Est. 1907.
Eligibility: NLS/BPH guidelines.
Area Served: Western
Pennsylvania.
Age Requirements: None.

Lends books and magazines
recorded on disks and cassettes,
large-print books, and special
cassette and record players for use
with recorded material. Provides
reference and information services.

Free Library of Philadelphia Library for the Blind and Physically Handicapped

919 Walnut Street
Philadelphia, PA 19107
(215) 925-3213 or toll-free in
Pennsylvania (800) 222-1754
FAX: (215) 928-0856
Vickie Lange Collins, Librarian
Richard A. Riddell, Machine
Lending Information

Funded by: Public funds.
History/Date: Est. 1899.
Area Served: Eastern
Pennsylvania.

Regional library supplying talking,
braille and large type books, tapes
and cassettes. Computer access.

MEDIA PRODUCTION SERVICES

Allegheny Intermediate Unit Vision Program

Pathfinder School
Donati Road
Bethel Park, PA 15102
(412) 963-0452
Dr. Gillian Meieran, Vision
Program Administrator

County/District Where Located:
Allegheny County.
Area Served: 42 school districts in
Allegheny County.

Groups Served: K-12.

Types/Content: Textbooks;
recreational; career/vocational;
assistive technoogy material.
Title Listings: No title listings
available.

Association of Pleasant Hills Community Church

102 East Bruceton Road
Pittsburgh, PA 15236
(412) 655-4379
Mrs. A. J. Brown, Chairperson,
Vision Aid Project

County/District Where Located:
Allegheny County.
Groups Served: Any person with
vision problems.

Types/Content: Textbooks; any
requests.
Media Formats: Braille books,
talking books/cassettes.
Title Listings: No title listings
available.

Bower Hill Braille Foundation

70 Moffett Street
Pittsburgh, PA 15243
(412) 279-7316
Sylvia Procyk, President

Groups Served: K-12, college
students, other adults.

Types/Content: Textbooks,
recreational, career/vocational,
religious.
Media Formats: Braille books.
Title Listings: Print and braille
lists available at no charge.

Capital Area Intermediate Unit

55 Miller Street
P.O. Box 489
Summerdale, PA 17093-0489
(717) 732-8400
Vi Shearer, Materials Specialist

Area Served: None specified.
Groups Served: K-12.

Types/Content: Textbooks.
Media Formats: Braille books,
talking books/cassettes, large print
books.
Title Listings: Print and braille for
a charge.

Central Instruction Support Center

6340 Flank Drive
Suite 600
Harrisburg, PA 17112
(717) 541-4960 or (800) 360-7282
FAX: (717) 541-4968
Dan Sella, Program Manager

County/District Where Located:
Dauphin County.
Area Served: Pennsylvania.
Groups Served: Blind, visually
impaired, and deaf-blind persons,
birth-21 years.

Media Formats: Braille and large-
print books.
Title Listings: Title listings
available via APH-CARL.

Coordinates/provides
consultation and technical
assistance to LEAs, associated
service providers and parents.

Lehigh Valley Braille Guild

614 North 13th Street
Allentown, PA 18102
(610) 264-2141
FAX: (610) 433-4856
Elsie Andrews
Lois Rader, Chairperson

County/District Where Located:
Lehigh County.
Area Served: International.
Groups Served: K-12; college
students; other adults.

Types/Content: Textbooks;
recreational; vocational; religious.
Media Formats: Braille books;
cassettes.
Title Listings: No title listings
available.

Northland Public Library
300 Cumberland Road
Pittsburgh, PA 15237
(412) 366-8100
FAX: (412) 366-2064
Laura Shelley, Director
Pat McCarthy, Director, Volunteer
Services

County/District Where Located:
Allegheny County.
Area Served: Ross, McCandless,
Franklin Park, Bradford Woods
and Marshall townships;
Allegheny County.
Groups Served: K-12, college
students, other adults.

Types/Content: Textbooks,
recreational.
Media Formats: Talking books/
cassettes, large-print books.
Title Listings: Printed at no
charge.

**Recording for the Blind and
Dyslexic**
101 South Bryn Mawr Avenue
Suite 110
Bryn Mawr, PA 19010
(610) 527-2222
FAX: (610) 526-2758
Elise Dormond, Executive Director

County/District Where Located:
Montgomery County.

See Recording for the Blind and
Dyslexic in U.S. national listings.

**Rodef Shalom Temple
Sisterhood**
4905 Fifth Avenue
Pittsburgh, PA 15217
(412) 621-6566
FAX: (412) 621-5475

County/District Where Located:
Allegheny County.
Groups Served: K-12, college
students, other adults.

Types/Content: Textbooks.

Media Formats: Braille/large
print books.
Title Listings: No title listings
available.

Temple Sinai Sisterhood
5505 Forbes Avenue
Pittsburgh, PA 15217
(412) 421-9715
Kathy March, Chairperson

County/District Where Located:
Allegheny County.
Area Served: Pittsburgh.
Groups Served: None specified.

Types/Content: None specified.
Media Formats: Talking books/
cassettes.
Title Listings: None specified.

RADIO READING

**Harrisburg Area Radio Reading
Service**
1800 North Second Street
Harrisburg, PA 17102
(717) 238-2531
Melissa F. Stachacz, Executive
Director

County/District Where Located:
Dauphin County.
Hours of Operation: Mon.-Fri.
8:30 AM-4:30 PM.
History/Date: Est. 1984.
Area Served: Dauphin,
Cumberland and Perry Counties.

**Keystone Radio Information
Service**
**Blair County Association for the
Blind and Visually Handicapped**
300 Fifth Avenue
Altoona, PA 16602-2730
(814) 944-2021
FAX: (814) 944-3197
Marty Sekerak, Executive Director

County/District Where Located:
Blair County.
Hours of Operation: Mon.-Fri.
2:30 PM-4:30 PM.

History/Date: Est. 1970.
Age Requirements: None.

North Central Sight Services
901 Memorial Avenue
P.O. Box 3292
Williamsport, PA 17701
(717) 323-9401
FAX: (717) 323-8194
E-mail: rgarrett@sunlink.net
Robert B. Garrett, President and
CEO

County/District Where Located:
Lycoming County.
Funded by: Contributions and
foundations.
Hours of Operation: Mon.-Fri.
8:30 AM-4:30 PM.
Staff: 1.
History/Date: Est. 1987.
Area Served: Clinton, Sullivan
and Lycoming Counties.
Age Requirements: None.

**Pennsylvania Association for
the Blind and Handicapped**
228 Adams Avenue
Scranton, PA 18503
(717) 348-1812
FAX: (717) 348-1813
Paul Trama, Station Manager

Hours of Operation: Mon.-Fri.
8:30 AM-6:00 PM.
History/Date: Est. 1981.
Area Served: Scranton/Wilkes-
Barre area, including 17 counties in
northeastern Pennsylvania.

**Radio Information Center for the
Blind (RICB)**
Associated Services for the Blind
919 Walnut Street
P.O. Box 1559
Philadelphia, PA 19105
(215) 627-0600
FAX: (215) 922-0692
E-mail: asbinfoalibertynet.org
John Corrigan, Manager

Funded by: Grants and donations.
Hours of Operation: 24 hours daily.
Staff: 5 full time, 70 volunteers.
History/Date: Est. 1974.
Area Served: Greater Philadelphia area, including portions of New Jersey and Delaware.

Radio Information Services
2100 Warton Street
Suite 140
Pittsburgh, PA 15203
(412) 434-6023
FAX: (412) 488-3953
Patricia Ligetti, General Manager

County/District Where Located: Allegheny County.
Funded by: Public/private monies.
Hours of Operation: 24 hours, 7 days a week, 365 days.
Staff: 3 full-time staff, 4 part-time staff members.
History/Date: Est. 1976.
Area Served: Pittsburgh greater metropolitan area (12 counties of southwestern Pennsylvania).
Age Requirements: 16 years of age to volunteer, listeners range in age from 14 to 100+.

WRKC-Radio Home Visitor
Kings College
1602-D
Wilkes-Barre, PA 18711-0801
(717) 826-5811
Thomas Carten, Manager

County/District Where Located: Luzerne County.
Hours of Operation: Mon.-Sun. 10:00 AM-12:00 noon.
Staff: 2.
History/Date: Est. 1974.
Area Served: 25-mile radius from Wilkes-Barre.

WRRS/RADPRIN of Lehigh Valley
3835 Green Pond Road
College Center 335
Bethlehem, PA 18017
(610) 861-5583
FAX: (610) 861-4125
Thomas Eberts, Studio Manager
Vesta Kear, Administrative Manager

County/District Where Located: Northampton County.
Hours of Operation: 24 hours a day.
History/Date: Est. 1978.
Area Served: Northhampton, Lehigh, Berks, Bucks, Carbon and Monroe Counties.

York County Blind Center Radio Reading Service
1380 Spahn Avenue
York, PA 17403
(717) 848-1690
Rodger Simmons, Radio Program Director

County/District Where Located: York County.
Hours of Operation: 6:00 AM - 2:00 AM, 7 days a week.
History/Date: Est. 1976.
Area Served: York County.

Local programming is augmented by programs taken from In Touch Networks.

INFORMATION AND REFERRAL

The Foundation Fighting Blindness
Philadelphia Affiliate
P.O. Box 17300
Philadelphia, PA 19105
(800) 477-2220
Barbara Marks, Contact Person
Maria Moen, President

See The Foundation Fighting Blindness in U.S. national listings.

See also in national listings:

American Blind Bowling Association

Associated Services for the Blind

Braille Authority of North America (BANA)

National Organization for Albinism and Hypopigmentation (NOAH)

Overbrook International Overbrook School for the Blind

◆ Rehabilitation Services

STATE SERVICES

Bureau of Blindness and Visual Services
Pennsylvania Department of Public Welfare
1401 North Seventh Street
P.O. Box 2675
Harrisburg, PA 17105-2675
(717) 787-6176 or toll-free in Pennsylvania (800) 622-2842
FAX: (717) 787-3210
Robert M. Eschbach, Director

Type of Agency: State.
County/District Where Located: Dauphin County.
Mission: To provide vocational rehabilitation services to the blind and visually impaired consumers of the Commonwealth.
Funded by: Federal and state funds.
Hours of Operation: 8:30 AM-5:00 PM.
Staff: 149 full time.
History/Date: Est. 1925.
Eligibility: Legally blind or visually impaired; resident of Pennsylvania.
Area Served: Pennsylvania.
Age Requirements: None.

Counseling/Social Work/Self-Help: Social casework; counseling; consultation and referral; group work.

Professional Training: Regular in-service training program, open to enrollment by other organizations.

Rehabilitation: Orientation/ mobility; personal management; home economics; communications; independent living; training; physical restoration; placement; and counselling.

Employment: Evaluation, prevocational and vocational training; placement; vending facility training; supported employment.

Local Offices:

Altoona: Executive House I, 615 Howard Avenue, Altoona, PA 16601, (814) 946-7330.

Erie: 448 West 11th Street, Erie, PA 16501, (814) 871-4401.

Harrisburg: 2923 North Seventh Street, Suite B, Harrisburg, PA 17110, (717) 787-7500.

Philadelphia: State Office Building, Rm 206, 1400 Springgarden Street, Philadelphia, PA 19123, (215) 560-5700.

Pittsburgh: G-10 Kossman Building, Forbes and Stanwix Streets, Pittsburgh, PA 15222, (412) 565-5240.

Wilkes-Barre: 111 North Pennsylvania Avenue, Third Floor, Wilkes-Barre, PA 18701, (717) 826-2361.

REHABILITATION

Associated Services for the Blind
919 Walnut Street

Philadelphia, PA 19107
(215) 627-0600
FAX: (215) 922-0692
E-mail: asbinfo@libertynet.org
Patricia C. Johnson, Chief Executive Director

Type of Agency: Private; non-profit.
Mission: Provide resource and training center for blind persons and those losing useful vision.
Funded by: Foundations and trusts; corporations; and the public, including Lions and Lioness Clubs, and special friends. Contracts with federal and state agencies, for-profit and non-profit corporations.
Budget: $3,000,000.
Hours of Operation: 9:00 AM-4:30 PM.
Program Accessibility: Totally accessible.
Staff: Approximately 100. Uses volunteers.
History/Date: Est. 1984 from the merger of Volunteer Services for the Blind, Nevil Institute for Rehabilitation and Service, and Radio Information Center for the Blind.
Eligibility: Varies.
Area Served: Philadelphia metropolitan area.
Transportation: Y.

Health: Blindness prevention through informational programs at senior centers; speakers for corporate, community, and professional organizations; and distribution of information on eye care and blindness prevention at employer and community health fairs.
Counseling/Social Work/Self-Help: Support groups; educational and vocational evaluation; escort service to medical appointments and shopping; volunteer visitors for

housebound persons; telephone peer counselors.
Educational: Youth transitional program.
Reading: Volunteer reader service; fills requests for specific braille and large-print books. Radio Information Center broadcasts for 4,000 listeners.
Rehabilitation: Rehabilitation Center, a prevocational center-based program, evaluates client skills and provides blindness adjustment training, orientation and mobility training, and communication instruction.
Recreational: Supports social and recreational activities.
Employment: Resume preparation assistance; skills assessment and counseling; job search assistance; job coaching; job-seeking skills seminars. Employer awareness training.
Computer Training: Electronic Aids Program for training with electronic enhancement devices.
Low Vision: Monthly clinics for eligible clients.
Low Vision Aids: Sense Sations, a retail and catalogue store, sells white canes, braille writing materials, talking clocks, calculators, and other aids.

Association for the Blind and Visually Impaired of Lehigh County
Pennsylvania Association for the Blind
614 North 13th Street
Allentown, PA 18102-2199
(610) 433-6018
FAX: (610) 433-4856
Frank Smith, Executive Director

Type of Agency: Private; non-profit.
Mission: To help blind or visually impaired people and their families with problems that are caused by or associated with visual

impairment; to develop and maintain educational programs; to conduct screenings for the early detection of vision problems.
Funded by: United Way, government grants, endowment, individual and corporate giving.
Budget: $412,000.
Hours of Operation: Mon.-Fri. 8:30 AM-4:30 PM.
Staff: 10 full time; 6 part time.
History/Date: Est. 1928.
Number of Clients Served: 1997: 512.
Eligibility: Visual eligibility for rehabilitation and social services: 20/70 or less in better eye with correction. Prevention and education: all are eligible.
Area Served: Lehigh County.
Transportation: Y.
Age Requirements: 18 years for rehabilitation and social services; prevention and education: all ages.

Health: Vision screening and public education.
Counseling/Social Work/Self-Help: Information and referral; casework; peer support groups.
Educational: Life skills training.
Reading: Braille transcribing; readers; tape recording.
Rehabilitation: Rehabilitation teaching and mobility instruction; supportive services.
Recreational: Therapeutic recreation; social activities.
Low Vision: Magnifier evaluations.
Low Vision Aids: Lends low vision devices.
Low Vision Follow-up: Y.

Beaver County Association for the Blind
616 Fourth Street
Beaver Falls, PA 15010
(412) 843-1111 or (412) 728-5555
FAX: (412) 843-8886
Jean G. Keller, Director

Type of Agency: Private; non-profit.
County/District Where Located: Beaver County.
Mission: Provide services relating to the general welfare of blind/visually impaired clients and the prevention of blindness.
Funded by: United Way, state contract, workshop, sales, contributions.
Hours of Operation: Mon.-Fri. 8:30 AM-4:00 PM.
Staff: 8 full time, 300 volunteers.
History/Date: Est. 1947.
Number of Clients Served: 1995/1996: 350.
Eligibility: Blind/visually impaired.
Area Served: Beaver County.
Transportation: Y.
Age Requirements: None.

Health: Remedial eye care; screenings; eye safety programs in schools.
Counseling/Social Work/Self-Help: Transport/escort; chore services; social recreation; educational activities.
Reading: Braille; large type; talking book machines; radio receivers; readers.
Rehabilitation: Life skills; education; personal management; housing assistance.
Recreational: Social activities; crafts; field trips.
Employment: Sales; caning.

Bedford Branch
Pennsylvania Association for the Blind
242 East John Street
Bedford, PA 15522
(814) 623-8214
Joanne Smith, Administrative Secretary

Type of Agency: Private; non-profit.

Mission: Services for totally blind, legally blind, and visually impaired persons.
Funded by: Volunatry contributions.
Hours of Operation: 8:30 AM-12:00 noon and 1:00 PM-4:30 PM.
Program Accessibility: Serve those of all ages who are print handicapped.
Staff: 1 full time, 2 part time. Uses volunteers.
History/Date: Est. 1948.
Number of Clients Served: Approximately 600.
Eligibility: Visually handicapped.
Area Served: Bedford, Fulton, and Somerset counties.
Transportation: Y.
Age Requirements: None.

Reading: Arrange for talking books and large print books for clients.
Low Vision Aids: Provide low vision aids to clients.

Berks County Association for the Blind
Pennsylvania Association for the Blind
2020 Hampden Boulevard
Reading, PA 19604
(610) 375-8407
FAX: (610) 375-6467
David R. Neideigh, Executive Director

Type of Agency: Private; non-profit.
County/District Where Located: Berks County.
Funded by: Workshop sales, sub-contracts, endowment, and contributions.
Budget: 1992: $675,000.
Hours of Operation: Mon.-Fri. 8:00 AM-4:00 PM.
Staff: 6 full time, 8 part time.
History/Date: Est. 1929.
Number of Clients Served: 1996: 750.

Eligibility: Blind or visually impaired.
Area Served: Berks County.

Health: Diagnostic; public education.
Counseling/Social Work/Self-Help: Consultation and referral.
Educational: Educational films available for loan; speakers available on request.
Preschools: Vision screeing.
Reading: Braille and large-type books; recorders and talking book machines; readers.
Rehabilitation: Home mechanics; personal management; orientation/mobility.
Recreational: Crafts; cooking classes; field trips.
Employment: Prevocational training; workshop.
Low Vision: Vision screening.

Blair County Association for the Blind and Visually Handicapped

300 Fifth Avenue
Altoona, PA 16602-2730
(814) 944-2021
FAX: (814) 944-3197
Marty Sekerak, Executive Director

Type of Agency: Private; non-profit.
County/District Where Located: Blair County.
Mission: To act as a member agency of the Pennsylvania Association for the Blind for the support, care, training, and rehabilitation of blind persons, prevention of blindness, and conservation of sight.
Funded by: Fees for service, workshop sales, sub-contracts, contributions and grants.
Budget: $150,000.
Hours of Operation: Mon.-Fri. 8:00 AM-4:30 PM.
Program Accessibility: Y.
Staff: 5 full time, 10 part-time. Uses volunteers.

History/Date: Est. 1952.
Number of Clients Served: 100.
Eligibility: Legally blind (acuity not more than 20/70 in best corrected eye); income guidelines, under sub-contract.
Area Served: Blair County.
Transportation: Y.
Age Requirements: Adult age.

Health: Public education, preschool vision screenings, adult visual acuity and intraocular pressure screenings, industrial screenings, in-service training for care givers.
Counseling/Social Work/Self-Help: Consultation and referral; sight loss support group; social services (transportation, chores, educational programs).
Educational: Eye health and safety programs–all ages; programs to aid independent living.
Preschools: Eye health and safety programs; vision screening.
Professional Training: In-service training of employees in caregiver facilities, i.e. nursing home.
Reading: Braille and large-type books; recorders; talking books and machines; readers; aids and appliances.
Recreational: Social activities.

Blind Relief Fund of Philadelphia

3600 Market Street
Suite 320
Philadelphia, PA 19104
(215) 222-7613
FAX: (215) 222-7624
A. Victor Cancelmo III, Executive Director

Type of Agency: Private; non-profit.
Mission: Services for blind.
Funded by: Private contributions.
Hours of Operation: Mon.-Fri. 9:00 AM-4:00 PM.

Staff: 3 full time and 1 part time.
History/Date: Est. 1909.
Number of Clients Served: 485.
Eligibility: Philadelphia resident; legally blind.
Area Served: Philadelphia.
Age Requirements: 18 years and over.

Counseling/Social Work/Self-Help: Individual counseling; information and referral service; limited financial aid available.
Recreational: Refers for residential summer camp; annual summer outing.

Bucks County Association for the Blind
Pennsylvania Association for the Blind

400 Freedom Drive
Newtown, PA 18940
(215) 968-9400
FAX: (215) 968-2127
Elaine R. Welch, Executive Director

Type of Agency: Private; non-profit.
County/District Where Located: Bucks County.
Mission: Services for totally blind; legally blind; visually impaired.
Funded by: Endowments; government grants; Community fund raising; contributions;
Budget: $388,000.
Hours of Operation: Mon.-Fri. 8:00 AM-4:00 PM.
Program Accessibility: Fully accessible.
Staff: 11 full time, 4 part time. Uses volunteers.
History/Date: Est. 1945.
Number of Clients Served: 1,400.
Eligibility: Resident of Bucks County; visually impaired.
Area Served: Bucks County.
Transportation: Y.
Age Requirements: None.

Health: Refers for health services.
Counseling/Social Work/Self-Help: Social evaluation; individual/group counseling; case management; support groups; chore service in the home; advocacy.
Professional Training: Internship/fieldwork placement in rehabilitation counseling; vocational rehabilitation.
Reading: Talking book and cassette players distribution and instruction.
Rehabilitation: Instruction in home management and personal management; braille; handwriting; typing; rehabilitation teaching in client's home and community; remedial education. Refers for other rehabilitation services.
Recreational: Summer day camp for blind children; adult recreation programs; summer teen recreation program.
Low Vision: Magnifier evaluations.
Low Vision Aids: Carries a full line of non-prescription low vision aids for demonstration and sale. Vision and hearing screenings.

Butler County Association for the Blind
Pennsylvania Association for the Blind
308 West Cunningham Street
P.O. Box 468
Butler, PA 16003-0468
(412) 287-4059
FAX: (412) 287-4888
Maddie Riddell, Director

Type of Agency: Private; non-profit.
County/District Where Located: Butler County.
Funded by: Public funds, contributions, workshop sales, sub-contracts, and endowments.
History/Date: Est. 1932.

Area Served: Butler County.
Transportation: Y.

Health: Vision screening; examination; eyeglasses; eye bank; industrial eye safety program.
Counseling/Social Work/Self-Help: Consultation and referral.
Reading: Braille and large type books; recorders and talking book machines; readers.
Rehabilitation: Orientation/mobility.
Employment: Sheltered workshop.

Cambria County Association for the Blind and Visually Handicapped
Pennsylvania Association for the Blind
211 Central Avenue
Johnstown, PA 15902
(814) 536-3531
FAX: (814) 539-3270
E-mail: ccabh@twd.net
Richard C. Bosserman, President

Type of Agency: Private; non-profit.
County/District Where Located: Cambria County.
Mission: Services for totally blind, legally blind, visually impaired, deaf-blind, learning disabled, mentally retarded, and physically disabled persons.
Funded by: Fees; workshop sales.
Budget: $5.3 million.
Hours of Operation: Mon.-Fri. 8:30 AM-5:00 PM.
Staff: 41 full time. Uses volunteers.
History/Date: Est. 1927.
Number of Clients Served: 1995-96: 650.
Eligibility: Visually impaired; visual acuity of 20/70 or less. For vocational or educational services, mental or physical disabling conditions determine eligibility.

Area Served: Cambria County.
Transportation: Y.
Age Requirements: 18 and older.

Health: Prescribes and provides low vision aids; evaluates eye treatment or prescription. Refers for other health services.
Counseling/Social Work/Self-Help: Social evaluation; individual, group, family/parent, couple counseling; placement in school; referral to community service. Refers for other counseling/social work services.
Educational: Accepts emotionally disturbed, learning disabled, and mentally retarded persons. Programs for vocational/skill development; prevocational skill development; social/personal development.
Reading: Lends talking book records and cassette players; talking book records and cassettes; large-print books; recorded magazines. Information and referral.
Rehabilitation: Personal management; handwriting; electronic mobility aids; home management; orientation/mobility; rehabilitation teaching in client's home and community; remedial education. Refers for other rehabilitation services.
Recreational: Arts and crafts; hobby groups; swimming. Refers for other recreational services.
Employment: Prevocational evaluation; career and skill counseling; occupational skill development; job retention; work centers. Vocational placement; follow-up service; personal work adjustment training.
Low Vision Aids: Provides low vision aids.
Low Vision Follow-up: Provides low vision follow-up.

Central Susquehanna Sight Services, Inc.
241 Chestnut Street
Sunbury, PA 17801
(717) 286-1471
Donna Wilkinson, Office Manager

Type of Agency: Private; non-profit.
County/District Where Located: North Umberland County.
Mission: Services for totally blind, legally blind, visually impaired, and deaf-blind persons.
Funded by: Workshop sales, capital income, direct mail appeal.
Hours of Operation: Mon.-Fri. 8:00 AM-3:30 PM.
Staff: Uses volunteers.
History/Date: Est. 1949.
Number of Clients Served: More than 1,000.

Health: Refers and contracts for other health services.
Counseling/Social Work/Self-Help: Social evaluations; individual counseling; referral to community services. Refers and provides consultation to other agencies for other counseling/social work services.
Reading: Lends talking book record and cassette players; braille and large-print books; recorded magazines. Information and referral.
Rehabilitation: Refers for and provides consultation to other agencies for rehabilitation services.
Recreational: Contracts and refers for recreation services.
Employment: Sheltered workshops. Refers for other employment-oriented services.
Low Vision: Low vision service; provides free low vision aids.

Chester County Association for the Blind
Pennsylvania Association for the Blind
71 South First Street
P.O. Box 1440
Coatesville, PA 19320
(610) 384-2767
FAX: (610) 384-8005
Anita Cavuto, Executive Director

Type of Agency: Private; non-profit.
County/District Where Located: Chester County.
Mission: Services for totally blind; legally blind; visually impaired.
Funded by: Donations and small workshop.
Hours of Operation: Mon.-Fri. 8:00 AM-4:00 PM.
Staff: 5 full time. Uses volunteers.
History/Date: Est. 1948.
Number of Clients Served: 625.
Eligibility: Blindness or visual impairment.
Area Served: Chester County.

Health: Diagnosis and evaluation of eye health; treatment of eye conditions; follow-up evaluation of eye treatment or prescription.
Reading: Lends talking book record and cassette players; talking book records and cassettes. Information and referral; transcription to braille. Tape recording services on demand.
Rehabilitation: Personal management; braille; typing; home management; orientation/mobility; rehabilitation teaching in client's home. Referral to other agencies.
Employment: Handicapped employment.
Low Vision: Low vision service; prescription of spectacles or aids.

Delco Blind/Sight Center
100 West 15th Street

Chester, PA 19013
(610) 874-1476
FAX: (610) 874-6454
E-mail: dbsc@apond.com
Robert M. Nelson, Executive Director

Type of Agency: Private; non-profit.
County/District Where Located: Delaware County.
Mission: To enrich the quality of life for persons with visual impairments or blindness and to reduce the incidence of vision loss through prevention-of-blindness activities.
Funded by: United Way; contracts, donations, bequests, grants.
Budget: 1995-1996: $1,900,000.
Hours of Operation: Mon.-Fri. 8:00 AM-5:00 PM.
Program Accessibility: Fully accessible.
Staff: Uses volunteers.
History/Date: Est. 1941.
Number of Clients Served: 1995-1996: 3,800, including 585 blind clients.
Eligibility: Determined by program area and service offered.
Area Served: Pennsylvania, Delaware, and New Jersey.
Transportation: Y.
Age Requirements: Determined by program area and service offered.

Health: Low vision service. Indigent eye care; eye safety training. Refers for and provides consultation to other agencies for health services.
Counseling/Social Work/Self-Help: Social evaluation; casework management; life skills groups; psychological testing, evaluation and counseling; referral to community services.
Educational: Vocational and blindness skills evaluation and

training, transitional services, referral services, public education.
Professional Training: In-service training to professionals with blind patients.
Reading: Lends talking book machines, cassette players and makes referrals to the Radio Information Center for the Blind for the client to receive radio services.
Residential: On-site supervised dormitory for residential students in training. Close association with Stinson Tower, an apartment building, specially equipped and designed for independent living for blind, physically disabled, and elderly persons.
Rehabilitation: Personal adjustment to blindness training; communication skills; home management; orientation/ mobility; sensory training; vocational evaluation; psychological testing, individual counseling services; work adjustment training, computer access technology training, job placement services. Summer transitional program for high school students with vision loss. Refers, provides consultation to other agencies for other rehabilitation services.
Recreational: Newly blinded group; field trips; bell choir; day camp; refers and provides consultation to other agencies for other recreation services.
Employment: Prevocational evaluation; career and skill counseling; occupational skill development; job retention; vocational placement; follow-up service.
Computer Training: Training for computer novices in the use of computers, accompanying adaptive equipment, and popular software packages used in today's computer workspace; guidance in

job placement or further training. Advanced training course in computer access technology related to career goals.
Low Vision: Eye care professionals, specially trained in the field of low vision, will perform a complete clinical assessment of the medical diagnosis and visual impairment. Optical/non-optical devices or techniques, may be prescribed if it is determined that they will be beneficial.
Low Vision Aids: Obtained for clients, as needed.
Low Vision Follow-up: Provided as needed.

Edith R. Rudolphy Residence for the Blind

3827 Powelton Avenue
Philadelphia, PA 19104
(215) 382-6412
FAX: (215) 382-1231
Shirley Brockman, Executive Director
Francine Lingham, Director

Type of Agency: Private, non-profit residence for blind men and women.
Mission: To provide a full-service residence and sheltered employment for adult blind persons.
Funded by: United Way, trusts, grants, contributions, and fees of residents.
Budget: 1992: $860,000.
Hours of Operation: 24.
Staff: 32. Uses volunteers.
History/Date: Est. 1868.
Number of Clients Served: Licensed for 50 residents.
Eligibility: 20/200 visual acuity or less; must pass physical examinations.
Area Served: Northeastern United States.
Transportation: Y.

Age Requirements: 18 years and older.
Health: General medical services. Refers for eye treatment/ evaluation, physical therapy.
Counseling/Social Work/Self-Help: Refers for social evaluation, individual/group counseling, community services.
Professional Training: In-service training programs.
Reading: In-house distribution of talking book records/tapes; braille books/magazines; recorded magazines; large print books.
Residential: Boarding home for blind adults.
Rehabilitation: Refers for rehabilitation services as needed.
Recreational: In-house entertainment programs and local area day trips.
Employment: Provides sheltered workshop.

Erie Center for the Blind and Visually Handicapped Pennsylvania Association for the Blind

2402 Cherry Street
Erie, PA 16502
(814) 455-0995
FAX: (814) 455-0997
Tyco V. Swick, Executive Director

Type of Agency: Private; non-profit.
Mission: Services for totally blind, legally blind, and visually impaired persons.
Funded by: United Way, endowment, fees, and contributions.
Budget: $350,000.
Hours of Operation: Mon.-Fri. 8:00 AM-4:30 PM.
Program Accessibility: Fully accessible.
Staff: 6 full time, 4 part time. Uses volunteers.

History/Date: Est. 1938.
Eligibility: Any person with functional vision loss is eligible.
Area Served: Erie County.
Transportation: Y.

Health: Diagnostic and medical treatment; public education programs.
Counseling/Social Work/Self-Help: Casework and referral services.
Reading: Talking book machines; voice mail information service.
Rehabilitation: Personal management; orientation/mobility; home management.
Recreational: Social group for elderly blind persons.
Low Vision Aids: Low vision aid evaluations and prescriptions. Aids and appliances.

Fayette County Association for the Blind
Pennsylvania Association for the Blind
48 Bierer Lane
Uniontown, PA 15401
(412) 437-2791
Nancy C. Shockey, Executive Director

Type of Agency: Private; non-profit.
County/District Where Located: Fayette County.
Mission: Services for totally blind, legally blind, and visually impaired persons.
Funded by: Service clubs; contributions.
Budget: 1991: $110,000.
Hours of Operation: Mon.-Fri. 8:30 AM-4:00 PM.
Staff: 4 full time. Uses volunteers.
History/Date: Est. 1946.
Number of Clients Served: 1996: 702.
Eligibility: Resident of Fayette County.

Area Served: Fayette County.
Health: Follow-up evaluation of eye treatment or prescription. Refers for other health services.
Educational: Eye safety; aids and appliances demonstrations to clients and public.
Preschools: Preschool visual screenings and follow-up.
Professional Training: Regular in-service training programs, open to enrollment from other agencies.
Reading: Lends talking book record players. Information and referral.
Rehabilitation: Refers for rehabilitation services.
Recreational: Adult social parties. Refers for other recreational services.
Employment: Refers for employment-oriented services.
Low Vision: Low vision clinic and consultation.
Low Vision Aids: Prescribes and provides spectacles and low vision aids.

Greater Pittsburgh Guild for the Blind (now known as Pittsburgh Vision Services)
311 Station Street
Bridgeville, PA 15017
(412) 221-2200
FAX: (412) 257-8574
Richard L. Welsh, Ph.D., President
Jack C. Lydic, Director of Rehabilitation

Type of Agency: Private; non-profit.
County/District Where Located: Allegheny County.
Mission: Personal adjustment training for totally blind, legally blind, visually impaired, and visually impaired multiply disabled adolescents and adults. In-home training to elderly blind persons as needed.

Funded by: Fees, contributions, grants.
Budget: 1991: $1.4 million.
Hours of Operation: Mon.-Fri. 8:00 AM-4:00 PM.
Program Accessibility: Fully accessible.
Staff: 33 full time, 19 part time. Uses volunteers.
History/Date: Est. 1959.
Number of Clients Served: 1991: 1,100.
Eligibility: Severe visual impairment that causes a functional disability; ophthalmological or optometric report.
Area Served: Unlimited.
Age Requirements: Primarily adolescents and adults with additional disabilities. Specialized service for elderly persons.

Health: Audiological and low vision screening; psychiatric consultation; general medical screening; health education.
Counseling/Social Work/Self-Help: Psychosocial evaluations; psychological testing and evaluations; individual, group, family/parent, couple counseling.
Educational: General academics; college prep; GED prep; literacy training; summer programming for school-age children.
Professional Training: Internship/field work placement in orientation/mobility; rehabilitation counseling; social work; special education; vocational rehabilitation; low vision; adaptive technology training.
Reading: Talking book record and cassette players; braille and large-print books and magazines; trancription to braille; translation to other languages; tape recording services on demand; Optacon; Kurzweil Reading Machine; closed-circuit television training.

Residential: Available during training and on weekends.
Rehabilitation: Personal management; handwriting; listening skills; typing; electronic aids; home management; orientation/mobility; remedial education; sensory training; household mechanics.
Recreational: Bowling; swimming; calisthenics; theater; museums; many other activities.
Employment: Prevocational evaluations; career and skill counseling. Computer-related skill training.
Computer Training: Evaluations and training on a wide range of adapted hardware and software.
Low Vision: Low vision service. Available for personal adjustment clients and separately on an outpatient basis.
Low Vision Aids: Evaluations, training, and loans.
Low Vision Follow-up: As needed.

Greater Wilkes-Barre Association for the Blind

63 North Franklin Street
Wilkes-Barre, PA 18701
(717) 823-1161
FAX: (717) 823-4841
Ronald V. Petrilla, Ph.D., Executive Director

Type of Agency: Private; non-profit.
County/District Where Located: Luzerne County.
Mission: Serve the needs and interests of blind and visually impaired persons and prevent blindness.
Funded by: Public funds, endowments and contributions; some state/county contracts.
Budget: $270,000.
Hours of Operation: Mon.-Fri. 8:30 AM-4:30 PM.

Staff: 3 professional, 5 service workers.
History/Date: Est. 1918.
Number of Clients Served: 600.
Area Served: Serves Luzerne County, except Hazleton area.

Health: Vision and glaucoma screening; remedial eye care.
Counseling/Social Work/Self-Help: Support group, consultation and referral.
Educational: Life skills education.
Preschools: Vision screenings and educational programs.
Reading: Talking book machines; radio reading service; braille transcription.
Rehabilitation: Communications; support services for independent living; informational and socialization counseling; home visitation.
Recreational: Social and recreational activities.
Employment: Support services.
Low Vision Aids: Magnifiers.
Low Vision Follow-up: Yes.
Professional Training: In-service training; speakers bureau.

Guiding Light for the Blind

919 Walnut Street
Philadelphia, PA 19107
(215) 627-0600
FAX: (215) 922-0692
James P. Swed, Director

Type of Agency: Non-profit.
Mission: To promote the use of and partially subsidize electronic travel guides.
Funded by: Trusts, foundations, corporations, friends.
Budget: $117,000.
Hours of Operation: Mon., Tues., Wed., Thurs. 9:00 AM-3:30 PM.
Staff: One part time plus 5 volunteer workers.
History/Date: Inc. 1990.
Number of Clients Served: 500.

Eligibility: Need for travel aid to and from work and school, some income limitations.
Area Served: Nationwide.

Counseling/Social Work/Self-Help: Self help.
Educational: Provides free classes through Lens Crafters; income requirement.

Hazleton Blind Association Pennsylvania Association for the Blind

1201 N. Church Street
Building 13, Suite 409
Hazelton, PA 18201-1457
(717) 455-0421
FAX: (717) 459-2046
Ronald V. Petrilla, Acting Director

Type of Agency: Private; non-profit.
County/District Where Located: Luzerne County.
Mission: To provide services to blind and visually impaired persons of Lower Luzerne County and provide prevention of blindness services to the community.
Funded by: Contributions and special fund-raising events.
Budget: $90,000.
Hours of Operation: Mon.-Fri. 9:00 AM-4:30 PM.
Staff: 2 full time; 2 part time.
History/Date: Est. 1946.
Number of Clients Served: 200.
Eligibility: Varies according to service requested.
Area Served: Hazleton and Luzerne County.
Transportation: Y.

Health: Free public education programs; free preschool vision screening. Provides aids, appliances at cost, and eyeglasses at low cost.
Counseling/Social Work/Self-Help: Personal management;

home management;
communications.
Educational: Elementary school
education program for blindness
and eye safety.
Preschools: Vision screening
program.
Professional Training: In-service
programs on blindness.
Reading: Brailled material
available.
Rehabilitation: Referrals to other
agencies.
Recreational: Bowling; crafts; bus
trips; parties; life skills classes.
Employment: Refers to other
agencies.

Indiana County Blind Association

31 South Tenth Street
Indiana, PA 15701
(412) 465-5549
Hazel M. (Rusty) Lomman,
Executive Director

Type of Agency: Private; non-
profit.
County/District Where Located:
Indiana County.
Mission: Services for totally blind;
legally blind; visually impaired;
learning disabled; mentally
retarded; physically handicapped;
hearing impaired; visually
impaired in concert with any of the
preceding.
Funded by: United Way;
workshop sales; sub-contracts;
grants; fund raisers; contributions.
Hours of Operation: Mon.-Fri.
8:30 AM-4:30 PM.
Staff: 3 full time. Uses volunteers.
History/Date: Est. 1952.
Eligibility: Medically diagnosed
visual disability that constitutes a
handicap to social and economic
self-sufficiency, or a progressive
condition expected to result in
such a handicap.
Area Served: Indiana County.

Transportation: Y.
Age Requirements: None.

Health: Preschool vision
screening. Refers for health
services.
**Counseling/Social Work/Self-
Help:** Psychosocial evaluation;
individual, group, family/parent,
couple counseling; referral to
community service. Refers and
provides consultation to other
agencies for other counseling/
social work services.
Educational: Referrals.
Educational: Vision screening;
prevention education; refers to
preschools.
Professional Training: Vocational
rehabilitation.
Reading: Lends talking book
record and cassette players; talking
book records and cassettes; braille
and large-print books; braille and
recorded magazines. Information
and referral; tape recording
services on demand.
Rehabilitation: Personal
management; video magnifier;
orientation/mobility;
rehabilitation in client's home and
community. Refers and provides
consultation to other agencies for
other rehabilitation services.
Recreational: Limited.
Employment: Sheltered
workshops; follow-up service.
Refers and provides consultation
to other agencies for other
employment-oriented services.
Low Vision: Low vision service;
low vision aids or appliances.

Juniata Association for the Blind

658 Valley Street
Lewistown, PA 17044
(717) 242-1444
FAX: (717) 242-1445
Charles O. Nale, Executive
Director

Type of Agency: Private; non-
profit.
County/District Where Located:
Mifflin County.
Mission: To help blind and
visually impaired individuals and
their families cope with sight loss
and provide them with the
necessary training and support to
maintain their independence.
Funded by: Workshop sales, sub-
contracts, United Way, and public
funds.
Budget: $800,000.
Hours of Operation: Mon.-Fri.
8:00 AM-4:30 PM.
Staff: 7 full time.
History/Date: Est. 1945.
Number of Clients Served: Social
Service Department: 63.
Eligibility: Blind or visually
impaired; meets requirements of
needs assessment and financial
guidelines.
Area Served: Mifflin, Juniata, and
Huntingdon counties.
Transportation: Y.

Health: Prevention of blindness;
medical and financial services (for
Remedial Eye Care program only);
remedial eye care; vision
screening; eye safety; and health
education.
**Counseling/Social Work/Self-
Help:** Social and financial services
available.
Educational: Life skills education
classes.
Rehabilitation: Life skills and
chores.
Recreational: Sponsors a
Christmas party, picnic, and trip.
Employment: Refers to Blindness
and Visual Services Department
for vocational training if not
employed at agency workshop.
Low Vision: Refers to low vision
specialist and to Blindness and
Visual Services Department for
financial help with exams and aids.

Keystone Blind Association

1230 Stambaugh Avenue
Sharon, PA 16146
(412) 347-5501
FAX: (412) 347-2204
E-mail: kba@nauticom.net
URL: http://http:/
www.nauticom.net/www/kba
Jonathan Fister, President/C.E.O.

Type of Agency: Private; non-profit.
County/District Where Located:
Mercer County.
Mission: Improving quality of life
for blind persons preventing
blindness, and providing
employment for blind persons.
Funded by: United Way,
workshop sales.
Budget: 1997: $3 million.
Hours of Operation: Mon.-Fri.
8:30 AM -4:30 PM.
Staff: 20 full time. Uses
volunteers.
History/Date: Est. 1947.
Number of Clients Served: 800.
Eligibility: Legally blind, visually
impaired, disabled.
Area Served: Mercer and
Crawford counties.
Transportation: Y.

Health: Consultation and referrals
to other agencies. Prevention of
blindness services including
preschool vision screening,
glaucoma screenings, eye safety
programs; community education.
**Counseling/Social Work/Self-
Help:** Social evaluations;
individual, family, group
counseling; referrals to other
community services; housing
(includes form filing and moving);
chore service.
Professional Training:
Internship/fieldwork placement in
social work; in-service training
programs for other agencies.
Reading: Lends talking book
machines, cassette players, talking
book records and cassettes, large-

print books and magazines.
Information and referral; tape
recording services on demand;
radio reading service.
Rehabilitation: Rehabilitation
teacher on staff. Independent
living skills; personal and home
management. Training in personal
and home maintenance, nutrition
and adapted aids and appliances.
Recreational: Bowling; field and
shopping trips; audible darts;
social gatherings. Refers for other
recreational services.
Employment: Employment for
disabled persons; employment
referrals; follow-up.
Low Vision: Low vision aids and
services; prescription of spectacles
and aids.

Local Offices:

Meadville: Mercer County Blind
Association, Crawford County
Office: 287½ Chestnut Street,
Meadville, PA 16335.
Meadville: Keystone Blind
Association, Crawford County
Office, 312 Chestnut Street,
Meadville, PA 16335, (814) 333-
3121.

**Lackawanna Branch
Pennsylvania Association for
the Blind**

228 Adams Avenue
Scranton, PA 18503
(717) 342-7613
FAX: (717) 348-1813
Alfred B. Davis, III, Executive
Director

Type of Agency: Private; non-profit.
Mission: Services for totally blind,
legally blind, and visually
impaired persons.
Funded by: Sub-contracts; capital
income; Lions Club; gifts.
Hours of Operation: Mon.-Fri.
8:30 AM-4:30 PM.

Program Accessibility: Fully
accessible.
Staff: 8 full time. Uses volunteers.
History/Date: Est. 1913.
Eligibility: Legally blind, visually
impaired.
Area Served: Lackawanna
County.
Transportation: Y.

Health: Prevention of Blindness
Program; eye safety program;
preschool vision screening;
glaucoma screening clinics.
Supplies prevention information
via speakers' bureau; films; radio
and television. Refers for other
health services.
**Counseling/Social Work/Self-
Help:** Social evaluation;
individual counseling; referral to
community services. Refers for
other counseling/social work
services.
Educational: Life Skills Program.
Professional Training:
Internship/fieldwork placement in
orientation/mobility;
rehabilitation counseling; social
work.
Reading: Talking book record and
cassette players; talking book
records and cassettes; braille and
large-print books; braille and
recorded magazines. Transcription
to braille; tape recording services
on demand. Radio reading service.
Rehabilitation: Personal
management; home management;
orientation/mobility. Refers for
other rehabilitation services.
Recreational: Arts and crafts;
hobby groups; aerobics; bowling.
Refers for other recreational
services.
Employment: Refers for other
employment-oriented services.
Low Vision: Low vision service;
spectacles and low vision aids.

Lawrence County Branch
Pennsylvania Association for the Blind

319 North Jefferson Street
New Castle, PA 16101
(412) 652-4571
Larry R. Nord, Executive Director

Type of Agency: Private; non-profit.
County/District Where Located: Lawrence County.
Funded by: Workshop sales; United Way; sub-contracts and contributions.
Staff: 3 full time, 4 part time. Uses volunteers.
History/Date: Est. 1947.
Eligibility: Visually impaired. With need.
Area Served: Lawrence County.

Health: Diagnostic, medical and surgical treatment; eyeglasses; eye bank; public education.
Counseling/Social Work/Self-Help: Consultation and referral.
Reading: Braille and large type books; talking book machines.
Recreational: Social activities.
Employment: Workshop; home employment; placement; follow-up.

Montgomery County
Association for the Blind

212 North Main Street
North Wales, PA 19454-3117
(215) 661-9800
FAX: (215) 661-9888
Douglas A. Yingling, Executive Director

Type of Agency: Private; non-profit.
County/District Where Located: Montgomery County.
Mission: To enhance the quality of life of blind and visually impaired persons in Montgomery County through education, support, and advocacy programs

and to prevent blindness through education and screening programs.
Funded by: Community contributors; corporate/foundation grants; endowment; special events; bequests.
Hours of Operation: Mon.-Fri. 8:30 AM-4:30 PM.
Staff: 10 full time, 8 part time. Uses volunteers.
History/Date: Est. 1945.
Number of Clients Served: 1,200.
Eligibility: Montgomery County resident; blind or visually impaired.
Area Served: Montgomery County.
Transportation: Y.

Health: Preschool/adult vision screening.
Counseling/Social Work/Self-Help: Comprehensive social services; peer counseling; support groups.
Educational: Programs to community on education about blindness (schools, scouts, retirement centers).
Reading: Talking book machine distribution and instruction.
Rehabilitation: Mobility instruction, daily living skills.
Recreational: Recreation/socialization activities; children's summer day camp.
Computer Training: Technology training program.
Low Vision Aids: Some low vision aids distributed.

North Central Sight Services
Pennsylvania Association for the Blind

901 Memorial Avenue
P.O. Box 3292
Williamsport, PA 17701
(717) 323-9401
FAX: (717) 323-8194
E-mail: rgarrett@sunlink.net
Robert B. Garrett, President and CEO

Type of Agency: Private; non-profit.
Mission: To provide rehabilitation services and employment opportunities to people who are blind; prevention of blindness to children and adults.
Funded by: Workshop sales, sub-contracts, government contracts, endowment and Lions Club.
Budget: $1.8 million.
Hours of Operation: Mon.-Fri. 7:00 AM-4:30 PM.
Staff: 11 full time, 4 part time. Uses volunteers.
History/Date: Est. 1957.
Number of Clients Served: 600.
Eligibility: Visually impaired.
Area Served: Lycoming, Clinton, Sullivan counties.
Transportation: Y.
Age Requirements: None.

Health: Preschool vision screenings; eye examinations; prevention of blindness services (including intraocular pressure screenings and public education).
Counseling/Social Work/Self-Help: Consultation and referral; individual and group counseling.
Professional Training: Internship/fieldwork placement in social work; in-service training programs for volunteers and other agencies; radio reading service.
Reading: Talking book machines; large type; braille material; recording services.
Rehabilitation: Home management; communications; personal management; orientation/mobility.
Recreational: Field trips; social activities.
Employment: Sheltered workshop.
Computer Training: Access.
Low Vision: Purchase of eyeglasses; low vision aids.

Pennsylvania Association for the Blind

2843 North Front Street
Harrisburg, PA 17110-1284
(717) 234-3261
FAX: (717) 234-4733
Valerie N. Weiner, Executive Vice President
Albert Clark, Director of Services

Type of Agency: Private; non-profit.
Mission: To provide and secure comprehensive services for persons who are blind or visually impaired and to prevent blindness.
Funded by: State contracts, private contributions, grants, and trust income.
Budget: 1992/1993: $1,719,185.
Hours of Operation: Mon.-Fri. 8:30 AM-4:30 PM.
Program Accessibility: Mostly in-home/outreach service.
Staff: 7 full-time, 1 part time (administration/statewide operations); 3 (prevention of blindness), 8 (casework services).
History/Date: Est. 1910.
Number of Clients Served: 1,950 (Social Services), 20, 924 (prevention/screening), 21,424 (public education programs).
Eligibility: Visual impairment.
Area Served: Serves 27 counties in Pennsylvania through executive office, 4 satellites, and outstationed staff. Subcontracts with member agencies for social services in 42 additional counties.
Transportation: Y.

Health: Screening for visual acuity, intraocular pressure; eye health and safety programs for children/adults of all ages; diabetic eye care intervention.
Counseling/Social Work/Self-Help: Informational counseling, educational support groups, with referral for in-depth psychological counseling and support.
Educational: "Life Skills Education" to foster independence, community integration, and acquistion of practical adaptive skills.
Professional Training: In-service training for organizational/institutional personnel; certification program for prevention of blindness personnel; semi-annual conferences for membership.
Reading: Talking Book equipment distribution; information and referral for large print and Braille; sighted assistance for household paperwork.
Rehabilitation: Basic guidance in personal and household management techniques; referral for more intensive, individualized instruction.
Recreational: Limited group programs and activities for socialization and recreation.
Employment: Information and referral.
Low Vision: Information and referral.
Low Vision Aids: Information and referral.

Regional Offices:

Adams County Satellite: Pennsylvania Association for the Blind, 23 Buford Street, Gettysburg, PA 17325, (717) 334-8931.
Centre County Satellite: Pennsylvania Association for the Blind, 142 West Bishop Street, Bellefonte, PA 16823, (814) 355-0500.
Franklin County Satellite: Pennsylvania Association for the Blind, 181 Franklin Farm Lane, Chambersburg, PA 17201, (717) 263-5393.

Local Offices:

Lebanon: Lebanon County Satellite: Pennsylvania Association for the Blind, 738 Cumberland Street, Lebanon, PA 17042, (717) 274-6711.

Has 29 member agencies in Pennsylvania.

Pennsylvania Lions Beacon Lodge Camp

114 SR 103 South
Mt. Union, PA 17066-9601
(814) 542-2511
FAX: (814) 542-7437
Janet E. Snyder, Executive Director

Type of Agency: Private; non-profit.
County/District Where Located: Mifflin County.
Mission: Services for totally blind, legally blind, visually impaired, deaf-blind, learning disabled, mentally retarded, and physically disabled persons.
Funded by: Lions Club and fees.
Budget: $560,000.
Hours of Operation: 11-day sessions at residential camp; 6-day special needs sessions.
Staff: 6 full time; 100 summer paid staff.
History/Date: Est. 1948.
Number of Clients Served: 1996: 536.
Eligibility: Blind; visually impaired; mentally challenged; physically handicapped.
Area Served: Pennsylvania and surrounding states.
Age Requirements: 6 years and older.

Health: Nurse on duty 24 hours.
Counseling/Social Work/Self-Help: Self-help.
Reading: Talking book record and cassette players; talking book records and cassettes; braille and

large-print books; braille and recorded magazines.
Residential: Dormitories for adults; cabins for children.
Recreational: Residential summer camp; arts and crafts; bowling; swimming; wrestling; hiking; basketball; shuffleboard; bus trips; archery; canoeing; kayaking.

Pittsburgh Blind Association Pennsylvania Association for the Blind (now known as Pittsburgh Vision Services)
300 South Craig
Pittsburgh, PA 15213
(412) 682-5600
FAX: (412) 682-8104
Dennis J. Huber, President

Type of Agency: Private; non-profit.
County/District Where Located: Allegheny County.
Mission: Services for totally blind; legally blind; visually impaired; learning disabled; mentally retarded.
Funded by: Fees, United Way, workshop sales, sub-contracts, capital income, grants.
Budget: 1992-93: $3,225,000.
Hours of Operation: Mon.-Fri. 8:00 AM-5:00 PM.
Staff: 60 full time, 10 part time. Uses volunteers.
History/Date: Est. 1910.
Eligibility: Legally blind, visually impaired with acuity of 20/70 or less.
Area Served: Allegheny County.
Transportation: Y.

Health: Follow-up evaluation of eye treatment or prescription. Refers and provides consultation to other agencies for other health services.
Counseling/Social Work/Self-Help: Social evaluation; individual, group, family/parent, couple counseling. Referral to

community services. Refers for other counseling/social work services.
Professional Training: Internship/fieldwork placement in social work. Orientation/mobility and rehabilitation counseling. Regular in-service training programs.
Reading: Talking book record players and cassette players. Information and referral; transcription to braille; tape recording services upon request.
Rehabilitation: Personal management; braille; handwriting; listening skills; typing; video magnifier; home management; orientation/mobility; rehabilitation teaching in client's home and community. Provides consultation to other agencies for other rehabilitation services.
Recreational: Arts and crafts; hobby groups; special programs for the elderly; bowling. Refers for and provides consultation to other agencies for recreation services.
Employment: Career and skill counseling; occupational skill development; job retention; job retraining; sheltered workshops; vocational placement; work preparation training program; therapeutic activities center; supported work program; follow-up service. Refers for other employment-oriented service.
Low Vision: Evaluation and referral.
Low Vision Aids: Available on case basis.
Low Vision Follow-up: Y.

Pittsburgh Vision Services
300 South Craig Street
Pittsburg, PA 15213
(412) 682-5600 or (800) 706-5050
Dennis Huber, President

See Greater Pittsburgh Guild for the Blind and Pittsburgh Blind Association in U.S. state listings.

Susquehanna Association for the Blind and Vision Impaired
244 North Queen Street
Lancaster, PA 17603
(717) 291-5951
FAX: (717) 291-9183
E-mail: jazbeaux@lcab.pptnet.com
Stephen Patterson, President, CEO

Type of Agency: Private; non-profit.
County/District Where Located: Lancaster County.
Funded by: Contributions, sub-contracts, endowment, and bequests.
Budget: $1.5 million.
Hours of Operation: Mon.-Fri. 8:00 AM-4:00 PM.
Staff: 21 full time/6 part time. Uses volunteers.
History/Date: Est. 1926.
Number of Clients Served: Approximately 1,500.
Eligibility: Legally blind; visually impaired; unable to read newspaper print without correction; visual acuity of 20/70 or less; restricted fields.
Area Served: Lancaster County.
Transportation: Y.
Age Requirements: None.

Health: Diagnostic eye clinic with follow-up treatment; public education.
Counseling/Social Work/Self-Help: Consultation and referral. Group work.
Educational: Basic skills.
Preschools: Birth to school age.
Professional Training: Cooperates with colleges and universities on internships.
Reading: Radio reading service; braille transcribing and Library of Congress services.

Rehabilitation: Teaches daily living skills, communications, orientation & mobility; sells aids and appliances.
Recreational: Variety of center-based and community activities.
Employment: Industrial employment and vocational training.
Computer Training: Basic literacy, adaptive tools.
Low Vision: Low vision clinic.
Low Vision Aids: Y.
Low Vision Follow-up: Y.

Tri-County Branch
Pennsylvania Association for the Blind
1800 North Second Street
Harrisburg, PA 17102-2207
(717) 238-2531
FAX: (717) 238-0710
Melissa F. Stachacz, Executive Director

Type of Agency: Private; non-profit.
County/District Where Located: Dauphin County.
Mission: Services for totally blind; legally blind; visually impaired. Prevention of blindness services to the public at large.
Funded by: United Way, sub-contracts, workshop sales, government grants, fees, contributions, bequests.
Hours of Operation: Mon.-Fri. 8:30 AM-4:30 PM.
Program Accessibility: Program accessible.
Staff: 17 full time, 3 part time. Uses volunteers.
History/Date: Est. 1921.
Number of Clients Served: 1,949.
Eligibility: Visually impaired or legally blind.
Area Served: Cumberland, Dauphin, and Perry counties.
Transportation: Y.

Health: Refers for and provides consultation to other agencies for other health services.
Counseling/Social Work/Self-Help: Client and family counseling; information and referral; life skills education; chore service; case management services; support group.
Educational: Speakers' bureau, public education, eye safety programs, participation at health fairs.
Preschools: Preschool vision and hearing screening, eye safety education and information.
Professional Training: Internship/fieldwork in social work.
Reading: Lends talking book record players and cassette players; talking book records and cassettes; braille books; large-print books; braille magazines; recorded magazines. Information and referral; transcription to braille; tape recording services on demand; radio reading service (special receivers placed with print impaired persons).
Residential: Referral only.
Rehabilitation: Refers for rehabilitation services.
Recreational: Full range of social/recreational activities.
Employment: Sheltered workshops. Refers for other employment oriented-services.
Computer Training: Access.
Low Vision: Provides referrals for low vision evaluations.
Low Vision Aids: Provision of eyeglasses to low-income persons.

Venango County Branch
Pennsylvania Association for the Blind
406 West First Street

Oil City, PA 16301
(814) 676-1876
Mr. Robin D. Hart, Acting Executive Director

Type of Agency: Private; non-profit.
Mission: Provides services for totally blind, legally blind, and visually impaired persons and works for the prevention of blindness.
Funded by: United Way, endowment, private contributions, Lions Clubs, and grants.
Budget: 1992: $110,200.00.
Hours of Operation: Mon.-Fri. 8:30 AM-4:30 PM.
Staff: 1 full-time, 2 part-time.
History/Date: Est. 1927 and Inc. 1939.
Number of Clients Served: 184 blind clients; 4,961 through prevention programs.
Eligibility: Visually impaired.
Area Served: Venango County.
Transportation: Y.

Health: Comprehensive prevention of blindness program; vision screenings; follow-up; glasses.
Counseling/Social Work/Self-Help: Consultation and referral services.
Educational: Eye safety programs in all Venango County elementary schools.
Preschools: Vision screenings in daycare centers, nursery schools, and at the time of registration for kindergarten.
Professional Training: Refers for vocational rehabilitation.
Reading: As sub-lending agency for the Library of Congress, provides talking book record player and cassette player; talking book records and cassettes; braille books; large print books and magazines. Information and referral.

Rehabilitation: Refers for rehabilitation services.

Recreational: Adult continuing education; arts and crafts; summer camp; yoga; swimming; shopping trips and excursions.

Low Vision: Refers for low vision service; sells aids.

Low Vision Aids: Provides magnifiers; refers for other low vision services.

Visual Impairment and Blindness Services of Northampton County, Inc. (VIABL)

129 East Broad Street
Bethlehem, PA 18018
(610) 866-8049
FAX: (610) 866-8730
Jan F. Leon, Executive Director

Type of Agency: Private; non-profit.

County/District Where Located: Northampton County.

Mission: To promote the social, economic and physical self-sufficiency of blind, deaf blind and visually impaired by providing resources and skills needed to live rewarding, productive and independent lives.

Funded by: Private contributions, government contracts.

Budget: $215,000.

Hours of Operation: Mon.-Fri. 8:00 AM-4:00 PM.

Program Accessibility: Fully accessible.

Staff: 4 full time, 8 part time. Uses volunteers.

History/Date: Est. 1928.

Number of Clients Served: Approximately 600.

Eligibility: Visual impairment.

Area Served: Northampton County; Lehigh County residents with Bethlehem address.

Transportation: Y.

Age Requirements: None.

Health: Screenings and eye exams.

Counseling/Social Work/Self-Help: Adjustment to blindness counseling for individuals and their families; chore service in the home; housing assistance; life skills education (individual and group basis); personal advocacy. Assists clients to properly utilize public services and facilities; refers to community organizations for in-depth psychological counseling; rehabilitation service; drug/alcohol-related problems.

Educational: Community awareness programs; videos available for loan; resource room for client and community use.

Professional Training: Internship and field placement opportunities available.

Reading: Talking book equipment and large-print, braille, and recorded literature. Provides transcription service; assists in handling mail and home paperwork.

Rehabilitation: Instruction in home and personal management; orientation/mobility; referral for in-depth vocational rehabilitation.

Recreational: Weekly socialization programs designed to build appropriate communication skills, physical fitness, and adaptive abilities for crafts and homemaking; bowling; crafts, aerobics; lectures; concerts; community tours.

Computer Training: Computer access is availabe.

Low Vision: Vision screening for preschool children; purchases eyeglasses and special lenses for low-income people; low vision clinic; prescription of aids and appliances; training in the use of near and distance vision aids and lenses.

Low Vision Aids: Aids and training in use is provided. Devices are loaned for trial use prior to purchase.

Low Vision Follow-up: Y.

Washington-Greene Blind Association

566 East Maiden Street
Washington, PA 15301
(412) 228-0770
Jack W. Pilgun II, Executive Director

Type of Agency: Private; non-profit.

Funded by: Contributions and Government contracts.

Staff: 9 full time. Uses volunteers.

History/Date: Est. 1947.

Eligibility: Legally blind.

Area Served: Washington and Greene counties.

Transportation: Y.

Health: Preschool vision and remedial eye care and school safety program.

Counseling/Social Work/Self-Help: Consultation and referral; chore service.

Recreational: Group activities.

Employment: Sheltered workshop.

Westmoreland County Branch Pennsylvania Association for the Blind

911 South Main Street
P.O. Box 1048
Greensburg, PA 15601
(412) 837-1250
FAX: (412) 837-3135
Jim DiMichele, Executive Director
Howard Piper, Administrative Coordinator
Tim Miller, Director of Services

Type of Agency: Private; non-profit.

County/District Where Located: Westmoreland County.

Mission: Services for totally blind; legally blind; visually impaired; deaf-blind.
Funded by: Contributions.
Staff: 10 full time. Uses volunteers.
History/Date: Est. 1946.
Number of Clients Served: 200.
Eligibility: Blind or visually handicapped.
Area Served: Westmoreland County.
Transportation: Y.

Health: Vision screenings; remedial eye care.
Counseling/Social Work/Self-Help: Social evaluations; individual, and couple counseling; referral to community services. Refers and provides consultation to other agencies for other counseling/social work services.
Educational: Tuition fund.
Reading: Lends talking book record players and cassette players; talking book records and cassettes. Information and referral.
Rehabilitation: Personal management; braille; video magnifiers; rehabilitation teaching in client's home; community education; vocational evaluations. Refers for other rehabilitation services.
Recreational: Arts and crafts; hobby group; bowling; fishing; outdoor programs.
Employment: Sheltered workshops; follow-up services. Refers for other employment services.
Computer Training: On individual basis. Classroom potential.

Local Offices:

Somerset: Somerset County Blind Center, 322 South Lynn, Somerset, PA 15501, (814) 445-1310.

York County Blind Center
1380 Spahn Avenue
York, PA 17403
(717) 848-1690
FAX: (717) 845-3889
William H. Rhinesmith, President

Type of Agency: Private; non-profit.
County/District Where Located: York County.
Mission: Services for totally blind, legally blind, deaf-blind, and learning disabled persons. Advocacy services.
Funded by: Lions Club; United Way; community donations; capital income; sales of products.
Budget: 1992: $1,087,000.
Hours of Operation: Mon.-Fri. 8:30 AM-4:30 PM.
Program Accessibility: Fully accessible.
Staff: 22 full time; 3 part time. Uses volunteers.
History/Date: Est. 1932.
Number of Clients Served: 350.
Eligibility: Visually impaired.
Area Served: York County.
Transportation: Y.

Health: Screening services; preschool vision and hearing screening. Public health education; remedial eye care.
Counseling/Social Work/Self-Help: Individual, group, family/parent counseling; placement in rehabilitation training; referral to community services. Refers for other counseling/social work services.
Reading: Radio reading services; special receivers placed with visually impaired persons. Sublending agency for the Talking Book program; provides equipment, materials from the Philadelphia Public Library.
Rehabilitation: Personal management; handwriting; braille; typing; home management; rehabilitation teaching in client's

home and community; sensory training; orientation and mobility training. Refers for other rehabilitation services.
Employment: Occupational skills development; sheltered workshops; vocational placement; follow-up service. Refers for other employment-oriented services.
Computer Training: Y.
Low Vision: Low vision center providing evaluation and prescription of low vision aids by low vision specialist; follow-up training offered.
Low Vision Aids: Y.
Low Vision Follow-up: Y.

Local Offices:

Hanover: Hanover Industries for the Blind, 639 Frederick Street, Hanover, PA 17331, (717) 633-5831.

COMPUTER TRAINING CENTERS

Associated Services for the Blind
919 Walnut Street
Philadelphia, PA 19107
(215) 627-0600
FAX: (215) 922-0692
E-mail: asbinfo@libertynet.org
URL: http://www.libertynet.org/~asbinfo
Patricia C. Johnson, Chief Executive Officer
Frederick Noesner, Director

Type of Agency: Private; non-profit.
History/Date: Est. 1984.

Computer Training: Speech output systems; screen magnification systems; braille access systems; optical character recognition systems; closed-circuit television systems; word processing; database software; computer operating systems.

Greater Pittsburgh Guild for the Blind (now known as Pittsburgh Vision Services)
311 Station Street
Bridgeville, PA 15017
(412) 221-2200
FAX: (412) 257-8574
Richard L. Welsh, Ph.D., President
Brenda Loughrey, Coordinator

Computer Training: Speech output systems; screen magnification systems; braille access systems; optical character recognition systems; closed-circuit television systems; word processing; computer operating systems.

Evaluations, system recommendations, and training provided at center on the job.

Overbrook School for the Blind
6333 Malvern Avenue
Philadelphia, PA 19151-2597
(215) 877-0313
FAX: (215) 877-2709
E-mail: barbara@obs.org
Barbara Paton, Technology Specialist

Computer Training: Speech output systems; screen magnification systems; braille access systems; closed-circuit television systems; word processing; database software; computer operating systems; training for instructors.

♦ Low Vision Services

EYE CARE SOCIETIES

Pennsylvania Academy of Ophthalmology and Otolaryngology
4401 Penn Avenue
Suite 1560

Pittsburgh, PA 15224
(412) 687-1414
William C. Christie, M.D., President

Pennsylvania Optometric Association, Inc.
P. O. Box 3312
Harrisburg, PA 17105
(717) 233-6455
Terry O'H. Stark, C.A.E.

LOW VISION CENTERS

Center for Vision Rehabilitation
320 East North Avenue
Pittsburgh, PA 15212
(412) 359-6300
FAX: (412) 359-6768
Paul B. Freeman, O.D., Director

County/District Where Located: Allegheny County.
Mission: To enhance the visual quality of life.
Funded by: Client fees, county funds, federal and state funds.
Hours of Operation: Tues. and Fri. 9:00 AM-5:00 PM.
Staff: Low vision assistant; occupational therapist; orientation/mobility instructor; ophthalmic assistant; optometrist; optometry student/resident; ophtalmologist.
Number of Clients Served: 500-600 new patients per year.
Eligibility: None.
Area Served: Unlimited.
Age Requirements: None.

Computer Training: Training on computer aids and devices.
Low Vision: Full low vision evaluations.
Low Vision Aids: Provided on loan for trial; provided for purchase. On-site and in-home training provided.
Low Vision Follow-up: Return appointment, home visit or phone

interview; varies according to patient.

**The Eye Institute
Pennsylvania College of Optometry
William Feinbloom Vision Rehabilitation Center**
1201 West Godfrey Street
Philadelphia, PA 19141
(215) 276-6060 or (800) 433-3937 (433-EYES)
FAX: (215) 276-1329
Sarah Appel, Chief, Low Vision Service

Type of Agency: Private; non-profit.
County/District Where Located: Philadelphia County.
Mission: To provide comprehensive low vision services and offer rehabilitation teaching, orientation and mobility services, and computer training.
Funded by: Client fees.
Hours of Operation: Mon.-Fri. 8:30 AM-4:30 PM.
Staff: Optometrist; optometry student/resident; optician; social worker; special educator; mobility instructor; adaptive technology specialist; rehabilitation teacher; genetic counselor; consultation with ophthalmologist available.
History/Date: Est. 1978.
Number of Clients Served: 1,000 clients per year.
Area Served: Unlimited.

Health: Ocular health evaluations by optometrists and ophthalmologists.
Counseling/Social Work/Self-Help: Social service staff available to assist clients and their families. Older adults support group meets monthly.
Rehabilitation: Rehabilitation teaching and orientation and mobility services available.

Computer Training: Access; training on computer; adaptive technology and devices.
Low Vision: Comprehensive low vision rehabilitation services provided by an interdisciplinary staff.
Low Vision Aids: Provided on loan for trial; on-site training provided. Optical and nonoptical devices prescribed. Closed-circuit television magnification systems available for evaluations and instruction.
Low Vision Follow-up: 2 weeks, follow-up visit; 6 months, check-up; 2-year and 5-year recall.

Greater Pittsburgh Guild for the Blind

311 Station Street
Bridgeville, PA 15017
(412) 221-2200
FAX: (412) 257-8574
Richard L. Welsh, Ph.D., President
Kenneth Wojtczak, Coordinator

Type of Agency: Non-profit.
County/District Where Located: Allegheny County.
Mission: To provide for people with low vision clinical and functional evaluations; optometric prescriptions, loaner aids, and training.
Funded by: Client fees; foundation grants; general donations.
Hours of Operation: Mon.-Fri. 8:00 AM-4:00 PM.
Program Accessibility: Totally accessible.
Staff: Low vision specialist; orientation/mobility instructor; optometrist; rehabilitation counselor; rehabilitation teacher.
History/Date: Established for outpatients in 1992.
Eligibility: Severe visual problem that causes functional difficulty; current ophthalmological or optometric report.

Area Served: Unlimited.
Counseling/Social Work/Self-Help: Counseling regarding vision loss and use of vision. Refers for additional services.
Residential: Available on short-term basis if needed.
Computer Training: Training on computer aids and devices.
Low Vision: Assessment and training.
Low Vision Aids: Prescribed by O.D.; training provided; loaner aids available; dispensing of purchased aids.
Low Vision Follow-up: Return appointment or phone contact.

Moore Eye Foundation

2000 Old West Chester Pike
Havertown, PA 19083
(610) 449-0400
FAX: (610) 645-3951
Maryellen Bednarski, Director

Type of Agency: Public; non-profit.
County/District Where Located: Delaware County.
Mission: To provide comprehensive low vision assessment and rehabilitation services.
Funded by: Patient fees.
Hours of Operation: Two full days and one half day per week.
Staff: 3.
Eligibility: Visual problems which cannot be corrected by surgery, medication or eyeglasses.
Counseling/Social Work/Self-Help: Support group.
Rehabilitation: Referral to state agencies for orientation and mobility and rehabilitation teaching services.
Low Vision: Evaluation and referral when needed.
Low Vision Aids: Available on loan for home trial period; provided for purchase.

Low Vision Follow-up: Yes.

Northeast Eye Institute

200 Mifflin Avenue
Scranton, PA 18503
(717) 342-3145
Edward Reap, Director

Type of Agency: Non-profit.
County/District Where Located: Lackawana County.
Mission: Provides comprehensive eye care program, specializing in low vision.
Eligibility: By referral.

Low Vision: Evaluation; assessment; rehabilitation.
Low Vision Aids: Available on a case basis.
Low Vision Follow-up: Y.

Scheie Eye Institute Department of Ophthalmology
University of Pennsylvania Health System
Low Vision Research and Rehabilitation Center

51 North 39th Street
Philadelphia, PA 19104
(215) 662-9320
FAX: (215) 662-0985
E-mail: lovision@mail.med.upenn.edu
Janet DeBerry Steinberg, O.D., Chief of Service

Type of Agency: Non-profit.
County/District Where Located: Philadelphia County.
Mission: Comprehensive low vision evaluations and rehabilitation.
Funded by: Client fees, foundation grants, donations.
Hours of Operation: Tues., Wed., Fri. 9:00 AM-5:00 PM.
History/Date: Est. 1874.
Area Served: Unlimited.

Health: Optometry, ophthalmological consultations, genetics consultation.

Counseling/Social Work/Self-Help: Social services, psychiatry. Social worker available.

Professional Training: Referrals to community and university-based resources.

Rehabilitation: Orientation/mobility; occupational therapy.

Low Vision Aids: Available for purchase; on-site training provided.

Low Vision Follow-up: Telephone interviews; return appointment as needed.

Temple University Hospital Ophthalmology Department

3401 North Broad Street
6th Floor, Parkinson Pavilion
Philadelphia, PA 19140
(215) 707-3401
FAX: (215) 707-1684
Jay Kubacki, M.D.

County/District Where Located: Philadelphia County.

Funded by: Client fees, hospital practice plan, medical school.

Hours of Operation: Mon.-Fri. 9:00AM-5:00PM; Sat. 9:00AM-2:00PM.

Staff: Ophthalmology assistant/resident/technician; optician; psychologist; ophthalmologist; social worker available.

Area Served: Unlimited.

Computer Training: Access.

Low Vision Aids: Provided on loan at no charge; sold at cost; on-site training provided.

Low Vision Follow-up: Return appointment; phone interview.

Wills Eye Hospital Low Vision Service

Ninth and Walnut Streets
Philadelphia, PA 19107
(215) 928-3450
Susan E. Edmonds, O.D., Director
Scott A. Edmonds, O.D.

Type of Agency: Non-profit.

County/District Where Located: Philadelphia County.

Funded by: Client fees, foundation grants.

Hours of Operation: Mon.-Fri. 8:30 AM-4:30 PM.

Staff: Low vision assistant; ophthalmic resident; ophthalmologist; optometrist.

Eligibility: Referral; current ophthalmological report.

Area Served: Unlimited.

Low Vision Aids: Provided for purchase; prescribed and fitted for variable charge; on-site training provided.

Low Vision Follow-up: Return appointment; varies according to patient.

♦ Aging Services

STATE UNITS ON AGING

Pennsylvania Department of Aging

400 Market Street, 7th Floor
MSS Office Building
Harrisburg, PA 17101-2301
(717) 783-1550
FAX: (717) 783-6842
Richard Browdie, Secretary

Provides referrals to Area Agencies on Aging and information on other local aging services.

INDEPENDENT LIVING PROGRAMS

Pennsylvania Department of Public Welfare

P.O. Box 2675
Harrisburg, PA 17105
(717) 787-1069 or (800) 622-2842
Rose Putric, Administrator

Provides independent living services for persons age 55 and over. For further information, contact the Project Director or general phone number listed.

PUERTO RICO

♦ *Educational Services*

STATE SERVICES

Puerto Rico Department of Education
Special Education Program
P.O. Box 759
Hato Rey, PR 00919
(787) 759-2000
Marta Sanabria, Supervisor

For information about local programs, contact the above address.

EARLY INTERVENTION COORDINATION

Infants and Toddlers with Handicaps
Puerto Rico Department of Health
P.O. Box 15091
Old San Juan, PR 00902
(787) 274-7676
Carmen Aviles, Early Child Coordinator

SCHOOLS

Instituto Loaíza Cordero para Niños Ciegos
Fernandez Juncos 1312
Santurce, PR 00910
(787) 723-9610 or (787) 722-2498
FAX: (787) 722-3602
Shirley Raffucci, Director

Type of Agency: State residential school.
Mission: Services for totally blind; legally blind; mentally retarded, and multiply disabled persons.
Funded by: State and donations.

Hours of Operation: 24 hours (8:00 AM-3:00 PM school and rehabilitation service).
Program Accessibility: Preschool to 9th grade.
Staff: 91 full time. Uses volunteers.
History/Date: Est. 1919.
Number of Clients Served: 89.
Eligibility: Blind and visually impaired.
Area Served: Islandwide.
Transportation: Y.
Age Requirements: 3 to 21 years.

Health: Treatment of eye conditions; follow-up evaluations of eye treatment or prescription; general medical services; physical therapy. Refers and provides consultation to other agencies for health services.
Counseling/Social Work/Self-Help: Social evaluations; individual, family/parent, couple counseling; placement in school; referral to community services. Contracts and refers and provides consultation to other agencies for other counseling/social work services.
Educational: Preschool through grade 9. Programs for adult continuing education; general academic; vocational/skill development.
Preschools: Health, related services, and education.
Professional Training: Internship/fieldwork placement in orientation/mobility; special education. Regular in-service training programs, open to enrollment from other agencies.
Reading: Talking book record players and cassette players; talking book records and cassettes; braille books; large-print books; braille magazines; recorded magazines; information and referral; transcription to braille;

translation to other languages; tape recording services on demand.
Residential: Dormitories; food and board.
Recreational: Afterschool programs; arts and crafts; hobby groups; swimming; track; basketball. Refers and provides consultation to other agencies for other recreational services.
Employment: Prevocational evaluations. Refers for other employment-oriented services.
Computer Training: Computer education for 7th to 9th grade students. Elementary computer recreation and related training.
Low Vision: Refers and consults to other agencies.
Low Vision Aids: Refers and consults to other agencies.
Low Vision Follow-up: Refers.

STATEWIDE OUTREACH SERVICES

Instituto Loaíza Cordero para Niños Ciegos
Fernandez Juncos 1312
Santurce, PR 00910
(787) 724-0893
FAX: (787) 722-3602
Avilda Núñez, Director

Funded by: Instituto Loaíza Cordero.
Age Requirements: 3-21 years.

Assessment: Available from staff that includes an occupational therapist, speech pathologist, ophthalmologist and optometrist.
Consultation to Public Schools: Provided by the Department of Education.
Direct Service: To schools from preschool to Grade 9 programs; residential, recreation-related services, library, computers.
Parent Assistance: Available through Parent and Teachers Association.

Materials Production: Functional manual, brochures, norms provided.
Professional Training: In areas of visual impairment, mental retardation, multiple disabilities.

UNIVERSITY TRAINING PROGRAMS

University of Puerto Rico
P.O. Box 23355
San Juan, PR 00931-3355
(787) 764-2205
FAX: (787) 763-4130
Jose Santana, Director

◆ Information Services

LIBRARIES

Puerto Rico Regional Library for the Blind and Physically Handicapped
520 Ponce de Leon Avenue
San Juan, PR 00901
(787) 723-2519 or (800) 981-8008
FAX: (787) 721-8177

Type of Agency: State.
Mission: To provide talking and braille books and play-back machines to visually and physically impaired individuals in Puerto Rico.
Funded by: Puerto Rico Education Department in cooperation with the National Library Service for the Blind and Physically Handicapped.
Budget: $78,384.
Hours of Operation: Mon.-Fri. 7:30 AM-4:30 PM. Operates a 24-hour hot line.
Staff: 14.
History/Date: Est. 1975.
Number of Clients Served: 1,600.
Eligibility: Print-disabled individuals: blindness, visual impairment, physical disability, or reading disability.

Area Served: Puerto Rico.
Age Requirements: Preschoolers to senior citizens.

MEDIA PRODUCTION SERVICES

Puerto Rico Department of Education
Special Education Program
P.O. Box 190759
Hato Rey, PR 00919-0759
(787) 759-2000
FAX: (787) 250-0275
Maria Morales, Assistant

Groups Served: K-12.

Types/Content: Textbooks.
Media Formats: Braille/large print books.
Title Listings: Print and braille lists available at no charge.

Puerto Rico Regional Library for the Blind and Physically Handicapped
520 Ponce de Leon Avenue
Stop 8/12, Puerta de Tierra
San Juan, PR 00901
(809) 723-2519

Groups Served: K-12, college students, other adults.

Types/Content: Puerto Rican culture and history.
Media Formats: Talking books/cassettes.

INFORMATION AND REFERRAL

Puerto Rico Deaf-Blind Parents Association
Projecto Ninos Sordos-Ciegos
Edificio B/Antiguo Hospital Ruiz Soler
16 Santa Rosa Unit
Bayamon, PR 00619
(787) 793-8625
FAX: (787) 793-8625
Rachel George, Contact Person

◆ Rehabilitation Services

STATE SERVICES

Vocational Rehabilitation Program
Puerto Rico Department of Social Services
P.O. Box 191118
San Juan, PR 00919-1118
(787) 724-3120
FAX: (787) 721-6286
Francisco Vallejo, Assistant Secretary

Type of Agency: State.
Mission: Vocational rehabilitation services.
Funded by: Public funds.
Hours of Operation: Mon.-Fri. 8:00 AM-4:30 PM.
Program Accessibility: Fully accessible.
Staff: 1,040 full time.
History/Date: Est. 1936.
Eligibility: Vocational handicap.
Area Served: Islandwide.
Transportation: Y.

Health: General health services.
Educational: General academic.
Reading: Reader services for individuals studying for high school diploma or college.
Rehabilitation: Comprehensive services.
Recreational: Y.
Employment: Evaluations; vocational training; placements; vending facility program.
Computer Training: Limited.
Low Vision: Low vision aids training.

Local Offices:

Hato Rey: Home Teaching Program for Blind Adults, P.O. Box 1118, Hato Rey, PR 00919, (787) 725-1792, (787) 724-7400, ext. 2109.

Santurce: Corporation Industries for the Blind of Puerto Rico, San Rafael Street, Stop 20, Santurce, PR 00912, (787) 721-3266.

Santurce: Rehabilitation Center for the Blind of Puerto Rico, 1331 Las Palmas Street, Stop 19, Santurce, PR 00923, (787) 724-2497, (787) 724-7240.

REHABILITATION

Puerto Rico Blind Rehabilitation Center
U.S. Department of Veterans Affairs
VA Medical Center
One Veterans Plaza
San Juan, PR 00927-5800
(787) 758-7575
FAX: (787) 281-4973
Maria Neverez, Chief

Type of Agency: Federal.
Mission: Provides residential rehabilitation services to eligible legally blind veterans.
History/Date: Est. 1986.

Referral applications by Visual Impairment Services programs at VA Medical Centers and Outpatient Clinics in the geographical area served by the Blind Rehabilitation Center or Clinic.

See U.S. Department of Veterans Affairs in U.S. Federal Agencies listings.

◆ Low Vision Services

EYE CARE SOCIETIES

Puerto Rico Ophthalmological Society
P.O. Box 366274
San Juan, PR 00936
(787) 796-3746
Tere Bertran, Executive Director

◆ Aging Services

STATE UNITS ON AGING

Governor's Office for Elderly Affairs
Corbian Plaza, Stop 23
Ponce De Leon Avenue #1603
U.M. Office C
Santurce, PR 00908
(787) 721-5710 or Information & Referral (787) 721-4560
FAX: (787) 721-6510
Ruby Rodriguez, Executive Director

Provides referrals to Area Agencies on Aging and information on other local aging services.

RHODE ISLAND

◆ Educational Services

STATE SERVICES

Rhode Island Department of Education
22 Hayes Street
Providence, RI 02908
(401) 277-2031
Peter McWalters, Commissioner of
Elementary and Secondary
Education

Type of Agency: State.
Mission: Provides consultation
services.
Funded by: Public funds.
Area Served: Rhode Island.

Contact local school
superintendent for program
information or George Barros,
Consultant, or Robert Pryhoda,
Consultant, Special Education
Unit, 22 Hayes Street, Providence,
RI 02908, (401) 277-3505.

EARLY INTERVENTION COORDINATION

**Division of Family Health
Rhode Island Department of
Health**
3 Capitol Hill
Room 302
Providence, RI 02908-5097
(401) 277-2312
FAX: (401) 277-1442
William Hollinshead

County/District Where Located:
Providence County.

Early intervention services to
children aged 0-5.

◆ Information Services

LIBRARIES

**Rhode Island Regional Library
for the Blind and Physically
Handicapped**
300 Richmond Street
Providence, RI 02903
(401) 277-2726 or toll-free in Rhode
Island (800) 734-5141 or TDD
(401) 277-2726
FAX: (401) 277-4195
Kenneth Marold, Machine Lending
Information
Richard Leduc, Library Program
Specialist

County/District Where Located:
Providence County.
Funded by: Public funds.
Hours of Operation: Mon.-Fri.
8:30 AM-4:00 PM.
Staff: 5.
Area Served: Rhode Island.

Regional library of National
Library Service network supplying
talking books, braille and large-
type books, tapes, cassettes, and
machines. Cooperates in provision
of volunteer taping program; has
collection of regular print books
about handicaps.

RADIO READING

**IN-SIGHT Radio—Division of IN-
SIGHT**
43 Jefferson Boulevard
Warwick, RI 02888
(401) 941-3322
Carla Ferreira, Director, Radio
Reading
Judith T. Smith, President

Hours of Operation: Mon.-Fri.
8:00 AM-Midnight; Sat.-Sun.
8:30 AM-7:00 PM.
Staff: 2.
History/Date: Est. 1981.

Area Served: Rhode Island, also
nearby southeastern
Massachusetts and eastern
Connecticut.
Age Requirements: None.

INFORMATION AND REFERRAL

**The Foundation Fighting
Blindness
Rhode Island Affiliate**
18 Payan Street
West Warwick, RI 02893
(401) 828-0520
Diane Plante, Contact Person

See The Foundation Fighting
Blindness in U.S. national listings.

Saving Sight Rhode Island
1800 17th Post Road
Warwick, RI 02886
(401) 738-1150
Carolyn Hart, Executive Director

County/District Where Located:
Providence County.

◆ Rehabilitation Services

STATE SERVICES

**Services for the Blind and
Visually Impaired**
40 Fountain Street
Providence, RI 02903
(401) 277-2300 or TDD (401) 277-
3010
FAX: (401) 277-1328
Thomas J. Thompson, Deputy
Administrator

Type of Agency: State.
Mission: Administers the federal-
state vocational rehabilitation
program, Randolph-Sheppard
vending facilities program,
independent living program, social
service program.

Funded by: Federal, state grants.
Budget: 1996: $1,778,725.
Hours of Operation: 8:30 AM-4:00 PM.
Staff: 24 full time.
History/Date: Est. 1930; became part of Office of Rehabilitation Services, 1991.
Number of Clients Served: 1996: 1,572.
Eligibility: Legally blind; visually impaired (acuity of 20/60); deaf-blind.
Area Served: Statewide.
Age Requirements: None.

Health: Contracts for medical diagnoses; physical restoration and treatment.
Counseling/Social Work/Self-Help: Casework evaluation; individual, family/parent, group counseling; psychological testing; placement in training, institution; referral to community services; educational placements; vocational assessment and counseling.
Educational: Orientation and mobility; rehabilitation teaching.
Preschools: Consultation and casework services.
Professional Training: Internship/fieldwork placement in rehabilitation counseling; social work; vocational rehabilitation.
Rehabilitation: Personal management; braille; handwriting; typing; home management; orientation/mobility; sensory training; rehabilitation teaching in client's home and community; remedial education. Independent living, specialized program for those over 55 who are blind/visually impaired.
Recreational: Conducts a camp for blind/visually impaired children and teens.
Employment: Prevocational evaluation; career and skill counseling; job retention;

vocational placement; follow-up service; vending stand training.
Low Vision: Referrals to area specialists.
Low Vision Aids: Provided as needed (income requirements).

REHABILITATION

IN-SIGHT (Rhode Island Association for the Blind)
43 Jefferson Boulevard
Warwick, RI 02888
(401) 941-3322 or Workshop (401) 941-6607
Judith T. Smith, President
Phillip F. Janes, Workshop Director

Type of Agency: Private; non-profit.
Mission: To provide comprehensive services to persons who are blind or severely visually impaired.
Funded by: Contributions, fees for service, grants; endowment; workshop enterprise; annual fund-raising appeals.
Budget: $1,000,000.
Hours of Operation: Mon.-Fri. 8:30 AM-4:30 PM.
Staff: 65 full and part time; 400 volunteers.
History/Date: Est. 1923.
Number of Clients Served: 3,500.
Area Served: Rhode Island and southeastern Massachusetts.

Health: Special training for persons with diabetes by registered nurse in health component of Life Skills Program.
Counseling/Social Work/Self-Help: Casework; individual, group and family counseling; information and referral; peer support groups.
Educational: Parent seminars; orientation/mobility instruction.
Professional Training: Internship/fieldwork placement in low vision. Regular in-service

training programs; seminars for professionals in allied fields.
Reading: Uses volunteers for taping and recording services and as guides; readers; braille transcribers; computerized braille center provides ready access to brailled materials for area students. Operates IN-SIGHT Radio, a radio information service.
Rehabilitation: Activities of daily living; communication; home management; orientation/mobility; and other training. PRIDE (Path to Rehabilitation through Information, Discovery and Education) program (ages 55 and over); aids and appliances; life skills-diabetic rehabilitation program; regional support groups.
Recreational: Arts and crafts.
Employment: Industrial workshop and chair reseating, (401) 727-1111.
Low Vision: Low vision clinic providing examinations and evaluations and dispensing aids and devices.

Local Offices:

Providence: IN-SIGHT, 57 Porter Street, Providence, RI 02905, (401) 941-6666, Phillip F. Janes, Workshop Director.

COMPUTER TRAINING CENTERS

Assistive Technology Center
Meeting Street Center
667 Waterman Avenue
East Providence, RI 02914
(401) 438-9500
FAX: (401) 438-3760
Danielle King, Coordinator

County/District Where Located: Providence County.

Computer Training: Speech output systems; screen magnification systems; word processing; computer operating systems; training for individuals and instructors; consultation to schools.

Rhode Island Services for the Blind and Visually Impaired

40 Fountain Street
Providence, RI 02903
(401) 277-2382
Susan Shapiro, Supervisor

County/District Where Located:
Providence County.

Computer Training: Speech output systems; braille access systems; closed-circuit television systems; word processing; database software; computer operating systems.

◆ Low Vision Services

EYE CARE SOCIETIES

Rhode Island Society of Eye Physicians and Surgeons
Ophthalmology Consultants
106 Francis Street
Providence, RI 02903
(401) 331-1501
Edwin Rego, President

County/District Where Located:
Providence County.

Rhode Island Optometric Association
P.O. Box 8400
Warwick, RI 02888-0400
(401) 461-7550 or (800) 491-7550
FAX: (401) 941-5979
Rhoda Kelly, Executive Director

LOW VISION CENTERS

IN-SIGHT (Rhode Island Association for the Blind)
43 Jefferson Boulevard

Warwick, RI 02888
(402) 941-3322
Helene Bradley, O.D., Director, Low Vision Service

Type of Agency: Non-profit.
Hours of Operation: Mon., Wed. 9:00 AM-12:00 noon.
Eligibility: Ophthalmological report.
Area Served: Rhode Island.

Low Vision Aids: Provided on loan for trial; no rental fee; on-site training provided.
Low Vision Follow-up: By return appointment with optometrist in 1 month; home visit by social worker as needed.

◆ Aging Services

STATE UNITS ON AGING

Rhode Island Department of Elderly Affairs
160 Pine Street
Providence, RI 02903-3708
(401) 277-2858
FAX: Information and Referral in State (800) 322-2880 or (401) 277-1490
Barbara Ruffino, Director

Provides referrals to Area Agencies on Aging and information on other local aging services.

INDEPENDENT LIVING PROGRAMS

Rhode Island Services for the Blind and Visually Impaired Rhode Island Department of Human Services
40 Fountain Street
Providence, RI 02903-1898
(401) 277-2300 or (800) 752-8088
FAX: (401) 277-1328
Thomas J. Thompson, Deputy Administrator

Provides independent living services for persons age 55 and

over. For further information, contact the Project Director or general phone number listed.

SOUTH CAROLINA

◆ *Educational Services*

STATE SERVICES

Office of Programs for Exceptional Children
South Carolina Department of Education
Rutledge Office Building
1429 Senate Street
Columbia, SC 29201
(803) 734-8222
FAX: (803) 734-4824
Dr. Ora Spann, Director, Office of Programs for Exceptional Children
Dr. Bill Chaiken, Director, Office of Technical Assistance
Suzanne Swaffield, Education Associate

Type of Agency: State.
County/District Where Located: Richland County.
Mission: To provide consultation to school districts about the needs of their visually impaired students.
Funded by: Public funds.
Hours of Operation: Mon.-Fri. 8:30 AM-5:00 PM.
Program Accessibility: Fully accessible.
Staff: 1 full time for blind and visually impaired children.
Number of Clients Served: 500 legally blind children.
Eligibility: 20/50 or less activity.
Area Served: South Carolina.
Age Requirements: Legal school age (3-21 years).

Educational: Consultations to public schools.
Preschools: Program for 3 year olds.

Professional Training: In-service training for special education teachers and other professionals.

For information about educational services for children with visual disabilities, consult the director or education associate for the Office of Programs for Exceptional Children, or the superintendent of schools in the area.

EARLY INTERVENTION COORDINATION

Baby Net
South Carolina Department of Health and Environmental Control
2600 Bull Street
Columbia, SC 29201
(803) 737-4047
FAX: (803) 734-4459
Kathryn F. Hart, Baby Net Program Director

County/District Where Located: Richland County.

Evaluations, service coordination, parent-to-parent support, individualized family service plans.

SCHOOLS

South Carolina School for the Deaf and the Blind
355 Cedar Springs Road
Spartanburg, SC 29302-4699
(864) 594-3212
FAX: (864) 585-3555
Linda A. Mackechnie, Principal, School for the Blind
Dr. Sheila Breittweiser, President

Type of Agency: State.
County/District Where Located: Spartanburg County.
Funded by: State funds; foundation grants; private donations.
Budget: 1996: $19.7 million.

Program Accessibility: Barrier-free building.
Staff: 39 full time; 3 part time.
History/Date: Est. 1849.
Number of Clients Served: 1996: 67 (residential and day programs); 102 (outreach).
Eligibility: Visual impairment that prevents participation in regular school program without resource room assistance.
Area Served: South Carolina.
Transportation: Y.
Age Requirements: 3-22 years. Adult postsecondary.

Health: Diagnosis and evaluation of eye health; treatment of eye condition; audiology evaluations; general medical services; speech therapy. Refers and contracts for other eye health services. Occupational therapist and physical therapist.
Counseling/Social Work/Self-Help: Social evaluations; psychological testing and evaluations; individual counseling; placement in school.
Educational: Preschool through 12th grade. Programs for adult continuing education; college prep; general academic studies; vocational/skill development; technology preparation; computer lab.
Preschools: Kindergarten preparation (age 3-5) and early intervention (age 0-6).
Professional Training: Internship/fieldwork placement in special education. Regular in-service training programs, short-term or summer training.
Reading: Lends talking book cassette players; talking book cassettes; braille books; large-print books; braille magazines. Library on campus. Descriptive videos. Extensive computer, special access references.

Residential: Dormitories; small apartments; Independent Living House.
Rehabilitation: Personal management; braille; handwriting; listening skills; keyboarding; home management; orientation/ mobility. Refers for other rehabilitation services.
Recreational: Afterschool programs; arts and crafts; weight lifting; horsebackriding; bowling; swimming; track; wrestling; football; roller skating. Cheerleading; volleyball; cross-country; paraolympics; goal ball. Refers for other recreational services.
Employment: Prevocational evaluations; career and skill counseling; occupational skill development; vending stand training. Job coaches. Contracts for vocational placement.
Computer Training: Keyboarding skills; IBM and MAC word processing; educational software; adaptive devices.
Low Vision: Assessments; training weekly.
Low Vision Aids: Closed-circuit television; Apollo; VTEK; magnifiers; adapted computers.
Low Vision Follow-up: Training and re-evaluation.

Provides extensive support to public schools through consultation and direct service in orientation/mobility; itinerant service to public schools available on request. Provides training in braille skills. Technology evaluations and summer programs.

Consultant for Visually Handicapped Programs, South Carolina Department of Education, 1429 Senate Street, Columbia, SC 29201, (803) 734-8222.

INFANT AND PRESCHOOL

South Carolina Commission for the Blind
1430 Confederate Avenue
Columbia, SC 29201
(803) 734-7520
FAX: (803) 734-7885
Donald Gist, Commissioner

Type of Agency: State.
County/District Where Located: Richland County.
Mission: To afford blind and visually impaired children the opportunity to develop maximum growth; to teach the skills necessary for optimal independent functioning; and to develop competencies for mainstreaming blind and visually impaired children effectively within community programs.
Funded by: State funds.
History/Date: Est. 1967.
Eligibility: Legally blind, with or without other disabilities.
Area Served: South Carolina.

Health: Low vision exams; medical social services (dependent on financial eligibility).
Counseling/Social Work/Self-Help: Family counseling; parent workshops.
Educational: Orientation/ mobility, positioning and handling training available on consultant or referral basis; instruction in most developmental areas.

STATEWIDE OUTREACH SERVICES

South Carolina School for the Deaf and the Blind
355 Cedar Springs Road
Spartanburg, SC 29302
(864) 594-3212
Craig Jacobs, Director, Support Services and Outreach
Elizabeth McKown, Outreach Coordinator

Funded by: State funds; foundation grants; private donations.

Assessment: Psychological; low vision; braille, orientation and mobility; speech and language; audiology. Occupational therapist and physical therapist available.
Consultation to Public Schools: On request.
Direct Service: Parent-infant program; tours; referrals, resources.
Professional Training: Braille and sign language classes.

UNIVERSITY TRAINING PROGRAMS

Programs in Special Education
University of South Carolina
Columbia, SC 29208
(800) 777-7000
FAX: (803) 777-3045
Annette Skellenger, Director of Programs for the Visually Impaired, (803) 777-6732

Programs Offered: Graduate (master's) program for teachers of the visually handicapped; master's program in rehabilitation counseling; doctoral-level program in counselor education.

◆ Information Services

LIBRARIES

South Carolina State Library Department for the Blind and Physically Handicapped
301 Gervais Street
P.O. Box 821

Columbia, SC 29202
(803) 737-9970 or toll-free in South
Carolina (800) 922-7818
E-mail: guynell@leo.scsl.state.
sc.us
URL: http://www.state.sc.us/
scsl/
Guynell Williams, Director

Type of Agency: State.
County/District Where Located:
Richland County.
Mission: To provide library
services to print disabled residents
of South Carolina.
Funded by: Federal/state funds.
Hours of Operation: Mon-Fri
8:30 AM-5:00 PM.
Staff: 9.
Number of Clients Served: 7,650.
Eligibility: Certification of print-
handicap condition.
Area Served: State of South
Carolina.

Provides talking books, tapes,
cassettes, and large-print books on
loan. Provides playback equipment
on loan. Reader advisory service.
Provides descriptive videotapes on
loan.

MEDIA PRODUCTION SERVICES

Charleston County School District
Pupil Personnel Services
4720 Jenkins Avenue
North Charleston, SC 29405
(803) 745-7150
FAX: (803) 566-7799
Jan Lichtenstein, Coordinator

Groups Served: Preschool-high
school.

Types/Content: Textbooks;
recreational; workbooks; dittos.
Media Formats: Braille books;
talking books/cassettes; large print
books.

South Carolina Commission for the Blind
1430 Confederate Avenue
Columbia, SC 29201
(803) 734-7577
Norman J. Verigood, Media Center
Manager

County/District Where Located:
Richland County.
Area Served: South Carolina.
Groups Served: K-12, college
students, other adults.

Types/Content: Textbooks,
recreational, career/vocational,
religious.
Media Formats: Braille books,
talking books/cassettes, large print
books.
Title Listings: No title listings
available.

South Carolina School for the Deaf and the Blind
355 Cedar Springs Road
Spartanburg, SC 29302
(864) 585-7711
FAX: (864) 585-3555
Jack Todd, Contact Person

Area Served: South Carolina.
Groups Served: K-12 and
postsecondary.

Types/Content: Textbooks;
career/vocational; fiction for
children; descriptive videos.
Media Formats: Braille, large-
print and cassette books.
Title Listings: Available on
request.

South Carolina State Library Department for the Blind and Physically Handicapped
301 Gervais Street
P.O. Box 821

Columbia, SC 29202
(803) 737-9970 or (800) 922-7818
FAX: (803) 737-9983
E-mail: guynell@leo.scsl.state.
sc.us
URL: http://www.state.sc.us/
scsl/
Guynell Williams, Director

County/District Where Located:
Richland County.
Area Served: Statewide.
Groups Served: Pre-school
through adult.

Types/Content: Wide variety of
fiction and non-fiction titles.
Media Formats: Talking books/
cassettes, large print books,
recorded magazines, braille books,
descriptive videotypes.
Title Listings: None specified.

Theodore Lester Elementary School
3501 East Palmetto Street
Florence, SC 29506
(803) 665-0695
FAX: (803) 679-6753
Carol Roy, Resource Teacher for
the Visually Handicapped

County/District Where Located:
Florence County.
Area Served: PeeDee region of
South Carolina.
Groups Served: Students aged 3-
21.

Types/Content: Textbooks.
Media Formats: Braille/large-
print books.
Title Listings: None specified.

RADIO READING

South Carolina Educational Radio for the Blind
1430 Confederate Avenue

Columbia, SC 29201
(803) 734-7555
FAX: (803) 734-7885
E-mail: b.jones122@genie.geis.
com
Beth Jones, Station Manager

County/District Where Located:
Richland County.
Funded by: South Carolina
Commission for the Blind.
Hours of Operation: Mon.-Sun.
6:00 AM-Midnight.
Staff: 3 full-time, 4 part-time; 85
volunteers.
History/Date: Est. 1973.
Area Served: South Carolina.
Age Requirements: None.

See also in national listings:

**National Association of Radio
Reading Services**

♦ Rehabilitation Services

STATE SERVICES

**South Carolina Commission for
the Blind**
1430 Confederate Avenue
Columbia, SC 29201
(803) 734-7520 or toll-free in South
Carolina (800) 922-2222
FAX: (803) 734-7885
Donald Gist, Commissioner

Type of Agency: State.
County/District Where Located:
Richland County.
Funded by: Public funds.
History/Date: Est. 1967.
Area Served: South Carolina.

Health: Diagnosis, medical and
surgical treatment; prescribes
eyeglasses and optical aids; public
education.
Educational: Tuition support.

Rehabilitation: Orientation/
mobility; home economics;
communications.
Employment: Evaluation;
prevocational and vocational
training; placement; vending stand
program; home employment;
follow-up.

Local Offices:

Charleston: Fairfield Office Park,
Suite 109, Charleston, SC 29407,
(803) 766-5556.
Conway: 311 Beaty Street,
Conway, SC 29526, (803) 248-2017.
Florence: 825 West Evans Street,
Florence, SC 29501, (803) 661-4788.
Greenville: 669 North Academy
Street, Greenville, SC 29601,
(864) 241-1111.
Greenwood: 1 Park Plaza, Suite
15, Greenwood, SC 29646,
(864) 223-3334.
Orangeburg: The Moore Building,
1180 Boulevard, Suite A,
Orangeburg, SC 29115, (803) 531-
6885.
Rock Hill: 339 East Main Street,
Suite 3, Rock Hill, SC 29730,
(803) 324-1845.
Spartanburg: 269 South Church
Street, Suite 312, Spartanburg, SC
29306, (864) 594-4911.
Walterboro: 776-A North Jeffries
Boulevard, Walterboro, SC 29488,
(803) 549-1501.

REHABILITATION

Association for the Blind
2209 Mechanic Street
Charleston, SC 29405-9320
(803) 723-6915
Roy M. Proffitt, Executive Director

Type of Agency: Private; non-
profit.
County/District Where Located:
Charleston County.
Mission: To improve the lives of
blind and visually impaired
persons in the tri-county area.

Funded by: United Way;
workshop sales; endowment;
contributions; membership.
Budget: $550,000.
Hours of Operation: Mon.-Fri.
8:30 AM-4:30 PM.
Staff: 6 (management and
general); 6 cane workshop; 4
medical transcriptionists; 2 others.
History/Date: Est. 1936.
Number of Clients Served: 1996:
5,000.
Eligibility: Legally blind.
Area Served: Charleston,
Dorchester, and Berkeley counties.
Transportation: Y.

Health: White canes provided and
eyeglasses purchased for needy
clients as fimds are available.
**Counseling/Social Work/Self-
Help:** On-going counseling
groups, varied informal
educational classes for self-
improvement.
Educational: Medical
transcription training.
Reading: Braille; talking books;
talking book machines; readers.
Rehabilitation: Braille instruction
and crafts classes.
Recreational: Social activities:
beep ball, walking, and bowling.
Recreational: Social activities.
Employment: Cane workshop;
medical transcriptions.
Employment: Affiliated with
National Industries for the Blind.

♦ Low Vision Services

EYE CARE SOCIETIES

**South Carolina Society of
Ophthalmology**
1331 Laurel Street
Columbia, SC 29202
(803) 254-6964
Ronald Scott, Executive Director

South Carolina Optometric Association, Inc.
2730 Devine Street
Columbia, SC 29205
(803) 799-6721 or (803) 799-2305
Claire Haltiwanger, Executive Director

LOW VISION CENTERS

South Carolina Commission for the Blind
355 Cedar Springs Road
Spartanburg, SC 29302-4699
(864) 594-3370
William Spearman, O.D.
Joy F. Rodgers, Clinic Coordinator

Type of Agency: State.
County/District Where Located: Spartanburg County.
Funded by: Client fees; state funds.
Hours of Operation: One Friday each month, 8:30 AM-4:00 PM.
Staff: Optometrist/low vision specialist.
Eligibility: Referral by agency representative after ophthalmological examination is provided.
Area Served: South Carolina.
Transportation: Y.

Low Vision Aids: Provided by agency or purchased by patient; on-site training provided.
Low Vision Follow-up: By return appointment as applicable.

South Carolina Commission for the Blind
Columbia Office
1430 Confederate Avenue
Columbia, SC 29201
(803) 734-7876
Scott B. Johnson, Coordinator

County/District Where Located: Richland County.
Funded by: State funds.
Staff: Ophthalmologist; low vision assistant; optometrist.

Eligibility: Referral by agency representative after ophthalmological examination is provided.
Area Served: South Carolina.
Transportation: Y.

Low Vision Aids: Provided by agency or purchased by patient; on-site training provided.
Low Vision Follow-up: By return appointment as applicable.

Local Offices:

Charleston: Fairfield Office Park, Suite 109, Charleston, SC 29407, (803) 766-5556.
Florence: 825 West Evans Street, Florence, SC 29501, (803) 661-4788.
Walterboro: 776-A North Jeffries Boulevard, Walterboro, SC 29488, (803) 549-1501.

South Carolina Eye Institute
Department of Ophthalmology
University of South Carolina
School of Medicine
4 Richland Medical Park
Suite 100
Columbia, SC 29203
(803) 434-6836
FAX: (803) 434-2387
Dr. Ramesh Tripathi, Chairman, Ophthalmology Dept.
Earl Loftis, Low Vision Specialist

County/District Where Located: Richland County.
Funded by: Client fees.
Hours of Operation: Mon.-Fri. 8:30AM-5:30PM.
Staff: Ophthalmologist; low vision specialist; cornea specialist; retina specialist; glaucoma specialist; neuro-ophthalmologist; ophthalmic assistant; ophthalmic technician; ophthalmology resident; orthoptist; ophthalmic photographer; pediatric ophthalmologist.
Eligibility: Referral from ophthalmologist.

Area Served: Unlimited.

Low Vision Aids: Provided for purchase or prescribed; fitted; sold at cost; on-site training provided.
Low Vision Follow-up: As needed.

♦ Aging Services

STATE UNITS ON AGING

South Carolina Commission on Aging
202 Arbor Lake Drive
Suite B 500, #301
Columbia, SC 29223
(803) 737-7500 or Information & Referral In State (800) 868-9095 or In Columbia (800) 735-0210
FAX: (803) 737-7501
Constance Rinehart, Director

Provides referrals to Area Agencies on Aging and information on other local aging services.

INDEPENDENT LIVING PROGRAMS

South Carolina Commission for the Blind
1430 Confederate Avenue
Columbia, SC 29201
(803) 734-7566
Jim Stuart, Director

Provides independent living services for persons age 55 and over. For further information, contact the Project Director or general phone number listed.

SOUTH DAKOTA

♦ *Educational Services*

STATE SERVICES

Office of Special Education
South Dakota Division of
Education and Resources
700 Governors Drive
Pierre, SD 57501-2291
(605) 773-3678 or TDD (605) 773-6139
FAX: (605) 773-6139
Deborah Barnett, Director of Special Education

Type of Agency: State, a division of the State Department of Education and Cultural Affairs.
Funded by: Public funds.
Hours of Operation: Mon.-Fri. 8:00 AM-5:00 PM.
Area Served: South Dakota.

In cooperation with the Division of Service to the Blind and Visually Impaired, maintains staff responsible for the education of students with disabilities.

For further information, consult the Director of the Office of Special Education. For information about local facilities, consult the superintendent of schools in the area.

EARLY INTERVENTION COORDINATION

Office of Special Education
South Dakota Division of
Education and Resources
700 Governors Drive
Pierre, SD 57501-2291
(605) 773-3678 or TDD (605) 773-6302
FAX: (605) 773-6139
Barbara Lechner, Part H Early Childhood Coordinator

County/District Where Located: Hughes County.

Coordinates early intervention programs for preschoolers in South Dakota.

SCHOOLS

South Dakota School for the Visually Handicapped
423 S.E. 17th Avenue
Aberdeen, SD 57401-7699
(605) 626-2580 or TDD (605) 626-7829 or toll-free (888) 275-3814
FAX: (605) 626-2607
E-mail: kaiserm@sdsvh.northern.edu
URL: http://www.ris.sdbor.edy/sdsvh/main.htm
Marjorie Kaiser, Superintendent

Type of Agency: State.
Mission: Educational programs and services for totally blind; legally blind; visually impaired; and deaf-blind students.
Funded by: State general funds.
Budget: 1997FY: $1,721,690.
Staff: 54 full time. Uses volunteers.
History/Date: Est. 1900.
Number of Clients Served: 180 total, on campus and outreach.
Eligibility: Visually impaired.
Area Served: State of South Dakota; out-of-state tuition students.
Age Requirements: 21 years and under.

Health: Nursing; speech therapy. Contracts occupational therapy and physical therapy and refers for other health services.
Counseling/Social Work/Self-Help: Social evaluation; psychological testing and evaluation; individual, group, counseling. Contracts, refers and provides consultation to other agencies.
Educational: Grades K through 12; also non-graded. General academic studies; vocational/skill development. Diagnostic program provides comprehensive, multidisciplinary educational evaluations, including braille and functional vision.
Professional Training: Internship/fieldwork placement; low vision; orientation/mobility; special education. Regular in-service training programs, open to enrollment from other agencies.
Reading: Braille, large print.
Residential: Dormitories.
Rehabilitation: Cooperative services with Service to the Blind and Visually Handicapped (state vocational rehabilitation).
Recreational: Afterschool programs; arts and crafts; bowling; swimming; track; wrestling; rifle club; cross country skiing.
Employment: Transition services statewide; prevocational evaluation; career and skill counseling; occupational skill development; job retention; vocational placement; follow-up service.
Computer Training: Adaptations for screen readers and screen enlargement.
Low Vision: Low vision service.
Low Vision Aids: Functional applications in classroom and community.

Outreach offices in Aberdeen, Sioux Falls and Rapid City.

Outreach consultants assist parents and local schools in providing appropriate educational programs; on-site visits; in-service training and educational materials and resources.

STATEWIDE OUTREACH SERVICES

South Dakota School for the Visually Handicapped

423 S.E. 17th Avenue
Aberdeen, SD 57401
(605) 626-2580
FAX: (605) 626-2607
E-mail: kaiserm@sdsvh.northern.edu
URL: http://www.ris.sdbor.edu/sdsvh/main.htm
Dawn LaMee, Liaison for Services

Age Requirements: Birth-21 years.

Assessment: Multidisciplinary assessments conducted.
Consultation to Public Schools: Provided by outreach consultants.
Direct Service: Regional consultants perform on-site visits and in-service training to assist parents and local schools.

INSTRUCTIONAL MATERIALS CENTERS

South Dakota State Library for the Handicapped

800 Governors Drive
Pierre, SD 57501-2295
(605) 773-3131 or toll-free
(800) 423-6665
FAX: (605) 773-4950
E-mail: danb@stlib.state.sd.us
Daniel W. Boyd, Director

Area Served: South Dakota.
Groups Served: K-12, college students, other adults.

Types/Content: Textbooks, recreational, career/vocational.
Media Formats: Braille books, talking books/cassettes, large print books.
Title Listings: Printed at no charge, supplied in braille with a charge.

UNIVERSITY TRAINING PROGRAMS

Northern State College Special Education Program

P.O. Box 645
Aberdeen, SD 57401
(605) 626-2621
FAX: (605) 626-3102
Dr. Marva Gelhaus, Contact Person

County/District Where Located: Brown County.

Programs Offered: Undergraduate program for teachers of the visually handicapped.

♦ Information Services

LIBRARIES

South Dakota State Library for the Handicapped

800 Governors Drive
Pierre, SD 57501-2295
(605) 773-3514 or (800) 423-6665
FAX: (605) 773-4950
E-mail: danb@stlib.state.sd.us
Daniel W. Boyd, Director

Type of Agency: Library for the blind and physically handicapped.
Mission: Provide access to print materials in braille, recorded, or large-print formats.
Funded by: Public funds.
Budget: $325,000.
Hours of Operation: Mon.-Fri. 8:00 AM-5:00 PM.
Program Accessibility: Fully accessible.
Staff: 7.
History/Date: Est. 1966.
Number of Clients Served: 5,000.
Eligibility: Application required certifying visual impairment physical handicap that prevents holding book and/or turning pages, or reading/learning

disability caused by organic disfunction.
Area Served: South Dakota.
Age Requirements: All ages.

Low Vision: Y.
Low Vision Aids: Y.

MEDIA PRODUCTION SERVICES

South Dakota Industries for the Blind

800 West Avenue North
Sioux Falls, SD 57104-5796
(605) 367-5266
FAX: (605) 367-5263
Frank Greet, Braille Print Coordinator

Area Served: U.S.
Groups Served: Schools, the public and private businesses.

Types/Content: All types of print materials.
Media Formats: Braille supplied at $.30/pg.; $15.00/min.

RADIO READING

Services to the Blind and Visually Impaired

East Highway 34, c/o 500 East Capitol
Pierre, SD 57501-5070
(605) 773-4644
FAX: (605) 773-5483
E-mail: theresag@dhs.state.sd.us
Grady Kickul, Director

County/District Where Located: Hughes County.
Funded by: Federal funds.
Hours of Operation: 8:00AM - 5:00PM.
Staff: 50.
Area Served: Statewide.
Age Requirements: 14 and up.

♦ Rehabilitation Services

STATE SERVICES

**Division of Service to the Blind and Visually Impaired
South Dakota Department of Human Services**
East Highway 34
c/o 500 East Capitol
Pierre, SD 57501-5070
(605) 773-4644 or TDD (605) 773-4544
FAX: (605) 773-5483
Grady Kickul, Director, Division of Service to the Blind and Visually Impaired

Type of Agency: State.
Mission: To provide individualized rehabilitation services which result in optimal employment and independent living outcomes for citizens who are blind and visually impaired.
Funded by: Federal and state funds.
Budget: 1997: $2,800,000.
Hours of Operation: Mon.-Fri. 8:00 AM-5:00 PM.
Program Accessibility: Fully accessible.
Staff: 40 full time. Uses volunteers.
History/Date: Est. 1943.
Number of Clients Served: 1,000 annually.
Eligibility: Legally blind or visually impaired and residing in South Dakota.
Area Served: Statewide.
Age Requirements: 14 years and older.

Health: Diagnosis, evaluation, and physical restoration services resulting in increased visual functioning, including low vision services.
Counseling/Social Work/Self-Help: Personal adjustment, vocational, peer, and family counseling. Information and referral services. Consultation.
Educational: Assistance with vocational and academic training leading to employment.
Professional Training: Regular in-service training program open to enrollment by other organizations.
Rehabilitation: Orientation/mobility; communications; independent living skills; leisure time activity; self-advocacy; and in-home rehabilitation teaching services.
Employment: Vocational evaluation, exploration; work adjustment; and job-seeking skills services. Job placement follow-up; and supported employment services.
Computer Training: Evaluation regarding access devices, job-specific training, employment consultation and placement; training in word processing, database and spreadsheets.
Low Vision: One state-run low vision clinic and 16 rural low vision clinics annually.
Low Vision Aids: All aids recommended provided, subject to agency financial need criteria.
Low Vision Follow-up: Low vision specialist and rehabilitation teacher provide in-home training and follow-up.

Local Offices:

Aberdeen: Service to the Blind and Visually Impaired, 315 South Wilson, Aberdeen, SD 57401-5055, (605) 626-2395.
Pierre: Service to the Blind and Visually Impaired, c/o 912 East Sioux, Pierre, SD 57501-5070, (605) 773-4921.

Rapid City: Service to the Blind and Visually Impaired, Time Square Plaza, 111-A New York Street, Rapid City, SD 57701-1156, (605) 394-2253.
Sioux Falls: Rehabilitation Center for the Blind, 800 West Avenue North, Sioux Falls, SD 57104-5796, (605) 367-5260.
Sioux Falls: Service to the Blind and Visually Impaired, 817 West Russell, Suite 102, Sioux Falls, SD 57104-1360, (605) 367-5260.

REHABILITATION

South Dakota Industries for the Blind
800 West Avenue North
Sioux Falls, SD 57104-5796
(605) 367-5266
FAX: (605) 367-5263
Martin M. Luebke, Administrator
Steve Bruggeman, Sales/Production Manager

Type of Agency: State.
Mission: Services for individuals who are totally blind, legally blind, visually impaired, deaf-blind, multiply disabled.
Funded by: Public funds; workshop sales; federal grants.
Hours of Operation: Mon.-Fri. 7:30 AM-4:00 PM.
Staff: 9.
History/Date: Est. 1969.
Number of Clients Served: 1996.: 70.
Eligibility: Visually impaired; other disabilities.

Health: Referred to community resources.
Counseling/Social Work/Self-Help: Individual counseling, referrals to community resources.
Rehabilitation: Work adjustment training; World of Work Classes; job placement; job coaching; life coaching.
Employment: Development of work skills; job placement and

retention; situational community-based evaluation; braille services; job coaching services; employment services.

South Dakota Rehabilitation Center for the Blind

800 West Avenue North
Sioux Falls, SD 57104-5796
(605) 367-5260
FAX: (605) 367-5263
E-mail: martin l@hssfi.state.
sd.us
Martin M. Luebke, Administrator

Type of Agency: State.
Mission: Services for individuals who are totally blind, legally blind, visually impaired, deaf-blind, multiply disabled.
Funded by: Public funds, fees for services.
Hours of Operation: Mon.-Fri. 8:00 AM-4:30 PM.
Staff: 10 full time, 2 part time. Volunteers used.
History/Date: Est. 1969.
Number of Clients Served: 1996: 65.
Eligibility: Visually impaired.
Area Served: Midwest.

Health: Referred to community resources.
Counseling/Social Work/Self-Help: Individual and group counseling, referrals to community resources.
Professional Training: Field rehabilitation teacher training.
Rehabilitation: Personal management; braille; handwriting; typing; money management; home management; orientation/mobility; independent living experience; computer training; remedial education.
Recreational: Individualized evening/weekend programs; arts and crafts; camping; canoeing; hiking; bowling; swimming; table games; beepball; goal ball; cross country skiing.
Employment: Vocational evaluation; career/skill counseling; referral to South Dakota Vocational Resources for work adjustment training; job placement; job coaching services; employment services.
Computer Training: IBM compatible systems.
Low Vision: Low vision clinic.

COMPUTER TRAINING CENTERS

Service to the Visually Impaired/Business and Education Institute

Dakota State University
Madison, SD 57042
(605) 256-5555
FAX: (605) 256-5174
Rick Sterling

Computer Training: Speech output systems; screen magnification systems; braille access systems; closed-circuit television systems; word processing; database software; computer operating systems; voice activated applications.

◆ Low Vision Services

EYE CARE SOCIETIES

South Dakota Academy of Ophthalmology

1025 Strawberry
P.O. Box 803
Helena, MT 59624
(605) 449-2334
Gloria Hermanson, Executive Director

South Dakota Optometric Society

P. O. Box 1173
Pierre, SD 57501
(605) 224-8199
Cathie Ellis, Director

LOW VISION CENTERS

South Dakota Low Vision Services
Service for the Blind and Visually Impaired

800 West Avenue North
Sioux Falls, SD 57104-5796
(605) 367-5262 or (605) 367-5260
FAX: (605) 367-5263
Dawn Backer, Low Vision Specialist

Type of Agency: State.
County/District Where Located: Minnehaha County.
Funded by: State funds and client fees.
Staff: Optometrist; low vision specialist.
Eligibility: Referral by agency representative after ophthalmological examination is provided. Referral from other state agencies.
Area Served: South Dakota.

Low vision clinics conducted across the state and at the South Dakota Rehabilitation Center for the Blind.

◆ Aging Services

STATE UNITS ON AGING

Office of Adult Services and Aging

700 Governor's Drive
Pierre, SD 57501
Information and Referral
(605) 773-3656 or Department of Human Services (800) 265-9684
FAX: (605) 773-4855
Gail Ferris, Executive Director

Provides referrals to Area Agencies on Aging and information on other local aging services.

INDEPENDENT LIVING PROGRAMS

**Division of Service to the Blind
and Visually Impaired
South Dakota Department of
Human Services**
East Highway 34
c/o 500 East Capitol
Pierre, SD 57501-5070
(605) 773-4644 or (800) 265-9684
Grady Kickul, Director
Gaye Mattke, Project Director

Provides independent living
services for persons age 55 and
over. For further information,
contact the Project Director or
general phone number listed.

TENNESSEE

◆ *Educational Services*

STATE SERVICES

Tennessee Department of Education
132 Cordell Hull Building
Nashville, TN 37219
(615) 741-2851
FAX: (615) 532-9412
Dr. Jane Walters, Commissioner
Joseph Fisher, Executive Director, Division of Special Education
Dr. Cleo J. Harris, Coordinator of Vision Services

Type of Agency: State.
Mission: Administers supplemental state funds for visually handicapped children attending local schools.
Funded by: Public funds.
History/Date: Est. 1947.

Provides consultation in educational services for local schools and agencies. Distributes braille and large type books, tapes, tape recorders, and talking books.

For information about local programs consult the superintendent of schools in the area.

EARLY INTERVENTION COORDINATION

Office for Special Education Tennessee Department of Education
8th Floor, Andrew Johnson Tower
710 James Robertson Parkway
Nashville, TN 37243-0380
(615) 741-2851
FAX: (615) 532-9412
Dr. Jane Walters, Commissioner
Sarah Willis, Part H Early Childhood Coordinator

County/District Where Located: Davidson County.

SCHOOLS

Tennessee School for the Blind
115 Stewarts Ferry Pike
Nashville, TN 37214
(615) 231-7300
FAX: (615) 231-7307
E-mail: brewerr01@ten-nash.ten.k12.tn.us
Ralph A. Brewer, Superintendent

Type of Agency: State.
County/District Where Located: Davidson County.
Mission: Services for totally blind; legally blind; deaf-blind; learning disabled; mentally retarded.
Funded by: State funds.
Hours of Operation: Mon.-Fri. 8:00AM-4:30PM.
Staff: 181 full time. Uses volunteers.
History/Date: Est. 1844.
Number of Clients Served: Approximately 165.
Eligibility: Legally blind; resident of Tennessee.
Area Served: Tennessee.
Transportation: Y.
Age Requirements: 3-21 years.

Health: Clinic provided for students.
Counseling/Social Work/Self-Help: Provides counseling and psychological evaluations.
Educational: Preschool-grade 12, and nongraded. Programs for college prep; general academic; prevocational.
Preschools: Programs for 3 and 4 year olds.
Professional Training: Internship/field work placement in low vision; orientation/mobility; special education.
Residential: Y.
Recreational: Arts and crafts; hobby groups; residential summer camp; bowling; swimming; track; wrestling. Refers for other recreational service.
Employment: Prevocational evaluation; career and skill counseling; occupational skill development; office occupations; work experience (community).
Computer Training: Access; training on computer aids and devices.
Low Vision: Evaluation of students.

Contact local school superintendent or Ms. Rebecca Reddy, Preschool Counselor, (615) 231-7300.

INFANT AND PRESCHOOL

Memphis City Schools
2597 Avey Avenue
Memphis, TN 38112
(901) 325-5614
Genevieve De Priest, Director of Special Education
Lev Williams, Consultant for Visually Limited

Type of Agency: Public school preschool program.
County/District Where Located: Shelby County.
Funded by: P.L. 89-313 and 94-142 monies, state funds, Handicapped Children's Early Education Program grants.
Hours of Operation: Mon.-Fri. 8:00AM-4:00PM.
Staff: For vision program: 31 full time (includes visually handicapped teachers); various therapists and specialists available as consultants. Uses volunteers.
History/Date: Est. 1980.
Area Served: Memphis.

Health: Adaptive equipment; health services available on consultant or referral basis.

Counseling/Social Work/Self-Help: Parent and other counseling.
Educational: Provides instruction in all developmental areas. Classes for visually handicapped and multihandicapped children, 3-5 years old. Consultant services to other programs.

Local Offices:

Memphis: Visually Limited Center, 1360 Colonial Road, Memphis, TN 38117, (901) 761-8940.

Metropolitan Nashville Public Schools
Visually Impaired Multihandicapped Program

2601 Bransford Avenue
Nashville, TN 37204
(615) 259-8698
FAX: (615) 259-8708
Margaret Horsnell, Director of Special Education
Karen White, Lead Vision Teacher

County/District Where Located: Davidson County.
Funded by: P.L. 94-142 monies and local school funds.
Staff: 2 full time (visually handicapped/multiply handicapped teacher); 6 part time (includes physical therapist); occupational therapist available as consultant. Uses volunteers, practicum students.

Health: Adaptive equipment; low vision exams.
Counseling/Social Work/Self-Help: Parent counseling and financial assistance available on referral.
Educational: Provides instruction in all developmental areas. Multihandicapped classroom in special public school.

Services for the Blind
Tennessee Division of Rehabilitation Services

Citizens Plaza Building, 11th Floor
400 Deaderick Street
Nashville, TN 37248-6200
(615) 313-4914
FAX: (615) 741-6508
Terry C. Smith, Director

Type of Agency: State, a division of the Department of Human Services.
Mission: Services to visually impaired children, with or without other disabilities.
Funded by: State funds.
Hours of Operation: Mon.-Fri. 8:00 AM-4:30 PM.
Staff: 13 full time (rehabilitation teachers).
History/Date: Est. 1943.
Eligibility: Visually impaired.
Area Served: Entire state.

Health: Adaptive equipment.
Counseling/Social Work/Self-Help: Parent counseling.
Educational: Instruction in some developmental areas.

Local Offices:

Chattanooga: Tennessee Services for the Blind, 1501 Riverside Drive, Fifth Floor, Chattanooga, TN 37406, (423) 493-6056, Reed White, Regional Supervisor.
Columbia: Tennessee Services for the Blind, P.O. Box 457, 6011 Mount Pleasant Pike, Columbia, TN 38401, (615) 388-4015, Linda Fleming, Regional Supervisor.
Jackson: Tennessee Services for the Blind, 225 Martin Luther King Boulevard, Suite 104-A, Jackson, TN 38301, (901) 423-5620, John R. Warmath, Regional Supervisor.
Johnson City: Tennessee Services for the Blind, 905 Buffalo Street, Johnson City, TN 37604, (423) 929-9142, Clyde T. Bible, Regional Supervisor.

Knoxville: Tennessee Services for the Blind, 531 Hemley Street, Suite 204, Knoxville, TN 37902, (423) 594-6054, Cal Gilespie, Regional Supervisor.
Memphis: Tennessee Services for the Blind, 170 North Main Street, Room 802, Memphis, TN 38103, (901) 543-7309, Roger Boeving, Regional Supervisor.
Nashville: Tennessee Services for the Blind, 88 Hermitage Avenue, Nashville, TN 37210, (615) 741-2111, Stephen Pruitt, Regional Supervisor.

Home-based, consultant services to other programs.

Tennessee School for the Blind

115 Stewarts Ferry Pike
Nashville, TN 37214
(615) 231-7300
FAX: (615) 231-7307
Rebecca Reddy, Director of Outreach Services

Type of Agency: State school.
Mission: Parent training for families with preschool children who are visually impaired or blind.
Funded by: State funds.
Hours of Operation: 12-month program operating within school hours.
Staff: 3 regional coordinators.
History/Date: Est. 1844.
Eligibility: Visually impaired children with or without other disabilities.
Area Served: Tennessee.
Transportation: Y.
Age Requirements: 0-5 years.

Health: Provides adaptive equipment; genetic counseling; various health services, including low vision exams.
Counseling/Social Work/Self-Help: Parent counseling.
Educational: Instruction in all developmental areas.

Center- and home-based programs for visually impaired children; consultation services to other programs.

STATEWIDE OUTREACH SERVICES

Tennessee School for the Blind

115 Stewarts Ferry Pike
Nashville, TN 37214
(615) 231-7300
FAX: (615) 231-7307
Rebecca Reddy, Director of
Outreach Services

County/District Where Located:
Davidson County.
Funded by: State funds.
History/Date: Est. 1884.
Age Requirements: Birth through school age.

Assessment: Preschool diagnostic program.
Consultation to Public Schools:
On request.
Direct Service: Through Media Center.
Parent Assistance: Parent training available for parents of preschool children.

INSTRUCTIONAL MATERIALS CENTERS

Tennessee Department of Education
Resource Center for the Visually Impaired

115 Stewarts Ferry Pike
Nashville, TN 37214
(615) 231-7340
FAX: (615) 231-7307
Carol McCarroll, Director

County/District Where Located:
Davidson county.
Groups Served: All ages.

Types/Content: Textbooks, tangible aids equipment.
Media Formats: Braille, large print.

UNIVERSITY TRAINING PROGRAMS

Peabody College of Vanderbilt University

Box 328, Peabody College
Nashville, TN 37203
(615) 322-2249
FAX: (615) 343-1570
Dr. Ann Kaiser, Chairperson

Programs Offered: Undergraduate and graduate (master's, doctoral) programs for teachers of visually impaired.

◆ Information Services

LIBRARIES

Tennessee Library for the Blind and Physically Handicapped

403 Seventh Avenue North
Nashville, TN 37243-0313
(615) 741-3915 or toll-free in
Tennessee (800) 342-3308
E-mail: mmarkham@mail.state.tn.us
Mary Lou Markham, Director

Type of Agency: Public library service.
Mission: To provide free public library to residents of Tennessee, who cannot read a regular print book due to a visual or physical impairment.
Funded by: State and federal monies.
Hours of Operation: Mon.-Fri. 8:00 AM-4:30 PM.
Program Accessibility: Fully accessible.
Staff: 15.
History/Date: Est. 1970.
Number of Clients Served: More than 6,700.
Eligibility: Anyone who cannot read, hold, or turn the pages of a regular print book due to visual or physical impairment.

Area Served: State of Tennessee.

MEDIA PRODUCTION SERVICES

Clover Bottom Developmental Center

275 Stewarts Ferry Pike
Nashville, TN 37214
(615) 231-5000
Steve Roth, Superintendent

County/District Where Located:
Davidson County.
Groups Served: None specified.

Types/Content: None specified.
Media Formats: Talking books/cassettes, large print books.
Title Listings: None specified.

Middle Tennessee Reception Center

7177 Cockrill Bend Industrial
Nashville, TN 37243-0470
(615) 741-4840
Mike Slaughter, Unit Manager

Groups Served: K-12, college students, other adults.

Types/Content: Textbooks, recreational, career/vocational, religious, general.
Media Formats: Braille books.

Recording for the Blind and Dyslexic

205 Badger Road
Oak Ridge, TN 37830
(423) 482-3496
FAX: (423) 483-9934
E-mail: tennessee@rfbd.org
Sherrie Shuler, Executive Director

County/District Where Located:
Anderson County.

See Recording for the Blind and Dyslexic in U.S. national listings.

Temple Israel Sisterhood

1376 East Massey Street

Memphis, TN 38120
(901) 761-3130
FAX: (901) 761-1448
Doris S. Kiersky, Chairperson,
Services to the Blind

County/District Where Located:
Shelby County.
Groups Served: K-12; college
students; other adults.

Types/Content: Textbooks;
recreational; career/vocational;
religious; personal requests.
Media Formats: Braille books.
Title Listings: Braille lists
supplied at no charge.

Tennessee Library for the Blind and Physically Handicapped

403 Seventh Avenue North
Nashville, TN 37243-0313
(615) 741-3915 or toll-free in
Tennessee (800) 342-3308
E-mail: mmarkham@mail.state.tn.
us
Mary Lou Markham, Librarian

Area Served: Tennessee.
Groups Served: Visually and
physically handicapped residents
of Tennessee.

Types/Content: Recreational and
informational reading.
Media Formats: Braille books,
talking books/cassettes and large-
print books.
Title Listings: No title listings
available.

RADIO READING

The Talking Library
700 Second Avenue
Nashville, TN 37210
(615) 862-5874
FAX: (615) 862-5796
Jim Stanford, Manager, Talking
Library

County/District Where Located:
Davidson County.

Hours of Operation: 24 hours a
day, 7 days a week.
History/Date: Est. 1975.
Area Served: 100-mile radius from
Nashville (43 counties in middle
Tennessee).

WYPL-FM

1850 Peabody Avenue
Memphis, TN 38104
(901) 725-8833
FAX: (901) 725-8814
E-mail: wypl@memphis.lib.tn.us
URL: http://
www.memphislibrary.lib.tn.us
Steven C. Terry, Sr., Station
Manager

County/District Where Located:
Shelby County.
Hours of Operation: Mon.-Sun.
6:00 AM-12:00 midnight.
Staff: 4 full-time, 9 part-time,
volunteer readers.
History/Date: Est. 1980.
Area Served: 21 counties in west
Tennessee.

INFORMATION AND REFERRAL

Prevent Blindness Tennessee
95 White Bridge Road
Suite 513
Nashville, TN 37205
(615) 352-0450
FAX: (616) 352-5750
E-mail: 104706.1101@compuserve.
com
Alice Orr, Executive Director

County/District Where Located:
Davidson County.

See Prevent Blindness America in
U.S. national listings.

◆ Rehabilitation Services

STATE SERVICES

**Services for the Blind and
Visually Impaired
Tennessee Division of
Rehabilitation Services**
Citizens Plaza Building, 11th Floor
400 Deaderick Street
Nashville, TN 37248-6200
(615) 313-4914
FAX: (615) 741-6508
Terry C. Smith, Director, Services
for the Blind and Visually
Impaired

Type of Agency: State, a division
of the Department of Human
Services.
Mission: Services for totally blind,
legally blind, visually impaired
and deaf-blind persons.
Funded by: Fees; state and federal
funds.
Hours of Operation: Mon.-Fri.
8:00 AM-4:30 PM.
Staff: 81 full-time staff working
with visually impaired clients.
Uses volunteers.
History/Date: Est. 1943.
Number of Clients Served: 1,750.
Eligibility: Severely visually
impaired or with bilaterally
progressive vision.
Area Served: State of Tennessee.
Transportation: Y.

Health: Diagnosis and evaluation
of eye health; treatment of eye
condition; follow-up evaluation of
eye treatment or prescription.
**Counseling/Social Work/Self-
Help:** Social evaluation;
individual, group, family/parent,
couple counseling; placement in
school, training; referral to
community services. Contracts,
refers and provides consultation to
other agencies for other
counseling/social work services.

Educational: Non-graded. Accepts deaf-blind; learning disabled; mentally retarded. Programs for adult continuing education; college prep; general academic; vocational/skill development.
Preschools: Direct services provided by rehabilitation teachers.
Professional Training: Internship/fieldwork placement in low vision; orientation/mobility; rehabilitation counseling; vocational rehabilitation. Regular in-service training programs, short-term or summer, open to enrollment from other agencies.
Reading: Reader services provided to clients who are in college or other training programs. Some services may be coordinated with state library.
Residential: Dormitories available at Tennessee Rehabilitation Center.
Rehabilitation: Vocational rehabilitation services; personal management; braille; handwriting; listening skills; typing; low vision services; technology-related services; vocational training; orientation/mobility; rehabilitation teaching in client's home and community. Refers for other rehabilitation services.
Recreational: Provided at Tennessee Rehabilitation Center. Refers for other recreational services.
Employment: Prevocational evaluation; career and skill counseling; sheltered workshops; vocational placement; follow-up service; vending facility training. Contracts and provides consultation to other agencies for other employment services.
Computer Training: Evaluation and training on computer aids and devices.
Low Vision: Prescription and provision of spectacles or low vision aids.

Low Vision Aids: Glasses and aids available.
Low Vision Follow-up: Y.

Local Offices:

Chattanooga: 311 Martin Luther King, Jr. Boulevard, Chattanooga, TN 37403, (423) 634-6735, Sandy Booher, Regional Supervisor.
Columbia: 209 Waynes Street, P.O. Box 457, Columbia, TN 38401, (615) 380-2563, Patti Bell, Regional Supervisor.
Cookeville: 444 Neal Street, Cookeville, TN 38561, (615) 526-9783, Sandy Booher, Regional Supervisor.
Dyersburg: 1979 St. John Avenue, Dyersburg, TN 38024, (901) 285-4220, Kathy Edwards, Regional Supervisor.
Jackson: 225 Martin Luther King Boulevard, Suite 104-A, Jackson, TN 38301, (901) 423-5606, Kathy Edwards, Regional Supervisor.
Johnson City: 905 Buffalo Street, Johnson City, TN 37604, (423) 434-6937, Clyde T. Bible, Regional Supervisor.
Knoxville: 531 Henley Street, Suite 204, Knoxville, TN 37902, (423) 594-6054, Cher Bosch, Regional Supervisor.
Memphis: 170 North Main Street, Memphis, TN 38103, (901) 543-7578, Angie Respess, Regional Supervisor.
Nashville: 88 Hermitage Avenue, Nashville, TN 37210, (615) 532-4851, Stan Long, Regional Supervisor.
Shelbyville: P.O. Box 496, 1304 Railroad Avenue, Shelbyville, TN 37160, (615) 685-5019, Patti Bell, Regional Supervisor.
Smyrna: Tennessee Rehabilitation Center, 460 Ninth Avenue, Smyrna, TN 37167, (615) 741-4921, Gale Demmick, Supervisor of Visually Impaired Services.

REHABILITATION

Alliance for the Blind and Visually Impaired
220 Overton Avenue
P.O. Box 111274
Memphis, TN 38111-1274
(901) 577-7800
FAX: (901) 577-3613
Deborah Cotney, President, Senior Services
Kim Bishop, Program Director

Type of Agency: Private; non-profit.
Mission: Primary, vocational and non-vocational services to blind and visually impaired persons.
Funded by: Community grants and donations; state funding.
Budget: $350,000.
Hours of Operation: Mon.-Fri. 8:15 AM-4:30 PM.
Staff: 5.5. Uses volunteers.
History/Date: Est. 1983.
Number of Clients Served: More than 200.
Eligibility: Severe visual impairment that limits independence.
Area Served: Greater Memphis and surrounding counties.
Age Requirements: Serves all ages.

Health: Refers for health services.
Counseling/Social Work/Self-Help: Individual, group and family counseling; referral to community services. Refers for other counseling/social work services. Provides consultation to other agencies.
Educational: Provides in-service tranining. Contracts with public schools.
Preschools: Consultation and contract assessment and instruction.
Professional Training: Orientation and mobility; rehabilitation teaching.

Reading: Tutorial assistance.
Rehabilitation: Provides vocational rehabilitation services. Provides consultation to other agencies.
Recreational: Refers for recreation services. Provides consultation to other agencies. Periodically provides planned group activities.
Employment: Refers for employment services.
Computer Training: Computer Training Center.
Low Vision: Assessment; dispense nonprescription devices.
Low Vision Aids: Aids recommended and dispensed.
Low Vision Follow-up: Provided as necessary.

Local Offices:

Memphis: 4700 Poplar Avenue, Suite 100, Memphis, TN 38117.

Ed Lindsey Industries for the Blind

4110 Charlotte Avenue
Nashville, TN 37209
(615) 741-2251
FAX: (615) 741-5024
W. Allen Broughton, Executive Vice President
Tonya Craft, Rehabilitation Manager

Type of Agency: Non-profit.
Mission: To provide employment for visually impaired persons.
Funded by: Lions Club, donations, state of Tennessee.
Budget: $1,394,991.
Hours of Operation: Mon.-Fri. 7:30 AM-4:30 PM.
History/Date: Est. 1982.
Number of Clients Served: 82.
Eligibility: Central visual acuity does not exceed 20/200 in the better eye with correcting lenses or whose visual acuity if better than 20/200 is accompanied by a limit to the field of vision in the better eye to such a degree that its widest diameter subtends an angle no greater than 20°.
Area Served: Tennessee.
Age Requirements: 18 years and older.

Rehabilitation: Rehabilitation program to train and place visually impaired persons.
Employment: Provides employment to the blind and legally blind persons.

Lions Volunteer Blind Industries

758 West Morris Boulevard
Morristown, TN 37815
(423) 586-3922
FAX: (423) 586-1479
Fred Overbay, Executive Director

Type of Agency: Private; non-profit.
County/District Where Located: Washington County.
Mission: Provides gainful employment for blind workers.
Funded by: Sales.
Budget: $300,000.
Hours of Operation: Mon.-Fri. 8:00 AM-4:30 PM.
Staff: 31.
History/Date: Est. 1987.
Eligibility: Legally blind.
Area Served: Tennessee.
Transportation: Y.
Age Requirements: 18-65 years.

Local Offices:

Donalson: 115 Stewarts Ferry Pike, Donalson, TN 37214.
Johnson City: 2232 Watauga Road, Johnson City, TN 37601, (423) 927-7008.

Tennessee Rehabilitation Center Visually Impaired Services

460 Ninth Avenue
Smyrna, TN 37167-2010
(615) 741-4921
FAX: (615) 355-1373
Gayle Demmik, Director

Type of Agency: State.
Mission: Comprehensive rehabilitation and referral services.
Funded by: Federal and state funds.
Hours of Operation: Residential facility.
Staff: 10.
History/Date: Est. 1985.
Number of Clients Served: Fiscal year 1991-92: approximately 145 clients.
Eligibility: Blind or visually impaired; Tennessee resident.
Area Served: Entire state of Tennessee.
Transportation: Y.
Age Requirements: 17 years or older.

Health: Occupational/physical/speech therapy.
Counseling/Social Work/Self-Help: Psychological testing and evaluation; individual/group counseling.
Educational: Adult continuing education; vocational/skill development.
Preschools: Child care for clients who are day students.
Residential: Dormitory for multiply handicapped adults.
Rehabilitation: Daily living/communication skills; orientation/mobility; sensory training; low vision; braille.
Recreational: Arts/crafts; hobbies; bowling; swimming; evenings/weekends.
Employment: Evaluation; counseling; training; refers for placement in sheltered workshops and vocational placements.
Computer Training: Adaptive technology for visually impaired persons to access computers.
Low Vision Aids: Spectacles and aids loaned, issued.
Low Vision Follow-up: Referred as needed.

VITAL (Visually Impaired Training and Learning) Center

1302 South Willow Street
P.O. Box 3467
Chattanooga, TN 37404
(423) 624-0025
FAX: (423) 624-1226
Michael Bliss, Executive Director

Type of Agency: Private; non-profit.
Mission: To provide professional rehabilitation services to blind and visually impaired individuals.
Funded by: Fees, state and local funds, foundations, fund raising, and bequests.
Budget: $270,000.
Hours of Operation: Mon.-Fri. 8:30 AM-4:30 PM.
Program Accessibility: Accessible for all disabilities.
Staff: 6.
History/Date: Founded 1987.
Eligibility: Blind or visually impaired individuals.
Area Served: Middle Tennessee and northern Kentucky.
Transportation: Y.
Age Requirements: All ages.

Health: Low vision clinic. Sells low vision devices, independent living aids and appliances.
Counseling/Social Work/Self-Help: Sight loss discussion groups, family program, information and referral.
Educational: Contract services available for area schools and agencies.
Preschools: Contract services available for area schools and agencies.
Professional Training: University intern program. Low vision training for ophthalmology residents.
Reading: Talking book information and referral.
Residential: Day facility.
Rehabilitation: Orientation and mobility, adapted living skills, and communications.
Recreational: Social activities. Sports program.
Employment: Adaptive Employment Program (AEP), progressive program to train and assist in the placement of visually impaired individuals in jobs in the community. On-site job analysis for employers.
Computer Training: Access; training on adaptive computers.
Low Vision: Low vision evaluation by appointment.
Low Vision Aids: Available for training and purchase.
Low Vision Follow-up: 6 month follow-up or as needed.

VITAL (Visually Impaired Training and Learning) Center of Nashville

P.O. Box 121498
Nashville, TN 37212-1498
(615) 321-3773
FAX: (615) 321-4092
Carlene Lebous, President

Type of Agency: Private; non-profit.
County/District Where Located: Davidson County.
Mission: To provide professional rehabilitation services to blind and visually impaired individuals.
Funded by: Fees and contractual services.
Budget: $325,000.
Hours of Operation: Mon.-Fri. 8:30 AM-4:30 PM.
Program Accessibility: Accessible for all disabilities.
Staff: 7.
History/Date: Est. 1992.
Number of Clients Served: 250 annually.
Eligibility: Blind or visually impaired individuals.
Area Served: Middle Eastern Tennessee and Southern Kentucky.
Transportation: Y.
Age Requirements: All ages.

Health: Low vision clinic. Sells low vision devices, independent living aids and appliances.
Counseling/Social Work/Self-Help: Sight loss discussion groups, family program, information and referral.
Educational: Contract services available for area schools and agencies.
Preschools: Contract services available for area schools and agencies.
Professional Training: University intern program.
Reading: Talking book and radio reading service information and referral.
Residential: Day facility.
Rehabilitation: Orientation and mobility, adapted living skills, and communications.
Employment: Adaptive Employment Program (AEP), progressive program to train and assist in the placement of visually impaired individuals in jobs in the community. On-site job analysis for employers.
Computer Training: Access; training on adaptive computers.
Low Vision: Low vision evaluation by appointment.
Low Vision Aids: Available for training and purchase.
Low Vision Follow-up: 6 month follow-up or as needed.

Volunteer Blind Industries

758 West Morris Boulevard
Morristown, TN 37815-0706
(615) 586-3922
Fred Overbay, Executive Director

Type of Agency: Private; non-profit.

County/District Where Located:
Hamblen County.
Mission: Offer rehabilitation
services and gainful employment.
Funded by: Fees; workshop sales;
capital income.
Budget: $300,000 (Rehabilitation
Department).
Hours of Operation: Mon.-Fri.
8:00 AM-4:30 PM.
Program Accessibility: Y.
Staff: 13 full time.
History/Date: Est. 1951.
Number of Clients Served: More
than 100 (rehabilitation); 150
workshop employers.
Eligibility: Legally blind or
visually impaired.
Area Served: Tennessee.
Transportation: Y.
Age Requirements: 18 and older.

Health: Referrals to eye health
services.
Educational: Programs for deaf-
blind persons; for adult continuing
education; vocational/skill
development.
Reading: Distributes talking book
record players and cassette
players; talking book records and
cassettes; braille books; large print
books; braille magazines.
Information and referral.
Residential: Y.
Rehabilitation: Personal
management; braille; gesticulation;
handwriting; Optacon; typing;
video magnifiers; home
management; rehabilitation
teaching in client's home and
community; remedial education;
orientation/mobility.
Employment: Prevocational
evaluation; occupational skill
development; job retention; job
retraining; sheltered workshops;
vocational placement.
Computer Training: Basic skills;
sensory aids technology.
Low Vision: Evaluation; training
in use of low vision aids.

Low Vision Aids: Y.

COMPUTER TRAINING CENTERS

Tennessee Rehabilitation Center
460 Ninth Avenue
Smyrna, TN 37167-2010
(615) 741-4921
FAX: (615) 355-1373
Cynthia Andersen, Sensory Aids
Specialist

Computer Training: Speech
output systems; screen
magnification systems; braille
access systems; optical character
recognition systems; closed-circuit
television systems; word
processing; computer operating
systems; assessments for
educational and vocational
programs.

Tennessee School for the Blind
115 Stewarts Ferry Pike
Nashville, TN 37214
(615) 231-7300
Ralph A. Brewer, Superintendent

Computer Training: Speech
output systems; screen
magnification systems; braille
access systems; closed-circuit
television systems; word
processing; database software.

♦ Low Vision Services

EYE CARE SOCIETIES

**Tennessee Academy of
Ophthalmology**
P.O. Box 681806
Franklin, TN 37068-1806
(615) 794-1851
James C. Fleming, M.D., President
Sue Chasteen, Executive Director

**Tennessee Optometric
Association, Inc.**
3200 West End Avenue, Suite 402
Nashville, TN 37203
(615) 269-9092 or (800) 451-2438
Gary Odom

LOW VISION CENTERS

**Erlanger Medical Center
Lions Low Vision Service**
970 East Third Street
Chattanooga, TN 37403
(423) 778-4000
FAX: (423) 778-4050
Deborah D. DiStefano, M.D.,
Department Director

Type of Agency: Non-profit.
County/District Where Located:
Hamilton County.
Funded by: Lions Club.
Hours of Operation: Mon.-Fri.
8:00 AM-5:00 PM.
Staff: Low vision assistant;
ophthalmic resident;
ophthalmologist.

Low Vision Aids: Assistance for
patients ordering from optical
shop.

Southern College of Optometry
1245 Madison Avenue
Memphis, TN 38104
(901) 725-0180 or (901) 722-3200,
ext. 274
FAX: (901) 722-3275
E-mail: teubank@sco.edu
Tressa Eubank, O.D., Low Vision
Clinic

Type of Agency: Non-profit.
County/District Where Located:
Shelby County.
Mission: To provide low vision
rehabilitation services for persons
of all ages.
Funded by: Client fees.
Hours of Operation: Mon.-Fri.
10:00AM-4:00PM.
Staff: Optometrist; optometry
student/resident.

Number of Clients Served: 200 annually.
Eligibility: None.
Area Served: Unlimited.
Age Requirements: None.

Computer Training: Access; training on computer aids and devices.
Low Vision: Comprehensive low vision evaluation performed by optometrist with student assistance.
Low Vision Aids: Provided on loan for trial period at no charge; sold at cost; prescribed and fitted for variable charge. On-site and in-home training provided.
Low Vision Follow-up: By return appointment.

White Station Lions Foundation
P.O. Box 240123
Memphis, TN 38124
(901) 767-5466
Gene Williams, Acting Executive Director

Type of Agency: Private; non-profit.
County/District Where Located: Shelby County.
Mission: Serves as a clearinghouse to provide low vision and visually impaired persons with referrals to medical and service organizations.

Low Vision: Evaluation and referral.

♦ *Aging Services*

STATE UNITS ON AGING

Commission on Aging
500 Deaderick Street
Ninth Floor
Andrew Jackson Building

Nashville, TN 37243-0860
(615) 741-2056
FAX: (615) 741-3309
Emily Wiseman, Executive Director

Provides referrals to Area Agencies on Aging and information and other local aging services.

INDEPENDENT LIVING PROGRAMS

Tennessee Department of Human Services
Division of Rehabilitation Services
400 Deaderick Street
Nashville, TN 37248
(615) 313-4921 or (800) 628-7818
Julia Hinds, Program Director

Provides independent living services for persons age 55 and over. For further information, contact the Project Director or general phone number listed.

TEXAS

◆ *Educational Services*

STATE SERVICES

Texas Education Agency
1701 North Congress Avenue
Austin, TX 78701
(512) 463-9414
FAX: (512) 475-9560
URL: http://
www.tea.state.tx.us/special.ed/
spec~main.ahtm
Ms. Marty Murrell, Director of
Programs for Students with Visual
Impairments

Type of Agency: State.
County/District Where Located:
Travis County.
Mission: Administers state funds
for education and related services
to students with visual,
impairments from birth through
age 21. Provides consultation, and
other support for education
programs. Interfaces with other
public education services and
other agencies serving disabled
persons. Provides state adopted
braille, large print textbooks to
students with visual impairment.
Funded by: Public funds.
Hours of Operation: 8:00 AM-
5:00 PM.
Area Served: Statewide.

EARLY INTERVENTION COORDINATION

**Early Childhood Program
Texas Department of Health**
4900 North Lamar Boulevard
Austin, TX 78756
(512) 424-6745
FAX: (512) 424-6833
Mary Elder, Executive Director

Type of Agency: State.
Mission: Services for children:
screening and assessment;
physical, occupational, speech, and
language therapy; activities to
develop cognitive and (adaptive)
skills; adaptive equipment;
transportation. Families are served
through: case management;
training on how to help their
children; counseling; support
groups.
Funded by: State funds.
Eligibility: Children under age 3
with a developmental delay or a
medically diagnosed condition
known to lead to delay.
Area Served: Texas.
Transportation: Y.
Age Requirements: Under age 3.

SCHOOLS

**Texas School for the Blind and
Visually Impaired**
1100 West 45th Street
Austin, TX 78756
(512) 454-8631
FAX: (512) 454-3395
Philip Hatlen, Superintendent

Type of Agency: State.
County/District Where Located:
Travis County.
Funded by: Public funds.
Budget: 1997: $11,073,314.
Hours of Operation: 24 hours/
day.
Staff: 416 full time and part time.
History/Date: Est. 1856.
Number of Clients Served: 96:
420.
Eligibility: Visually impaired,
resident of Texas.
Area Served: Texas.
Transportation: Y.
Age Requirements: 5-22 years.

Health: Medical,
ophthalmological, and dental
treatment for students.

**Counseling/Social Work/Self-
Help:** Family counseling;
psychological testing; consultation
and referral.
Educational: Elementary through
secondary level for blind children,
including those who are multiply
disabled and deaf-blind; summer
school programs. Vocational
evaluations for public school
students; educational assessments
for all visually impaired students;
early childhood outreach program
statewide.
Professional Training: Summer
programs; college-level
coursework on campus.
Residential: Home-style living
facilities and group homes for
elementary, secondary and deaf-
blind students.
Rehabilitation: Orientation/
mobility; home management;
personal management;
communications; occupational
therapy; physical therapy.
Recreational: Afterschool and
weekend activities.
Employment: Evaluation;
prevocational and vocational
training.
Computer Training: Speech
output systems, screen
magnification systems, braille
access systems, and word
processing.
Low Vision: Low vision clinic.

INFANT AND PRESCHOOL

**Dallas Services for Visually
Impaired Children**
4242 Office Parkway
Dallas, TX 75204
(214) 828-9900
FAX: (214) 828-9901
Robert Berger, Executive Director
Carol Danielson, Education
Director

Type of Agency: Private; non-
profit.

County/District Where Located: Dallas County.

Mission: To provide comprehensive family-focused services to families who have a child with developmental delays, including visual impairment.

Funded by: Private donations, state, federal funds, United Way.

Hours of Operation: 7:00 AM-6:00 PM.

Staff: 16 full time (visually handicapped, early childhood, severely handicapped teachers; physical therapist; orientation/mobility specialists); occupational therapists, speech pathologists, social workers. Uses volunteers. Advisory board with parent members.

History/Date: Est. 1950.

Eligibility: Visually handicapped children ages 0-3, with or without other handicaps.

Area Served: Dallas, Tarrant, and surrounding counties.

Transportation: Y.

Age Requirements: 0-5 years.

Health: Adaptive equipment; functional vision exams; medical evaluations; immunizations.

Counseling/Social Work/Self-Help: Parent and other counseling; financial assistance; case management; family-focused early childhood intervention parent component.

Educational: Provides instruction in all developmental areas; consultant services to other specialized programs, and inclusive settings.

Preschools: Home- and center-based programs for developmentally delayed, including visually handicapped, children, 0-5 years. Inclusive day care facility.

Professional Training: Professional development and parent workshops on working with preschool aged visually impaired children.

Low Vision: Clinic on-site.

Low Vision Aids: Training in use of aids available.

Low Vision Follow-up: Yes.

Developmental Education Birth through Two (DEBT Project)

1628 19th Street
Lubbock, TX 79401
(806) 766-1172
FAX: (806) 766-1286
Laura Kender, Coordinator

Type of Agency: Public school program.

County/District Where Located: Lubbock County.

Funded by: Local funds, state funds for Early Education. Federal Part H IDEA funds, Early Education Program Outreach grant, Title IV-B, private donations.

Staff: 45 full-time equivalents. Various therapists and specialists available as consultants. Uses volunteers. Advisory board with parent members.

History/Date: Est. 1973.

Number of Clients Served: 330.

Eligibility: Developmentally delayed children aged 0-2 years.

Area Served: Lubbock Independent School District. Expanded program serving 12-county rural areas in western Texas.

Transportation: Y.

Age Requirements: 0-2 years.

Health: Adaptive equipment; medical evaluations; nutrition; services necessary to enable a child to benefit from the other early intervention services.

Counseling/Social Work/Self-Help: Parent counseling; financial assistance; skill-building opportunities for parents; service coordination.

Educational: Provides instruction in developmental areas. Home-based activities and consultant services for visually impaired, multihandicapped, and other disabled children, 0-2 years.

STATEWIDE OUTREACH SERVICES

Texas School for the Blind and Visually Impaired

1100 West 45th Street
Austin, TX 78756
(512) 206-9242
FAX: (512) 206-9320
E-mail: cmiller@tenet
Cyral Miller, Director of Outreach

Funded by: State and federal funds.

History/Date: Est. deaf-blind program in 1981; expanded to a separate Outreach Department in 1990 to serve all students with visual impairments.

Age Requirements: Students from 0-22 years, their families, and related service providers.

Assessment: Technology evaluation; assistance in training assessment personnel on appropriate evaluation techniques.

Consultation to Public Schools: On-site consultation regarding programming for identified students as well as organization of overall delivery of services.

Direct Service: Technical assistance to local personnel rather than direct provision of educational instruction.

Parent Assistance: Parent training; resources and information; support for parent groups; financial assistance to attend workshops.

Professional Training: Offer local, regional, and statewide workshops and conferences both as sponsor and in coordination with other organizations.

INSTRUCTIONAL MATERIALS CENTERS

Texas Instructional Materials Center for Students with Visual Handicaps/Texas Education Agency
Texas School for the Blind and Visually Impaired
1100 West 45th Street
Austin, TX 78756
(512) 206-9335
FAX: (512) 206-9320
E-mail: necaise@tenet.edu
Nick Necaise, Visually Handicapped Program Consultant

County/District Where Located: Travis County.
Area Served: Texas.
Groups Served: Local school districts.

Title Listings: Titles available through quota funds listed in catalogs from the American Printing House for the Blind.

UNIVERSITY TRAINING PROGRAMS

Stephen F. Austin State University
SFA Station, Box 13019
Nacogdoches, TX 75962
(409) 468-2906
FAX: (409) 468-1342
Robert Bryant, Orientation and Mobility, (409) 468-1220
William Bryan, Visually Handicapped, Dual Competency, (409) 468-1036

County/District Where Located: Nacogdoches County.

Programs Offered: Undergraduate programs for teachers of the visually impaired, orientation and mobility specialists, dual competency teachers of the visually impaired/orientation and mobility.

Texas Tech University
College of Education
Box 41071
Lubbock, TX 79409-1071
(806) 742-2320 or (806) 742-2345
FAX: (806) 742-2179 or (806) 742-1331
E-mail: vpvms@ttacs.ttu.edu
Dr. Virginia Sowell, Orientation and Mobility and Visual Impairment
Dr. Alan Koenig, Coordinator of Programs
Dr. Roseanna Davidson, Dual Sensory Impairment
Dr. Nora Griffin-Shirley, Orientation and Mobility
Dr. Pat Kelley, Orientation and Mobility and Visual Impairment

Programs Offered: Graduate (master's, doctoral) programs for teachers of students with visual impairments and multiple disabilities and students with dual sensory impairments and for orientation and mobility specialists. Certification-only and summer coursework also offered.
Distance Education: Y.

University of Texas at Austin
Special Education Department, EDB 306
Austin, TX 78712
(512) 471-4161
FAX: (512) 471-4061
URL: http://www.utexas.edu/depts/oandm/
Dr. Brad Walker, Orientation and Mobility

Programs Offered: Certification (post bachelor's) and graduate (master's, doctoral) programs for teachers of the visually impaired or multiply disabled students. Additional coursework in early childhood available. Other areas of special education and rehabilitation and transitional programming.

Distance Education: Y.

◆ Information Services

LIBRARIES

Texas State Library
Talking Book Program
Capitol Station
P.O. Box 12927
Austin, TX 78711
(512) 463-5458 or toll-free in Texas (800) 252-9605
FAX: (512) 463-5436
E-mail: tbp.services@tsl.state.tx.us
URL: http://link.tsl.state.tx.us
Dale Propp, Director

County/District Where Located: Travis County.
Mission: Provide free library service to Texans who, because of a visual, physical, or learning disability, are unable to read standard print material.
Funded by: Public funds.
Hours of Operation: Mon.-Fri. 8:00 AM-5:00 PM.
Program Accessibility: Y.
Staff: 52 full-time.
History/Date: Est. 1931.
Number of Clients Served: 25,000.
Eligibility: Certified application required.
Area Served: Texas.

Disability Reference Center available to provide information and make referrals.

Regional library providing talking books, braille and large type books, cassette books.

MEDIA PRODUCTION SERVICES

Dallas Services for the Visually Impaired
4242 Office Parkway
Dallas, TX 75204
(214) 828-9900
FAX: (214) 828-9901
Mike Palise, Braille Manager

County/District Where Located: Dallas County.
Area Served: Texas.
Groups Served: None specified.

Types/Content: None specified.
Media Formats: Braille books.
Title Listings: None specified.

Lighthouse of Houston
3530 West Dallas Avenue
P.O. Box 130435
Houston, TX 77219-0435
(713) 527-9561 or (713) 527-8165
FAX: (713) 527-8165
Brenda Parsell, Director of Braille Services
Gibson M. DuTerroil, President

Area Served: Greater Houston and southwestern Texas.
Groups Served: K-12, college students, other adults.

Types/Content: Textbooks, career/vocational, menus, cards, general.
Media Formats: Braille/large print books.
Title Listings: No title listings available.

North Texas Taping and Radio for the Blind
3001 Bookhout
Dallas, TX 75201
(214) 871-7668
FAX: (214) 871-7669
Betty Hersey, Executive Director
Sharon Komorn, Recorded Books Manager

County/District Where Located: Dallas County.
Area Served: Statewide.
Groups Served: K-12, college students, other adults, educational institutions.

Types/Content: Textbooks, career/vocational, general books other than recreational.
Media Formats: Talking books/cassettes.
Title Listings: Catalogs available.

Reading agency for Library of Congress Talking Book program.

Recording for the Blind and Dyslexic
404 West 30th Street
Austin, TX 78705
(512) 323-9390
FAX: (512) 323-9399
E-mail: rfbdtex@io.com
URL: http://www.satori3.com/rfbd
Kathy Keegan-Davis

County/District Where Located: Travis County.

See Recording for the Blind and Dyslexic in U.S. national lisitings.

Recording Library for the Blind and Physically Handicapped
2012 Cuthbert Street
Midland, TX 79701
(915) 682-2731
Sandy Davis, Executive Director

Area Served: Texas.
Groups Served: K-12, college students and adults.

Types/Content: Textbooks, recreational, career/vocational, religious, as requested.
Media Formats: Talking books/cassettes.
Title Listings: None specified.

Region IV Education Service Center
7145 West Tidwell
Houston, TX 77092
(713) 744-8144
FAX: (713) 744-8148
E-mail: dspence@tenet.edu
Diane Spence, Director, Computer Braille Center

Groups Served: K-12.

Types/Content: Textbooks, tests, supplementary materials.
Media Formats: Braille books.
Title Listings: Computer disk listing at no charge.

Texas State Library Talking Book Program
P.O. Box 12927
Austin, TX 78711-2927
(512) 463-5458 or toll-free in Texas (800) 252-9605
FAX: (512) 463-5436
E-mail: tbp.services@tsl.state.tx.us
Donald Brower, Audio Operations
Sara Stiffler, Recording Studio
Patsy Alvarez, Recording Studio

County/District Where Located: Travis County.
Area Served: Texas.
Groups Served: K-12, college students, other adults.

Types/Content: Recreational.
Media Formats: Talking books/cassettes.
Title Listings: Print and braille lists available at no charge.

Braille production and recordings at cost.

RADIO READING

El Paso Radio Reading Service
200 Washington Street
El Paso, TX 79905
(915) 532-4495
FAX: (915) 532-6338
Grant Downey, Executive Director

County/District Where Located:
El Paso County.
Hours of Operation: Mon.-Fri.
11:00 AM-7:00 PM.
History/Date: Est. 1980.
Area Served: 60-mile radius from
El Paso serving western Texas and
south central New Mexico.

**Houston Taping for the Blind
Radio**
3935 Essex Lane
Houston, TX 77027
(713) 622-2767
FAX: (713) 622-2767
E-mail: 102677.2656@compuserve.
com
Beth O'Callaghan, Executive
Director
Bill Albers, Manager of Radio

County/District Where Located:
Harris County.
Funded by: Private donations.
Hours of Operation: 24 hours,
daily.
Staff: 3.
History/Date: Est. 1978.
Area Served: 33 counties in
southeast Texas.

KUT 90.5FM
Communications Building B
University of Texas at Austin
Austin, TX 78712
(512) 471-4683
Michael Lee, Producer
David Alvarez, Director

County/District Where Located:
Travis County.
Hours of Operation: Mon.-Sat.
9:00 AM-1:00 PM; Sun. 8:00 AM-
12:00 noon.
History/Date: Est. 1980.
Area Served: 42-mile radius from
Austin; 87-mile radius from central
Texas.

**North Texas Taping and Radio
for the Blind**
3001 Bookhout
Dallas, TX 75201
(214) 871-7668
FAX: (214) 871-7669
Betty Hersey, Executive Director
Dick Jenkins, Station Manager

County/District Where Located:
Dallas County.
Funded by: United Way; private
donations.
Hours of Operation: 7 days a
week, 5:00 AM-11:00 PM.
History/Date: Est. 1976.
Area Served: 100-mile radius from
Dallas.

INFORMATION AND REFERRAL

**American Foundation for the
Blind Southwest**
260 Treadway Plaza
Exchange Park
Dallas, TX 75235
(214) 352-7222
FAX: (214) 352-3214
E-mail: afbdallas@afb.org
URL: http://www.afb.org

See American Foundation for the
Blind in U.S. national listings.

**The Foundation Fighting
Blindness
Dallas Affiliate**
2053 Vatican Circle
Dallas, TX 75224
(214) 331-5304
Larry Hansen, President

See The Foundation Fighting
Blindness in U.S. national listings.

**The Foundation Fighting
Blindness
Texas Panhandle Affiliate**
Texas Tech University Health and
Sciences Center
Department of Ophthalmology

Lubbock, TX 79430
(806) 743-2412
D. R. Rockefeller Young, Contact
Person

See The Foundation Fighting
Blindness in U.S. national listings.

**Prevent Blindness Texas
Austin Branch**
5555 North Lamar Street, K103
Austin, TX 78751
(512) 459-8936
Diane Ingram, Executive Director
Mary Burion, Program Director

County/District Where Located:
Travis County.

See Prevent Blindness America in
U.S. national listings.

**Prevent Blindness Texas
Dallas Branch**
3610 Fairmont Street
Dallas, TX 75219
(214) 528-5521
FAX: (214) 521-5248
Marilyn Zeok, Executive Director
Linda Ziegler, Program Director

See Prevent Blindness America in
U.S. national listings.

**Prevent Blindness Texas
East Texas Branch**
824 South Beckham
Suite 209
Tyler, TX 75701
(903) 592-2664
FAX: (903) 592-6641
Donna Luker, Executive Director
Amy Gould, Program Director

See Prevent Blindness America in
U.S. national listings.

**Prevent Blindness Texas
El Paso Branch**
7500 Viscount
Suite 108

El Paso, TX 79925
(915) 775-1200
FAX: (915) 779-0643
Carmen Pacheco, Branch Executive
Director

See Prevent Blindness America in
U.S. national listings.

Prevent Blindness Texas
Fort Worth Branch

329 South Henderson
Fort Worth, TX 76104
(817) 332-8125
Debra Johnson, Executive Director
Len Langham, Program Director

See Prevent Blindness America in
U.S. national listings.

Prevent Blindness Texas
Galveston/Gulf Coast Branch

P.O. Box 2050
Galveston, TX 77553
(409) 762-9074
FAX: (409) 765-8475
Janyce Blozinski, Executive
Director

See Prevent Blindness America in
U.S. national listings.

Prevent Blindness Texas
Lubbock Branch

3008 50th Street, Suite E
Lubbock, TX 79413
(806) 797-6701
Lyn Garcia, Program Director

See Prevent Blindness America in
U.S. national listings.

Prevent Blindness Texas
Midland Branch

2303 West Wall, Suite 628
P.O. Box 5325
Midland, TX 79705-5325
(915) 683-0003
Peggy Hards, Program Director
Robin Frerich, Executive Director

See Prevent Blindness America in
U.S. national listings.

Prevent Blindness Texas
San Antonio Branch

10205 Oasis Drive
Suite 202
San Antonio, TX 78216
(210) 342-3292
FAX: (210) 342-3293
Nancy Fassnidge, Executive
Director

See Prevent Blindness America in
U.S. national listings.

Prevent Blindness Texas
State Office

3211 West Dallas Avenue
Houston, TX 77019-3400
(713) 526-2559
FAX: (801) 322-3647
E-mail: 104706.2523@compuserve.
com
Elaine Barber, President and CEO

See Prevent Blindness America in
U.S. national listings.

See also in national listings:

**Austin Junior Women's
Federation**

Christian Education for the Blind

Taping for the Blind

Visual Aid Volunteers, Inc.

◆ *Rehabilitation Services*

STATE SERVICES

Texas Commission for the Blind

Administration Building
4800 North Lamar Boulevard
P.O. Box 12866

Austin, TX 78711
(512) 459-2500 or (800) 252-5204
(voice/TDD)
FAX: (512) 459-2685
Pat D. Westbrook, Executive
Director
Terry Murphy, Deputy Director for
Programs

Type of Agency: State.
Mission: To work in partnership
with Texans who are blind or
visually impaired to reach their
goals.
Funded by: Public funds.
Hours of Operation: Mon.-Fri.
8:00 AM-5:00 PM.
History/Date: Est. 1931.
Area Served: Texas.

Health: Contracts for diagnostic,
medical, and surgical treatment;
low vision clinic.
**Counseling/Social Work/Self-
Help:** Psychological testing;
consultation and referral.
Rehabilitation: Orientation/
mobility; home management;
personal management;
communications.
Employment: Evaluation;
prevocational and vocational
training; placement; vending stand
program; business enterprises
program; follow-up.

Local Offices:

Abilene: 100 Chestnut, Suite 101,
Abilene, TX 79602, (915) 672-1385
(voice/TDD).
Amarillo: Park West, Building B,
7132 Interstate 40 West, Amarillo,
TX 79106, (806) 353-9568 (voice/
TDD).
Austin (North): Administration
Building, 4800 North Lamar,
(Mailing: P.O. Box 12866, Austin,
TX 78711), Austin, TX 78756,
(512) 459-2544 (voice/TDD).
Austin (South): 3001 South
Lamar, Austin, TX 78704,
(512) 326-1441 (voice/TDD).

Beaumont: 3515 Fannin Street, Suite 105, Beaumont, TX 77701, (409) 838-5201 (voice/TDD).

Bryan-College Station: Southwest Professional Building, Suite 110, 1701 Southwest Parkway, College Station, TX 77840, (409) 696-9610 (voice/TDD).

Corpus Christi: 410 South Padre Island Drive, Suite 103, Corpus Christi, TX 78405, (512) 289-1128.

Dallas: 1555 W. Mockingbird Lane, Suite 219, Dallas, TX 75235, (214) 688-7007 (voice/TDD).

El Paso: 1314 Lomaland Drive, El Paso, TX 79935, (915) 590-7388 (voice/TDD).

Fort Worth: 4200 South Freeway, Suite 307, Fort Worth, TX 76115-1404, (817) 926-4646 (voice/TDD).

Galveston: 4607 Fort Crockett Boulevard, #A, Galveston, TX 77551, (409) 763-4441 (voice/TDD).

Harlingen: 513 East Jackson, Harlingen, TX 78550, (210) 423-9411 (voice/TDD).

Houston: Heights Medical Tower, Suite 407, 427 West 20th, Houston, TX 77008, (713) 880-0721 (voice) or TDD (713) 880-8002.

Laredo: 1718 E. Calton Road, Suite 1, Laredo, TX 78041, (210) 723-2955 (voice/TDD).

Lubbock: 5121 69th Street, Suite A-5, Lubbock, TX 79424, (806) 798-8181 (voice/TDD).

Lufkin: 3201 South Medford, Suite 5, Lufkin, TX 75901, (409) 634-7733 (voice/TDD).

Odessa: Building A, Suite 103, 2817 John Ben Sheppard Parkway, Odessa, TX 79762, (915) 368-0881 (voice/TDD).

Pharr: 1899 North Cage, Pharr, TX 78577, (210) 787-7364.

Richardson: 1200 Executive Drive East, #130, Richardson, TX 75081, (972) 889-2500 (voice/TDD).

San Angelo: 2201 Sherwood Way, Suite LL8, San Angelo, TX 76901, (915) 949-4601.

San Antonio: 4204 Woodcock Drive, Suite 274, Trinity Building, San Antonio, TX 78228, (210) 732-9751 (voice/TDD).

Texarkana: 410 Baylor Street, Suite C, Texarkana, TX 75501, (903) 831-3846 (voice/TDD).

Tyler: 1121 East Southeast Loop, 323, Building 1, #106, Woodgate Office Park, Tyler, TX 75701-9638, (903) 581-9945 (voice/TDD).

Victoria: Town Plaza Mall, 1502 E. Airline, #13, Victoria, TX 77901, (512) 575-2352.

Waco: Raleigh Building, 7th Floor, 801 Austin, Waco, TX 76701, (817) 753-1552 (voice/TDD).

Wichita Falls: 3123 Lawrence Road, Suite D, Wichita Falls, TX 76308, (817) 691-8675 (voice/TDD).

REHABILITATION

Beacon Lighthouse for the Blind
300 Seventh Street
Wichita Falls, TX 76301
(817) 767-0888
FAX: (817) 767-0893
A. W. Edgemon, President

Type of Agency: Non-profit.
County/District Where Located: Wichita County.
Funded by: Product sales.
Staff: 5 full time; uses volunteers.
History/Date: Est. 1975.
Eligibility: Legally blind.
Area Served: North central Texas.

Rehabilitation: Independent living rehabilitation provides counseling, daily living skills instruction, self-help groups, casework services, and recreational opportunities for blind, legally blind, deaf-blind and multiply disabled blind adults. Vocational rehabilitation includes vocational evaluation, work adjustment counseling, on-the-job training, therapeutic mobility training, and casework services. Clients should

be referred by the Texas Commission for the Blind.
Employment: Sheltered workshop offers job opportunities in manufacturing plant. Volunteer, intern, and practicum opportunities are available. Supportive employment.

Blind Rehabilitation Center U.S. Department of Veterans Affairs
Central Texas Veterans Health Care System
4800 Memorial Drive
Waco, TX 76711
(817) 752-6581, ext. 7492
FAX: (817) 755-8768
Stan Poel, Chief

Type of Agency: Federal.
Mission: Provides comprehensive residential blind rehabilitation services to eligible legally blind veterans in the central portion of the country.
Hours of Operation: Mon.-Fri. 8:00 AM-4:30 PM.

Referral applications by Visual Impairment Services programs at VA Medical Centers and Outpatient Clinics in the geographical area served by the Blind Rehabilitation Center or Clinic.

See U.S. Department of Veterans Affairs in U.S. Federal Agencies listings.

Dallas Lighthouse for the Blind, Inc.
4245 Office Parkway

Dallas, TX 75204
(214) 821-2375 or TDD (800) 735-2989
FAX: (214) 824-4612
Jeffrey J. Battle, President
Kerry L. Goodwin, Vice President, Rehabilitation Services
Jerry Holcknecht, Vice President, Industrial Division
Richard T. Smith, Vice President, Finance and Administration

Type of Agency: Private; non-profit; NAC accredited.
County/District Where Located: Dallas County.
Mission: To provide opportunities for people with sight disabilities to achieve personal, social and economic independence.
Funded by: Revenues from sales of products; federal and state grants and fees; private contributions; United Way.
Budget: $6.6 million.
Hours of Operation: Mon.-Fri. 8:00 AM-5:00 PM.
Program Accessibility: Bilingual (Spanish/English) and sign language interpreters; readers; brailled, large-print, and taped materials; Kurzweil Reader. Facilities are fully accessible.
Staff: 43 full-time equivalents. Uses volunteers.
History/Date: Est. 1931.
Number of Clients Served: 950 per year.
Eligibility: Totally blind, legally blind, deaf-blind, multiply disabled blind, or severely visually impaired persons.
Area Served: Primarily the following counties in northern central Texas: Collin, Cooke, Dallas, Denton, Ellis, Fannin, Grayson, Hunt, Kaufman, Navarro, and Rockwall.
Transportation: Y.
Age Requirements: At least 16 years old.

Counseling/Social Work/Self-Help: Independent living services include information and referral; assessment and intake; participant support; staff counseling; peer counseling; emergency assistance; home visits; daily living skills instruction; orientation and mobility training; support groups; follow-up.
Residential: Dormitory and transitional housing programs.
Rehabilitation: Vocational rehabilitation services include vocational evaluation; psychological assessment; neuro-psychological evaluation; work adjustment training; on-the-job training; work activities training; extended rehabilitation training; employment readiness training; personal/social adjustment training; supported employment; placement assistance; Kurzweil Reader instruction; school-to-work transition; orientation and mobility training. Clients should be referred by the Texas Commission for the Blind.
Recreational: Instructional classes; fitness activities; social activities; special events; outdoor activities.
Employment: Industrial Division offers training and employment opportunities from hand packaging/assembly to complex machine operations. Agency gives priority to people with sight disabilities in clerical, staff, and managerial positions. Volunteer, intern, and practicum opportunities available.
Computer Training: Technology evaluations and basic technology training services.

Dallas Services for Visually Impaired Children

4242 Office Parkway
Dallas, TX 75204
(214) 828-9900
FAX: (214) 828-9901
Robert H. Berger, Executive Director

Type of Agency: Private; non-profit.
County/District Where Located: Dallas County.
Funded by: United Way; Early Childhood Intervention; Texas Commission for the Blind; contributions; grants; memorials; sliding fee scale.
Budget: $1,750,000.
Hours of Operation: 7:00 AM-6:00 PM.
Staff: 34.
History/Date: Est. 1950.
Eligibility: Visual impairment.
Area Served: Dallas County and surrounding areas.
Age Requirements: 0-21 years.

Health: Low vision training.
Counseling/Social Work/Self-Help: Individual and group counseling; referral.
Reading: Braille transcription.
Rehabilitation: Orientation/mobility; braille; mother-infant class.
Recreational: Summer program for children, 6-22 years.
Low Vision: Evaluations.
Low Vision Aids: Aids, devices and training.
Low Vision Follow-up: Y.

East Texas Lighthouse for the Blind

500 North Bois D'Arc
Tyler, TX 75702
(903) 595-3444
FAX: (903) 595-3447
J. Gordon Bryson, President

Type of Agency: Private; non-profit.
Mission: Services for totally blind and legally blind.

Funded by: Workshop sales; sub-contracts; income from capital funds; fees; donations.

Budget: 1996: $1,400,000.

Hours of Operation: Mon.-Fri. 7:00 AM-5:00 PM.

Staff: 12 full time.

History/Date: Est. 1976.

Number of Clients Served: 1996: 45.

Eligibility: Legally blind.

Area Served: 35 counties of Eastern Texas.

Transportation: Y.

Age Requirements: Over 18 years.

Professional Training: Regular in-service training; short-term or summer training.

Reading: Talking book record players and cassette players; talking book records and tapes; braille books; large-print books; braille magazines; closed-circuit television.

Residential: Dormitory for adults and multiply disabled persons.

Rehabilitation: Personal management; video magnifier.

Recreational: Beep baseball.

Employment: Prevocational evaluation; job retention; job retraining; sheltered workshops. Provides consultation to other agencies on other employment services.

Computer Training: Access.

Low Vision Aids: Low vision clinic available twice monthly.

Local Offices:

Tyler: Client Services Center, 1716 Forest Avenue, Tyler, TX 75702, (214) 595-3444.

El Paso Lighthouse for the Blind
200 Washington
El Paso, TX 79905
(915) 532-4495
FAX: (915) 532-6338
Grant Downey, Executive Director

Type of Agency: Private; non-profit.

County/District Where Located: El Paso County.

Mission: Employment, training, rehabilitation, and technical services for totally blind, legally blind, visually impaired, and deaf persons.

Funded by: Fees; donations; workshop sales; grants.

Budget: $650,000.

Hours of Operation: Mon.-Fri. 8:00 AM-4:30 PM, or by appointment.

Staff: 15 full time. Uses volunteers.

History/Date: Est. 1934.

Number of Clients Served: 2,400 per year (all programs).

Eligibility: Legally blind; vocationally handicapped; by referral.

Area Served: Western Texas, southern New Mexico, northern Mexico.

Transportation: Y.

Age Requirements: None.

Health: Refers for health services.

Counseling/Social Work/Self-Help: Psychological testing and evaluations; individual, family/parent, couple counseling; placement in training; referral to community services.

Professional Training: Internship/fieldwork placement in orientation/mobility; vocational rehabilitation; rehabilitation teaching.

Reading: Lends talking book record players and cassette players. Information and referral. Operates radio reading service in English and Spanish.

Rehabilitation: Personal management; braille; gesticulation; handwriting; listening skills; typing; home management; orientation/mobility; refers for other rehabilitation services;

extensive rehabilitation program for elderly blind persons.

Employment: Full supported employment services. Occupational skill development; sheltered workshops; work activity center. Refers for other employment services.

Computer Training: Complete training program in low vision and speech systems. Training in 14 software packages. Assists in low vision computer vocational evaluations.

Low Vision: Complete low vision clinic with fitting and training.

Low Vision Aids: Loaned for period of 6 weeks. Available for purchase at cost.

Low Vision Follow-up: As needed.

Helen Keller National Center for Deaf-Blind Youths and Adults South Central Region Office
4455 LBJ Freeway, LB#3
Suite 814
Dallas, TX 75244-5998
(972) 490-9677 (voice/TDD)
FAX: (972) 490-6042
C. C. Davis, Regional Representative
Martha Bagley, Services to Older Adults

County/District Where Located: Dallas County.

See Helen Keller National Center for Deaf-Blind Youths and Adults in U.S. national listings.

Lighthouse for the Blind of Fort Worth
912 West Broadway
Fort Worth, TX 76104
(817) 332-3341
FAX: (817) 332-3456
Robert W. Mosteller, President

Type of Agency: Private; non-profit.

County/District Where Located: Tarrant County.
Funded by: Workshop sales, sub-contracts, contributions, endowment, and fees for service.
Budget: $1,000,001.
Hours of Operation: Mon.-Fri. 8:00 AM-5:00 PM.
Program Accessibility: Fully accessible.
Staff: 17 full time. Uses volunteers.
History/Date: Est. 1935.
Number of Clients Served: 1996: 896.
Eligibility: Visually impaired.
Area Served: Tarrant County, northwest central Texas region.
Transportation: N.

Health: Public education.
Counseling/Social Work/Self-Help: Consultation and referral.
Residential: Co-educational living facilities for blind multiply disabled persons.
Rehabilitation: Personal management; orientation/mobility.
Employment: Evaluation; vocational training; placement; work adjustment; manufacturing operation.
Computer Training: Speech output systems; database software.

Lighthouse of Houston

3530 West Dallas Avenue
P.O. Box 130435
Houston, TX 77219-0435
(713) 527-9561
FAX: (713) 527-8165
Gibson M. DuTerroil, President
Shelagh Moran, Vice President of Programs & Services

Type of Agency: Private; non-profit.
County/District Where Located: Harris County.
Mission: Provides vocational rehabilitation evaluations, training, and education programs. Community Services include residential program, skills training, low vision clinic, senior services.
Funded by: Industrial sales; sub-contracts; United Way; fees for service; grants; contributions.
Budget: 1997: $8.6 million.
Hours of Operation: Mon.-Fri. 7:30 AM-4:00 PM.
Staff: 117 full time. Uses volunteers.
History/Date: Est. 1939.
Number of Clients Served: 1996: 4,800.
Eligibility: Blind, legally blind, or deaf-blind.
Area Served: Greater Houston area and southwestern Texas.
Transportation: Y.

Counseling/Social Work/Self-Help: Evaluation; psychological testing; counseling; consultation and referral.
Preschools: Daycare centers.
Professional Training: Internships at the Lighthouse of Houston, University of Houston, and Low Vision Clinic.
Reading: Braille, tape, and large-type books. CCTVs, speech output.
Residential: Deaf-blind group homes, training apartments, 240-unit apartment facilities.
Rehabilitation: Personal management; independent living; clerical, word processing, and medical transcription training; computer programming and literacy; multi-care for elderly blind; orientation/mobility; residential services for deaf-blind adults and children.
Recreational: Outdoor activities; music; arts and crafts; sports and games; special events; cultural arts.
Employment: Vocational assessments and training; employment skills development; placement; high school equivalency.
Computer Training: Access; training on computer aids and devices. Full-service technology training unit.
Low Vision: Low vision clinic.
Low Vision Aids: Provided on loan for trial; on-site training provided.
Low Vision Follow-up: Phone interview.

San Antonio Lighthouse

2305 Roosevelt Avenue
San Antonio, TX 78210
(210) 533-5195
FAX: (210) 533-4230
Bob R. Plunkett, President

Type of Agency: Private; non-profit.
County/District Where Located: Bexar County.
Mission: Services for totally blind; legally blind; visually impaired.
Funded by: Fees; donations; bequests; sales.
Budget: Mon.-Fri. 7:30 AM-4:30 PM.
Staff: 34 full time.
History/Date: Est. 1933.
Number of Clients Served: 500 annually.
Eligibility: Totally blind; legally blind; visually impaired; multiply disabled; self-referral through local state agency.
Area Served: San Antonio and surrounding area.
Age Requirements: High school and up.

Counseling/Social Work/Self-Help: Refers for counseling and other social work services.
Educational: Programs for vocational/skill development.
Reading: Talking book record player and cassette player; talking book records and cassettes; braille

books; large print books; braille magazines; recorded magazines.
Rehabilitation: Vocational evaluation; occupational skill development; job retention; job retraining; personal management; handwriting; typing; orientation/mobility. Refers and contracts for other rehabilitation services.
Employment: Sheltered workshops. Competitive job training and client employment assistance, job readiness, job placement.
Computer Training: Skills training.

South Texas Lighthouse for the Blind

1907 Leopard Street
Corpus Christi, TX 78469
(512) 883-6553 or (512) 883-1041
Eileen Butler, Director of Human Resources

Type of Agency: Private; non-profit.
County/District Where Located: Necues County.
Mission: Services for totally blind; legally blind; visually impaired; deaf-blind; and multiply disabled persons.
Funded by: Fees; workshop sales; sub-contracts; contributions.
Budget: 1997: $13,000,000.
Staff: 35 full-time.
History/Date: Est. 1964.
Eligibility: Legally blind.
Age Requirements: 18 years and older.

Rehabilitation: Sells special aids and appliances at cost; computer training.
Employment: On-the-job training and sheltered workshop employment.
Computer Training: Available.

Texas Commission for the Blind Criss Cole Rehabilitation Center

4800 North Lamar
Austin, TX 78756
(512) 467-6300
FAX: (512) 467-6432
Ed Kunz, Director

Type of Agency: State.
County/District Where Located: Travis County.
Mission: Services for totally blind, legally blind, deaf-blind, learning disabled, and orthopedically disabled persons.
Funded by: Primarily federal funds.
Budget: $3 million.
Hours of Operation: 24 hours a day, 7 days a week.
Program Accessibility: Program accessible in accordance with ADA.
Staff: 100.
History/Date: Est. 1971.
Number of Clients Served: 60.
Eligibility: Clients of the Texas Commission for the Blind; legally or totally blind.
Area Served: Texas.
Transportation: Y.
Age Requirements: 18 years old.

Health: Diagnosis and evaluation of eye health; treatment of eye condition; follow-up evaluation of eye treatment or prescription; audiology therapy; general medical services; occupational therapy and sensory integration; physical therapy. Refers for speech therapy.
Counseling/Social Work/Self-Help: Vocational rehabilitation counseling services; psychiatric evaluation; psychological testing and evaluation; individual, group, family/parent counseling. Refers for other counseling/social work services.
Educational: Accepts all multiply disabled students. Programs for

adult GED; college prep; English as a second language.
Professional Training: Internship/fieldwork placement in orientation/mobility; rehabilitation counseling; social work; special education; teaching; nursing and general rehabilitation. Regular in-service training programs; rehabilitation teacher training.
Reading: Talking book cassette player; talking book cassettes; braille books; large-print books; braille magazines; recorded magazines; information and referral; special collection.
Residential: Dormitories for adults; elderly; multiply handicapped; and on-site apartments for independent living experience.
Rehabilitation: Personal management; braille; sign language; handwriting; listening skills; typing; video magnifier; home and money management; orientation/mobility; sensory training; remedial education; sex education; independent living experience. Refers for rehabilitation teaching in client's home and community.
Recreational: Adult continuing education; evening/weekend programs; arts and crafts; hobby groups; camping; canoeing; hiking; bowling; swimming; track; table games. Community recreation services.
Employment: Prevocational evaluation; career guidance; prevocational skill development. Refers for other employment services. Feasibility studies; business plan development.
Low Vision: Low vision service; prescription and provision of spectacles and low vision aids.

Travis Association for the Blind

P.O. Box 3297

Austin, TX 78764
(512) 442-2329
FAX: (512) 442-5498
Fred M. Weber, Sr., President

Type of Agency: Private; non-profit.
County/District Where Located: Travis County.
Mission: Services for totally blind, legally blind, visually impaired, deaf-blind, learning disabled, and mentally retarded persons.
Funded by: Fees; workshop sales.
Budget: $2 million.
Hours of Operation: 8:00 AM-4:30 PM.
Staff: 13 full time; 1 part time.
History/Date: Est. 1934.
Eligibility: Visual impairment; supported by state agency; ambulatory.
Area Served: Austin area.
Age Requirements: 16 years and older.

Health: Provides low vision aids. Contracts and refers for other eye health services.
Rehabilitation: Orientation/mobility.
Employment: Prevocational evaluation; job retention; job retraining; sheltered workshops.

West Texas Lighthouse for the Blind

2001 Austin Street
San Angelo, TX 76903
(915) 653-4231
FAX: (915) 657-9367
Robert B. Porter, Executive Director

Type of Agency: Private; non-profit.
County/District Where Located: Tom Green County.
Mission: Services for totally blind, legally blind, learning disabled, and mentally retarded persons.

Funded by: Workshop sales; sub-contracts; training fees; and donations.
Budget: $1.5 million.
Hours of Operation: Mon.-Fri. 7:30 AM-4:00 PM.
Program Accessibility: Wheelchair accessibility.
Staff: 3 full time. Uses volunteers.
History/Date: Est. 1963.
Number of Clients Served: 30.
Eligibility: Visually impaired; referral from state agency.
Area Served: 42 counties in western Texas.
Transportation: Y.
Age Requirements: 18 years and older.

Health: Refers for health services.
Counseling/Social Work/Self-Help: Refers for other counseling/social work services. Provides consultation to other agencies.
Educational: Accepts emotionally disturbed, learning disabled, and wheelchair-bound clients.
Professional Training: Regular in-service training programs; open to enrollment from other agencies.
Employment: Sheltered workshops. Refers for other employment services.

COMPUTER TRAINING CENTERS

Center for Computer Assistance to the Disabled

1950 Stemmons Freeway
Suite 4041
Dallas, TX 75207
(214) 800-2223 or (214) 800-2225
FAX: (214) 800-2224
Mary Ann Schroeder, Director

County/District Where Located: Dallas County.

Computer Training: Speech output systems; optical character recognition systems; closed-circuit television systems; word processing; database software; computer operating systems.

Lighthouse for the Blind of Fort Worth

912 West Broadway
Fort Worth, TX 76104
(817) 332-3341
FAX: (817) 332-3456
James Baggott, Rehabilitation Services

County/District Where Located: Tarrant County.

Computer Training: Speech output systems; database software.

Lighthouse of Houston

3530 West Dallas Avenue
P.O. Box 130435
Houston, TX 77219-0435
(713) 527-9561
FAX: (713) 527-8165
Gibson M. Du Terroil, President
Shelagh Moran, Vice President

Type of Agency: Private; non-profit.
County/District Where Located: Harris County.
Hours of Operation: Mon.-Fri. 7:30 AM-4:00.
Eligibility: Blind; legally blind; deaf-blind.
Area Served: Greater Houston area and southwestern Texas.

Computer Training: Speech output systems; screen magnification systems; braille access systems; optical character recognition systems; closed-circuit television systems; word processing; database software; computer operating systems; full-service technology training unit.

Texas Commission for the Blind

4800 North Lamar
Suite 110

Austin, TX 78756
(512) 459-2568
Mary Anne Longenecker,
Supervisor, Adaptive Technical
Unit

Computer Training: Speech
output systems; screen
magnification systems; braille
access systems; optical character
recognition systems; closed-circuit
television systems; word
processing; database software;
computer operating systems;
training for instructors.

Texas School for the Blind and Visually Impaired

1100 West 45th Street
Austin, TX 78756
(512) 454-8631
URL: http://www.tsbvi.edu
James Allan, Education Technical
Specialist

Computer Training: Speech
output systems; screen
magnification systems; braille
access systems; word processing;
Internet access.

William Judson Center
San Antonio Lighthouse

2305 Roosevelt Avenue
San Antonio, TX 78210
(210) 533-5195
FAX: (210) 533-4230
Cindy Miller, Vice President,
Rehabilitation Services

County/District Where Located:
Bexar County.

Computer Training: Speech
output systems; screen
magnification systems; braille
access systems; closed-circuit
television systems; word
processing; database software;
computer operating systems;
notetakers; reading/scanning
programs.
Career guidance; industrial
training; job readiness/placement

services; literacy-BE, GED, ESL,
Braille; orientation and mobility
training; support group/low
vision club; and low vision
products store.

◆ Low Vision Services

EYE CARE SOCIETIES

Texas Ophthalmological Association

401 West 15th Street, 825
Austin, TX 78701-1665
(512) 370-1440
FAX: (512) 370-1637
E-mail: toa@flash.net
Jay W. Propes, Executive Director
David G. Shulman, Contact Person

Texas Optometric Association, Inc.

1503 South IH-35
Austin, TX 78741
(512) 707-2020
Diane Lake, Executive Director

LOW VISION CENTERS

Dallas Services for the Visually Impaired
Low Vision Clinic

4242 Office Parkway
Dallas, TX 75204
(214) 828-9900
FAX: (214) 828-9901
Nancy Hinkley, Director

Type of Agency: Private, non-
profit, multidisciplinary clinic.
County/District Where Located:
Dallas County.
Hours of Operation: Mon.-Fri.
8:30 AM-4:30 PM.
Area Served: Unlimited.

Low Vision: Low vision
evaluation; private and group
counseling; low vision aid training;
orientation/mobility instruction.

Low Vision Aids: Provided on
loan; no rental fee; on-site training
available.

El Paso Lighthouse for the Blind
Low Vision Center

200 Washington
El Paso, TX 79905
(915) 532-4495
FAX: (915) 532-6338
Grant Downey, Executive Director

Type of Agency: Non-profit.
County/District Where Located:
El Paso County.
Mission: Employment, training,
rehabilitation, and technical
services for blind and visually
impaired persons.
Funded by: Client fees;
foundation grants; donations.
Budget: $650,000.
Hours of Operation: Mon.-Fri.
8:00 AM-4:30 PM, or by
appointment.
Staff: Low vision assistant;
orientation/mobility instructor;
ophthalmologist; optometrist.
History/Date: Est. 1934.
Number of Clients Served: 2,400
per year. All programs.
Eligibility: Referral; current
ophthalmological report.
Area Served: El Paso and
surrounding areas of western
Texas, southern New Mexico and
northern Mexico.
Transportation: Y.

Low Vision Aids: Provided on
loan for trial period at no charge;
provided for purchase; prescribed
and fitted at no charge. On-site and
in-home training provided.
Low Vision Follow-up: Return
appointment; phone interview;
varies according to patient.

Lighthouse of Houston
Low Vision Clinic

3602 West Dallas Avenue

Houston, TX 77019
(713) 284-8402
FAX: (713) 527-8165
Stanley Woo, O.D., Director of
Clinical Services
Debbie Repka, Clinic
Administrator

County/District Where Located:
Harris County.
Funded by: Client fees; state
funds.
Hours of Operation: Mon.-Fri.
8:00 AM-5:00 PM.
Staff: Optometrist; optometry
student/resident; social worker;
mobility instructor; special
education instructor.
Eligibility: None.
Area Served: Unlimited.

Low Vision: Provided on loan for
trial; on-site training provided.
Low Vision Follow-up: Phone
interview, as needed.

Low Vision Unit
Hermann Eye Center
6411 Fannin Street
Houston, TX 77030-1697
(713) 704-1777
FAX: (713) 704-0617
Judianne Kellaway, Director
Kathleen Saathoff, C.O., Low
Vision Coordinator

County/District Where Located:
Harris County.
Hours of Operation: Mon.-Fri.
8:30 AM-4:30 PM.
Staff: Ophthalmologist; low vision
specialists; ophthalmic assistant/
technician; ophthalmology
residents; optician; rehabilitation
counselor; contact lens technician;
orthoptist.
Eligibility: Ophthalmologic
report.
Area Served: Unlimited.
Age Requirements: 6 years and
older.

Professional Training: Refers for
in-service programs.
Rehabilitation: Rehabilitation
counseling for individuals for
home, school, and on the job.
Low Vision: Low vision services.
Low Vision Aids: On-site training
provided. Loan for trial purpose at
no charge; available for purchase
after evaluation. CCTVs and
computer-related devices on site
for demonstration.
Low Vision Follow-up: By return
appointment.

Santa Rosa Low Vision Clinic
315 North San Saba
Suite 1220
San Antonio, TX 78207
(210) 228-0030
FAX: (210) 228-0277
Dr. Kathleen E. Fraser, O.D.,
F.A.A.O., Director

Type of Agency: Private.
Funded by: Client fees.
Hours of Operation: Mon.-Fri.
8:00 AM-6:00 PM.
Staff: Orientation/mobility
instructor; ophthalmology
resident; opthalmic technician;
optometrist.
History/Date: Est. 1985.
Number of Clients Served: 1,200
annually.
Eligibility: Visual impairment.
Area Served: Unlimited.
Age Requirements: None.

**Counseling/Social Work/Self-
Help:** Peer counseling.
Low Vision: On-site/in-home
training provided.
Low Vision Aids: Provided on
loan at no charge and/or purchase.
Low Vision Follow-up: Return
appointment; home visit; phone
interviews.

Orientation/mobility specialist
trains for use of all optical aids,
including reading lenses and
telescopes for public

transportation. Access and
training on computer aids and
devices.

Texas Tech University
School of Medicine
Health Sciences Center
Department of Ophthalmology
and Visual Sciences
Thompson Hall
Lubbock, TX 79430
(806) 743-2020
FAX: (806) 743-1782
E-mail: eyesmm@ttuhsc.edu
URL: http://www.eye.ttu.edu
Dr. Steven Matthews, O.D., Ph.D.,
Director of Low Vision Service

Type of Agency: University
medical school.
County/District Where Located:
Lubbock County.
Mission: To help patients with
decreased acuity improve the
usefulness of their vision.
Funded by: Client fees; state
funds.
Hours of Operation: Wed.
1:00 PM-5:00 PM.
Staff: Optometrist; ophthalmology
resident; ophthalmic assistant/
technician.
History/Date: Est. 1980.
Number of Clients Served: 3 per
week.
Eligibility: Prefer ophthalmologic
report, but will accept all patients.
Area Served: Southwest Texas,
western Texas, and eastern New
Mexico.

Low Vision Aids: Provided on
loan for trial; no rental fee; on-site
training provided.
Low Vision Follow-up: By return
appointment in 6 months.

University of Texas
Health Science Center at Dallas
Department of Ophthalmology
Low Vision Clinic
5303 Harry Hines

Dallas, TX 75235-8866
(214) 648-3835
Dr. Edward Mendelson, O.D., Low
Vision Clinic Director

Type of Agency: Non-profit.
Funded by: Client fees and Texas
Commission for the Blind.
Hours of Operation: Mon.-Fri.
8:30 AM-5:00 PM.
Staff: Optometrist.
Eligibility: Referral.
Area Served: Unlimited.

Low Vision Aids: Half glasses,
magnifiers and telescopes
provided for purchase; on-site
training not provided.
Low Vision Follow-up: Return
appointment.

University of Texas, Health Science Center

Department of Ophthalmology
7703 Floyd Curl Drive
San Antonio, TX 78284-6230
(210) 567-8400
FAX: (210) 567-8413
W. A. J. van Heuven, M.D.,
Professor and Chairman

Type of Agency: Non-profit.
County/District Where Located:
Bexar County.
Funded by: Client fees, and Texas
Commission for the Blind.
Hours of Operation: By
appointment.
Staff: Ophthalmology resident;
ophthalmologist.
Eligibility: None.
Area Served: Unlimited.

Low Vision: Evaluation.
Low Vision Follow-up: By
appointment.

◆ Aging Services

STATE UNITS ON AGING

Texas Department on Aging

Capitol Station
1949 IH 35 South
P.O. Box 12786
Austin, TX 78741-3702
(512) 424-6840 or (800) 252-2412 or
Information & Referral In State
(800) 252-9240
FAX: (512) 424-6890
Mary Sapp, Executive Director

Provides referrals to Area Agencies
on Aging and information on other
local aging services.

INDEPENDENT LIVING PROGRAMS

Texas Commission for the Blind

Administration Building
4800 North Lamar
Austin, TX 78711
(512) 459-2500 or (800) 252-5204
FAX: (512) 459-2685
Pat D. Westbrook, Executive
Director
Charles Burtis, Project Director,
(512) 459-2589

Provides independent living
services for persons age 55 and
over. For further information,
contact the Project Director or
general phone number listed.

UTAH

◆ *Educational Services*

STATE SERVICES

Utah State Office of Education Special Education Section
250 East 500 South
Salt Lake City, UT 84111
(801) 538-7706 or (801) 538-7708
Dr. Stevan Kukic, Coordinator, Services for At Risk Students and Director, Special Education
John Killoran, Specialist, Preschool Program for Special Education

Type of Agency: State.
Funded by: Public funds.
Area Served: Utah.

Local school districts administer supplemental state funds for visually impaired students in local schools. For information about local facilities, consult the superintendent of schools in the area or the coordinator of special education programs.

EARLY INTERVENTION COORDINATION

Early Intervention Program Division of Family Services Utah Department of Health
P.O. Box 16650-BCSHS
Salt Lake City, UT 84116-0650
(801) 538-6922
FAX: (801) 538-6510
Jennifer Haake, Acting Early Childhood Coordinator

Developmental services for disabled and developmentally delayed 0-2 year olds. Family support/educational services relevant to the child's disability.

SCHOOLS

Utah Schools for the Deaf and the Blind
742 Harrison Boulevard
Ogden, UT 84404
(801) 629-4700
FAX: (801) 629-4896
Dr. Lee Robinson, Superintendent

Type of Agency: State.
County/District Where Located: Weber County.
Mission: Services for totally blind; legally blind; visually impaired; deaf-blind; children who might also be learning disabled; mentally retarded; emotionally disturbed; orthopedically handicapped.
History/Date: Est. 1896.
Number of Clients Served: 1996: 1,130.
Eligibility: Visually impaired; unable to receive appropriate education in regular public school classroom.

Counseling/Social Work/Self-Help: Parent/infant program.
Educational: Full program of general academic studies; prevocational skill development; daily living skills; orientation/mobility classes. Teacher consultant program serving public school students.
Preschools: Preschool classes offered to visually impaired children between ages 3 and 5, with transportation provided.
Professional Training: Internship programs; in-service training, fieldwork with public schools.
Residential: Dormitories for visually impaired students ages 4 1/2-21 provided during the week.

INFANT AND PRESCHOOL

Center and Homebound Preschool Intervention Program
Center for Persons with Disabilities
UMC 6800, Utah State University

Logan, UT 84322
(801) 797-2002
FAX: (801) 797-2044
E-mail: sebst@cpd2.usu.edu
Dr. Sebastian Striefel, Director of Services
Dr. Phyllis Cole, Coordinator of Clinical Services
Karen Hansen, Early Intervention

Type of Agency: University-affiliated facility.
Mission: To provide services via interdisciplinary teams.
Funded by: State funds, Titles XIX and XX and fees.
Hours of Operation: Mon.-Fri. 8:00AM-5:00PM.
Staff: 31 full time (early childhood/visually handicapped, psychologists, occupational therapist); 17 part time (various specialists, graduate assistants). Advisory board with parent members for overall program.
History/Date: Est. 1974.
Number of Clients Served: 140 families.
Eligibility: Visually handicapped; multihandicapped and disabled.
Area Served: Cache, Box Elder and Rich Counties.
Transportation: Y.
Age Requirements: 3 years and under.

Health: Provides adaptive equipment; genetic counseling; low vision exams; immunizations; blood tests; acute illness/emergency sick care; school physicals.
Counseling/Social Work/Self-Help: Parent counseling and training.
Educational: Provides instruction in all developmental areas.
Professional Training: Train students from various disciplines.

Home-based program for visually handicapped, multihandicapped, and other handicapped infants, 0-3 years. Consultant services to other programs. Conducts research and training.

Utah Schools for the Deaf and the Blind
Parent-Infant Program (PIP)
742 Harrison Boulevard
Ogden, UT 84404
(801) 629-4700
FAX: (801) 629-4896
E-mail: bsogd1.jnielsen@email.state.ut.us
Judi Nielsen, Director

Type of Agency: State residential school.
County/District Where Located: Weber County.
Mission: Services for visually impaired and hearing impaired, multiply disabled, and deaf-blind children.
Funded by: P.L. 89-313 and 94-142 funds, state funds, and limited donations.
Staff: 1 full-time, 45 part-time.
History/Date: PIP est. 1979.
Eligibility: Visually or hearing impaired, with or without other impairments.
Area Served: Entire state.
Transportation: N.

Health: Adaptive equipment, audiological testing and functional vision evaluations.
Counseling/Social Work/Self-Help: Parent counseling.
Educational: Provides instruction in developmental areas. Home-based program for visually or hearing impaired infants, 0-2 years, with or without other impairments (includes deaf-blind); home teaching, preschool classes, consultant services to other programs for visually handicapped, multihandicapped, and hearing impaired.

STATEWIDE OUTREACH SERVICES

Utah Schools for the Deaf and the Blind
742 Harrison Boulevard
Ogden, UT 84404
(801) 629-4735
FAX: (801) 629-4896
URL: http://www.usdb.k12.ut.us
Dorothy Smith

County/District Where Located: Weber County.
Funded by: State funds.
History/Date: Est. 1983.
Age Requirements: 3-21 years of age.

Counseling/Social Work/Self-Help: Teacher consultant program for the rural districts of Utah. Liaison for itinerant teachers for visually impaired students employed by districts.
Assessment: Growing up, INSITE, Barraga Assessment of Visual Development tests.
Direct Service: Instruction on skills particular to blindness.
Materials Production: Braille and large-print when other sources are not available.
Professional Training: Vision certification; Multi-University Consortium Teacher Training Program, Sensory Impaired.

INSTRUCTIONAL MATERIALS CENTERS

Utah Educational Resource Center
742 Harrison Boulevard
Ogden, UT 84404
(801) 629-4810
FAX: (801) 629-4896
Lori Quigley, Contact Person

Area Served: Statewide.

Types/Content: Textbooks; teaching aids; instructional materials.

Media Formats: Braille; large print; descriptive videos.

◆ *Information Services*

LIBRARIES

Utah State Library
Division for the Blind and Physically Handicapped
2150 South 300 West
Suite 16
Salt Lake City, UT 84115
(801) 468-6789
FAX: (801) 468-6767
Gerald A. Buttars, Librarian
Bessie Oaks, Librarian

Type of Agency: Public library for the blind and physically handicapped.
Mission: To provide books and other information to the blind and physically handicapped in a format they can use.
Funded by: Public funds.
Budget: $700,000.
Hours of Operation: Mon.-Fri. 8:00 AM-5:00 PM.
Staff: 18 full time equivalents.
History/Date: Est. 1961.
Number of Clients Served: 10,000.
Eligibility: Must be certified by a competent authority, defined by law as being blind, physically or reading disabled.
Area Served: Utah and Wyoming with total library service. Serves Montana, New Mexico, Colorado, Idaho, Nevada, Kansas, Nebraska, the Dakotas, Alaska and Arizona with braille service only.
Transportation: N.

Reading: All reading to patrons is done on magnetic tape and circulated to them.

Regional library supplying talking books, braille and large-type books, and cassette books.

MEDIA PRODUCTION SERVICES

National Federation of the Blind of Utah

10 West Broadway
Suite 500
Salt Lake City, UT 84101
(801) 364-9007 or (800) 876-9007
Nick Schmittroth

County/District Where Located: Salt Lake County.
Area Served: Primarily Utah but other states as well.
Groups Served: Blind and visually impaired.

Types/Content: Text materials other than music, including computer-related materials.
Media Formats: Braille, cassette and print.

Utah Schools for the Deaf and the Blind

742 Harrison Boulevard
Ogden, UT 84404
(801) 629-4700
FAX: (801) 629-4896
E-mail: lrobin@email.state.ut. us
Dr. Lee Robinson, Superintendent

County/District Where Located: Weber County.
Groups Served: K-12.

Types/Content: Textbooks, recreational.
Media Formats: Braille books, talking books/cassettes, large print books.
Title Listings: No title listings available.

RADIO READING

Utah State Radio Reading Service

2150 South 300 West
Suite 16
Salt Lake City, UT 84115
(801) 468-6798
FAX: (801) 468-6767
Bob Wall, Manager

County/District Where Located: Salt Lake County.
Hours of Operation: Mon.-Fri. 7:00 AM-Midnight; Sat.-Sun. 6:00 PM-8:00 PM.
History/Date: Est. 1976.
Area Served: Wasatch Front and St. George area.

INFORMATION AND REFERRAL

The Foundation Fighting Blindness Utah Chapter

746 South 475 East
Centerville, UT 84014
(801) 299-8767
Martha Lapetina, President
Steve Andrews, Contact Person

See The Foundation Fighting Blindness in U.S. national listings.

Prevent Blindness Utah

661 South 200 East
Salt Lake City, UT 84111
(801) 524-2020
FAX: (801) 322-3647
E-mail: 76710.2267@compuserve. com
Colleen Malouf, President

County/District Where Located: Salt Lake County.

See Prevent Blindness America in U.S. national listings.

See also in national listings:

American Council on Rural Special Education (ACRES)

Church of Jesus Christ of Latter-Day Saints
Special Curriculum

♦ Rehabilitation Services

STATE SERVICES

Utah Division of Services for the Blind and Visually Impaired

309 East 100 South
Salt Lake City, UT 84111
(801) 323-4343
FAX: (801) 323-4396
E-mail: vflake@usoe.k12.ut.us
William Gibson, Director

Type of Agency: State.
Mission: To assist blind and visually impaired people in living as fully and independently as possible.
Funded by: Public funds.
Hours of Operation: Mon.-Fri. 8:00 AM-5:00 PM.
Staff: 45 full-time, 2 part-time.
History/Date: Est. 1919.
Eligibility: Legally blind or visually impaired.
Area Served: Utah.
Age Requirements: 16 and older.

Counseling/Social Work/Self-Help: Consultation and referral; group work; individual counseling.
Educational: Public education concerning blindness. Orientation and training program for blind and visually impaired adults. Outreach training in homes and businesses.
Preschools: Vision screening clinics for pre-school and kindergarten children throughout the state.
Professional Training: Internship/fieldwork for social work and rehabilitation counseling.

Reading: Braille and computer access.

Residential: Apartments provided for out-of-town students.

Rehabilitation: Orientation/ mobility; home management; personal management; communications; adjustment to blindness; social skills; braille; college preparation; computer skills.

Recreational: Weekly activities as part of orientation and training program.

Employment: Evaluation; prevocational and vocational training; placement; vending facility training; follow-up.

Computer Training: Access; training on computer aids and devices.

Low Vision: Low vision clinic; pre-clinic evaluations and post-clinic follow-up and training.

Low Vision Aids: Sold at cost.

Low Vision Follow-up: By low vision advisor.

Local Offices:

Ogden: Ogden Center for the Blind, 150 North Washington Boulevard, Ogden, UT 84404, (801) 393-0166.

Provo: Provo District Office, 150 East Center Street, Suite 3300, Provo, UT 84603, (801) 374-7724.

REHABILITATION

Utah Industries for the Blind
1595 West 500 South
Salt Lake City, UT 84104
(801) 975-4025 or (800) 933-5191
FAX: (801) 975-0279
Jan Quinn, Acting Executive Director
David Yonkstedtter, Director

Type of Agency: Integrated employment.

County/District Where Located: Salt Lake County.

Mission: To provide employment and employment placement services for blind and visually impaired adults.

Funded by: Self-generated revenues and fund raising.

Budget: $1.9 million.

Hours of Operation: Mon.-Fri. 7:30 AM-4:30 PM.

Program Accessibility: Fully accessible.

Staff: 1.

History/Date: Est. 1909; Converted from public to private, nonprofit in 1991.

Number of Clients Served: 40.

Eligibility: Blind adults.

Area Served: Utah.

Age Requirements: 18 years and older.

Rehabilitation: In cooperation with state of Utah rehabilitation program.

Employment: Job placement; employment and job skills.

COMPUTER TRAINING CENTERS

Computer Center for Citizens with Disabilities
2056 South, 1100 East
Salt Lake City, UT 84106
(801) 485-9152
FAX: (801) 485-8675
E-mail: cboogaar@usoe.k12.ut.us
Craig Boogaard, Director

Computer Training: Speech output systems; word processing; database software.

Introduction to adaptive computer devices also provided.

◆ Low Vision Services

EYE CARE SOCIETIES

Utah Ophthalmological Society
540 East 500 South
Salt Lake City, UT 84102
(801) 355-7477
Sue Vicchrilli, Executive Director

Utah Optometric Association
230 West 200 South
Salt Lake City, UT 84101
(801) 364-9103
Clive Watson, Executive Director

LOW VISION CENTERS

Low Vision Services
Utah Division of Services for the Blind and Visually Impaired
309 East 100 South
Salt Lake City, UT 84111
(801) 323-4373 or (800) 284-1823
FAX: (801) 323-4396
Robert M. Christiansen, M.D., Staff Ophthalmologist
Bryan R. Gerritsen, Coordinator

Type of Agency: State.

County/District Where Located: Salt Lake County.

Mission: Comprehensive low vision services to visually impaired persons throughout the state of Utah.

Funded by: State funds; vocational rehabilitation; and payment (at cost) by clients for low vision aids purchased.

Hours of Operation: Daily, 8:00 AM-4:30 PM, by appointment.

Staff: Ophthalmologist; low vision specialist; low vision advisors; social worker; rehabilitation teacher; orientation/mobility instructor.

History/Date: Est. 1959.

Number of Clients Served: 1996: 1,045.

Eligibility: Referral by an optometrist or ophthalmologist; visually impaired.
Area Served: All areas of Utah.

Counseling/Social Work/Self-Help: Adjustment to blindness and vision loss by social worker, or in a class/group. Provides link to support groups in Utah.
Low Vision: Provides help for near vision tasks, distance vision tasks, improved lighting, reduced glare, improved functioning, and suggestions for modification in the home, work site, and school.
Low Vision Aids: Available for sale at cost. Provided on loan for trial upon request. Post-clinic training provided.
Low Vision Follow-up: Visits to home, job site, and/or school within one week of clinic appointment, by a low vision advisor.

Outreach clinics conducted regularly in hospitals throughout the state. Call for schedule and appointment.

University Medical Center Department of Ophthalmology/ John A. Moran Eye Center
50 North Medical Drive
Salt Lake City, UT 84132
(801) 581-2352
FAX: (801) 581-3357
Randall J. Olson, M.D., Chairman and Director

Type of Agency: Non-profit.
County/District Where Located: Salt Lake County.
Funded by: Client fees, Medicaid/Medicare.
Staff: Ophthalmologist, counselor.
Eligibility: Referral and current ophthalmological report.
Area Served: Unlimited.

Counseling/Social Work/Self-Help: Counseling for visually impaired individuals and families;

support groups; orientation to vision loss program.
Low Vision Aids: Prescribed and fitted for variable charge; on-site training provided.
Low Vision Follow-up: Return appointments.

◆ Aging Services

STATE UNITS ON AGING

Division of Aging and Adult Services
Utah Department of Social Services
120 North 200 West
P.O. Box 45500
Salt Lake City, UT 84145-0500
(801) 538-3910
Helen Goddard, Director

Provides referrals to Area Agencies on Aging and information on other local aging services.

INDEPENDENT LIVING PROGRAMS

Utah State Office of Rehabilitation
250 East 500 South
Salt Lake City, UT 84111
(801) 538-7530 or (800) 473-7530
FAX: (801) 538-7522
R. Blaine Petersen, Executive Director
William Gibson, Project Director, (801) 323-4343

Provides independent living services for persons age 55 and over. For further information, contact the Project Director or general phone number listed.

VERMONT

◆ *Educational Services*

STATE SERVICES

Special Education Unit
Vermont Department of
Education
State Office Building
120 State Street
Montpelier, VT 05620
(802) 828-3067
FAX: (802) 828-3140
E-mail: fjones@doe.state.vt.us
Dennis Kane, Executive Director
Kathy Andrews, Early Education
Consultant
Fred Jones, Consultant

Type of Agency: State, a unit of
the Department of Education.
Mission: Administers
supplemental state funds for
visually impaired children
attending local schools. Provides
special educational services for
visually impaired children.
Funded by: Public funds.
Hours of Operation: Mon.-Fri.
7:30 AM-4:30 PM.
Area Served: Vermont.

Counseling/Social Work/Self-
Help: Provides parental
counseling and preschool services.
Educational: Offers tuition and
fellowships.
Reading: Distributes braille and
large-type books, tapes and tape
recorders.

For information about local
facilities, consult the
superintendent of schools in the
area or the Vermont Association
for the Blind and Visually
Impaired, 37 Elmwood Avenue,
Burlington, VT 05401.

EARLY INTERVENTION COORDINATION

Special Education Unit
Vermont Department of
Education
State Office Building
120 State Street
Montpelier, VT 05620
(802) 828-3067
FAX: (802) 828-3140
Fred Jones, Consultant

County/District Where Located:
Washington County.

Educational support team for
families.

INSTRUCTIONAL MATERIALS CENTERS

Vermont Association for the
Blind and Visually Impaired
37 Elmwood Avenue
Burlington, VT 05401
(802) 863-1358
FAX: (802) 863-1481
E-mail: vabvi@aol.com
Jules Cote, Executive Director

County/District Where Located:
Chittenden County.
Area Served: Vermont.
Groups Served: All consumers
with visual impairments.

Types/Content: Durable
equipment and consumable
supplies.
Media Formats: Braille, large-
print, tape.
Title Listings: Call for up-to-date
listings.

◆ *Information Services*

LIBRARIES

Vermont Department of
Libraries
Special Services Unit
RD #4, Box 1870
Montpelier, VT 05602
(802) 828-3273 or toll-free
(800) 479-1711
FAX: (802) 828-2199

Type of Agency: Vermont State
Library.
County/District Where Located:
Washington County.
Mission: Talking book and large
print service to the blind, visually
impaired, and physically disabled.
Funded by: State and federal
government.
Budget: $156,450.
Hours of Operation: Mon.-Fri.
7:45 AM-4:30 PM.
Program Accessibility:
Handicapped accessible.
Staff: 4.
Number of Clients Served: 2,000.
Eligibility: Blind, visually
impaired and physically disabled.
Area Served: State of Vermont
(most service by mail, postage-
free).

Regional library in a cooperating
network administered by the
National Library Service for the
Blind and Physically Handicapped,
Library of Congress.

Book collection: Talking books on
disc and cassette, and large-print
books.

Special collections: Reference
materials on blindness and other
handicaps; children's print/braille
books; and descriptive videos.

INFORMATION AND REFERRAL

**The Foundation Fighting Blindness
Vermont Affiliate**
37 Elmwood Avenue
Burlington, VT 05401
(802) 863-1358
FAX: (802) 863-1481
Michael Richman, Contact Person

See The Foundation Fighting Blindness in U.S. national listings.

♦ Rehabilitation Services

STATE SERVICES

**Division for the Blind and Visually Impaired
Vermont Agency of Human Services**
Osgood Building
103 South Main Street
Waterbury, VT 05671-2304
(802) 241-2210
FAX: (802) 241-3359
E-mail: steve@dad.state.vt.us
Steve Stone, Director

Type of Agency: State.
Mission: Administers the federal-state rehabilitation program; provides services for totally blind, legally blind, and visually impaired persons.
Funded by: Federal and state monies.
Budget: 1996: $1,500,000.
Hours of Operation: 7:45 AM-4:30 PM.
Program Accessibility: Fully accessible.
Staff: 13.
History/Date: Est. 1927.
Number of Clients Served: 1996: 1200.
Eligibility: Medically diagnosed visual impairment that constitutes a handicap to social and economic self-sufficiency.
Area Served: Statewide.
Transportation: Y.

Health: Contracts and refers for health services.
Counseling/Social Work/Self-Help: Individual, group, family/parent, couple counseling; placement in school; referral to community services. Contracts for and provides consultation to other agencies for other counseling/social work services.
Educational: Limited.
Preschools: Limited.
Professional Training: Internship/fieldwork placement in rehabilitation counseling; vocational rehabilitation.
Reading: Y.
Rehabilitation: Contracts and refers for rehabilitation services.
Recreational: Contracts and refers for recreational services.
Employment: Prevocational evaluation; career and skill counseling; job development; vocational placement; follow-up service; vending stand training. Contracts for other employment-related services.
Computer Training: Training on computer aids and devices.
Low Vision: Y.
Low Vision Aids: Y.
Low Vision Follow-up: Y.

Local Offices:

Barre: 255 North Main Street, Barre, VT 05641, (802) 479-4278.
Burlington: 108 Cherry Street, Suite 202, P.O. Box 3347, Burlington, VT 05401, (802) 863-7530.
Rutland: 190 ASA Bloomer Building, Rutland, VT 05701-9408, (802) 786-5822.
Springfield: 260 River Street, Springfield, VT 05156-2306, (802) 885-9133.

REHABILITATION

Vermont Association for the Blind and Visually Impaired
37 Elmwood Avenue
Burlington, VT 05401
(802) 863-1358 or (800) 639-5861
FAX: (802) 863-1481
E-mail: vabvi@aol.com
Jules Coté, Executive Director

Type of Agency: Private; non-profit.
County/District Where Located: Chittenden County.
Mission: Services for blind, visually impaired, multiply disabled persons.
Funded by: Capital income; state appropriation; fees for service; fund raising; federal and state grants.
Budget: $1.2 million.
Hours of Operation: Mon.-Fri. 8:00 AM-4:00 PM.
Staff: 27 full time equivalents.
History/Date: Est. 1926.
Number of Clients Served: 1991: 1,500.
Eligibility: Visual impairment.
Area Served: Vermont.
Transportation: Y.

Counseling/Social Work/Self-Help: Information and referral; outreach; peer counseling.
Educational: Special education programs.
Rehabilitation: Orientation/mobility; rehabilitation teaching, low vision.

Local Offices:

Brattleboro: 8 Park Place, Brattleboro, VT 05301, (802) 254-8761.
Montpelier: 73 Main Street, Montpelier, VT 05602, (802) 223-5618.
Rutland: 10 Burnham Avenue, Rutland, VT 05701, (802) 775-6452.

Vermont Association of Business, Industry, and Rehabilitation
Champlain Mill, #60
Winooski, VT 05404
(802) 655-7215
FAX: (802) 655-7216
Kevin Veller, Executive Director

Type of Agency: Private; non-profit.
Mission: To place people with disabilities into jobs and to help employers retain people who become disabled while working.
Funded by: Federal grants, contracts, fees for service.
Budget: 1997: $500,000.
Hours of Operation: 8:00 AM-5:00 PM.
Staff: 10 full time.
History/Date: Est. 1979.
Number of Clients Served: 250.
Eligibility: Job-ready disabled persons referred by the State Division of Vocational Rehabilitation.
Age Requirements: Set by the State Division of Vocational Rehabilitation.
Educational: Job-seeking skills training.
Employment: Vocational counseling, job development, job placement, and follow-up. Consultation and training to employers on disability-employment issues.

COMPUTER TRAINING CENTERS

Division for the Blind and Visually Impaired
Vermont Agency of Human Services
103 South Main Street
Waterbury, VT 05671
(802) 241-2245
E-mail: geoff@dad.state.vt.us
URL: http://www.cit.state.vt.us/dad/dbvi.htm
Geoff Howard, Consultant

Computer Training: Speech output systems; screen magnification systems; braille access systems; optical character recognition systems; closed-circuit television systems; word processing; database software; computer operating systems.

◆ Low Vision Services

EYE CARE SOCIETIES

Vermont Ophthalmological Society
P.O. Box 1457
Montpelier, VT 05601
(802) 223-7898
Ada Bagalio, Executive Director

Vermont Optometric Association
168 North Street
Bennington, VT 05201-1874
(802) 442-2115
Alexander Tenentes, O.D.

County/District Where Located: Bennington County.

◆ Aging Services

STATE UNITS ON AGING

Vermont Department of Aging and Disabilities
Osgood Building
103 South Main Street
Waterbury, VT 05676
(802) 241-2400 or Information & Referral In State, Senior Helpline Service (800) 642-5119
FAX: (802) 241-2324
David Yavacone, Commissioner

Provides referrals to Area Agencies on Aging and information on other local aging services.

INDEPENDENT LIVING PROGRAMS

Division for the Blind and Visually Impaired
Vermont Agency of Human Services
Osgood Building
103 South Main Street
Waterbury, VT 05671
(802) 241-2210
FAX: (802) 241-3359
Steven Stone, Director

Provides independent living services for persons age 55 and over. For further information, contact the Project Director or general phone number listed.

VIRGINIA

◆ Educational Services

STATE SERVICES

Virginia Department for the Visually Handicapped Program for Infants, Children, and Youth
395 Azalea Avenue
Richmond, VA 23227-3697
(804) 371-3140
FAX: (804) 371-3351
W. Roy Grizzard, Commissioner
Glen R. Slonneger, Jr., Program Director, Educational Services

Type of Agency: State.
County/District Where Located: Henrico County.
Mission: Services to infants, children, and youths, from birth through 21 years of age, who have a visual disability.
Funded by: State funds, Section 110 funds.
Budget: $440,000.
Hours of Operation: Mon.-Fri. 8:15 AM-5:00 PM.
Program Accessibility: Y.
Staff: 7 full time.
History/Date: Est. 1936.
Number of Clients Served: 1,500.
Eligibility: Visual impairment.
Area Served: Virginia.
Age Requirements: 0-21 years.

Health: Adaptive equipment; low vision aids.
Counseling/Social Work/Self-Help: Parent counseling.
Educational: Works cooperatively with public schools to develop and maintain itinerant and resource room programs for visually impaired children/youths. Provides technical assistance.

Reading: Braille and large-print textbooks, special equipment, and adapted material are available for loan to schools through the agency's instructional material and resource center.
Rehabilitation: Vocational training.
Recreational: Summer camp.
Computer Training: Instructional and technical assistance for students and teachers.

For Agency information, see our listing under Rehabilitation Services.

EARLY INTERVENTION COORDINATION

Infant and Toddler Program Virginia Department of Mental Health, Mental Retardation and Substance Abuse Services
P.O. Box 1797
Richmond, VA 23219
(804) 786-3710
FAX: (804) 371-7959
Anne Lucas, Part H Early Childhood Coordinator

Coordination of statewide early intervention services for infants and toddlers with disabilities and their families in accordance with Part H of the Individuals with Disabilities Education Act.

SCHOOLS

Virginia School for the Deaf and Blind at Hampton
700 Shell Road
Hampton, VA 23661
(757) 247-2075
FAX: (757) 247-2224
Frank R. Bryan, Superintendent

Type of Agency: State.
County/District Where Located: Hampton County.
Funded by: Public funds.
Hours of Operation: 8:00 AM-4:30 PM.

Program Accessibility: Fully accessible.
Staff: 17 full time. Uses volunteers.
History/Date: Est. 1906.
Number of Clients Served: 1996: 20.
Eligibility: Blind; Virginia resident living east of I-95.
Area Served: Virginia.
Transportation: Y.
Age Requirements: 2-21 years (day school); 5-21 years (residential school).

Health: Well-staffed infirmary open 24 hours per day, Monday to Friday.
Counseling/Social Work/Self-Help: Counseling available for students.
Educational: Preschool through secondary level for blind children, including multiply disabled children.
Residential: 5 days per week.
Rehabilitation: Orientation/mobility; home management; personal management; communications.
Recreational: Athletics.
Employment: Evaluation; prevocational and vocational training; placement; follow-up.
Low Vision: Low vision exams.
Low Vision Aids: Aids available.
Low Vision Follow-up: Y.

Virginia School for the Deaf and the Blind
P.O. Box 2069
Staunton, VA 24402
(540) 332-9046
FAX: (540) 332-9042
Dr. Joseph Panko, Superintendent

Type of Agency: State.
Mission: Services for totally blind, legally blind, and visually impaired persons.
Funded by: State funds.

Budget: $5 million.
Hours of Operation: 8:00 AM-4:30 PM.
Staff: 22 full time; 2 part time. Uses volunteers.
History/Date: Est. 1839.
Number of Clients Served: 40 annually.
Eligibility: Blind; Virginia resident living west of I-95.
Area Served: Virginia.
Transportation: Y.
Age Requirements: 5-22 years.

Health: Audiology therapy; general medical services; speech therapy. Refers for other health services.
Counseling/Social Work/Self-Help: Social evaluations; individual, group, family/parent, couple counseling; placement in school. Refers for other counseling/social work services.
Educational: Grades K through 12. Programs for general academic studies.
Professional Training: Internship/fieldwork placement in special education. Regular in-service training programs, open to enrollment from other agencies.
Reading: Talking book record players and cassette players; talking book records and cassettes; braille books; large-print books; braille magazines; recorded magazines; information and referral; special collection; transcription to braille; tape recording services on demand.
Residential: Dormitories and day students.
Rehabilitation: Personal management; braille; handwriting; listening skills; video magnifier; home management; orientation/mobility; remedial education; sensory training. Refers for rehabilitation teaching in client's home and community.

Recreational: Afterschool programs; arts and crafts; hobby groups; swimming; physical education. Refers for other recreational services.
Employment: Prevocational evaluation; career and skill counseling; follow-up service.
Low Vision: Evaluation and referral.
Low Vision Aids: Aids available.
Low Vision Follow-up: Y.

INFANT AND PRESCHOOL

Children's Rehabilitation Center University of Virginia Hospital

2270 Ivy Road
Charlottesville, VA 22903
(804) 924-5161
FAX: (804) 924-2780
Sharon L. Hostler, M.D., Medical Director
Susan Anderson, M.D., Pediatrician

Type of Agency: State.
County/District Where Located: Albemarle County.
Funded by: P.L. 89-313 monies, income from capital funds, state funds, and other sources.
Staff: 190 full time (includes visually handicapped, early childhood, severely handicapped teachers; occupational and physical therapists; various other specialists), 30 part time. Uses volunteers. Has advisory board for overall program.
History/Date: Est. 1973.

Health: Adaptive equipment, genetic counseling, health immunizations, and blood tests. Low vision exams, other health services available on consultant or referral basis.
Counseling/Social Work/Self-Help: Parent counseling; financial assistance.
Educational: Provides instruction in all developmental areas.

Center-based programs and consultant services to other programs for visually handicapped/multihandicapped, other handicapped infants, 0-2 years. Multihandicapped and noncategorical classrooms, resource room, consultant services to other programs for visually handicapped/multihandicapped, other handicapped children, 3-5 years.

Virginia Department for the Visually Handicapped

395 Azalea Avenue
Richmond, VA 23227-3623
(804) 371-3140
FAX: (804) 371-3351
Glen R. Slonneger, Educational Services Program Director

Type of Agency: State.
Mission: Provides services to visually impaired persons aged 0-21.
Funded by: State funds; IDEA (Part B).
Hours of Operation: Mon.-Fri. 8:15 AM-5:00 PM.
Program Accessibility: Fully accessible.
Staff: 17 full time.
History/Date: Est. 1936.
Eligibility: Visual impairment.
Area Served: Virginia.
Transportation: N.
Age Requirements: 0-5 years.

Health: Adaptive equipment; low vision exams.
Counseling/Social Work/Self-Help: Parent counseling.
Educational: Provides technical assistance in all developmental areas.
Professional Training: Y.
Low Vision: Y.
Low Vision Aids: Y.
Low Vision Follow-up: Y.

Contact local school superintendent for program information in local areas. For regional offices in which educational coordinators and orientation and mobility specialists can be found, see Virginia Department for the Visually Handicapped in the Rehabilitation Services listings.

Virginia School for the Deaf and Blind at Hampton
700 Shell Road
Hampton, VA 23661
(757) 247-2075
Amelia Mondok-Pearson, Educational Director

Type of Agency: State residential school.
Mission: Provides essential services for children who are deaf or blind or have sensory-impaired multiple disabilities by providing quality day and residential programs to children referred by local school divisions and by serving as a resource for similar children educated throughout the commonwealth.
Funded by: State funds and other sources.
Hours of Operation: 8:00 AM-4:30 PM.
Program Accessibility: Fully accessible.
Staff: Includes teachers of visually impaired students and staff dually certified as teachers and orientation/mobility specialists; various specialists and therapists available as part-time staff or consultants. Uses volunteers. Has advisory board (parent members) for overall program.
History/Date: Est. 1906.
Number of Clients Served: 1991-92: 21.
Eligibility: Blind; Virginia resident living east of I-95.

Area Served: Virginia.
Transportation: Y.
Age Requirements: Day students–2 to 21 years of age. Residential students–5 to 21 years of age.
Health: Well-staffed infirmary open 24 hours per day, Monday to Friday.
Counseling/Social Work/Self-Help: Guidance counselors, social worker, psychologist, and clinical psychologist available.
Educational: Provides instruction in all developmental areas.
Residential: Dormitories.
Employment: Vocational training.
Low Vision: Low vision exams.
Low Vision Aids: Aids available.
Low Vision Follow-up: Y.

STATEWIDE OUTREACH SERVICES

Virginia School for the Deaf and Blind at Hampton
700 Shell Road
Hampton, VA 23661
(757) 247-2284
Amelia Mondok-Pearson, Lead Teacher for the Blind

Funded by: State funds.
History/Date: Est. 1906.
Age Requirements: Birth to 21.

Assessment: Y.
Consultation to Public Schools: Y.
Direct Service: In conjunction with Department for the Visually Handicapped.
Parent Assistance: Y.

INSTRUCTIONAL MATERIALS CENTERS

Virginia Department for the Visually Handicapped Instructional Materials and Resource Center
395 Azalea Avenue

Richmond, VA 23227-3623
(804) 371-3661 or (800) 552-7015
FAX: (804) 371-3508
Barbara McCarthy, Director
Laura Rhodes, Manager

Area Served: State of Virginia.
Groups Served: Ages 0-22 who are still enrolled in a public, private, or parochial secondary program.
Types/Content: Developmental and educational materials.
Media Formats: Braille, large-print textbooks.

◆ *Information Services*

LIBRARIES

Fredericksburg Area Subregional Library
Central Rappahannock Regional Library
1201 Caroline Street
Fredericksburg, VA 22401
(703) 372-1144 or toll-free in Virginia (800) 628-4807 or TDD (703) 372-1144
FAX: (703) 373-9411
Nancy Schiff, Librarian

Subregional library.

Hampton Subregional Library for the Blind and Physically Handicapped
4207 Victoria Boulevard
Hampton, VA 23669
(757) 727-1900 or TDD (757) 727-1900
FAX: (757) 727-1151
Mary Sue Newman, Librarian

Subregional library.

Library and Resource Center Virginia Department for the Visually Handicapped
395 Azalea Avenue

Richmond, VA 23227-3623
(804) 371-3661 or toll-free in
Virginia (800) 552-7015 (voice/
TDD)
FAX: (804) 371-3508
E-mail:
mccarthybn@dvhmail.state.
va.us
Barbara McCarthy, Director

Type of Agency: State program of
the Virginia Department for the
Visually Handicapped.
Mission: To provide free library
service to all eligible print-
handicapped individuals in
Virginia; braille and large print
textbooks and adaptive equipment
to students.
Funded by: State general funds;
federal grants.
Budget: $1 million.
Hours of Operation: Mon.-Fri.
8:15 AM-5:00 PM.
Staff: 25.
History/Date: Est. 1958.
Number of Clients Served:
Average 9,000 statewide.
Eligibility: Blind, visually
impaired, physically handicapped,
or learning disabled not able to use
conventional print; certification of
disability required; Virginia
residents only.
Area Served: Virginia.
Transportation: N.
Age Requirements: None.

Library for the Blind and Physically Handicapped Newport News Public Library System

110 Main Street
Newport News, VA 23601
(757) 591-4855 or (757) 886-2828 or
TDD (757) 591-7418
FAX: (757) 591-4680
Julie M. Hewin, Librarian

Subregional library.

Roanoke City Public Library Outreach Services

2607 Salem Turnpike N. W.
Roanoke, VA 24017
(540) 981-2648
Rebecca Cooper, Librarian

Subregional library.

Special Services Fairfax County Public Library

2501 Sherwood Hall Lane
Alexandria, VA 22306
(703) 660-6943 or TDD (703) 660-
8524
FAX: (703) 765-5893
Jeanette A. Studley, Librarian

Subregional library.

Special Services Division Virginia Beach Public Library

930 Independence Boulevard
Virginia Beach, VA 23455
(757) 464-9175 or TDD (757) 464-
9136
FAX: (757) 464-6741
Aleen Wicher, Librarian

Subregional library.

Talking Book Center Staunton Public Library

1 Churchville Avenue
Staunton, VA 24401-3229
(540) 885-6215
Oakley Pearson, Librarian

Subregional library.

Talking Book Service Alexandria Library

826 Slaters Lane
Alexandria, VA 22314
(703) 838-4298 or TDD (703) 838-
4568
Patricia Bates, Librarian

Subregional library.

Talking Book Service Arlington County Department of Libraries

1015 North Quincy Street
Arlington, VA 22201
(703) 358-6333 or TDD (703) 358-
6320
FAX: (703) 358-5998
Roxanne Barnes, Librarian

Subregional library.

MEDIA PRODUCTION SERVICES

Recording for the Blind and Dyslexic

1021 Millmont Street
Charlottesville, VA 22901
(804) 293-4797
Janet Ewert, Director

See Recording for the Blind and
Dyslexic in U.S. national listings.

RADIO READING

Hampton Roads Voice of the Print Handicapped

5200 Hampton Boulevard
Norfolk, VA 23508
(757) 889-9400
FAX: (757) 489-0007
Peter Pine, Coordinator

Funded by: United Way; State
funds and voluntary contributions.
Hours of Operation: 24 hours,
seven days.
History/Date: Est. 1961.
Area Served: Southwest Virginia.
Age Requirements: None.

Valley Voice Radio Reading Service

WMRA-FM
James Madison University
Harrisonburg, VA 22807
(703) 568-3811
Elizabeth A. Rubush

County/District Where Located:
Rockingham County.

Hours of Operation: Mon.-Sun. 5:00 AM-Midnight.
Staff: 3.
History/Date: Est. 1982.
Area Served: 35-mile radius from Harrisonburg, including Staunton, Waynesboro, New Market, and Charlottesville.
Age Requirements: None.

Virginia Tech Radio Reading Service

4235 Electric Road, S.W.
Suite 105
Roanoke, VA 24014
(540) 989-8900
FAX: (540) 776-2727
Ben Martin, Director

County/District Where Located: Roanoke County.
Funded by: WVTF Public Radio, Virginia Tech Foundation, Voice of the Blue Ridge.
Hours of Operation: 24 hours a day.
Staff: 1.
History/Date: Est. 1979.
Area Served: 80-mile radius from Roanoke, southwestern Virginia.
Age Requirements: None.

Virginia Voice for the Print Handicapped

401 Azalea Avenue
P.O. Box 15546
Richmond, VA 23227
(804) 266-2477
FAX: (804) 266-2478
Nick Morgan, Executive Director

Hours of Operation: Mon.-Fri. 7:15 AM-11:00 PM; Sat. 9:00 AM-5:00 PM; Sun. 2:00 PM-5:00 PM.
History/Date: Est. 1979.
Area Served: Richmond metropolitan areas and, via network, Charlottesville, Yorktown, and Harrisonburg areas.

Voice of the Peninsula

9600 George Washington Highway
P.O. Box 1469
Yorktown, VA 23692
(757) 898-0357
Ambert Dail, Chairperson
William Swartz, Technical Advisor

County/District Where Located: York County.
Hours of Operation: 7 days a week, 7:30 AM-10:00 PM.
History/Date: Est. 1972.
Area Served: 50-mile radius from Yorktown, Tidewater areas.

INFORMATION AND REFERRAL

American Optometric Association

1505 Prince Street
Suite 300
Alexandria, VA 22314
(703) 739-9200
FAX: (703) 739-9497
Kelly Brand, Director of Professional Relations

County/District Where Located: Alexandria County.

See American Optometric Association in U.S. national listings.

The Foundation Fighting Blindness
Central Virginia Affiliate

9312 Huron Avenue
Richmond, VA 23294
(804) 270-2620
John Trageser, President
George P. Dolan, Contact Person

See The Foundation Fighting Blindness in U.S. national listings.

Prevent Blindness Virginia

9840 Midlothian Turnpike, Suite R
Richmond, VA 23235
(804) 330-3195
FAX: (804) 330-3198
E-mail: 104706.1107@compreserve.com
Tim Gresham, President

County/District Where Located: Chesterfield County.

See Prevent Blindness America in U.S. national listings.

See also in national listings:

American Diabetes Association National Center

American Society of Cataract and Refractive Surgery

Association for Education and Rehabilitation of the Blind and Visually Impaired

Better Vision Institute Vision Council of America

Council for Exceptional Children

National Association of State Directors of Special Education

National Industries for the Blind

Opticians Association of America

RESNA

◆ *Rehabilitation Services*

STATE SERVICES

Virginia Department for the Visually Handicapped

395 Azalea Avenue
Richmond, VA 23227-3623
(804) 371-3140
FAX: (804) 371-3351
URL: http://www.state.va.us%hhr/dvh-2.htm
W. Roy Grizzard, Jr., Commissioner

Type of Agency: State.

Mission: Services for totally blind, legally blind, visually impaired, and deaf-blind persons.

Funded by: Workshop sales; income from general funds; state and federal funds.

Budget: 1992-93: $16,970,942.

Hours of Operation: Mon.-Fri. 8:15 AM-5:00 PM.

Program Accessibility: Fully accessible.

Staff: 242 full time. Uses volunteers.

History/Date: Est. 1922.

Number of Clients Served: Unduplicated count not available.

Eligibility: Legally blind or visually impaired.

Area Served: Statewide.

Transportation: Y.

Health: Diagnosis and evaluation of eye health; follow-up evaluation of eye treatment or prescription; audiology therapy; general and eye medical services. Provides eye surgery and/or eye treatment. Contracts, refers, and provides consultation to other agencies for other health services.

Counseling/Social Work/Self-Help: Social evaluation; psychological testing and evaluation; individual, group, family/parent, couple counseling; placement in school, training; referral to community services. Contracts, refers, and provides consultation to other agencies for counseling/social work services.

Educational: Accepts persons who are deaf-blind, emotionally disturbed, learning disabled, mentally retarded, orthopedically disabled if visually impaired or have other multiple disabilities and are capable of meeting educational requirements. Programs for college prep; adapted tests, materials, and equipment; sponsorship for college training.

Professional Training: Internship/fieldwork placement in orientation/mobility; rehabilitation counseling; social work; vocational rehabilitation. Regular in-service training programs.

Reading: Lends talking book record player and cassette player; talking book records and cassettes; braille books; large-print books; braille magazines; recorded magazines. Information and referral; transcription to braille; tape recording services on demand. Department's library also serves physically disabled persons.

Residential: Dormitories for elderly and other adults, and multiply disabled persons; on-site apartments for adults and elderly persons while in training at the Virginia Rehabilitation Center for the Blind.

Rehabilitation: Personal management; braille; social skills; handwriting; listening skills; Optacon; typing; video magnifier; electronic mobility aids; home management; orientation/mobility; rehabilitation teaching in client's home and community; remedial education; sensory training.

Recreational: Afterschool programs; arts and crafts; hobby groups; special programs for elderly persons; bowling; swimming; track; basketball; pool. Contracts, refers, and provides consultation to other agencies for other recreational services.

Employment: Prevocational evaluation; career and skill counseling; occupational skill development; job retention; job retraining; sheltered workshops; vocational placement; follow-up service; vending stand training; supported employment; vocational training.

Computer Training: Computer adaptive skills training at Virginia Rehabilitation Center for the Blind.

Low Vision: Assessment of functional residual vision; evaluation for feasibility of specialized visual aids; prescription of spectacles or low vision aids or devices; provides specialized aids and follow-up training in use of aids and/or use of residual vision. Aids are distributed by in-house optical aids center. Low vision services are obtained by contacting regional offices.

Low Vision: Y.

Low Vision Aids: Y.

Low Vision Follow-up: Y.

Regional Offices:

Bristol Regional Office: 111 Commonwealth Avenue, Bristol, VA 24201, (703) 676-5457.

Fairfax Regional Office: 1150 Main Street, Suite 502, Fairfax, VA 22030, (703) 359-1100.

Norfolk Regional Office: 5505 Robin Hood Road, Suite F, Norfolk, VA 23513, (757) 858-6724.

Richmond Regional Office: 397 Azalea Avenue, Richmond, VA 23227, (804) 371-3353.

Roanoke Regional Office: Commonwealth of Virginia Building, 210 Church Avenue, S.W., Suite 308, Roanoke, VA 24011-1523, (540) 857-7122.

Stanton Regional Office: 620 East Beverly Street, Stanton, VA 24401, (540) 332-7729.

Local Offices:

Charlottesville: Virginia Department for the Visually Handicapped, Virginia Industries for the Blind, 1102 Monticello Road, Charlottesville, VA 22902, (804) 295-5168.

Richmond: Virginia Department for the Visually Handicapped, Virginia Industries for the Blind, 1535 High Street, Richmond, VA 23261, (804) 786-2056.

Special Sections:

Richmond: Virginia Rehabilitation Center for the Blind, 401 Azalea Avenue, Richmond, VA 23227, (804) 371-3151.

REHABILITATION

Virginia Association of Workers for the Blind
6400 Rigsby Road
Richmond, VA 23226
(804) 282-0813
Betty Meredith, Office Manager

Type of Agency: Private; non-profit.
County/District Where Located: Henrico County.
Funded by: Membership fees and contributions.
History/Date: Est. 1919.

Health: Prescribes eyeglasses.
Recreational: Summer camp.

**Virginia Industries for the Blind
Virginia Department for the Visually Handicapped**
1102 Monticello Road
Charlottesville, VA 22902
(804) 295-5168
FAX: (804) 977-0122
Janet Honeycutt, Plant Manager
Robert C. Berrang, General Manager

Type of Agency: Provides training and employment opportunities for blind persons.
County/District Where Located: Albemarle County.
Mission: To provide training, work evaluations and employment for blind and visually impaired Virginians to achieve their

maximum level of independence and participation in society.
Funded by: Self-supported by sales revenues.
Budget: $3,750,000.
Hours of Operation: Mon.-Fri. 7:30 AM-4:30 PM.
Staff: 1 vocational coordinator.
History/Date: Est. 1922.
Number of Clients Served: Approximately 100.
Eligibility: Eligibility determination made by Department for the Visually Handicapped Services Division.
Area Served: State of Virginia.
Age Requirements: Legal age to work.

Counseling/Social Work/Self-Help: Vocational counseling, training, evaluations.
Employment: Transitional and permanent.
Computer Training: Available.
Low Vision Aids: Available.
Low Vision Follow-up: Available.

**Virginia Industries for the Blind
Virginia Department for the Visually Handicapped**
1535 High Street
P.O. Box 27563
Richmond, VA 23220
(804) 295-6034 or (804) 295-5168
FAX: (804) 977-0122
Robert C. Berrang, General Manager

Type of Agency: State.
Mission: Provide a job program for blind and visually impaired persons.
Budget: $7,500,000.
Hours of Operation: Mon.-Fri. 7:30 AM-4:30 PM.
Staff: 10.
History/Date: Est. 1925.
Number of Clients Served: 100.
Eligibility: Eligibility determination made by the

Virginia Department for the Visually Handicapped.
Area Served: State of Virginia.
Age Requirements: 18 and over.

Rehabilitation: Training and vocational assistance for outward placement.
Employment: Training and employment opportunities.
Low Vision Aids: Available on case basis.
Low Vision Follow-up: Y.

COMPUTER TRAINING CENTERS

Virginia Rehabilitation Center for the Blind
401 Azalea Avenue
Richmond, VA 23227
(804) 371-3151
FAX: (804) 371-3092
Dennis Garza, Director

Computer Training: Speech output systems; screen magnification systems; braille access systems; closed-circuit television systems; word processing; computer operating systems; training for instructors.

◆ Low Vision Services

EYE CARE SOCIETIES

Virginia Society of Ophthalmology
P.O. Box 23027
Richmond, VA 23223
(804) 649-2407
Donna H. Scott, Executive Director

Virginia Optometric Association
118 North Eighth Street
Richmond, VA 23219-2305
(804) 643-0309
Bruce B. Keeney, Director

LOW VISION CENTERS

Virginia Department for the Visually Handicapped
395 Azalea Avenue
Richmond, VA 23227-3623
(804) 371-3140
FAX: (804) 371-3351
W. Roy Grizzard, Jr.,
Commissioner
Marge Owens, Coordinator

Type of Agency: State.
Mission: Provide an opportunity for all visually handicapped Virginians to maximize their visual abilities through community-based interdisciplinary low vision services.
Funded by: State, federal funds.
Budget: $232,000.
Hours of Operation: Mon.-Fri. 8:15 AM-5:00 PM.
Staff: 19 full time.
History/Date: Est. 1960.
Number of Clients Served: More than 1,000 annually.
Eligibility: Eye report.
Area Served: Virginia.
Transportation: N.

Low Vision: Available through local offices.
Low Vision Aids: Provided on loan for trial.
Low Vision Follow-up: As needed.

For office locations, see Virginia Department for the Visually Handicapped in the Rehabilitation Services listings.

Virginia Optometric Center
210 North James Street
Ashland, VA 23005
(804) 270-2020 or (804) 798-3010
Robert M. Malatin, O.D., Director

Type of Agency: Non-profit.
County/District Where Located: Henrico County.
Funded by: Client fees (sliding scale); state funds.

Hours of Operation: Mon.-Fri. 9:00 AM-1:00 PM.
Staff: Optometrist; low vision specialists.
Area Served: Unlimited.

Low Vision Aids: Provided on loan for trial; with deposit, no rental fee; on-site training provided.

Virginia Rehabilitation Center for the Blind
401 Azalea Avenue
Richmond, VA 23227
(804) 371-3151
FAX: (804) 371-3092
Lee Albright, O.D.
Gail Kinder, Assistant Director

Type of Agency: Public residential rehabilitation center.
County/District Where Located: Henrico County.
Mission: To provide an opportunity for all visually impaired Virginians to maximize their visual abilities through community and center-based interdisciplinary low vision services.
Funded by: State and federal funds.
Hours of Operation: Friday twice a month, 8:30 AM-5:00 PM, or as needed.
Staff: Social worker; orientation/mobility instructor; rehabilitation teacher; special educator; occupational therapist; rehabilitation counselor; consulting audiologist; work evaluator; consulting optometrist, low vision specialist; deaf-blind specialist.
History/Date: Est. 1975.
Number of Clients Served: 250 yearly.
Eligibility: Eye-care practitioner report.
Area Served: Virginia.

Age Requirements: 14 years and older.
Educational: Adult basic educational programs.
Employment: Adjustment training and some job-site training.
Computer Training: Y.
Low Vision: Y.
Low Vision Aids: Provided on loan for trial; no rental fee; on-site training provided.
Low Vision Follow-up: Varies.

♦ Aging Services

STATE UNITS ON AGING

Virginia Department for the Aging
700 Centre, Tenth Floor
700 East Franklin Street
Richmond, VA 23219-2327
(804) 225-2271 or Information & Referral In State (800) 552-3402
FAX: (804) 371-8381
Thelma Bland, Commissioner

Provides referrals to Area Agencies on Aging and information on other local aging services.

INDEPENDENT LIVING PROGRAMS

Virginia Department for the Visually Handicapped Services Division
395 Azalea Avenue
Richmond, VA 23227
(804) 371-3140 or (800) 622-2155
Jane Ward, Program Director

Provides independent living services for persons age 55 and over. For further information, contact the Project Director or general phone number listed.

VIRGIN ISLANDS

◆ *Educational Services*

STATE SERVICES

Virgin Islands Department of Education
State Office of Special Education
44-46 Kongens Gade
Charlotte Amalie
St. Thomas, VI 00802
(809) 774-4399
FAX: (809) 774-0817
Elsie Monsanto, Director of Special Education

Mission: To provide all appropriate educational and related services to eligible students, ages 3-21.
Funded by: Virgin Islands government and federal funds.
Area Served: St. Thomas, St. Croix, and St. John.
Age Requirements: 3-21 years.

Provides special classes for totally blind students. Partially sighted children attend regular classes. Provides reader service for students 15 years and over who qualify.

For information about local facilities, consult the head of schools in the area.

EARLY INTERVENTION COORDINATION

Division of Maternal and Child Health Care and Crippled Children Services
Virgin Islands Department of Health
Knud Hansen Complex
516 Strand Street
Charlotte Amalie
St. Thomas, VI 00802
(809) 772-5895 or (809) 774-0117
FAX: (809) 772-5895
Jose F. Poblete, Assistant Commissioner

◆ *Information Services*

LIBRARIES

Virgin Islands Regional Library for the Visually and Physically Handicapped
3012 Golden Rock
Christiansted
St. Croix, VI 00820
(809) 772-2250
FAX: (809) 772-3545
Laurie Cole, Regional Librarian

Hours of Operation: Mon.-Fri. 8:00 AM-5:00 PM.
Staff: 4.5 full time equivalents.
Number of Clients Served: 150.
Eligibility: As per National Library Service for the Blind and Physically Handicapped.

Regional library supplying talking books, braille, large-type books, cassette tapes, talking book machines, cassette players, and home visits.

◆ *Rehabilitation Services*

STATE SERVICES

Division of Disabilities and Rehabilitation Services
Virgin Islands Department of Human Services
Knud Hansen Complex
Building A, 1303 Hospital Ground
Charlotte Amalie
St. Thomas, VI 00802
(809) 774-0930
FAX: (809) 774-3466
Sadonie Halbert, Administrator of Disabilities

Type of Agency: Public.
Mission: Services to all disabled persons, including those who are blind or visually impaired.
Funded by: Federal and state funds.
Transportation: Y.

Counseling/Social Work/Self-Help: Counseling and guidance and personal adjustment services available.
Rehabilitation: Physical and mental restoration; mobility training; independent living services; vocational and college training; Randolph-Sheppard program; special equipment training.
Employment: Supported employment services.

Local Offices:

St. Croix: Vocational Rehabilitation and Division of Senior Citizens Affairs, P.O. Box 146, Christiansted, St. Croix, VI 00820, (809) 773-2333.
St. Thomas: Division of Senior Citizens Affairs, Barbel Plaza South, St. Thomas, VI 00802, (809) 774-5884.

◆ *Aging Services*

STATE UNITS ON AGING

Senior Citizen Affairs
Virgin Islands Department of
Human Services
19 Estate Diamond
Fredericksted
St. Croix, VI 00840
(809) 692-5950
FAX: (809) 692-2062
Bernice Hall, Administrator

Provides referrals to Area Agencies
on Aging and information on other
local aging services.

INDEPENDENT LIVING PROGRAMS

Virgin Islands Department of
Human Services
1303 Hospital Ground, Building A
Charlotte Amalie
St. Thomas, VI 00802
(809) 774-0930
Beverly Plankett, Administrator

Provides independent living
services for persons age 55 and
over. For further information,
contact the Project Director or
general phone number listed.

WASHINGTON

◆ *Educational Services*

STATE SERVICES

**Washington Office of Superintendent of Public Instruction
Special Education**
Old Capitol Building
P.O. Box 47200
Olympia, WA 98504-7200
(360) 753-6733
FAX: (360) 586-0247
Douglas H. Gill, Director of Special Education
Don L. Hanson, Supervisor, Special Education

Type of Agency: State education agency.
Mission: Provides program material and services for visually impaired children through state and federal funds.
Funded by: Public funds.
Area Served: Washington State.
Age Requirements: Primarily serve persons aged 3 through 21 (or high school graduation); children aged 0-2 are also eligible.

For information about local facilities, consult the local school district.

OSPI also funds the Washington Instructional Resource Center, a statewide project that serves blind and low vision students, and contributes support for Washington State Services for Children with Deaf-Blindness (which is partially federally supported). In addition, it funds the cooperative efforts of educational service districts and local school districts on the East side of the state.

EARLY INTERVENTION COORDINATION

**Birth to Three Early Intervention Program
Washington Department of Social and Health Services**
P.O. Box 45201
Olympia, WA 98504-5201
(360) 586-2810
FAX: (360) 902-8497
Sandy Loerch, Part H Early Childhood Coordinator

County/District Where Located: Thurston County.

Lead agency for the Individuals with Disabilities Education Act (Part H).

SCHOOLS

Washington State School for the Blind
2214 East 13th Street
Vancouver, WA 98661-4120
(360) 696-6321
FAX: (360) 737-2120
Dr. Dean O. Stenehjem, Superintendent

Type of Agency: State.
County/District Where Located: Clark County.
Mission: Provides specialized 24-hour quality educational services to visually impaired youths ages 0-21 within the state of Washington. A statewide demonstration and resource center, the school provides direct and indirect services to students both on campus and in each child's local community. Provides services to families, educators, and others interested in assisting visually impaired youths to become independent, contributing citizens.
Budget: 1995-97: $7,214,404.
Hours of Operation: Mon.-Fri. 7:30 AM-4:30 PM.

Staff: 72 full time; 2 part time. Uses volunteers and foster grandparents.
History/Date: Est. 1886.
Number of Clients Served: 233 monthly average 1995-96; 74 on campus, 159 off campus.
Eligibility: Visually impaired or blind.
Area Served: Washington residents accepted without tuition. Students from other states or countries accepted on a tuition basis if space is available.
Transportation: Y.
Age Requirements: Birth to 21 years.

Health: School health center staffed by RNs.
Educational: Preschool through post-high school. College prep; general academic studies; vocational/skill development. Major emphasis in community integration and intensive specialized skill development. All students enrolled with a 24-hour Individualized Education Program (IEP) and Individual Transition Plan (ITP). Summer school provided for students from local education areas (LEAs) from throughout the state of Washington who are not currently enrolled at the school. Emphasis on specialized skill training.
Professional Training: Internship/student teaching in a wide variety of areas: classroom vision, orientation and mobility, special education-related services, and low vision. Regular in-service workshops for state and region.
Residential: Five cottages and one independent living center. Major emphasis in the cottage program is placed on students developing skills that will lead toward independence.
Recreational: Afterschool programs; arts and crafts; snow

skiing, swimming, integration with community recreational sources.

Employment: Assistance for students in smooth transition to adult placement/careers.

Computer Training: Training on computer aids and devices.

Low Vision: Clinic funded by Lions Clubs. Provides comprehensive low vision evaluations at no charge. Clinic open two days a week during the school year.

Low Vision Aids: Depository funded by Lions Clubs. Lends low vision aids after evaluation and training. Provides follow-up on low vision evaluation and use of low vision aids.

Braille Access Center - Public and private braille production center. Operates on a fee-for-services basis. (360) 696-6321, ext. 158#.

Computer Technology Center - Statewide services provided to local public schools, staff and students. (360) 696-6321, ext. 157#.

Instructional Material Center - Statewide resources provided - materials, aids, applicance, material acquisition, and consultative services. (360) 696-6321, ext. 183#.

Provides consultative outreach services throughout the state. Also provides long-term contracted consultant services and contracted itinerant services.

STATEWIDE OUTREACH SERVICES

Washington State School for the Blind
2214 East 13th Street
Vancouver, WA 98661-4120
(360) 696-6321, ext. 124
FAX: (360) 737-2120
Rod Humble, Outreach Services Coordinator

Funded by: State of Washington.
History/Date: Outreach services; est. 1978.
Age Requirements: 0-21 years.

Assessment: Assessment of needs in public schools, throughout state and more comprehensive assessments at School for the Blind.
Consultation to Public Schools: Entire school and residential staff available to consult with local schools and families.
Direct Service: Provide direct service to 23 districts within the state.
Parent Assistance: On request, visits with parents in their homes.
Materials Production: Braille materials and instructional resource center.
Professional Training: Numerous yearly workshops for teachers, para-professionals and parents. Summer institute for staff throughout the state who have no training with visually impaired children.

INSTRUCTIONAL MATERIALS CENTERS

Washington Instructional Resource Center
Washington State School for the Blind
2120 East 13th Street
Vancouver, WA 98661
(360) 696-6321, ext. 183 or 184
FAX: (360) 737-2120
Joan Christensen, Coordinator

Area Served: Washington State.
Groups Served: Blind or partially sighted persons; public and private schools.

Types/Content: Textbooks.
Media Formats: Braille and large print.
Title Listings: Available on request.

◆ *Information Services*

LIBRARIES

Washington Library for the Blind and Physically Handicapped
821 Lenora Street
Seattle, WA 98129
(206) 464-6930 or toll-free in Washington (800) 542-0866 or TDD (206) 464-6930
FAX: (206) 464-0247
E-mail: wtbbl@spl.lib.wa.us
URL: http://www.spl.lib.wa.us/wtbbl.html
Jan Ames, Librarian
Phyllis Cairns, Machine Lending Information

Type of Agency: Regional library for individuals with disabilities.
Mission: To provide library services to citizens who are unable to utilize print materials.
Funded by: Public funds.
Budget: $1,246,758.
Hours of Operation: Mon.-Fri. 8:30 AM-5:00 PM, Sat. 9:00 AM-1:00 PM.
Staff: 22.4.
History/Date: Est. 1931.
Number of Clients Served: 12,000 annually.
Eligibility: Blind, visually or physically disabled, deaf/blind, reading disabled.
Area Served: Washington.

Low Vision: Closed-circuit televisions on a loan basis.

Regional library supplying braille, large type, audio cassette books, talking book records and cassette machines; offers braille and taping service.

Has radio reading service (special programming for blind and physically disabled persons) in Seattle, Spokane and most of eastern Washington.

MEDIA PRODUCTION SERVICES

Father Palmer Memorial Braille Service
Lilac Blind Foundation
North 1212 Howard Street
Spokane, WA 99201
(509) 325-1442 or (800) 422-7893
Caroline Means, President

County/District Where Located:
Spokane.
Area Served: Statewide.

Types/Content: Textbooks, recreational, career/vocational, religious, any requests.
Media Formats: Braille books; thermoform - computer.
Title Listings: No title listings available.

Seattle Area Braillists, Inc.
13746 Corliss Avenue North
Seattle, WA 98133
(206) 362-3764
Jeanne Horsey, President

County/District Where Located:
King County.
Area Served: State of Washington.
Groups Served: K-12; assignments from Washington State Special Education Materials Clearinghouse and Depository.

Types/Content: Textbooks.
Media Formats: Braille books.
Title Listings: Available through the Special Education Materials Clearinghouse and Depository, (360) 696-6321, ext. 158.

University of Washington
448 Schmitz Hall
Box 355839
Seattle, WA 98195
(206) 543-8924
FAX: (206) 616-8379
E-mail: uwdss@u.washington.edu
Dyane Haynes, Director

Groups Served: College students.
Types/Content: Textbooks.
Media Formats: Braille books, talking books/cassettes, large-print books.
Title Listings: No title listings available.

Washington State Braille Access Center
Washington State School for the Blind
2214 East 13th Street
Vancouver, WA 98661-4120
(360) 696-6321, ext. 158
FAX: (360) 737-2120
Colleen Heiden, Coordinator

Area Served: Washington State.
Groups Served: 3-21 years, college students. Other adults.

Types/Content: Textbooks, career/vocational, general fiction, nonfiction.
Media Formats: Braille books, talking books/cassettes, large-print books.
Title Listings: No title listings available.

RADIO READING

Evergreen Radio Reading Service
821 Lenora Street
Seattle, WA 98129
(206) 464-6930
FAX: (206) 464-6930
E-mail: wtbbl@spl.lib.wa.us
Donna Amos, Assistant Manager

Hours of Operation: Mon.-Fri. 7:00 AM-10:00 PM; Sat. 9:00 AM-5:00 PM; Sun. 1:00 PM-7:00 PM.
History/Date: Est. 1973 (Seattle), 1983 (Spokane), 1986 (eastern Washington), 1994 (24-hour reading).
Area Served: Western Washington; all major population centers in eastern Washington.

INFORMATION AND REFERRAL

The Foundation Fighting Blindness
Seattle Affiliate
300 Queen Anne Avenue North
Seattle, WA 98109-4599
(206) 946-1433
Gerald Purdy, Contact Person

See The Foundation Fighting Blindness in U.S. national listings.

♦ Rehabilitation Services

STATE SERVICES

Washington State Department of Services for the Blind
1400 S. Evergreen Park Drive
Suite 100
Olympia, WA 98504-0933
(360) 586-1224
FAX: (360) 586-7627
E-mail: ssmi315@dsb.wa.gov
Shirley Smith, Director

Type of Agency: Public.
Mission: Services for totally blind, legally blind, visually impaired, and deaf-blind persons.
Funded by: State and federal funding.
Budget: $6 million.
Hours of Operation: Mon.-Fri. 8:00 AM-5:00 PM.
Program Accessibility: All offices accessible.
Staff: 70.
Number of Clients Served: 3,000 annually.
Area Served: Statewide.

Counseling/Social Work/Self-Help: Counselors for vocational rehabilitation and adjustment.
Educational: Family program to educate parents.
Rehabilitation: Independent living program; vocational rehabilitation.

Employment: Vocational counseling, training, placement. Business enterprise program.
Computer Training: Individualized training at job site.
Low Vision: Complete program of evaluation, referral and rehabilitation.
Low Vision Aids: Available.
Low Vision Follow-up: Y.

Local Offices:

Seattle: 3411 South Alaska Street, Seattle, WA 98118, (206) 721-4422.
Spokane: West 55 Mission Street, Suite 3, Spokane, WA 99201, (509) 456-4458.
Tacoma: 10209 Bridgeport Way, S.W., Suite 1A, Tacoma, WA 98499, (206) 589-7227.
Vancouver: 500 West Eighth Street, Suite 18, Vancouver, WA 98660, (360) 696-6238.
Yakima: 1600 West Perry Building 1, Suite D, Yakima, WA 98902, (509) 575-2014.

REHABILITATION

American Lake Blind Rehabilitation Clinic
U.S. Department of Veterans Affairs
VA Puget Sound Health Care System
9900 Veterans Drive S.W.
Tacoma, WA 98493
(206) 582-8440, ext. 6203
FAX: (206) 589-4112
Mike Weatherly, Chief
Kent Wardell, Assistant Chief

Type of Agency: Federal.
County/District Where Located: King County.
Mission: Provides residential and rehabilitation services to eligible legally blind veterans.
History/Date: Est. 1971.

Referral applications by Visual Impairment Services programs located at VA Medical Centers and Outpatient Clinics in the geographical area served by the Blind Rehabilitation Center or Clinic.

See U.S. Department of Veterans Affairs in U.S. Federal Agencies listings.

Community Services for the Blind and Partially Sighted
9709 Third Avenue N.E.
Suite 100
Seattle, WA 98115-2027
(206) 525-5556 or toll-free in Washington (800) 458-4888
FAX: (206) 525-0422
E-mail: csbps@csbps.com
URL: http://www.csbps.com
June W. Mansfield, President/CEO

Type of Agency: Private; non-profit.
Mission: Services for totally blind and visually impaired persons.
Funded by: United Way; contributions; bequests; used merchandise; solicitation; fees.
Budget: 1996: $1,100,000.
Hours of Operation: Mon.-Fri. 8:00 AM-5:00 PM.
Staff: 34 full time, 49 part time. Uses volunteers.
History/Date: Est. 1965.
Number of Clients Served: 1996: 1,600.
Eligibility: Legally blind, blind, visually impaired.
Area Served: King, Snohomish, and Skagit Counties.

Health: Low vision clinic includes evaluation of functional vision; prescription of low vision aids and training in their use; trial loan of aids before purchase before purchase.
Counseling/Social Work/Self-Help: Psychological assessment; individual, group, family/parent, couple counseling; referral to community resources. Workshops, classes, support groups. Provides consultation to other agencies for other counseling/social work.
Educational: Information and referral; quarterly newsletter; statewide srsource guide; classes. Consultation about Americans with Disabilities Act.
Professional Training: Internship/fieldwork placement in orientation/mobility; social work.
Reading: Volunteers available to assist at home with mail reading and grocery shopping.
Rehabilitation: Orientation/ mobility; rehabilitation teaching in client's home and community; activities of daily living services, personal management; braille and other communication; adaptive aids; diabetes management; brailler repair.
Employment: Refers for employment-oriented services.
Computer Training: Individual tutorials offered in agency's assistive technology center.
Low Vision: Low vision clinic.
Low Vision Aids: Operates a "teaching store" where persons purchase and learn to use a variety of adaptive products.
Low Vision Follow-up: Y.

Operates a volunteer service to meet client requests for assistance; service includes reading, grocery shopping, and bill paying.

Emil Fries Piano Hospital and Training Center
2510 East Evergreen Boulevard
Vancouver, WA 98662
(360) 693-1511
FAX: (360) 693-6891
Kenneth D. Serviss, Executive Vice President and Manager

Type of Agency: Private; non-profit.
County/District Where Located: Clark County.

Mission: Teaching men and women, primarily those with visual limitations, to be self-sufficient as piano tuner-technicians.

Funded by: Tuition, piano sales and service, donations.

Budget: $485,000.

Hours of Operation: Mon.-Fri. 8:00 AM-5:00 PM; Sat. 9:00 AM-4:00 PM.

Staff: 7 full time. Uses volunteers.

History/Date: Est. 1949.

Eligibility: Totally or legally blind; high school graduate or equivalent.

Area Served: Unlimited.

Age Requirements: 18 years or older.

Health: Refers for health services.

Counseling/Social Work/Self-Help: Advice on site, refers for counseling.

Educational: Program for vocational/skill development.

Professional Training: Regular full-time training program; short-term or summer training.

Reading: Talking book record and cassette players; talking book records and tapes; braille and large-print books; braille and recorded magazines. Tape recording services on request.

Residential: Off-site apartments and boarding homes.

Employment: Occupational skill development; job retention; job retraining; job referral; follow-up service.

Low Vision Aids: Vistek; braille writers, talking computer.

Helen Keller National Center for Deaf-Blind Youths and Adults Northwest Region Office

2366 Eastlake Avenue East
Suite 209
Seattle, WA 98102-3366
(206) 324-9120 (voice/TDD)
FAX: (206) 324-9159
Dorothy Walt, Regional Representative

County/District Where Located: King County.

See Helen Keller National Center for Deaf-Blind Youths and Adults in U.S. national listings.

The Lighthouse for the Blind, Inc.

2501 Plum Street
P.O. Box C-14119
Seattle, WA 98114
(206) 322-4200 or TDD (206) 324-1388
FAX: (206) 329-3397
George Jacobson, President
Paula Hoffman, Director of Vocational Rehabilitation Services

Type of Agency: Private; non-profit.

County/District Where Located: King County.

Mission: To be the premier manufacturer of products made by blind persons, offering a range of quality employment opportunities and services to people who are blind, deaf-blind, and blind/multiply disabled.

Funded by: Workshop sales; contributions; fees.

Budget: 1997: $17 million.

Hours of Operation: 8:00 AM-4:30 PM.

Program Accessibility: Fully accessible.

Staff: Approximately 30 administrative. Approximately 24 rehabilitation/services. Manufacturing division employs about 250.

History/Date: Est. 1918.

Number of Clients Served: Approximately 750 annually.

Eligibility: Visually impaired, blind, deaf-blind or blind with multiple disabilities.

Area Served: Pacific Northwest, particularly Seattle metropolitan area.

Age Requirements: 21 years and over.

Health: Occupational health nurse on-site.

Educational: Adult Continuing Education (ACE) program offered for part-time, individualized and self-paced study.

Professional Training: Internship/fieldwork placement in orientation/mobility; interpreter training; in-service training when requested by schools, institutions, hospitals, group homes and other facilities.

Rehabilitation: See "Employment."

Recreational: Week-long retreat for deaf-blind persons in August.

Employment: Vocational evaluation; orientation/mobility training; independent living classes/services; work-related counseling; competitive placement services; supported employment services; specialized support services for deaf-blind persons, including interpreting department. On-the-job training; employment in manufacturing company; prevocational training for developmentally disabled.

Computer Training: Computer basics, keyboarding, Windows software.

Lilac Blind Foundation

North 1212 Howard
Spokane, WA 99201
(509) 328-9116 or (800) 422-7893
FAX: (509) 328-8965
Nancy Domanico, Executive Director

Type of Agency: Private; non-profit.

Mission: To provide services and training to blind persons.
Funded by: Private donations.
Hours of Operation: Mon.-Fri. 8:30 AM-4:30 PM.
Staff: 8.
History/Date: Est. 1972.
Number of Clients Served: 800 clients served per year.
Eligibility: Visually impaired.
Area Served: Eastern Washington and northern Idaho.

Counseling/Social Work/Self-Help: Personal adjustment.
Rehabilitation: Independent living program.
Computer Training: Y.
Low Vision: Evaluation services available.
Low Vision Aids: Available.

COMPUTER TRAINING CENTERS

Olympia Educational Service District 114

105 National Avenue
Bremerton, WA 98312
(360) 478-6886
FAX: (360) 478-6869
Debra Knesal, Director

County/District Where Located: Kitsap County.

Computer Training: Speech output systems; screen magnification systems; optical character recognition systems; word processing; computer operating systems; training for instructors.

Special Education Technology Center

506 North Sprague

Ellensburg, WA 98926
(509) 925-8040
FAX: (509) 925-8025
Ann Black, Supervisor
Barbaralyn Harden, Technology Specialist
Jerry Connolly, Technology Specialist

County/District Where Located: Kittitas County.

Computer Training: Assistive technology; augmentative and alternative communication (A.A.C.); lending library.

Washington State School for the Blind
Technical Center for Blind and Visually Handicapped Students

2214 East 13th Street
Vancouver, WA 98661-4120
(360) 696-6321
FAX: (360) 737-2120
Bruce McClanahan, Instructor

Computer Training: Speech output systems; screen magnification systems; braille access systems; closed-circuit television systems; word processing; database software; training for instructors; computer operating systems; equipment with software loan program; evaluations on-site and off.

◆ Low Vision Services

EYE CARE SOCIETIES

Washington Academy of Eye Physicians and Surgeons

2033 6th Avenue
Suite 1100
Seattle, WA 98121
(206) 441-9762
FAX: (206) 441-5863
Kory Diemert, Executive Administrator

County/District Where Located: King County.

Washington Association of Optometric Physicians

555 116th Avenue N.E., #166
Bellevue, WA 98004-5274
(206) 455-0874
FAX: (206) 646-9646
Judy Balzer, Executive Director

LOW VISION CENTERS

Community Services for the Blind and Partially Sighted

9709 Third Avenue, N.E.
Suite 100
Seattle, WA 98115-2027
(206) 525-5556 or toll-free in Washington (800) 458-4888
FAX: (206) 525-0422
E-mail: csbps@csbps.com
URL: http://www.csbps.com
June W. Mansfield, President/CEO
Mark Mahnke, Vice President, Rehabilitation Services

Type of Agency: Private; non-profit.
County/District Where Located: King County.
Mission: To provide services for persons with low vision.
Funded by: Client fees; United Way; donations; third-party payers.
Hours of Operation: Mon.-Fri. 8:00 AM-5:00 PM.
Staff: Optometrist; low vision rehabilitation specialist; mobility instructor; social worker.
History/Date: Est. 1975.
Number of Clients Served: 600.
Eligibility: Low vision; ophthalmology report.
Area Served: Unlimited.

Low Vision: Evaluation of functional vision; prescription and training in use of low vision aids.
Low Vision Aids: Trial loan of low vision aids before purchase.

Low Vision Follow-up: Y.

Eye and Ear Clinic

600 Douglas Street
Wenatchee, WA 98801
(509) 662-7143
T. A. Sorom, M.D., Chairman

Funded by: Client fees.
Eligibility: None.
Area Served: Central Washington.

Low Vision Aids: Available on a
limited basis.

Group Health Cooperative of Puget Sound

Eastside Medical Center
2701 156th Avenue, N.E.
Redmond, WA 98052
(206) 883-5331
FAX: (206) 556-6110
John W. Barry, O.D., Optometrist

Type of Agency: Non-profit.
County/District Where Located:
King County.
Funded by: Client fees.
Hours of Operation: Mon.-Fri.
10:50 AM-2:50 PM.
Staff: Ophthalmologist;
optometrist.
Eligibility: Health plan member;
private patients also seen.
Area Served: Statewide.

Low Vision Aids: Provided on
loan for trial; no rental fee; on-site
training provided.
Low Vision Follow-up: Phone
interview in 1 month; return
appointment in 6 months.

Group Health Cooperative of Puget Sound

Central Hospital and Specialty
Center
200 15th Avenue East
Seattle, WA 98112
(206) 326-3133
Gregory L. Eisen, O.D.,
Optometrist

Type of Agency: Non-profit.
County/District Where Located:
King County.
Funded by: Client fees.
Hours of Operation: Mon.-Fri.
8:30 AM-5:30 PM.
Staff: Ophthalmologist;
optometrist; optician; ophthalmic
assistant/technician; optometric
assistant/technician; social
worker; occupational therapist;
psychologist/counselor.
Eligibility: Health plan member.
Area Served: King County and
northwestern Washington State.

Low Vision Aids: Provided on
loan for trial; no rental fee; on-site
training provided.
Low Vision Follow-up: By return
appointment in 6 months.

Lions Low Vision Clinic of the Inland Empire

4001 Cook
Spokane, WA 99207
(509) 484-4259
Karen Christensen, Director
Gene Teigen, O.D.,
Ophthalmologist

Type of Agency: Non-profit.
Funded by: Client fees and grants.
Hours of Operation: By
appointment.
Staff: Optometrist;
ophthalmologist; low vision
assistant; optometry student/
resident.
Eligibility: Referral.
Area Served: Unlimited.

Low Vision Aids: Provided on
loan for trial; rental fee charged;
on-site training provided.
Low Vision Follow-up: By return
appointment after 1 month.

Washington State School for the Blind

2214 East 13th Street
Vancouver, WA 98661-4120
(360) 696-6321, ext. 141#
FAX: (206) 737-2120
Dr. Dean O. Stenehjem,
Superintendent

Type of Agency: State.
Funded by: Lions State Sight
Conservation Program; Lions Club
MD#19 Sight Foundation.
Hours of Operation: 2 days per
week during school year.
Number of Clients Served: More
than 200 annually.
Eligibility: Visually impaired
students; referred.
Area Served: Washington.
Age Requirements: None.

Professional Training: Serves as a
training program for Pacific
University School of Optometry.
Low Vision Aids: Provided on
loan for trial; no rental fee; on-site
training provided.
Low Vision Follow-up: By return
appointment or school visit after 1
month.

Clinic provides examinations and
assessments at no cost to the
public. Summary reports include
diagnosis, recommended aids,
suggested additional therapy or
further examination, as needed.

♦ Aging Services

STATE UNITS ON AGING

**Aging and Adult Services
Administration
Washington State Department of
Social and Health Services**
P.O. Box 45050
Olympia, WA 98504-5050
(360) 586-8753 or Information &
Referral In State (800) 422-3263
FAX: (360) 902-7848
Ralph Smith, Assistant Secretary

Provides referrals to Area Agencies on Aging and information on other local aging services.

INDEPENDENT LIVING PROGRAMS

Washington Department of Services for the Blind
55 West Mission
Spokane, WA 99201
(509) 456-3165
Howard Kovasky, Program Manager

Provides independent living services for persons age 55 and over. For further information, contact the Project Director or general phone number listed.

WEST VIRGINIA

◆ *Educational Services*

STATE SERVICES

West Virginia Department of Education
State Capitol Building
Building #6, Room B-304/1900
Kanawha Boulevard East
Charleston, WV 25305
(304) 558-2696
FAX: (304) 558-3741
Dr. Michael Valentine, Director, Special Education
Annette Corey, Coordinator, Blind/Deaf-Blind

Type of Agency: State.
Mission: Administers supplemental state funds provided for blind children in local schools. Provides counseling on the education of visually impaired children.
Funded by: Public funds.
Hours of Operation: 8:15 AM-4:45 PM.
Program Accessibility: Fully accessible to all individuals with disabilities.
Number of Clients Served: 145 blind, or partially sighted students in public school programs; 65 blind students in state residential school for the blind.
Eligibility: State criteria; same as federal definition.
Area Served: State of West Virginia.
Age Requirements: 3-21 years.

Rehabilitation: By West Virginia Division of Rehabilitation Services.

For information about local facilities, consult the superintendent of schools in the area, or Superintendent, West Virginia Schools for the Deaf and Blind (304) 822-4801.

EARLY INTERVENTION COORDINATION

Office of Maternal and Child Health/Children with Special Health Care Needs Program West Virginia Department of Health and Human Resources
1116 Quarier Street
Charleston, WV 25301
(304) 558-3071
FAX: (304) 558-2866
Pamela Roush, Part H Early Intervention Director

County/District Where Located: Kanawha County.

Services include the following: audiology; service coordination; family training; counseling and home visits; health services; medical services for diagnostic or evaluation purposes; nursing; nutrition; physical therapy; psychological services; social work; special instruction; speech-language pathology; transportation; vision services; and assistive technology devices and technology services.

SCHOOLS

West Virginia Schools for the Deaf and the Blind
301 East Main Street
Romney, WV 26757
(304) 822-4800
FAX: (304) 822-3370
Jane K. McBride, Interim Superintendent
Thomas O. Workman, Principal, School for the Blind

Type of Agency: State.
County/District Where Located: Hampshire County.

Mission: Services for totally blind, partially sighted, deaf, hard of hearing, and deaf-blind persons.
Funded by: State funds.
Hours of Operation: 24 hours, 7 days.
Staff: Full-time educational and residential staff.
History/Date: Est. 1870.
Number of Clients Served: 179.
Eligibility: Visual or auditory impairment; West Virginia resident.
Area Served: Statewide.
Transportation: Y.
Age Requirements: 5 to 23 years.

Health: Audiology therapy; speech therapy. Refers for other health services.
Counseling/Social Work/Self-Help: Social evaluations; psychological testing and evaluation; placement in school, training. Contracts and refers for other counseling/social work services.
Educational: Grades K through 12. Programs for general academic study; vocational/skill development.
Professional Training: Internship/fieldwork placement in special education. Regular in-service training programs, short-term or summer training programs, open to enrollment from other agencies.
Reading: Talking book record players and cassette players; talking book records and cassettes; braille books; large-print books/braille magazines; recorded magazines; information and referral; transcription to braille.
Residential: Residential services as well as other necessary support services are provided.
Rehabilitation: Personal management; braille; gesticulation; handwriting; listening skills; Optacon; typing; video magnifier;

home management; orientation/mobility; sensory training; remedial education.

Recreational: Afterschool programs; arts and crafts; hobby groups; bowling; swimming; track; wrestling; cheerleading; band; chorus. Refers for residential summer camp.

Employment: Prevocational evaluation; career and skill counseling; occupational skill development. Refers for other employment services.

Computer Training: Training on computer aids and devices.

Contact local school superintendent for program availability.

INFANT AND PRESCHOOL

West Virginia Schools for the Deaf and the Blind
301 East Main Street
Romney, WV 26757
(304) 822-4800
FAX: (304) 822-3370
Jane K. McBride, Interim
Superintendent
Thomas O. Workman, Principal,
School for the Blind

Type of Agency: Residential school and state agency.
County/District Where Located: Hampshire County.
Mission: Services for totally blind, partially sighted, deaf, hard-of-hearing, and deaf-blind persons.
Funded by: State funds.
Staff: 4 full time (early childhood teachers/teachers of visually impaired students); 9 part time (includes orientation/mobility specialist, physical therapist). Various therapists and specialists available as consultants.
History/Date: Est. 1870.
Number of Clients Served: 146.
Eligibility: West Virginia resident with a visual or audio impairment.

Area Served: West Virginia.
Transportation: Y.
Age Requirements: Birth to 5 years.

Health: Genetic counseling; low vision exams; adaptive equipment; immunization; blood tests available on consultant or referral basis.
Counseling/Social Work/Self-Help: Parent and other counseling.
Educational: Provides instruction in all developmental areas.
Preschools: Home- and center-based programs, consultant services to other programs for visually impaired, hearing impaired, and multiply disabled infants, 0-2 years. Home teaching and consultant services to other programs for visually impaired, hearing impaired, and multiply disabled children, 3-5 years.

STATEWIDE OUTREACH SERVICES

West Virginia Schools for the Deaf and the Blind
301 East Main Street
Romney, WV 26757
(304) 822-4800
FAX: (304) 822-3370
Dan Oates, Outreach Specialist, Blind
Paul Athey, Outreach Specialist, Blind
Karen Cook, Outreach Specialist, Deaf

County/District Where Located: Hampshire County.
Funded by: State funds.
History/Date: Est. 1870.
Age Requirements: Under 21 years of age.
Assessment: Educational assessment, psychological assessment.
Consultation to Public Schools: On request.

Direct Service: On request.
Parent Assistance: On request.

INSTRUCTIONAL MATERIALS CENTERS

West Virginia Instructional Resource Center
West Virginia Schools for the Deaf and the Blind
301 East Main Street
Romney, WV 26757
(304) 822-4891
FAX: (304) 822-4898
Donna B. See, Director

Area Served: West Virginia.
Groups Served: K-12.

Types/Content: Textbooks and other educational materials.
Media Formats: Large-print books. Braille books.
Title Listings: No title listings available.

Braillers and other equipment are provided on a loan basis. Instructional aids and supplies are also available.

◆ Information Services

LIBRARIES

Services for Blind and Physically Handicapped
Kanawha County Public Library
123 Capitol Street
Charleston, WV 25301
(304) 343-4646, ext. 64
Dixie Smith, Librarian

Subregional library.

Services for the Blind and Physically Handicapped
Cabell County Public Library
455 Ninth Street Plaza

Huntington, WV 25701
(304) 528-5700
FAX: (304) 528-5701
Suzanne L. Coldiron, Librarian

Subregional library.

Services for the Blind and Physically Handicapped Ohio County Public Library

52 16th Street
Wheeling, WV 26003-3696
(304) 232-0244
FAX: (304) 232-6848
Lori Nicholson, Librarian

Type of Agency: Subregional library of the West Virginia Library for the Blind and Physically Handicapped.
Mission: To extend national services of the National Library Service for the Blind and Physically Handicapped.
Hours of Operation: Mon.-Fri. 9:00 AM-5:00 PM.
History/Date: Est. 1983.
Number of Clients Served: Approximately 240.
Eligibility: Print disabled.
Area Served: Wetzel, Brooke, Ohio, Hancock, Marshall Counties.
Age Requirements: None.

Educational: Distributes newsletter, posters, catalogs.
Computer Training: Basic DOS training.

Services for the Blind and Physically Handicapped Parkersburg and Wood County Public Library

3100 Emerson Avenue
Parkersburg, WV 26104-2414
(304) 420-4587
FAX: (304) 420-4589
Mike Hickman, Coordinator of Services for Blind and Physically Handicapped

Subregional library.

West Virginia Library Commission of Services for the Blind and Physically Handicapped

Science and Cultural Center
1900 Kanawha Boulevard East
Charleston, WV 25305
(304) 558-4061 or (304) 558-4062 or toll-free in West Virginia
(800) 642-8674
FAX: (304) 558-4066
E-mail:
fesenmf@mars.wvlc.wvnet.
edu
URL: http://
www.wvlc.wvnet.edu/blind/
bphhp.html
Dave Childress, Librarian
Quincy Adams, Machine Lending Information

Type of Agency: Regional library.
Mission: To serve library needs of blind and physically handicapped state residents.
Funded by: State and federal governments.
Hours of Operation: Mon.-Fri. 8:45 AM-5:00 PM.
Staff: 5 full-time equivalents.
Number of Clients Served: 4,000.
Eligibility: Persons who are certified by a professional to be unable to read regular print due to visual or physical limitations.
Area Served: State of West Virginia.

Regional library supplying large-print books and talking books on records and cassettes; operates radio reading service.

West Virginia Schools for the Deaf and the Blind

301 East Main Street
Romney, WV 26757
(304) 822-4800
Cynthia Johnson, Librarian

Subregional library.

RADIO READING

West Virginia Radio Reading Service

Cultural Center
1900 Kanawha Boulevard East
Charleston, WV 25305
(304) 558-1808
Dave Lewis, Coordinator

County/District Where Located: Kanawha County.
Hours of Operation: Mon.-Fri. 9:30 AM-4:30 PM.
History/Date: Est. 1977.
Area Served: Central and western West Virginia.

WJGF Radio Station

301 East Main Street
Romney, WV 26757
(304) 822-4838
FAX: (304) 822-3370
George Park, Director

County/District Where Located: Hampshire County.
Hours of Operation: 24 hours.
History/Date: Est. 1973.
Area Served: Romney.

♦ Rehabilitation Services

STATE SERVICES

Division of Rehabilitation Services West Virginia State Board of Rehabilitation

State Capitol Complex
P.O. Box 50890
Charleston, WV 25305-0890
(304) 766-4799
FAX: (304) 766-4671
William Tanzey, Director

Type of Agency: State; federal.
Mission: To enable West Virginians with disabilities to achieve independence and

integration within the work place, the family, and the community.
Funded by: State funds; foundation grants.
Budget: $45 million.
Hours of Operation: 8:30 AM-4:45 PM.
Program Accessibility: Meets all criteria of Title I, II, and IV of the Americans with Disabilities Act.
Staff: 7 full-time staff servicing visually impaired clients.
History/Date: Est. 1926.
Number of Clients Served: 1,456 blind and severely visually impaired clients.
Eligibility: Disability that is a handicap to employment.
Area Served: West Virginia.
Transportation: Y.
Age Requirements: Working age.

Health: Diagnosis and evaluation of eye health; treatment of eye condition; prescription of spectacles or aids; follow-up evaluation of eye treatment or prescription; audiology therapy; general medical service; occupational therapy; physical therapy; speech therapy.
Counseling/Social Work/Self-Help: Social evaluation; psychological testing and evaluation; individual, group, family/parent, couple counseling; placement in school, training, institution; referral to community services.
Educational: Accepts emotionally disturbed, learning disabled, mentally retarded, orthopedically disabled, other multiply disabled persons. Programs for vocational/skill development.
Professional Training: Internship/fieldwork placement in orientation/mobility; rehabilitation counseling; social work; vocational rehabilitation. Regular in-service training

programs, short-term or summer training.
Reading: Talking book record players and cassette players; talking book records and cassettes; braille books; large-print books; braille magazines; recorded magazines; information and referral; transcription to braille.
Rehabilitation: Personal management; braille; gesticulation; handwriting; listening skills; Optacon; typing; video magnifier; home management; orientation/mobility; sensory training; remedial education.
Employment: Prevocational evaluation; career and skill counseling; occupational skill development; job retention; job retraining; vocational placement; follow-up service; vending stand training. Contracts for sheltered workshops.
Low Vision: Low vision service.

Local Offices:

Beckley: Dvision of Rehabilitation Services, Beckley District Office, 402 Bair Building, Beckley, WV 25801, (304) 256-6900.
Charleston: Division of Rehabilitation Services, Charleston District Office, 515 Central Avenue, Charleston, WV 25302, (304) 558-3408.
Clarksburg: Division of Vocational Rehabilitation Services, Clarksburg District Office, John Davis Government Building, 153 West Main Street, Suite 406, Clarksburg, WV 26301-2913, (304) 624-0300.
Huntington: Division of Rehabilitation Services, Huntington District Office, 200 Keith-Albee Office Building, 929 1/2 Fourth Avenue, Huntington, WV 25701, (304) 528-5585.

Lewisburg: Division of Rehabilitation Services, Lewisburg District Office, 106 South Court Street, P.O. Box 426, Lewisburg, WV 24901, (304) 647-7515.
Martinsburg: Division of Rehabilitation Services, Martinsburg District Office, 106 Berkeley Plaza, Suite A, Martinsburg, WV 25401, (304) 267-0005.
Romney: Division of Rehabilitation Services, West Virginia Schools for the Deaf and the Blind, Romney Branch Office, Box 943, Romney, WV 26757, (304) 822-3957.
Wheeling: Division of Rehabilitation Services, Wheeling District Office, Central Union Building, 14th & Market Street, Wheeling, WV 26003, (304) 238-1092.

REHABILITATION

Cabell-Wayne Services for the Blind and Visually Impaired
910 Fourth Avenue, Room 300
P.O. Box 223
Huntington, WV 25707
(304) 522-6991
FAX: (304) 522-6924
Paul Slone, Executive Director

Type of Agency: Non-profit.
Mission: To provide quality comprehensive rehabilitation services to blind and severely visually impaired persons.
Funded by: Teubert Foundation, investments, and contributions.
Hours of Operation: Mon.-Fri. 8:00 AM - 4:30 PM.
Staff: 9 full time, 2 part time, uses volunteers.
History/Date: Est. 1975.
Number of Clients Served: Approximately 350.
Eligibility: Accuity of 20/100 in best eye.

Area Served: Cabell and Wayne Counties.
Transportation: Y.

Counseling/Social Work/Self-Help: Case finding; assessment; peer counseling; information and referral.
Educational: Public information and education programs to schools, civic groups and media; participates in school and community vision screening programs.
Reading: Eyeglass assistance program; provides transcriptions to tape, large print and braille.
Rehabilitation: Independent living evaluation; personal management; activities of daily living; braille; handwriting; orientation and mobility; sensory development; training in the use of aids and appliances; services provided in the home and community as appropriate.
Recreational: Beep baseball; bowling; dancing; golf; hiking; parties and picnics; theater and concerts; and trips.
Computer Training: Access; use of computer aids and devices; some customized programming.
Low Vision Aids: Evaluation and prescription of low vision aids; equipment loan and financial assistance programs.
Low Vision Follow-up: Y.

Seeing Hand Association

737 Market Street
Wheeling, WV 26003
(304) 232-4810
James Klages, Manager of Therapy Workshop

Type of Agency: Private.
Funded by: Sub-contracts; sales; United Way; donations.
History/Date: Est. 1935 and Inc. 1944.

Rehabilitation: Braille.
Recreational: Social and Recreational activities such as picnics, Christmas party, bowling, Easter party for children, boat rides.
Employment: Sheltered workshops, chair caning, rug weavings, subcontract work, and crafts.

West Virginia Society for the Blind and Severely Disabled

1427 Lee Street
Charleston, WV 25301
(304) 558-2373
David Naylor

Type of Agency: Private; non-profit.
County/District Where Located: Kawawha County.
Mission: To help blind persons secure gainful employment.
Funded by: Public funds, endowment, and fees for service.
Budget: $5 million.
Hours of Operation: Mon.-Fri. 8:30 AM-4:45 PM.
Staff: 13.
History/Date: Est. 1946.
Number of Clients Served: 100.
Eligibility: Blind or disabled.
Area Served: West Virginia.
Age Requirements: 18 and over.

Counseling/Social Work/Self-Help: Group work.
Professional Training: Training in food service management.
Employment: Vocational training; placement; vending stand and food service programs; follow-up.

COMPUTER TRAINING CENTERS

Division of Rehabilitation Services
West Virginia Division of Rehabilitation Services
State Capitol Complex
P.O. Box 50890
Charleston, WV 25305-0890
(304) 766-4600 or (304) 766-4799
Dan White, Program Supervisor

County/District Where Located: Kanawha County.

Computer Training: Speech output systems; screen magnification systems; braille access systems; closed-circuit television systems; word processing; database software; computer operating systems.

West Virginia Schools for the Deaf and the Blind
301 East Main Street
Romney, WV 26757
(304) 822-4800
Kathleen Johnson

County/District Where Located: Hampshire County.

Computer Training: Speech output systems; screen magnification systems; braille access systems; optical character recognition systems; closed-circuit television systems; word processing; database software; computer operating systems.

♦ *Low Vision Services*

EYE CARE SOCIETIES

West Virginia Academy of Ophthalmology
P.O. Box 5008

Charleston, WV 25361
(304) 343-5842
Thomas J. Stevens, Director

West Virginia Optometric Association
815 Quarier Street, Suite 215
Charleston, WV 25301-2641
(304) 345-4710
FAX: (304) 346-6416
Roger K. Price, Executive Director

LOW VISION CENTERS

Children's Vision Rehabilitation Project
West Virginia University, Department of Ophthalmology
Health Sciences Center North
P.O. Box 9193
Morgantown, WV 26506-9193
(304) 293-3757
FAX: (304) 293-7139
E-mail: tls@wvnvm.wvnet.edu
Terry L. Schwartz, MD

Type of Agency: Non-profit.
Mission: To provide comprehensive vision rehabilitation services to school-age children throughout West Virginia.
Funded by: State funds; Lions Sight Conservation Foundation.
Staff: Pediatric ophthalmologist; pediatric low vision specialist; orientation and mobility specialist; educational outreach specialist.
History/Date: Est. 1995.
Number of Clients Served: 30-40 children per year.
Eligibility: By referral.
Area Served: Statewide.
Age Requirements: School age.

Low Vision: Assessment, prescription of appropriate aids and training.
Low Vision Aids: Will be provided either through the state or local Lions organizations.

Low Vision Follow-up:
Completed 2-3 times per year for each child evaluated. Follow-up evaluations stress proper use of low vision aids and impact on education.

Low Vision Clinic
West Virginia University Department of Ophthalmology
Health Sciences Center North
P.O. Box 9193
Morgantown, WV 26506-6302
(304) 293-3757
John Linberg, M.D., Chairman, Department of Ophthalmology, Coordinator of Low Vision Clinic

Type of Agency: Non-profit.
Funded by: State funds.
Hours of Operation: Mon-Fri, 8:00 AM - 5:00 PM.
Staff: Ophthalmologists; low vision specialists; social workers; and psychologists.
Eligibility: Ophthalmology referral.
Area Served: Unlimited.

Low Vision Aids: Provided on loan for trial purposes.
Low Vision Follow-up: By return appointment as necessary.

West Virginia Rehabilitation Center
Low Vision Clinic
P.O. Box 1004
Institute, WV 25112-1004
(304) 766-4801
Sidney B. Boyce, Coordinator, Low Vision Clinic
Thomas E. Griffith, O.D., Low Vision Clinician

Type of Agency: Non-profit.
County/District Where Located: Kanawha County.
Funded by: Federal and state funds.
Hours of Operation: Mon.-Fri. 8:30 AM-4:45 PM.

Staff: Ophthalmologist; optometrist; low vision specialist/assistant; rehabilitation counselor; audiologist; optician; social worker; orientation/mobility instructor; rehabilitation teacher; special educator; occupational therapist; psychologist/counselor.
Eligibility: Current ophthalmological report; state residence.
Area Served: West Virginia.

Low Vision Aids: Sometimes provided on loan for trial; some on-site training can be provided.
Low Vision Follow-up: Varies according to patient.

◆ Aging Services

STATE UNITS ON AGING

Office of Aging
Holly Grove, State Capitol
Charleston, WV 25305
(304) 558-3317 or Information & Referral In State (800) 642-3671
FAX: (304) 558-0004
William L. Lytton, Jr., Interim Director

Provides referrals to Area Agencies on Aging and information on other local aging services.

INDEPENDENT LIVING PROGRAMS

West Virginia Division of Rehabilitation Services
State Capitol Complex
P.O. Box 50890
Charleston, WV 25305-0890
(304) 766-4601 or (800) 642-8207
FAX: (304) 766-4905
William Tanzey, Director
Daniel White, Program Supervisor, Blind and Visually Impaired Services, (304) 766-4799

Provides independent living services for persons age 55 and over. For further information, contact the Project Director or general phone number listed.

WISCONSIN

◆ *Educational Services*

STATE SERVICES

Wisconsin Department of Public Instruction
Exceptional Education Team
125 South Webster Street
P.O. Box 7841
Madison, WI 53707-7841
(608) 266-1781
FAX: (608) 267-3746
E-mail: papinas@mail.state.wi.us
Juanita Pawlisch, Assistant Superintendent
Andrew Papineau, State Consultant, Visually Impaired

Type of Agency: State, a division of the Wisconsin Department of Public Instruction.
County/District Where Located: Dane County.
Mission: Provides supervisory and consultation services to local educational agencies and private schools serving children with visual and dual sensory impairments. Administers supplemental state and federal funds for programs and services. Offers services in evaluation, consultation, low vision, and educational resources for preschool through high school students for multiply disabled students.
Funded by: Public funds.
Hours of Operation: Mon.-Fri. 7:15 AM-4:30 PM.
Number of Clients Served: 1,200.
Eligibility: Exceptional educational needs.
Area Served: Wisconsin.
Age Requirements: Birth-21 years.

Educational: 3-21 years.
Reading: Supplies braille, large-print books, tapes, and specialized equipment through the Educational Services Center for the Visually Impaired.

Provides parents and local educational agencies consultation in services and referral. Coordinates activities and services with the Wisconsin School for the Visually Handicapped and Educational Services Center for the Visually Impaired.

Provides supervisory and consultation services to local educational agencies serving visually impaired children. Administers supplemental state and federal funds for programs and services. Offers evaluation services. Provides educational resources for preschool through high school and multiply handicapped visually impaired students. Supplies braille, large type books, tapes, and specialized equipment; training on computer aids and devices. Offers consultation and referral services.

EARLY INTERVENTION COORDINATION

Birth to Three Early Intervention
Division of Supportive Living
Wisconsin Department of Health and Family Services
P.O. Box 7851
Madison, WI 53707-7851
(608) 267-3270
FAX: (608) 261-6752
E-mail: wroblbm@dhfs.state.wi.us
Beth Wroblewski, Early Childhood Specialist

Referral and identification; evaluation and assessment; development of service plan for eligible children birth to 3 who have a diagnosed disability or meet developmental criteria; ongoing service coordination and provision of all services in service/plan; procedural safeguards for parents.

Division of Health
Wisconsin Department of Health and Family Services
1414 East Washington Avenue
Room 96
Madison, WI 53703-3044
(608) 266-3822
FAX: (608) 267-3824
Meredith Washburn, Part H Early Childhood Coordinator

Technical assistance.

SCHOOLS

Center for Blind and Visually Impaired Children
5600 West Brown Deer Road
Milwaukee, WI 53223
(414) 355-3060
FAX: (414) 355-3547
Linda Bell, Executive Director

Mission: To help infants and preschoolers who are blind or visually impaired, including those with additional disabilities, to learn and develop in mind and body.
Funded by: Foundation grants; private donations; United Way; program service fees, civic organizations.
Budget: $463,000.
Hours of Operation: Mon.-Fri. 8:00AM to 3:00PM.
History/Date: Founded in; est. 1967.
Number of Clients Served: 60-70 Annually.
Eligibility: Birth-age 5 years, children with blindness, vision impairment, including the multi handicapped.
Area Served: Greater Milwaukee area and surrounding counties.

Transportation: Y.
Age Requirements: Birth through five years.

Northcentral Technical College
1000 Campus Drive
Wausau, WI 54401
(715) 675-3331, ext. 4087
FAX: (715) 675-9776
E-mail:
mielczarekntc@mail.northcentral.
tec.wi.us
Joe Mielczarek, Counselor,
Program for Visually Impaired

Type of Agency: Public.
Mission: Rehabilitation and education of blind and visually impaired people.
Funded by: College, state, private monies.
Budget: $350,000.
Hours of Operation: 8:00 AM-4:00 PM.
Program Accessibility: Y.
Staff: 10 full time.
History/Date: Est. 1971.
Number of Clients Served: Approximately 200.
Eligibility: Totally blind; legally blind; multidisabled blind, deaf/blind.
Area Served: Primarily Wisconsin.
Transportation: Y.

Counseling/Social Work/Self-Help: Career counseling; refers and provides consultation to other agencies for counseling/social work services.
Educational: One-year diploma programs. Two-year associate's degree programs. Certificates of competencies. Programs for adult continuing education. Vocational and skill development.
Professional Training: Internship/fieldwork placement in special education. Regular in-service training programs, short-term or summer training, open to enrollment from other agencies.

Residential: Dormitory.
Rehabilitation: Communicative typing; occupational typing; job-seeking skills; low vision; orientation/mobility; techniques of communications; foods; home management; career exploration; access technology; assistive technology for diabetics.
Employment: Prevocational evaluation; career and skill counseling; vocational placement; follow-up service.
Computer Training: Access; training on computer aids and devices.
Low Vision: Complete evaluation.
Low Vision Aids: Many varieties available to evaluate.
Low Vision Follow-up: Y.

Program for Visually Impaired Milwaukee Area Technical College
700 West State Street
Milwaukee, WI 53233
(414) 297-6838
FAX: (414) 297-8142
URL: http://
www.milwaukee.tec.wi.us/
spneeds
Chuck Kevil, Manager

Type of Agency: Public.
Mission: To provide quality occupational, academic and lifelong education for improving personal and employment potential for the handicapped and disabled.
Funded by: State, local and federal funds.
Budget: $2.8 Million.
Hours of Operation: Mon.-Fri. 8:00 AM-7:00 PM.
Staff: 33 full time; 2 part time.
History/Date: Est. 1979.
Number of Clients Served: 550 annually.
Eligibility: Totally blind, legally blind, deaf-blind, learning disabled, mentally retarded, or

orthopedically handicapped disabled persons.
Transportation: Y.
Age Requirements: 18 years and older.

Health: Refers for health services.
Counseling/Social Work/Self-Help: Social evaluation; individual and group counseling; placement in school; training. Refers and provides consultation to other agencies for other counseling/social work services.
Educational: First and second year of college. Programs for adult continuing education; college prep; vocational/skill development. Associate's degree.
Professional Training: Internship/fieldwork placement in special education. Regular in-service training programs; short-term or summer training; open to enrollment from other agencies.
Reading: Lends talking book cassettes; braille books. Talking book record players and cassette players; information and referral; transcription to braille; tape recording services on demand.
Rehabilitation: Personal management; braille; handwriting; listening skills; keyboarding; CCTVs; typing; video magnifier; electronic mobility aids; home management; orientation/mobility; remedial education.
Recreational: Adult continuing education; afterschool programs; bowling; swimming; track; adapted physical education for blind persons.
Employment: Prevocational evaluation; career and skill counseling; vocational placement; follow-up service. Refers for other employment-oriented services.
Computer Training: Access; training on computer aids and devices.

Low Vision: Evaluation and referral.
Low Vision Aids: Available for loan.

Wausau School District

415 Seymour Street
Wausau, WI 54402-0359
(715) 261-2545
FAX: (715) 261-2556
David Damgaard, Administrator, Exceptional Education
Karen Schultz, Teacher of Visually Impaired

Type of Agency: Public school.
Funded by: P.L. 94-142 monies, state funds, and local taxes.
Budget: 1992 (vision program): $80,000.
Hours of Operation: 8:15 AM-3:00 PM.
Staff: 2 full time (teacher of visually impaired students, aide). 17 part time (social worker, psychologist, occupational and physical therapists). Specialists and therapists available as consultants. Has advisory board (parent members) for overall program.
History/Date: Est. 1974.
Number of Clients Served: 8.
Eligibility: Wisconsin Department of Public Instruction requirements regarding visual impairment.
Area Served: Central and northern Wisconsin.
Transportation: Y.
Age Requirements: 3-21 years.

Health: Adaptive equipment; genetic counseling; low vision exams; immunization; blood tests available on consultant or referral basis.
Counseling/Social Work/Self-Help: Parent and other counseling; financial assistance; other social services.
Educational: Provides instruction in all developmental areas.

Orientation/mobility. Home teaching and resource room programs for visually impaired/multiply disabled persons, 3-21 years.

Wisconsin School for the Visually Handicapped and Educational Services Center for the Visually Impaired

1700 West State Street
Janesville, WI 53546
(608) 758-6100
FAX: (608) 758-6161
William S. Koehler, Superintendent
Dr. Susan Hunt, Education Director

Type of Agency: State.
Mission: Services for totally blind, legally blind, visually impaired, learning disabled, mentally retarded, emotionally disturbed, orthopedically handicapped.
Funded by: State and federal funds.
Budget: $4.1 million.
Hours of Operation: Office: Mon.-Fri. 8:00 AM-4:30 PM.
Program Accessibility: Wheelchair accessible.
Staff: 95 full time, 25 part time. Uses volunteers.
History/Date: Est. 1849.
Number of Clients Served: 900.
Eligibility: Wisconsin resident; visually impaired; school-age referrals must be through local school district.
Area Served: Statewide.
Transportation: Y.
Age Requirements: 3-21.

Health: Physical therapy; speech therapy. Contracts and provides consultation to other agencies for other health services.
Counseling/Social Work/Self-Help: Social evaluations; psychological testing and evaluation; individual, group, family/parent, couple counseling.

Provides consultation to other agencies for other counseling/social work services, especially local school districts.
Educational: Grades K through 12. Programs for adult continuing education; college prep; general academic studies; vocational/skill development. Provides instructional materials and equipment to children throughout Wisconsin. Services to local school districts; Individualized Education Program (IEP) assistance.
Preschools: Day student enrollment only.
Professional Training: Internship/fieldwork placement in industrial arts; orientation/mobility; special education. Regular in-service training programs, open to enrollment from other agencies.
Reading: Talking book record players and cassette players; talking book records and cassettes; braille books; large-print books; braille magazines; recorded magazines; information and referral; special collection; translation to braille; tape recording services on demand.
Residential: Dormitories; independent living apartments.
Rehabilitation: Personal management; braille; handwriting; listening skills; Optacon; typing; video magnifier; electronic mobility aids; home management; orientation/mobility; sensory training; remedial education; transition training and vocational guidance.
Recreational: Adult continuing education; afterschool programs; arts and crafts; hobby groups; swimming; track; wrestling; cross country skiing. Contracts for bowling.
Employment: Prevocational evaluation; career and skill counseling; occupational skill

development; job training and placement.

Low Vision: Low vision service; low vision aids.

Low Vision Follow-up: Yes.

INFANT AND PRESCHOOL

Center for Blind and Visually Impaired Children

5600 West Brown Deer Road
Milwaukee, WI 53223
(414) 355-3060
FAX: (414) 355-3547
Linda Bell, Executive Director

Type of Agency: Private; non-profit.

Funded by: Donations from foundations, civic organizations, individuals. Insurance coverage and program service fees. United Way.

Budget: $463,000.

Hours of Operation: Mon.-Fri. 8:00 AM-3:00 PM.

Staff: 15 part time.

History/Date: Est. 1967.

Number of Clients Served: 60-70 annually.

Eligibility: Visually impaired; multiply disabled.

Area Served: Greater Milwaukee and surrounding area.

Transportation: Y.

Age Requirements: Birth-5 years.

Counseling/Social Work/Self-Help: Informational meetings, parent and family support group meetings.

Educational: Provides early intervention, including early childhood special education, education for the visually impaired, orientation and mobility and therapies. Center-based programs. Home visits and consultation services are available.

Wisconsin School for the Visually Handicapped and Educational Services Center for the Visually Impaired

1700 West State Street
Janesville, WI 53546
(608) 758-6100
FAX: (608) 758-6161
William S. Koehler, Superintendent

Type of Agency: Public residential school.

County/District Where Located: Rock County.

Mission: To provide educational and related services to school age children with visual impairments.

Budget: $4 million.

Program Accessibility: Fully accessible.

Staff: Includes administrators; teachers certified in visual impairment and early childhood and dually certified teachers; various therapists; orientation/mobility and other specialists. Various therapists and specialists also available as consultants.

History/Date: Est. 1849.

Number of Clients Served: 900.

Area Served: Wisconsin.

Educational: Provides instruction in developmental areas. Home-based programs and consultant services to other programs for visually impaired children, with or without other disabilities, 0-5 years.

Program serves as resource to local education agencies statewide; numerous support and related services available through school system.

Contact local school superintendent for program availability or Andrew Papineau, State Consultant, Visually Impaired, Wisconsin Department of Public Instruction, 125 South Webster Street, Madison, WI 53707 (608) 266-3522.

STATEWIDE OUTREACH SERVICES

Wisconsin School for the Visually Handicapped and Educational Services Center for the Visually Impaired

1700 West State Street
Janesville, WI 53546
(608) 758-6100
FAX: (608) 758-6161
William Anthony King, Coordinator

Funded by: State and federal monies.

History/Date: Est. 1858.

Age Requirements: 3-21 years.

Assessment: Asessment site determined by child's needs. Provided at no cost.

Consultation to Public Schools: In-service training for teachers, parent education, preschool and early childhood conferences.

Parent Assistance: Informational services.

Materials Production: Produces braille and large-print textbooks. Statewide depository for American Printing House for the Blind materials.

INSTRUCTIONAL MATERIALS CENTERS

Wisconsin Educational Services Center for the Visually Impaired

1700 West State Street
Janesville, WI 53546
(608) 758-6146
FAX: (608) 758-6161
William Anthony King, Coordinator

Area Served: Wisconsin.

Groups Served: 3-21 years.

Types/Content: Text books.

Media Formats: Braille books, talking books/cassettes, large-print books.

♦ *Information Services*

LIBRARIES

Wisconsin Regional Library for the Blind and Physically Handicapped
813 West Wells Street
Milwaukee, WI 53233
(414) 286-3045 or toll-free in
Wisconsin (800) 242-8822 or TDD
(414) 278-3062
FAX: (414) 278-2137
E-mail: pirtle@omnifest.uwm.edu
Marsha Valance, Regional
Librarian

Type of Agency: Talking Book
program.
Mission: To provide recreational
reading to print-handicapped
residents of Wisconsin.
Funded by: Public funds.
Budget: $533,900.
Hours of Operation: Mon.-Fri.
9:00 AM-4:45 PM.
Staff: 14.
History/Date: Est. 1961.
Number of Clients Served: 8,000
individuals; 2,000 institutions.
Eligibility: Print-handicapped
residents of Wisconsin.
Area Served: Wisconsin.
Transportation: N.

Reading: Popular titles, levels
preschool-adult.
Recreational: Books and
magazines in braille and recorded
forms; audiodescribed videos.
Computer Training: Special needs
center, with Apple and IBM-PC,
Arkenstone Reader and Adaptor.
Low Vision: Closed-circuit
television to magnify text.

Regional library lending free books
and magazines in braille and
recorded on disk and cassette tape
as well as the special equipment
and accessories to utilize the
recorded materials.

MEDIA PRODUCTION SERVICES

Green Bay Public Schools
200 South Broadway
Green Bay, WI 54303
(414) 448-2000
Surita Hall-Smith, Director
Nancy Kraft, Resource Teacher for
the Visually Impaired

County/District Where Located:
Brown County.
Groups Served: K-12.

Types/Content: Textbooks,
recreational, career/vocational,
religious, tests, handouts.
Media Formats: Braille books,
talking books/cassettes, large print
books.
Title Listings: Printed at no
charge.

Volunteer Services for the Visually Handicapped
803 West Wells Street
Milwaukee, WI 53233-1436
(414) 278-3039
FAX: (414) 286-5450
Carol Chew, Executive Director

Area Served: Primarily Wisconsin
but requests are honored from
across the country.
Groups Served: K-12, college
students, other adults.

Types/Content: Textbooks,
recreational, career/vocational.
Media Formats: Braille books,
talking books/cassettes.
Title Listings: Available on
computer disk.

Wisconsin Educational Services Center for the Visually Impaired
1700 West State Street
Janesville, WI 53546
(608) 758-6146
FAX: (608) 758-6161
William Anthony King,
Coordinator

Area Served: Wisconsin.
Groups Served: 3-21 years.

Types/Content: Textbooks.
Media Formats: Braille books,
talking books/cassettes, large print
books.
Title Listings: None specified.

RADIO READING

Education and Reading Service (EARS)
3520 30th Avenue
Kenosha, WI 53144
(414) 656-8950
FAX: (414) 656-7264
Peter Atkinson, Coordinator

County/District Where Located:
Kenosha County.
Hours of Operation: Mon.-Fri.
10:00 AM-6:00 PM.
History/Date: Est. 1978.
Area Served: Racine and Kenosha
Counties.

INSIGHT/WYMS

5225 West Vliet Street
Milwaukee, WI 53208
(414) 475-8488
FAX: (414) 475-8413
Russ Rapczyk, Technical Support

Hours of Operation: 10:00 AM-
12:00 PM and 5:30 PM-7:00 PM
(local program); 8:00 AM-
10:00 AM, 12:00 PM-10:00 PM
(national network).
History/Date: Est. 1978.
Area Served: Milwaukee
metropolitan area.

INFORMATION AND REFERRAL

Prevent Blindness Wisconsin
759 North Milwaukee Street
Milwaukee, WI 53202-3745
(414) 765-0505
FAX: (414) 765-0377
Kathleen Nelson, Executive
Director

County/District Where Located: Milwaukee County.

See Prevent Blindness America in U.S. national listings.

See also in national listings:

Volunteer Braillists and Tapists

♦ Rehabilitation Services

STATE SERVICES

Bureau for Sensory Disabilities Wisconsin Division of Supportive Living
2917 International Lane
P.O. Box 7852
Madison, WI 53707-7852
(608) 243-5622 or (608) 243-5656
FAX: (608) 243-5680
John Conway, Director
Michael Nelipovich, Director, Office for the Blind

Type of Agency: State.
Hours of Operation: Mon.-Fri. 7:45 AM-4:30 PM.
Staff: 31 full time.
Eligibility: Legally blind; visually impaired; deaf-blind.

Counseling/Social Work/Self-Help: Individual counseling; referral to community services.
Professional Training: Internship/fieldwork placement in rehabilitation counseling and mobility.
Rehabilitation: Independent living; personal management; technology; braille; handwriting; listening skills; typing; video magnifier; electronic mobility aids; home management; orientation/mobility; rehabilitation teaching in client's home and community; sensory training.
Computer Training: Access statewide technology loan center.

For information about related services, contact Wisconsin Division of Vocational Rehabilitation, 2917 International Lane, Madison, WI 53707, (608) 243-5600, Judy Norman-Nunnery, Administrator.

REHABILITATION

Badger Association for the Blind
912 North Hawley Road
Milwaukee, WI 53213
(414) 258-9200
FAX: (414) 256-8744
Patrick Brown, Executive Director

Type of Agency: Private; non-profit.
Mission: Services for totally blind; legally blind; visually impaired.
Funded by: Room and board fees; capital income; contributions; membership dues.
Budget: 1996: $1,000,000.
Hours of Operation: Mon.-Fri. 8:30 AM-5:00 PM.
Staff: 16 full time, 13 part time. Uses volunteers.
History/Date: Est. 1919.
Number of Clients Served: 5,000 annually.
Eligibility: Totally blind; legally blind; visually impaired.
Area Served: Southeastern Wisconsin.
Age Requirements: 18 years or older.

Residential: Operates a home for the adult blind.
Recreational: Activity center program providing social and recreational activities for adult blind.
Low Vision: Sales of appliances and low vision aids.

Volunteers in Visual Assistance (VIVA) program recruits volunteers to assist visually impaired persons throughout the Milwaukee metropolitan area.

Focus for Newly Blind and Family
P.O. Box 17575
Milwaukee, WI 53217
(414) 964-6661
Gordon Haldiman, Director

Type of Agency: Non-profit.
County/District Where Located: Milwaukee County.
Mission: Services to newly blind adult individuals and their families.
Funded by: Private contributions and donations.
History/Date: Est. 1971.

Counseling/Social Work/Self-Help: Counseling available on Saturday mornings. Hotline services available. Information and referrals. Speakers service.

Industries for the Blind, Inc.
3220 West Vliet Street
Milwaukee, WI 53208
(414) 933-4319
FAX: (414) 933-4316
Chuck Lange, president

Type of Agency: Private; non-profit.
County/District Where Located: Milwaukee County.
Mission: Employ people who are totally blind; legally blind; deaf-blind; and blind with other disabilities.
Funded by: Workshop sales.
Budget: 1992: $7.2 million.
Staff: 60 full time.
History/Date: Est. 1952.
Area Served: Wisconsin.
Age Requirements: Adults age 16 and older.

Employment: Sheltered workshop providing employment for blind and visually impaired people.

Local Offices:

Jamesville: 1713 R. West State Street, Jamesville, WI 53546, (608) 754-3208.

Sunrise Care Center Inc.
3540 South 43rd Street
Milwaukee, WI 53220
(414) 933-6977
FAX: (414) 933-9118
Michael J. Kern

Type of Agency: Non-profit; nursing home for aging and disabled persons.
Mission: To provide quality health care services with specialization in the prevention and rehabilitation of blindness, recognizing each person as an individual with special physical and emotional needs.
Funded by: Residents, families, state and federal government, donations.
Budget: $5 million.
Staff: 110.
History/Date: Est. 1963.
Number of Clients Served: 99.
Eligibility: Blind; visually impaired. Aging sighted persons are also admitted.
Area Served: Primarily Milwaukee; entire state.

Health: Medical and therapeutic care administered by staff physicians.
Counseling/Social Work/Self-Help: Referrals available.
Rehabilitation: Physical, occupational, and speech therapy.
Recreational: Many physical activities available.

Wisconsin Council for the Blind
354 West Main Street

Madison, WI 53703-3115
(608) 255-1166
FAX: (608) 255-3301
Jack Malin, Director
Marshall Flax, M.S., Low Vision Rehabilitation Specialist

Type of Agency: Private; non-profit.
Mission: To advance the interests of the blind of Wisconsin in every way possible.
Funded by: Contributions from mail appeal campaign; royalties and endowment.
Hours of Operation: Mon.-Fri. 8:30 AM-4:30 PM.
History/Date: Est. 1952.
Eligibility: Blind; visually impaired.
Area Served: Wisconsin.

Health: Subsidizes eye research projects; gives free white canes.
Educational: College and vocational school scholarships.
Reading: Subsidizes organizations engaged in production of reading materials for blind persons.
Residential: Operates low-interest business and home improvement loan program.
Rehabilitation: Distributes on a nonprofit basis special aids, appliances, and visual aids. Rehabilitation teacher on staff for in-home visits.
Recreational: Subsidizes recreational projects.
Employment: Grants to organizations engaged in promotion of the general welfare of blind persons. Low-interest business loans.
Low Vision: Evaluations available by appointment. Fee charged for services; financial support available for some clients. Follow-up visits by appointment.

Service officer available to investigate cases of alleged discrimination.

Wiscraft
Wisconsin Enterprises for the Blind
5316 West State Street
Milwaukee, WI 53208
(414) 778-5800
FAX: (414) 778-5805
John Baumgart, President

Type of Agency: Private; non-profit.
County/District Where Located: Milwaukee County.
Mission: Services for totally blind, legally blind, and deaf-blind persons.
Funded by: Production sales revenues; private donations.
Budget: $3 million.
Hours of Operation: 7:30 AM-5:00 PM.
Program Accessibility: Fully accessible.
Staff: 13 full time.
History/Date: Est. 1903 as a state agency; converted to a private, non-profit organization in 1985.
Number of Clients Served: 42.
Eligibility: Legally blind.
Area Served: Wisconsin; especially Milwaukee metropolitan area.
Age Requirements: 18 years and older.

Counseling/Social Work/Self-Help: Refers for counseling/social work services.
Rehabilitation: Sheltered employment. Refers for other rehabilitation services.
Recreational: Refers for recreation services.
Employment: Job retraining; sheltered workshops. Provides employment opportunities and refers for other employment services.

COMPUTER TRAINING CENTERS

Computers to Help People

825 East Johnson Street
Madison, WI 53703
(608) 257-5917
Carl Durocher, Instructor/
Consultant
John Boyer, Braille Specialist

Computer Training: Screen magnification, speech-output systems, systems for computers.

Assessment, consultation, set-up, and familiarization training available for DOS, Windows, Win95, and Macintosh.   Low vision and blind-access strategies. Also provides a print-to-braille service.

Milwaukee Area Technical College

700 West State Street
Milwaukee, WI 53233-1443
(414) 297-6838
FAX: (414) 297-7990
E-mail: spcneeds@milwaukee.tec.
wi.us
Chuck Kevil, Manager

Computer Training: Speech output systems; screen magnification systems; braille access systems; closed-circuit television systems; word processing; database software; computer operating systems; training for instructors.

Northcentral Technical College

1000 Campus Drive
Wausau, WI 54401
(715) 675-3331, ext. 4087
FAX: (715) 675-9776
E-mail:
mielczarekntc@mail.northcentral.
tec.wi.us
Joe Mielczarek, Vocational
Counselor/Instructor

Computer Training: Speech output systems; screen magnification systems; braille access systems; optical character recognition systems; closed-circuit television systems; word processing; database software; computer operating systems; training for instructors.

Technology Loan Center offers equipment available to rent.

Wisconsin School for the Visually Handicapped and Educational Services Center for the Visually Impaired

1700 West State Street
Janesville, WI 53546
(608) 758-6100
FAX: (608) 758-6161
Margaret Wenzel, Teacher

Computer Training: Speech output systems; screen magnification systems; optical character recognition systems; closed-circuit television systems; word processing; database software; computer operating systems.

◆ Low Vision Services

EYE CARE SOCIETIES

Wisconsin Academy of Ophthalmology

Ten West Phillips Road
Vernon Hills, IL 60061
(847) 680-1666
Richard H. Paul, Executive
Director

Wisconsin Optometric Association, Inc.

5721 Odana Road

Madison, WI 53719
(608) 274-4322
FAX: (608) 274-8646
E-mail: brownlowod@aol.com
Charles B. Brownlow, O.D.,
Executive Director

County/District Where Located:
Dane County.

LOW VISION CENTERS

Low Vision Rehabilitation Service
University Station Clinics

2880 University Avenue
P.O. Box 5902
Madison, WI 53705
(608) 263-7171
Stephen D. Kessler, O.D., Staff
Optometrist

County/District Where Located:
Dane County.
Funded by: Client fees; state funds; private donations.
Hours of Operation: Thurs., AM.
Staff: Ophthalmologist; optometrist; optician.
Eligibility: Referral; ophthalmologic report.
Area Served: Unlimited.

Health: Can provide ocular health exams by clinic ophthalmologist.
Low Vision Aids: Provided on loan for trial; on-site training provided.
Low Vision Follow-up: 1-year unlimited follow-up at no additional charge.

Programs for the Blind and Visually Impaired
Wisconsin Division of Vocational Rehabilitation Low Vision Services

6830 West Villard Avenue
Milwaukee, WI 53218-3936
(414) 438-4888
FAX: (414) 438-4885
Rodney Kossick, Low Vision
Technology Specialist

Type of Agency: State.
Funded by: Federal funds; state funds.
Hours of Operation: Mon.-Fri. 7:45 AM-4:30 PM.
Eligibility: State residence.
Area Served: Wisconsin.

Low Vision: Low vision assessment; services of orientation/mobility instructor available.
Low Vision Aids: Provided on loan for trial period at no charge. On-site training provided.
Low Vision Follow-up: Varies according to patient.

Veterans Administration Center

5000 West National
Milwaukee, WI 53295
(414) 384-1832
Leon Haith, Visual Impairment Team Coordinator

County/District Where Located: Milwaukee County.
Funded by: Federal funds.
Hours of Operation: Mon.-Fri. 8:00 AM-4:30 PM.
Staff: Ophthalmologist; ophthalmology residents; social worker; rehabilitation teacher; rehabilitation counselor; audiologist.
Eligibility: Blind or visually impaired veterans.

Low Vision Aids: Provided on loan for trial purposes; on-site training provided.
Low Vision Follow-up: When necessary.

Vision Rehabilitation Service
Wisconsin Council of the Blind

354 West Main Street
Madison, WI 53703-3115
(608) 255-6178
URL: http://www.wcblind.org
Marshall Flax, Director

Type of Agency: Private; non-profit.
County/District Where Located: Dane County.
Mission: To promote the dignity and independence of people in Wisconsin who are blind and visually impaired by providing services, advocating legislation and educating the general public.
Funded by: Client fees; private donations; no government funding.
Hours of Operation: Mon.-Fri. 8:00 AM-4:30 PM.
Staff: Low vision therapist; orientation and mobility specialist, rehabilitation teacher.
History/Date: Est. 1952.
Number of Clients Served: 200 annually.
Eligibility: Eye report.
Area Served: Wisconsin.
Age Requirements: None.

Counseling/Social Work/Self-Help: Support group references for visually impaired.
Educational: Braille instruction.
Professional Training: Internships for graduate students in related fields.
Rehabilitation: Home management, Braille, orientation and mobility, assistive devices.
Recreational: Subsidies, planned outings, activity coordination.
Low Vision: Services in Madison, and at eye care centers in southern and central Wisconsin.
Low Vision Aids: Provided on loan for trial, and available for sale on an at-cost basis.
Low Vision Follow-up: Follow-up visits included.

◆ Aging Services

STATE UNITS ON AGING

Bureau of Aging
Wisconsin Division of Community Services

217 South Hamilton Street
Suite 300
Madison, WI 53707
(608) 266-2536
FAX: (608) 267-3203
Donna McDowell, Director

Provides referrals to Area Agencies on Aging and information on other local aging services.

INDEPENDENT LIVING PROGRAMS

Division of Supportive Living
Wisconsin Department of Health and Family Services

2917 International Lane
P.O. Box 7852
Madison, WI 53707-7852
(608) 243-5600 or Office for the Blind (608) 243-5656
FAX: (608) 243-5680
Gerald Born, Administrator
Michael Nelipovich, Director

Provides independent living services for persons age 55 and over. For further information, contact the Project Director or general phone number listed.

WYOMING

◆ *Educational Services*

STATE SERVICES

Services for the Visually Impaired
Wyoming Department of Education
2300 Capitol Avenue
Hathaway Building, 2nd Floor
Cheyenne, WY 82002-0050
(307) 777-6257
FAX: (307) 777-6234
E-mail: jwood@educ.state.wy.us
Janet Wood, Contact Person

Type of Agency: State.
County/District Where Located: Laramie County.
Mission: Coordinates educational services for all visually impaired individuals in the state.
Funded by: State funds; P.L. 94-142 monies; and other sources.
Staff: Six consultants, 1 director, seven part-time secretaries.
Area Served: Wyoming.
Age Requirements: 0-adults.

Health: Adaptive equipment.
Counseling/Social Work/Self-Help: Parent and other counseling; other social services.
Educational: Provides instruction in developmental areas; orientation/mobility and other instruction.
Preschools: Direct service, consultation.

Local Offices:

Casper: Services for Visually Impaired, 539 South Payne Avenue, Casper, WY 82609, (307) 234-9741, Paul Newman, Educational Consultant.

Cheyenne: Services for Visually Impaired, Hathaway Building, Room 144, Cheyenne, WY 82002, (307) 777-7274, C. Jill Mathis, Consultant.
Powell: Services for Visually Impaired, P.O. Box 947, Powell, WY 82435, (307) 754-2147, Gary Olson, Consultant.
Rawlins: Services for Visually Impaired, Carbon Building, Room 325, Rawlins, WY 82301, (307) 324-5333, Joanne Whitson, Educational Consultant.
Riverton: Services for Visually Impaired, 205 North Fifth East, Riverton, WY 82501, (307) 856-5652, Ron Warpness, Consultant.
Sheridan: Services for Visually Impaired, 2161 Coffeen Avenue, Sixth Floor, Sheridan, WY 82801, (307) 672-6129, Jerry Baker, Consultant.

For information about local services, contact the school district's special education director.

EARLY INTERVENTION COORDINATION

Division of Developmental Disabilities
Wyoming Department of Health
Herschler State Office Building West
Cheyenne, WY 82002
(307) 777-5246
FAX: (307) 777-6047
David Haines, Ed.D., Children's Services Manager

County/District Where Located: Laramie County.

Early intervention services to children from birth to age 3 with developmental disabilities. Special education and related services for children with developmental disabilities from age 3 to 5.

◆ *Information Services*

TALKING BOOK MACHINE DISTRIBUTORS

Services for the Visually Impaired
Wyoming Department of Education
2300 Capitol Avenue
Hathaway Building, Room 144
Cheyenne, WY 82002-0050
(307) 777-7274
Jill Mathis, Contact Person

Distributor of talking book machines.

◆ *Rehabilitation Services*

STATE SERVICES

Division of Vocational Rehabilitation
Wyoming Department of Employment
First Floor, East Wing
1100 Herschler Building
Cheyenne, WY 82002
(307) 777-7385
FAX: (307) 777-5939
Gary W. Child, Administrator

Type of Agency: State.
County/District Where Located: Laramie County.
Funded by: 80% federal, 20% state.
Staff: 70 full time.
History/Date: Est. 1920.
Eligibility: Physically or mentally disabled with vocational handicap.
Area Served: Wyoming.

Health: Diagnostic, medical, and surgical treatment.
Counseling/Social Work/Self-Help: Counseling services.
Professional Training: Internships.

Employment: Evaluation; prevocational and vocational training; placement; vending stand business enterprise programs; follow-up.
Computer Training: Access; training on computer aids.

REHABILITATION

Montgomery Home for the Blind Wyoming Pioneer Home
141 Pioneer Home Drive
Thermopolis, WY 82443
(307) 864-3151
Ralph Barnes, Facility Manager

Type of Agency: State residential facilities for Wyoming residents.
County/District Where Located: Hot Springs County.
Funded by: Appropriated funds.
History/Date: Est. 1948.
Number of Clients Served: 108.
Eligibility: Retiree; ambulatory; resident of Wyoming.
Area Served: Wyoming.
Age Requirements: 55 years and older.

Reading: Large type and tape books; recorders and talking book machines.

◆ Low Vision Services

EYE CARE SOCIETIES

Wyoming Ophthalmological Society
111 South Jefferson
Casper, WY 82601
(307) 237-2511
Matthew Taylor Dodds, M.D., Executive Director

Wyoming Optometric Association
520 Randall Avenue

Cheyenne, WY 82001
(307) 632-8819
FAX: (307) 634-0804
Dan Lex, Executive Director

County/District Where Located:
Laramie County.

◆ Aging Services

STATE UNITS ON AGING

Division on Aging
Hathaway Building, Room 139
Cheyenne, WY 82002-0710
(307) 777-7986 or Information & Referral In State (800) 442-2766
FAX: (307) 777-5340
Deborah Fleming, Director

Provides referrals to Area Agencies on Aging and information on other local aging services.

INDEPENDENT LIVING PROGRAMS

Division of Vocational Rehabilitation Wyoming Department of Employment
1100 Herschler Building
Cheyenne, WY 82002
(307) 777-7385
FAX: (307) 777-7155
Gary W. Child, Administrator
Woody Absher, Project Director,
(307) 777-7191

Provides independent living services for persons age 55 and over. For further information, contact the Project Director or general phone number listed.

CANADA
PROVINCIAL LISTINGS

ALBERTA

◆ *Educational Services*

PROVINCIAL SERVICES

Special Education Branch Alberta Department of Education

11160 Jasper Avenue
East Devonian Building, 10th Floor
Edmonton, AB T5K 0L2
(403) 422-6326
FAX: (403) 422-2039
Dr. Harvey Finnestad, Director

Monitors the provision of educational services to children and youths with disabilities.

INSTRUCTIONAL MATERIALS CENTERS

Materials Resource Centre for the Visually Impaired Alberta Education (AEEM)

12360 142nd Street N.W.
Edmonton, AB T5L 4X9
(403) 427-4681
FAX: (403) 427-6683
E-mail: kribeiro@edc.gov.ub.ca
URL: http://www.ednet.edc.gov.ub.ca/mrc
Kathryn Ribeiro, Manager

Type of Agency: Provincial government: educational.
Mission: Alberta Education, through the Materials Resource Centres for the Visually Impaired, loans alternate-format educational materials in braille, large print and audiotape, as well as specialized equipment and kits to Alberta schools or school jurisdictions for the use of visually impaired students in authorized educational programs, preschool through Grade 12.

Funded by: Alberta government.
Budget: 1996: $1,030,000.
Hours of Operation: Mon.-Fri. 8:15 AM-4:30 PM.
Staff: 18.
History/Date: Est. 1971.
Number of Clients Served: 633 registered visually impaired students in Alberta.
Eligibility: Blind or visually impaired students who have been assessed by educational consultants for the visually impaired.
Area Served: Alberta, with interlibrary loan agreements with the Canadian provincial resources center for the visually impaired.
Age Requirements: Students, 19 years of age and younger.

Educational: Supports authorized educational programs through the provision of alternate-format materials, kits, and equipment to visually impaired students and reading materials for professionals working with these students. Assists Alberta schools in the delivery of programs to print-disabled students by selling selected curriculum resources in audiotape format.
Preschools: Schools may borrow alternate-format materials, kits, and equipment for preschool children who are provincially funded and/or for whom individual program plans have been authorized by regional offices of education.
Reading: Loan and produce for loan alternate-format reading materials requested by schools and resources for professionals. Includes Braille books, large-print books and talking books.
Recreational: Provide recreational reading materials in special formats.
Low Vision Aids: Aids include CCTVs, speech synthesizers, 4-track cassette records, and talking calculators available for loan.

◆ *Information Services*

LIBRARIES

Library Services Alberta Community Development

10405 Jasper Avenue
Edmonton, AB T5J 4R7
(403) 427-6315
FAX: (403) 422-1105
E-mail: pjackson@mcd.gov.ab.ca
URL: http://www.gov.ab.ca/dept/mcd.html
Punch Jackson, Manager

Type of Agency: Provincial service agency.
Mission: To facilitate the development of public library services to all eligible print handicapped persons in the province.
Funded by: Province of Alberta.
Budget: $12.7 million.
Hours of Operation: Mon.-Fri. 8:30 AM-4:30 PM.
Staff: 10.
History/Date: Est. 1981.
Number of Clients Served: 3,000-4,000 registered patrons.
Eligibility: Visually or physically impaired; meets eligibility criteria; registered with local library.
Area Served: Province of Alberta.

Stanley A. Milner Public Library
7 Sir Winston Churchill Square

Edmonton, AB T5J 2V4
(403) 496-1888
FAX: (403) 496-1885
E-mail: epl@freenet.edmonton.
ab.ca
URL: http://
www.publib.edmonton.ab.ca
Linda Cook, Director
Judy Moore, Manager, Library
Access

Type of Agency: Library access
division.
Mission: To respond to the
information needs of people with
disabilities.
Budget: $308,000.
Hours of Operation: Mon.-Fri.
9:00 AM-5:00 PM.
Staff: 5 full-time.
History/Date: Est. 1973.
Eligibility: Not restricted to
legally blind persons.

Reading: Provides descriptive
videos, talking books and large
print. Volunteers available for
home visits.
Low Vision Aids: Magnifiers,
print enhancer, reading machines.

See also in national listings:

**Alberta Sports and Recreation
Association for the Blind**

**Operation Eyesight Universal
(OEU)**

♦ Rehabilitation Services

PROVINCIAL SERVICES

**Family and Social Services
Department**
10030-107th Street
Seventh Street Plaza
Edmonton, AB T5J 3E4
(403) 422-1150
Donna Wood, Director

Administers grant and
contributions program to help
fund services and integration
efforts for blind and visually
impaired and other disabled
persons.

REHABILITATION

**Canadian National Institute for
the Blind
Alberta–Northwest Territories
Division**
12010 Jasper Avenue
Edmonton, AB T5K 0P3
(403) 488-4871
FAX: (403) 482-0017
URL: http://www.cnib.ca
William J. McKeown, Executive
Director

Hours of Operation: Mon.-Fri.
8:30 AM - 4:30 PM.

District Offices:

Calgary: 15 Colonel Baker Place
N.E., Calgary, AB T2E 4Z3,
(403) 266-8831, FAX (403) 265-5029.
Grand Prairie: 408, 4-9728
Montrose Avenue, Aberdeen
Centre, Grand Prairie, AB T8V 5B6,
(403) 539-4719, FAX (403) 539-3331.
Lethbridge: 1119 3rd Avenue
South, Lethbridge, AB T1J 0J5,
(403) 327-1044, (403) 327-1044, FAX
(403) 380-2672.
Medicine Hat: 533 1 Street, SE,
Medicine Hat, AB T1A 0A9,
(403) 527-2211, FAX (403) 526-3548.
Red Deer: 11 McMillan Avenue,
Red Deer, AB T4N 5T6, (403) 346-
0037, FAX (403) 346-0037.
Yellowknife: Baker Community
Center, 5710 B 50th Avenue,
Yellowknife, NT X1A 1G1,
(403) 873-2647, FAX (403) 873-8447.

See Canadian National Institute for
the Blind, National Office, in
Canadian national listings.

♦ Low Vision Services

EYE CARE SOCIETIES

**Alberta Association of
Optometrists**
11830 Kingsway Avenue, #902
Edmonton, AB T5G 0X5
(403) 451-6824
FAX: (403) 452-9918
R. Glenn Campbell, Executive
Director

BRITISH COLUMBIA

◆ *Educational Services*

PROVINCIAL SERVICES

Special Programs Branch
633 Courtney Street, Suite 201
Victoria, BC V8V 2M4
(250) 356-2333
FAX: (250) 356-7631
Dr. Shirley McBride, Director

Monitors the provision of educational services to children and youths with disabilities.

INSTRUCTIONAL MATERIALS CENTERS

Provincial Resource Centre for the Visually Impaired Ministry of Education and Ministry Responsible for Multiculturalism and Human Rights
#106-1750 West 75th Avenue
Vancouver, BC V6P 6G2
(604) 266-3699
FAX: (604) 261-0778
URL: http://www.set.gov.bc.ca/provi
Fred Poon, Coordinator

Type of Agency: Government.
Mission: Provides alternate format materials and specialized equipment to school districts and independent schools enrolling eligible students with a visual impairment.
Funded by: Government.
Hours of Operation: 8:30 AM-4:30 PM.
Staff: 6 and 1 summer student worker.
History/Date: Est. 1978.

Number of Clients Served: 614 visually impaired; 605 print-handicapped.
Eligibility: Blind and visually impaired students; print handicapped students.
Area Served: British Columbia.

Alternate formats include braille books, large-print books, cassettes, electronic books, kits.

UNIVERSITY TRAINING PROGRAMS

University of British Columbia Educational Psychology and Special Education
Vancouver, BC V6T 1Z4
(604) 822-5538 or (604) 822-6446
FAX: (604) 822-3302

County/District Where Located: British Columbia Province.

Programs Offered: Programs offered: Master's degree in special education (education of children with blindness, visual impairment or visual/multiple disabilities). Graduate program for teachers of visually impaired children. Includes a component on orientation and mobility.

Students may qualify for certification in orientation and mobility. Advanced preparation in orientation and mobility offered (including mobility for young children and/or students with multiple disabilities).

◆ *Information Services*

LIBRARIES

British Columbia College and Institute Library Service for the Print Impaired
Vancouver Community College
Langara Campus Library
100 West 49th Avenue
Vancouver, BC V5Y 2X6
(604) 323-5237
FAX: (604) 323-5544
E-mail: cils@langara.bc.ca
Phyllis Mason, Janette Hellmuth

Type of Agency: Library; Clearinghouse.
County/District Where Located: British Columbia Province.
Mission: To provide educational materials and texts to college and institutions' students and staff who have print impairments.
Funded by: B.C. Ministry of Education, Skills and Training.
Budget: $400,000.
Hours of Operation: Mon.-Fri. 8:00 AM-4:15 PM.
Program Accessibility: Interlibrary loan.
Staff: 3.
History/Date: Founded 1984.
Number of Clients Served: 250.
Eligibility: Documented print impairment.
Area Served: Primarily British Columbia. Will lend worldwide.

Talking books, braille, and large print provided to clients.

British Columbia Library Services to the Handicapped
Lower Mainland Office
L50-4946 Canada Way
Burnaby, BC V5G 4H7
(604) 660-7343
Jim Looney

Talking books provided to clients of all ages.

Crane Resource Centre
University of British Columbia

1874 East Mall
Vancouver, BC V6T 1Z1
(604) 822-6111
FAX: (604) 822-6113
E-mail: crane@unixg.ubc.ca or pthiele@unixg.ubc.ca
Paul E. Thiele, Director

Type of Agency: University resource and student support centre.
Mission: To provide access to books, documents, adaptive technologies and electronic information to students, faculty, staff, and distance users who require alternates to print.
Funded by: University of British Columbia, public support, revenue services.
Budget: $300,000 annually.
Hours of Operation: Mon.-Fri. 9:00 AM-5:00 PM; some evening and Sat. hours during fall and winter academic terms.
Staff: 4 full time, 7 part time. 120 volunteers.
History/Date: Est. 1968 as reading room. Became branch of University of British Columbia libraries 1969. Became part of Student Services and UBC Disability Centre in 1995.
Number of Clients Served: 50-60 on campus; estimated 3-5,000 users nationally and internationally.
Eligibility: On-campus users: University of British Columbia students, staff, and faculty medically certified to require print alternatives. Distance users served via interlibrary/interagency loans or via other clearinghouses.
Area Served: University of British Columbia, Canada, and international.
Transportation: Y.

Counseling/Social Work/Self-Help: Primarily academic and career counseling, advice on financial assistance, assistive devices.
Reading: Assistance with braille and tape speed reading, retention, and efficiency.
Rehabilitation: Informal and peer group rehabilitation activities.
Computer Training: Training on information storage, retrieval, and management on adapted computers for visually impaired persons.
Low Vision Aids: Several assistive devices available.

Collection includes talking books, braille, large-print, computer disks, and regular print. Maintains sizeable reference collection, a variety of adaptive technical devices, and an 8-studio recording center. New fully digital recording facility.

Public Library InterLINK

Suite 110
6540 Bonsor Avenue
Burnaby, BC V5H 1H3
(604) 437-8441
FAX: (604) 430-8595
Colleen Smith

Type of Agency: Audiobook headquarters.
Mission: To provide full length books on cassette to people of all ages who have a diagnosed print handicap.
Hours of Operation: Mon.-Fri. 8:30AM-4:30 PM.
Number of Clients Served: 2,415.
Eligibility: Having any print handicap (visual, physical or perceptual).
Area Served: Lower mainland of British Columbia.

Low Vision Follow-up: Provided in some public libraries.

Braille, talking books, and large print provided to clients of all ages.

MEDIA PRODUCTION SERVICES

Audiobook Program
Province of British Columbia (BBLA) Library Services Branch
L50-4946 Canada Way
Burnaby, BC V5G 4H7
(604) 660-7343
FAX: (604) 660-0435
E-mail: gyusko@hq.marh.bc.ca
Gordon Yusko

Area Served: British Columbia, limited lending library to other North American locations.
Groups Served: Primarily adults.

Types/Content: Popular reading: mysteries, romances, biographies, travelogues.
Media Formats: 2-track audio cassettes.

See also in national listings:

Crane Resource Centre
University of British Columbia

I Can See Books

Ski for Light (Canada) Inc.

◆ *Rehabilitation Services*

PROVINCIAL SERVICES

Community Support Services Division
Ministry of Social Services
614 Humboldt Street
Victoria, BC V8V 1X4
(250) 387-1275
Paula Grant, Director

Administers grants and contributions program to help fund services and integration efforts for blind and visually impaired and other disabled persons.

REHABILITATION

Canadian National Institute for the Blind
British Columbia-Yukon Division
100-5055 Joyce Street
Vancouver, BC V5R 6B2
(604) 431-2121
FAX: (604) 431-2099
Mary Ann Roscoe, Executive Director

District Offices:

Kamloops: 101-635 Victoria Street, Kamloops, BC V2C 2B3, (604) 374-8080, FAX (604) 374-8033.

Kelowna: 1450 St. Paul Street, Kelowna, BC V1Y 2E6, (604) 763-1191, FAX (604) 763-1129.

Nanaimo: 225-285 Prideaux Street, Nanaimo, BC V9R 2N2, (604) 753-0233, FAX (604) 753-0651.

Prince George: 100-490 Quebec Street, Prince George, BC V2L 5N5, (604) 563-1702, FAX (604) 563-1787.

Vancouver: 100-5055 Joyce Street, Vancouver, BC V5R 6B2, (604) 431-2121, FAX (604) 431-2199.

Victoria: 2340 Richmond Avenue, Victoria, BC V8R 4R9, (604) 595-1100, FAX (604) 595-1129.

See Canadian National Institute for the Blind, National Office, in Canadian national listings.

MANITOBA

♦ Educational Services

PROVINCIAL SERVICES

**Special Materials Services
Manitoba Department of
Education and Training
(MWESM)**
215-1181 Portage Avenue
Winnipeg, MB R3G 0T3
(204) 945-7840
FAX: (204) 945-7914
Judy Rannard, Coordinator of
Services for the Visually Impaired

Type of Agency: Provincial
Department of Education.
County/District Where Located:
Manitoba Province.
Mission: Provides special format
materials (braille, large-print and
audio tape) and special learning
equipment (braillers, CCTVs,
adaptive devices).
Funded by: Province of Manitoba.
Hours of Operation: Mon.-Fri.
8:00 AM-4:30 PM.
History/Date: Est. 1973.
Eligibility: Determined by
educational consultants employed
by the department.
Area Served: Manitoba.
Age Requirements: Student age.
K-Sr.4 (Grade 12).

Educational: Support materials
and consultant/itinerant teachers.
Low Vision: Functional vision
assessment.
Low Vision Aids: CCTVs, large
prints, on loan to school students.

Monitors the provision of
educational services to children
and youths who are print
handicapped.

INSTRUCTIONAL MATERIALS CENTERS

**Special Materials Services
Manitoba Department of
Education and Training
(MWESM)**
215-1181 Portage Avenue
Winnipeg, MB R3G 0T3
(204) 945-7840
FAX: (204) 945-7914
Judy Rannard, Coordinator of
Services for the Visually Impaired

County/District Where Located:
Manitoba Province.
Area Served: Manitoba.
Groups Served: Blind and visually
impaired students.

Types/Content: Textbooks and
supplementary reading material.
Media Formats: Braille, large-
print, audiotape.

♦ Information Services

INFORMATION AND REFERRAL

**Manitoba Blind Sport
Association**
200 Main Street
Winnipeg, MB R3C 4M2
(204) 925-5694
FAX: (204) 925-5703
Michelle Barclay

Mission: Provides opportunities
for recreation and participation in
sports activities for blind and
visually impaired persons in the
province of Manitoba.

♦ Rehabilitation Services

PROVINCIAL SERVICES

**Department of Family Services
Community Living Division**
119-114 Garry Street, Room 119
Winnipeg, MB R3C 4V4
(204) 945-0172
Wes Henderson, Executive
Director, Adult Services

Administers grants and
contributions program to help
fund services and integration
efforts for blind and visually
impaired and other disabled
persons.

**Policy and Planning
Family Services**
114 Garry Street, Suite 219
Winnipeg, MB R3C 4V6
(204) 945-2324
Drew Perry, Director

Administers grants and
contributions program to help
fund services and integration
efforts for blind and visually
impaired and other disabled
persons.

REHABILITATION

**Canadian National Institute for
the Blind
Manitoba Division**
1080 Portage Avenue
Winnipeg, MB R3G 3M3
(204) 774-5421
FAX: (204) 775-5090
G. Dean Cousens, Executive
Director

District Offices:

Brandon: 354 Tenth Street,
Brandon, MB R7A 4G1, (204) 727-
0631, FAX (204) 727-1139.

See Canadian National Institute for
the Blind, National Office, in
Canadian national listings.

◆ *Low Vision Services*

EYE CARE SOCIETIES

**Manitoba Association of
Optometrists**
878-167 Lombard Avenue
Winnipeg, MB R3B 0V3
(204) 943-9811
Carol Loyd, Executive Director

NEW BRUNSWICK

♦ Educational Services

PROVINCIAL SERVICES

Atlantic Provinces Special Education Authority (APSEA) Department of Education
5940 South Street
Halifax, NS B3H 1S6
(902) 424-8500
FAX: (902) 424-0543
Deborah F. Pottie, Superintendent
P. Ann MacCuspie, Director of Services

Interprovincial agency responsible for services to visually impaired and hearing impaired children and youths in Atlantic Canada.

See listing under Nova Scotia Province for more information.

Student Services Branch
Kings Place
P.O. Box 6000
Fredericton, NB E3B 5H1
(506) 453-2816
FAX: (506) 453-3325
Karen Love, Director

County/District Where Located: New Brunswick.

Monitors the provision of educational services to children and youths with disabilities.

♦ Information Services

LIBRARIES

New Brunswick Library Service Department of Municipalities, Culture and Housing
P.O. Box 6000
Fredericton, NB E3B 5H1
(506) 453-2354
FAX: (506) 453-2416
Jocelyne LeBel, Director

Type of Agency: Library.

York Regional Library Talking Book Service
4 Carleton Street
Fredericton, NB E3B 5P4
(506) 453-5380
FAX: (506) 457-4878
E-mail: libyr@gov.nb.ca
Laurette Mackey
Jon Sears

Mission: To provide books recorded on cassette tape to patrons unable to read because of physical or visual disability.
Funded by: Province of New Brunswick.
Hours of Operation: Mon.-Fri. 8:00 AM-4:30 PM.
History/Date: Est. 1976.
Number of Clients Served: 186.
Eligibility: Physical or visual handicap. Signature of medical authority needed to register for service.
Area Served: York, Sunbury, Queens, Carlton, Victoria, and parts of Northumberland counties in New Brunswick.

Talking books provided for clients of all ages.

♦ Rehabilitation Services

PROVINCIAL SERVICES

Family and Community Social Services New Brunswick Department of Health and Community Services
P.O. Box 5100
Fredericton, NB E3B 5G8
(506) 453-2181
Gérard Doucet, Assistant Deputy Minister

County/District Where Located: New Brunswick Province.

Administers grants and contributions program to help fund services and integration efforts for blind and visually impaired and other disabled persons.

REHABILITATION

Canadian National Institute for the Blind New Brunswick Division
231 Saunders Street
Fredericton, NB E3B 1N6
(506) 458-0060
FAX: (506) 458-9219
Jean Ann Ledwell, Executive Director

District Offices:

Bathurst: 700 St. Peter Avenue, Bathurst, NB E2A 2Y7, (506) 546-9922, FAX (506) 546-8707.

Moncton: 118 Highfield Street, Moncton, NB E1C 5N7, (506) 857-4240, FAX (506) 857-3019.

Newcastle: 350 Morrison Lane, Newcastle, NB E1V 2C1, (506) 622-1513, FAX (506) 622-8137.

Saint John: 133 Prince William Street, Suite 306, Saint John, NB E2L 2B5, (506) 634-7277, FAX (506) 634-7202.

See Canadian National Institute for the Blind, National Office, in Canadian national listings.

NEWFOUND-LAND

♦ *Educational Services*

PROVINCIAL SERVICES

Atlantic Provinces Special Education Authority (APSEA) Department of Education
5940 South Street
Halifax, NS B3H 1S6
(902) 424-8500
FAX: (902) 424-0543
E-mail: maccuspiea@gov.ns.ca
Deborah F. Pottie, Superintendent
P. Ann MacCuspie, Director of Services

Interprovincial agency responsible for services to visually impaired and hearing impaired children and youths in Atlantic Canada.

See listing under Nova Scotia Province for more information.

Student Support Services Department of Education
P.O. Box 8700
St. John's, NF A1B 4J6
(709) 729-0709
FAX: (709) 729-2096
E-mail: bflight@edu.gov.nf.ca
Brenda Kelleher-Flight,
Consultant, Student Support Services Division

Type of Agency: Department of Education.
County/District Where Located: Newfoundland Province.
Mission: To provide services to children/youth with visual impairments.
Funded by: Government of Newfoundland and Labrador.
Budget: $2 million.

Hours of Operation: School year.
Program Accessibility: To all pre-school and school-age children.
Staff: 14.
Number of Clients Served: 159.
Eligibility: To students with 20/70 vision or less in the better eye or vision field of 20 degrees or less.
Area Served: Newfoundland and Labrador.
Transportation: Y.
Age Requirements: 0-21 years.

Preschools: Services are offered in child's home.
10 regional board offices.

Monitors the provision of educational services to children and youths with disabilities.

♦ *Information Services*

LIBRARIES

Newfoundland Provincial Public Libraries Board
Arts and Culture Centre
Allandale Road
St. John's, NF A1B 3A3
(709) 737-3966
FAX: (709) 737-3009
David Gale, Director

♦ *Rehabilitation Services*

PROVINCIAL SERVICES

Family and Rehabilitative Services Department of Social Services, Province of Newfoundland
Confederation Building

St. John's, NF A1B 4J6
(709) 729-2436
E-mail: dgallant@doss.gov.nf.ca
URL: http://www.gov.nf.ca/doss/progdev/famrehab.htm
Don Gallant, Director

Administers grants and contributions program to help fund services and integration efforts for blind and visually impaired and other disabled persons.

REHABILITATION

Canadian National Institute for the Blind Newfoundland and Labrador Division
70 Boulevard
St. John's, NF A1A 1K2
(709) 754-1180
FAX: (709) 754-2018
Elizabeth Hamilton, Executive Director

Regional Offices:

St. John's: 70 Boulevard, St. John's, NF A1A 1K2, (709) 754-1180, FAX (709) 754-2018.

Local Offices:

Corner Brook: 202-10 Main Street, Corner Brook, NF A2H 1B8, (709) 639-9167, FAX (709) 639-9290.
Grand Falls: 1A O'Neill Avenue, P.O. Box 442, Grand Falls, NF A2A 2J8, (709) 489-6515.

See Canadian National Institute for the Blind, National Office, in Canadian national listings.

NORTHWEST TERRITORIES

◆ Educational Services

Department of Education, Culture and Employment Early Childhood and School Services
P.O. Box 1320
Yellowknife, NT X1A 2L9
(403) 873-7678
Barbara Hall, Coordinator

County/District Where Located: Northwest Territories.

Monitors the provision of educational services to children and youths with disabilities.

◆ Information Services

**Northwest Territories Library Services
Department of Education, Culture and Employment**
62 Woodland Drive
Wright Center, Second Floor
Hay River, NT X0E 1G1
(403) 874-6531
FAX: (403) 874-3321
Suliang Feng, Librarian

◆ Rehabilitation Services

Stanton Regional House Board
550 Byrne Road
P.O. Box 10
Yellowknife, NT X1A 2N1
(403) 669-4102
FAX: (403) 669-4128
Dennis Cleaver, CEO
Donna Allen, Manager of Rehabilitation Services

Canadian National Institute for the Blind Alberta–Northwest Territories Division
12010 Jasper Avenue
Edmonton, AB T5K 0P3
(403) 488-4871
FAX: (403) 482-0017
URL: http://www.cnib.ca
William J. McKeown, Executive Director

See Canadian National Institute for the Blind, Alberta–Northwest Territories Division, in Alberta provincial listings.

NOVA SCOTIA

◆ *Educational Services*

PROVINCIAL SERVICES

Atlantic Provinces Special Education Authority (APSEA) Department of Education
5940 South Street
Halifax, NS B3H 1S6
(902) 424-8500
FAX: (902) 424-0543
E-mail: maccuspiea@gov.ns.ca
Deborah F. Pottie, Superintendent
P. Ann MacCuspie, Director of Services

Mission: To provide services for blind, visually impaired persons in home, community, school, or residential settings.
History/Date: Est. 1870.
Number of Clients Served: 722.
Eligibility: Visual acuity 20/70 or less with best correction or 20 degrees less field restriction.
Age Requirements: 21 years and under.

Health: General medical services for residential students. Referrals.
Rehabilitation: Living skills; remedial education; braille; orientation and mobility; sensory training.
Recreational: After-school programs.
Low Vision Aids: Training in use of aids.
Professional Training: Internship and fieldwork placements; regular in-service training.

Interprovincial agency responsible for services to visually impaired and hearing impaired children and youths in Atlantic Canada.

Student Services Division Department of Education
P.O. Box 578
Halifax, NS B3J 2S9
(902) 424-5839 or (902) 424-7454
FAX: (902) 424-0799
Ann Power, Director of Student Services

Monitors the provision of educational services to children and youths with disabilities.

SCHOOLS

Sir Frederick Fraser School Atlantic Provinces Special Education Authority
5940 South Street
Halifax, NS B3H 1S6
(902) 424-8500
FAX: (902) 424-0543
Dr. Ann MacCuspie, Director

Type of Agency: Resource center and school.
County/District Where Located: Nova Scotia Province.
Mission: Services for persons who are totally blind, legally blind, visually impaired, and those having additional disabilities, provided in their home, community school, or in a residential school setting.
Funded by: Atlantic provinces (New Brunswick, Nova Scotia, Newfoundland, and Prince Edward Island).
Staff: On campus: 21 teachers; 16 residence; 10 resource services and braille production; 27 other. Off campus: 25 itinerant teachers.
History/Date: Est. 1870 as Halifax School for the Blind; est. 1975 as APSEA Resource Center for the Visually Impaired.
Number of Clients Served: On campus: 35. Off campus: 450 direct service plus resources; 370 resources only.
Eligibility: Visually impaired, from birth to 21 years of age,

resident of Atlantic Canada. Visual acuity 20/70 or less with best correction or 20 degrees or less field restriction.
Area Served: Atlantic provinces in Canada.
Age Requirements: 0-21 years.

Health: Diagnosis, evaluation, medical care of eyes; general medical services; physical therapy; speech therapy; specialist medical services provided by local hospitals, physiotherapy.
Counseling/Social Work/Self-Help: Individual counseling; family counseling; psychological services; transition services; school placement.
Educational: On campus: preschool through 9th grade; general academic; prevocational/skill development; short-term placements. Off campus: itinerant service to public school programs, transition planning facilitators.
Preschools: Home visits; limited support for children enrolled in preschool programs.
Professional Training: Student teaching in special education; internship/fieldwork placements in orientation and mobility/classrooms/residence. Regular in-service training.
Reading: Braille books and magazines; large-print books; talking book cassettes; video tapes; professional library; transcription to braille; tape recording.
Residential: Apartments.
Rehabilitation: Daily living skills training; braille; electronic aids; technological aids; remedial education; sensory training, orientation and mobility; counseling, resource services.
Recreational: Afterschool programs; arts and crafts; music; bowling; goal ball; swimming; all recreational programs available in community.

Employment: Limited student employment opportunities.
Computer Training: On- and off-campus training provided.
Low Vision Follow-up: Educational vision assessments and training in the use of low vision aids.

♦ Information Services

LIBRARIES

Nova Scotia Provincial Library
3770 Kempt Road
Halifax, NS B3K 4X8
(902) 424-2457
FAX: (902) 424-0633
E-mail: admin@nshpl.library.ns.ca
URL: http://www.library.ns.ca
Marian Pape, Provincial Librarian
Ann Dunsworth, (902) 424-2473

Type of Agency: Provincial library.
Mission: To provide accessible reading material to Nova Scotia residents.
Funded by: Provincial government.
Budget: $1.4 million.
Hours of Operation: Mon.-Fri. 8:30 AM-4:30 PM.
Staff: 2.
History/Date: Est.1977.
Number of Clients Served: 500.
Area Served: Province of Nova Scotia; Canada and other countries through inter-library loan.
Age Requirements: None.

For more information about regional public libraries in Nova Scotia, contact the address above.

MEDIA PRODUCTION SERVICES

Ferguson Library for Print Handicapped Students
c/o Patrick Power Library
Saint Mary's University
Halifax, NS B3C 3C3
(902) 420-5553
FAX: (902) 420-5561

County/District Where Located: Nova Scotia.
Groups Served: Postsecondary students and professionals.
Media Formats: Audiotape.

Resource Services
Atlantic Provinces Special Education Authority
Sir Frederick Fraser School
5940 South Street
Halifax, NS B3H 1S6
(902) 424-8500
Francis Drake, Coordinator of Resource Services

Area Served: Atlantic provinces (Nova Scotia, New Brunswick, Newfoundland, and Prince Edward Island).
Groups Served: Totally blind and low vision students aged 0-21.
Media Formats: Braille, large-print, tape.

See also in national listings:

Atlantic Provinces Special Education Authority

♦ Rehabilitation Services

PROVINCIAL SERVICES

Strategic and Operational Planning and Policy Development
Department of Community Services, Province of Nova Scotia
Johnston Building, Fifth Floor
P.O. Box 696
Halifax, NS B3J 2T7
(902) 424-4455
FAX: (902) 424-0502
E-mail: coms.mcpheecm@gov.ns.ca
URL: http://www.gov.ns.ca
Cathy McPhee, Director

Administers grants and contributions program to help fund services and integration efforts for blind and visually impaired and other disabled persons.

REHABILITATION

Canadian National Institute for the Blind
Nova Scotia–Prince Edward Island Division
6136 Almon Street
Halifax, NS B3K 1T8
(902) 453-1480
FAX: (902) 454-6570
Guy M. Woodland, Executive Director

District Offices:

Charlottetown: 284 Graftson Street, Charlottetown, PE C1A 1L7, (902) 566-2580, FAX (902) 628-1445.

Sydney: 189 Townsend Street, Sydney, NS B1P 5E4, (902) 564-5711, (902) 564-9953, FAX (902) 562-9802.

Truro: 35 Commercial Street, Suite 316, Truro, NS B2N 3H8, (902) 893-9546, FAX (902) 893-4211.

See Canadian National Institute for the Blind, National Office, in Canadian national listings.

ONTARIO

♦ *Educational Services*

PROVINCIAL SERVICES

**Public Inquiries Unit
Communications Branch
Ministry of Education and
Training**
900 Bay Street
14th Floor-Mowat Block
Toronto, ON M7A 1L2
(416) 325-2929 or (800) 387-5512

County/District Where Located:
Ontario.

Monitors the provision of
educational services to children
and youths with disabilities.

SCHOOLS

Hollywood Public School
360 Hollywood Avenue
North York, ON M2N 3L4
(416) 395-2560
FAX: (416) 395-4485
Ms. Linda Beemer, Primary
Teacher
Brian Smith, Teacher, Junior
Grades

Type of Agency: Public school
program.
Mission: To provide braille
instruction on a daily basis to
young visually impaired children
(ages 4-11) within an integrated
classroom setting.
Hours of Operation: Mon.-Fri.
8:30 AM-3:15 PM.
Staff: 2 teachers of the blind, 1
orientation/mobility specialist. 2
braillists/classroom assistants.
History/Date: Est. 1977.
Number of Clients Served: 8-12.
Eligibility: Potential braille-using
students from senior kindergarten
to grade 5.

Area Served: Metropolitan
Toronto.
Age Requirements: 4-11 years.

Educational: Senior kindergarten
to grade 5.

**Metro Special Program (Vision)
(Itinerant Program-Public and
Special Schools)**
Northview Annex
550 Finch Avenue West
North York, ON M2R 1N6
(416) 395-2145
FAX: (416) 395-3711
E-mail: vis2020@torhookup.net
Sharyn Shell, Chief Consultant

Type of Agency: School support
service.
Funded by: Toronto school board.
Hours of Operation: School hours.
Number of Clients Served: 300.
Eligibility: Vision must be 20/70
or less.
Age Requirements: 21 years and
under.

W. Ross Macdonald School
350 Brant Avenue
Brantford, ON N3T 3J9
(519) 759-0730
FAX: (519) 759-4741
David Neill, Superintendent

Type of Agency: Public,
residential school.
Mission: School programs, grades
1 to 12, for visually impaired and
deaf-blind students. Resource
services to local school boards in
Ontario.
Funded by: Ontario Ministry of
Education and Training.
Hours of Operation: Office:
Mon.-Fri. 8:30 AM-4:45 PM.
Staff: 67.5 teachers; 135 other staff.
History/Date: Est. 1872.
Number of Clients Served: 185
blind pupils; 36 deaf-blind pupils.
Eligibility: Resident of Ontario.

Transportation: Y.
Age Requirements: 6-21 years of
age.

Preschools: Consulting service to
preschool deafblind families.
Professional Training:
Responsible for teacher education
in Ontario. For teachers of the
blind and deafblind.

Houses the Provincial Resource
Centre, which distributes audio
tapes, large-print and braille
educational books, provides
consultant services to educators in
local school board programs, and
is designated as an assessment and
loan center for high technology
communication equipment,
including computers as sight
substitution aids.

INFANT AND PRESCHOOL

**High Park Forest School
Ontario Foundation for Visually
Impaired Children Inc.**
P.O. Box 1116
Station D
Toronto, ON M6P 3K2
(416) 767-5977
April Cornell, Executive Director

Type of Agency: Non-profit.
Mission: Services to blind and
visually impaired children.
Funded by: Provincial
government and donations.
Age Requirements: 2-6 years.

**Counseling/Social Work/Self-
Help:** Counseling and support for
parents.
Educational: Assessment and
evaluations; activities in all areas.

INSTRUCTIONAL MATERIALS CENTERS

**W. Ross Macdonald School
Resource Services Library**
350 Brant Avenue

Brantford, ON N3T 3J9
(519) 759-2522
FAX: (519) 759-1036
E-mail: 10251.2100@compuserve.com
David Neill, Superintendent
Jane Field, Supervisor, Resource Services Library

Groups Served: Elementary, secondary schools in Ontario for print-disabled students.

Media Formats: Large print, braille, tape.

UNIVERSITY TRAINING PROGRAMS

Mohawk College of Applied Arts and Technology
Brant Campuses
411 Elgin Street
Brantford, ON N3T 5V2
(519) 758-6029
FAX: (519) 758-6043
E-mail: snookhm@operatns.mohawk.om.ca
John Schaeffer, Chair
Mary Maureen Snook-Hill, Coordinator

Programs Offered: Programs for orientation and mobility instructors and rehabilitation teachers.

◆ Information Services

MEDIA PRODUCTION SERVICES

Access 20/20
21 Inverness Road
Nepean, ON K2E 6N6
(613) 727-9508
Mark Joly, President

Media Formats: Braille, large-type, computer diskettes, and braille business cards at a reasonable cost.

Computer Braille Facility University of Western Ontario
Room UCC215
London, ON N6A 3K7
(519) 661-3061, ext. 6844
E-mail: kirk@braille.uwo.ca
Kirk Reiser, Manager

Area Served: Ontario.
Groups Served: Postsecondary students.

Types/Content: Textbooks, foreign language books, technical manuals, mathematical materials.
Media Formats: Braille.

Metropolitan Toronto Reference Library
Centre for People with Disabilities
789 Yonge Street
Toronto, ON M4W 2G8
(416) 393-7099 or (TTY) (416) 393-7100
FAX: (416) 393-7229
URL: http://www.mtrl.toronto.on.ca
Maureen Perez, Coordinator

Area Served: Metropolitan Toronto.
Groups Served: Provides talking book services to all eligible print handicapped persons in Metropolitan Toronto through public libraries. Provides a variety of adaptive technical devices as well as equipment training and individual assistance to clients of all ages to access information resources of this library.

Media Formats: Books on audiotape, some large print and braille books.

Ontario Audio Library Service Trent University
P.O. Box 4800
Peterborough, ON K9J 7B8
(705) 748-1240 or (705) 748-1383
FAX: (705) 748-1564
E-mail: kconway@trentu.ca
Lorna Hilborn, Executive Director

Area Served: Primarily Ontario; all of Canada.
Groups Served: Print disabled postsecondary students.

Types/Content: Postsecondary educational textbooks.
Media Formats: Four-track audio tape.

INFORMATION AND REFERRAL

Organization for the Education of the Visually Handicapped (OEVH)
350 Brant Avenue
Brantford, ON N3T 3J9
(519) 759-0730
FAX: (519) 759-4741
Don Bethune, Principal
David Neill, Superintendent

County/District Where Located: Brant County.
Mission: Network of educators that strives to enhance professional activities and relationships among persons working with blind and visually impaired students and children in the province of Ontario.

See also in national listings:

Alternate Media Canada
The National Broadcast Reading Service

Audio Vision Canada
The National Broadcast Reading Service, Inc.

Canadian Association of Optometrists

Canadian Blind Sports Association

Canadian Council for Exceptional
Children
Division for the Visually
Handicapped

Canadian Council of the Blind

Canadian National Institute for
the Blind
Department of Government
Relations and International
Services

Canadian National Institute for
the Blind
National Office

Canadian National Society of the
Deaf-Blind

Canadian Ophthalmological
Society

CDBRA (Canadian Deaf Blind
Research Association) National
Office

Christian Blind Mission
International

Christian Record Services

John Milton Society for the Blind
in Canada

Library for the Blind
Canadian National Institute for
the Blind

Low Vision Association of
Ontario

Multi-Lingual Braille and Large
Print Association

PAL Reading Services

People Helping People

Retinitis Pigmentosa Eye
Research Foundation

VIEWS for the Visually Impaired

VoicePrint
The National Broadcast Reading
Service, Inc.

◆ *Rehabilitation Services*

PROVINCIAL SERVICES

**Developmental Services Branch
Ministry of Community and
Social Services**
Hepburn Block, 80 Governor Street
Toronto, ON M7A 1E9
(416) 327-4962
FAX: (416) 325-5554
Brian Low, Director, (416) 325-5826

Administers grants and
contributions program to help
fund services and integration
efforts for blind and visually
impaired and other disabled
persons.

REHABILITATION

Balance
4920 Dundas Street West
Suite 302
Etobicoke, ON M9A 1B7
(416) 236-1796
FAX: (416) 236-4280
Sue Archibald, Executive Director

Type of Agency: Non-profit.
Mission: Provides a community-
based program to enhance
independent living skills to
visually impaired adults, while
they are living in their own
apartment.
Funded by: Ministry of
Community and Social Services,
Government of Ontario, Canada.
Budget: $375,000.
Hours of Operation: 9:00 AM-
9:00 PM.
Staff: 9 full time.
History/Date: Est. 1986.
Number of Clients Served: 73 to
date.
Eligibility: 18 years or over,
legally blind, living in
metropolitan Toronto, motivated
to learn independent living skills.

Area Served: Metropolitan
Toronto.
Age Requirements: 18 or over.

**Counseling/Social Work/Self-
Help:** Will provide support to our
participants to use community
services.
Educational: Refers for
educational courses.
Rehabilitation: Teaches
orientation and mobility, daily
living skills, community access
and awareness, and life skills.
Recreational: Referrals.
Employment: Referrals.
Computer Training: Referrals.
Low Vision: Referrals.
Low Vision Aids: Referrals.
Low Vision Follow-up: Referrals.

**Canadian National Institute for
the Blind
Ontario Division**
1929 Bayview Avenue
Toronto, ON M4G 3E8
(416) 486-2500
FAX: (416) 480-7503
Gary W. Magarrell, Executive
Director

District Offices:

Barrie: Simcoe/Muskoka Office,
49 Mary Street, Barrie, ON L4N
1T2, (705) 728-3352, FAX
(705) 722-5305.
Belleville: Hasting/Prince
Edward Office, 11 Victoria Avenue,
Belleville, ON K8N 1Z6, (613) 966-
8833, FAX (613) 966-2731.
Brantford: 67 King Street,
Brantford, ON N3T 5M8,
(519) 752-6831, FAX (519) 752-4920.
Cornwall: Eastern Counties, 222
Pitt Street, Cornwall, ON K6J 3P6,
(613) 936-2300, FAX (613) 936-2296.
Hamilton: Hamilton/Wentworth
Office, 1686 Main Street West,
Hamilton, ON L8S 1G4, (905) 528-
8555 (voice/TDD), FAX (905) 527-
9536.

Kingston: 826 Princess Street, Kingston, ON K7L 1G3, (613) 542-4975, FAX (613) 542-8639.

London: Southwest Office, 749 Baseline Road East, London, ON N6C 2R6, (519) 685-8420 (voice/TDD), FAX (519) 685-8419.

Mississauga: Halton/Peel Office 151 City Centre Drive, Suite 201, Mississauga, ON L5B 1H7, (905) 275-5332, FAX (905) 275-7710.

North Bay: Nipissing/Parry Sound Office, 483 Main Street West, North Bay, ON P1B 2V3, (705) 472-2710, FAX (705) 472-7269.

Oshawa: Dusham Office, 205 Bond Street East, Oshawa, ON L1G 1B4, (905) 436-7732, FAX (905) 436-1202.

Ottawa: Ottawa-Carlton and Lanark Office, 320 McLeod Street, Ottawa, ON K2P 1A3, (613) 563-4021 (voice/TDD), FAX (613) 563-1898.

Owen Sound: Bruce/Dufferin/Grey Office, 895 Third Avenue, East, Owen Sound, ON N4K 2K6, (519) 371-2721, FAX (519) 371-2741.

Pembroke: Renfrew County Office, Peter White Building, Suite 2, 217 Pembroke Street East, Pembroke, ON K8A 3J8, (613) 735-1921, FAX (613) 735-7010.

Peterborough: Haliburton/Kawartha/Pine Ridge Office, 236 King Street, Peterborough, ON K9J 7L8, (705) 745-6918, FAX (705) 745-9899.

Richmond Hill: York Office, 9050 Yonge Street, Suite 102, Richmond Hill, ON L4C 9S6, (905) 731-6307, FAX (905) 731-8979.

St. Catharines: Niagara Office, 63 Church Street, Suite 309, St. Catharines, ON L2R 3C4, (905) 688-0022, FAX (905) 688-9674.

Sault Ste. Marie: Saulte-Algoma Office, 763 Wellington Street East, Sault Ste. Marie, ON P6A 2M9, (705) 949-2610, FAX (705) 949-2291.

Scarborough: 1200 Markham Road, Suite 104, Scarborough, ON M1H 3C3, (416) 289-0019, FAX (416) 289-3942.

Sudbury: Sudbury/Manitonlin Office, 303 York Street, Sudbury, ON P3E 2A5, (705) 675-2468, FAX (705) 675-6635.

Thunder Bay: Northwest Office, 229 Camelot Street, Thunder Bay, ON P7A 4B2, (807) 345-3341, FAX (807) 345-0786.

Timmins: Northern Office, 303 Fifth Avenue, Timmins, ON P4N 5L5, (705) 264-2312, FAX (705) 264-9851.

Toronto: Etobicoke/York Office, 1243 Islington Avenue, Suite 900, Toronto, ON M8X 1Y9, (416) 234-9795, (416) 234-9796, FAX (416) 234-8018.

Toronto: North/York Office, 1929 Bayview Avenue, Toronto, ON M4G 3E8, (416) 480-7569, FAX (416) 480-7699.

Toronto: East York Office, 1929 Bayview Avenue, Toronto, ON M4G 3E8, (416) 480-7426, FAX (416) 480-7699.

Waterloo: Waterloo/Wellington Office, 160-180 King Street South, Suite 160, Waterloo, ON N2J 1P8, (519) 742-3536, FAX (519) 742-4003.

Windsor: Essex/Kent Office, 230 Strabane Avenue, Windsor, ON N8Y 4V2, (519) 945-2321, FAX (519) 945-9417.

See Canadian National Institute for the Blind, National Office, in Canadian national listings.

COMPUTER TRAINING CENTERS

Frontier Computing
250 Davisville Avenue
Suite 205
Toronto, ON M4S 1H2
(416) 489-6690
FAX: (416) 489-6693
E-mail: frontier@frontiercomputing.on.ca
URL: http://www.frontiercomputing.on.ca
Chris Chamberlin, President

Provides consultation, sales, set-up, and training on access technology as well as a braille transcription service.

DOG GUIDE SCHOOLS

Canadian Guide Dogs for the Blind
4120 Rideau Valley Drive North
P.O. Box 280
Manotick, ON K4M 1A3
(613) 692-7777
FAX: (613) 692-0650
Thomas Nesbitt, Executive Director

Type of Agency: Private; non-profit.
Funded by: Voluntary contributions from corporations, private individuals, service clubs, and special events.
Budget: $1 million.
Hours of Operation: 8:30 AM-5:00 PM.
Staff: 23.
History/Date: Est. 1984.
Number of Clients Served: 150.
Eligibility: Registered blind. All clients are interviewed in their home prior to acceptance for training.
Area Served: Canada.
Transportation: Y.
Age Requirements: Minimum 16 years of age.

Educational: Classes are held with 8 students and 2 or 3 staff members. All clients receive immediate postclass and routine follow-up, with a minimum of one visit per year.

Canine Vision Canada
Lions Foundation of Canada
P.O. Box 907
Oakville, ON L6J 5E8
(905) 842-2891
Elizabeth Thompson, Executive Assistant

Mission: Trains and supplies dog guides to blind persons. Provides consultation, follow-up, and orientation and mobility training.
Eligibility: Canadian citizen; minimum 17 years of age.
Area Served: All of Canada.

◆ Low Vision Services

LOW VISION CENTERS

Centre for Sight Enhancement
School of Optometry
University of Waterloo
Columbia Street West
Waterloo, ON N2L 3G1
(519) 888-4062
FAX: (519) 746-2337

Mission: Provides comprehensive clinical services for partially sighted persons, including assessing, prescribing and providing high-technology sight enhancement systems to visually impaired Ontario residents through the Assistive Devices Program.

Vision Institute
16 York Mills Road
Suite 110
North York, ON M2P 2E5
(416) 224-2273
FAX: (416) 224-9234
Dr. Mitch Samek, Executive Director

Hours of Operation: Mon.-Fri. 9:00 AM-5:00 PM.
Staff: 4 Doctors and staff of 3.
Area Served: Toronto and surrounding area.

Low Vision: Comprehensive services.
Low Vision Aids: Recommends optical and nonoptical aids.

PRINCE EDWARD ISLAND

♦ Educational Services

PROVINCIAL SERVICES

Atlantic Provinces Special Education Authority (APSEA) Department of Education
5940 South Street
Halifax, NS B3H 1S6
(902) 424-8500
Deborah F. Pottie, Superintendent
P. Ann MacCuspie, Director of Services

Interprovincial agency responsible for services to visually impaired and hearing impaired children and youths in Atlantic Canada.

See listing under Nova Scotia Province for further information.

Eastern School District Unit
P.O. Box 8600
Charlottetown, PE C1A 8V7
(902) 368-6990
FAX: (902) 368-6960
David McCabe, Superintendent of Education

Monitors the provision of educational services to children and youths with disabilities.

♦ Information Services

LIBRARIES

Provincial Library
Red Head Road
P.O. Box 7500

Morrell, PE C0A 1S0
(902) 961-7320
FAX: (902) 961-7322
Albert MacDonald, Provincial Librarian

Type of Agency: Public library.
Mission: To provide and promote an effective library service that supports the educational, recreational, and informational needs of residents of Prince Edward Island.
Funded by: Provincial government.
Budget: $1.684 million.
Hours of Operation: Main office: Mon.-Fri. 8:00 AM-4:30 PM.
Program Accessibility: Elevator for wheelchair users; large-print microfiche reader for visually impaired patrons.
Number of Clients Served: Approximately 300.
Eligibility: For talking books supplied by Canadian National Institute for the Blind, patrons must present a doctor's certificate verifying a visual impairment; for all other audio and large-print books, there are no eligibility requirements.
Area Served: Prince Edward Island.

Educational: Educational materials; workshops by professionals and information sessions by library staff.
Reading: Collection of large-print and recorded materials shared among branch libraries and book mobiles. Library has its own small collection; other titles are supplied by Canadian National Institute for the Blind.

Persons interested in registering for talking books should contact Confederation Centre Public Library, Box 7000, Charlottetown, PE CIA 8G8, Canada, Don Scott, (902) 368-4649.

♦ Rehabilitation Services

PROVINCIAL SERVICES

PEI Health and Community Services
4 Sydney Street
P.O. Box 2000
Charlottetown, PE C1A 7N8
(902) 368-6579
George O'Connor, Special Programs Consultant

Administers grants and contributions program to help fund services and integration efforts for blind and visually impaired and other disabled persons.

REHABILITATION

Canadian National Institute for the Blind
Nova Scotia–Prince Edward Island Division
6136 Almon Street
Halifax, NS B3K 1T8
(902) 453-1480
FAX: (902) 454-6570
Guy M. Woodland, Executive Director

See Canadian National Institute for the Blind, Nova Scotia–Prince Edward Island Division, in Nova Scotia provincial listings.

QUEBEC

◆ *Educational Services*

PROVINCIAL SERVICES

Direction de l'Adaption Scolaire et des Services Complémentaires
1035,de la Chevrotiere
Edifice Marie Guyart
Québec, PQ G1R 5A5
(418) 646-7000
FAX: (418) 528-2661
Dominique Fraser

Monitors the provision of educational services to children and youths with disabilities.

SCHOOLS

Montreal Association for the Blind
7000 Sherbrooke Street West
Montreal, PQ H4B 1R3
(514) 489-8201
FAX: (514) 489-3477
Ben Fagan, Elementary Principal

Type of Agency: Preschool, elementary and high school. Provides services both in agency and in public schools by itinerant teachers.
Mission: Offers training, education, and rehabilitation.
Funded by: Governments and private contributions.
Budget: $1,458,894.
Hours of Operation: 8:30 AM-4:30 PM.
Staff: 24.
History/Date: Est. 1908.
Number of Clients Served: 150.
Eligibility: Canadian citizens to age 21 years (also landed immigrants or special permit holders for nonCanadians).

Transportation: Y.
Age Requirements: Birth to 21 years.
Counseling/Social Work/Self-Help: Counseling and psychosocial training.
Preschools: Birth to 5 years.
Professional Training: Training for itinerant teachers for high school students.
Reading: Braille, large print, recordings, high-tech equipment.
Residential: Yes, as necessary.
Employment: Office for training and placement.
Computer Training: Training and equipment provided.
Low Vision: Low vision clinic.
Low Vision Aids: Aids are provided.
Low Vision Follow-up: Therapists and social workers maintain contact.

INFANT AND PRESCHOOL

Montreal Association for the Blind
7000 Sherbrooke Street West
Montreal, PQ H4B 1R3
(514) 489-8201
FAX: (514) 489-3477
E-mail: mabinfo@axess.com
URL: http://www.canpub.com/mab
Francis Rudkin, Preschool Principal

Mission: To offer services which will maximize the development of visually impaired children.
Funded by: Government grants; private donations.
Budget: $6,841,837.
Hours of Operation: Mon.-Fri. 8:30 AM-4:30 PM.
Staff: 6.
Number of Clients Served: 25-35 per year.
Eligibility: Blind or visually impaired.

Area Served: Province of Quebec.
Transportation: Y.
Age Requirements: Birth to 5 years.
Counseling/Social Work/Self-Help: Counseling, parent support groups.
Educational: Nursery school, parent/child interventions.
Preschools: Consultant services to community programs working with visually impaired preschoolers (nursery schools, daycares, other rehabilitation centres).
Rehabilitation: Orientation and mobility and other rehabilitation services as appropriate.
Low Vision: Pediatric low vision clinic.
Low Vision Aids: Provides a variety of visual aids.
Low Vision Follow-up: Y.

UNIVERSITY TRAINING PROGRAMS

University of Sherbrooke Faculty of Education
University of Sherbrooke
Sherbrooke, Quebec, PQ J1K 2R1
(819) 821-8000, ext. 2437
FAX: (819) 821-7950
Jean Toupin

County/District Where Located: Quebec Province.

Programs Offered: Graduate programs for orientation and mobility instructors.

♦ Information Services

LIBRARIES

Direction des Bibliothèques Publiques
Ministère des Affaires Culturelles
225 Grand Allèe Est
Quebec, PQ G1R 5G5
(418) 644-7206
FAX: (418) 643-4080
Michael Bonneau, Director

See also in national listings:

Institut Nazareth et Louis-Braille

Regroupement des Aveugles et Amblyopes du Quebec

♦ Rehabilitation Services

PROVINCIAL SERVICES

Service des Programmes aux Personnes Handicapées
Ministère de la Santé et des Services Sociaux,
Gouvernement du Québec
1075 Chemin Ste-Foy
3ième étage
Québec, PQ G1Z 2M1
(418) 643-6407
Julien Bourgeois, Conseillière en programmation

Administers grants and contributions program to help fund services and integration efforts for blind and visually impaired and other disabled persons.

REHABILITATION

Canadian National Institute for the Blind
Quebec Division
3622, rue Hochelega
Suite 420
Montrèal, PQ H1W 1J1
(514) 529-2040
FAX: (514) 529-4662
Ms. Penny Hartin, Executive Director

District Offices:

Matane: 235, St.-Jèrôme, Bureau 209, Matane, PQ G4W 3A7, (418) 562-4255.

See Canadian National Institute for the Blind, National Office, in Canadian national listings.

Centre Louis-Hébert
525 Boulevard Hamel Est, Aile J
Quebec, PQ G1M 2S8
(418) 529-6991
FAX: (418) 529-3450
Christiane Dion

Type of Agency: Rehabilitation center for visually impaired persons.
Mission: To offer adaptation/ rehabilitation and social integration services to visually impaired persons, residents of Quebec province.
Funded by: Provincial government.
Budget: $4.6 million.
Hours of Operation: 8:30 AM-4:30 PM (September to June); 8:00 AM-4:00 PM (July-August).
Staff: 56.
History/Date: Est. 1976.
Number of Clients Served: 2,391.
Eligibility: Resident of Quebec province who, after correction with appropriate ophthalmic lens, excluding special optical systems and correction superior to 4 dioptries, has a visual acuity of each eye inferior to 6/21 (20/70) or whose visual field in each eye is inferior to 60° in the meridian 180° or 90°.

Counseling/Social Work/Self-Help: Referrals to local centers; counseling for orientation in school and work.
Counseling/Social Work/Self-Help: Y.
Residential: Short-term.
Rehabilitation: Social and community integration; adaption to environment.
Employment: Works with outside agencies in job placement.
Computer Training: Education in special software for the visually impaired.
Low Vision: Clinic gives evaluations, referrals.
Low Vision Aids: Training in use of low vision aids.
Low Vision Follow-up: Y.

Institut Nazareth et Louis-Braille
1111 St. Charles West
Longueuil, PQ J4K 5G4
(514) 463-1710
FAX: (514) 463-0243
E-mail: gcollard@login.net
Gabriel Collard, Executive Director

Type of Agency: Services, research, and teaching center for visually impaired persons.
Mission: Rehabilitation, supported by information production and dissemination services in substitute media.
Funded by: Government of Québec.
Budget: $7 million.
Hours of Operation: Mon.-Fri. 8:00 AM-5:00 PM.
Staff: 121 people, 24 percent of whom are disabled.
History/Date: Result of the 1975 merger of two establishments, namely Institut Nazareth, founded in 1861, and the Institut Louis-Braille, opened in 1953 by the

Clercs de Saint-Viateur, with the support of Cardinal Léger and Mr. Jean Cypihot.

Number of Clients Served: 6,500.

Eligibility: All visually impaired individuals recognized as such according to the criteria of the Québec Health Insurance Board. These criteria include, after correction by means of appropriate ophthalmic lenses, except special optical systems and additions of more than four (4) dioptries, a visual acuity in each eye inferior to 6/21, or whose field of vision in each eye is inferior to 60° in the 180° or 90° meridian, and who in either event is unable to read, write, or negotiate unfamiliar surroundings.

Area Served: Part of Québec for rehabilitation services and all Canada for French braille services.

Transportation: Y.

Professional Training: Provided with the University of Sherbrooke.

Reading: For Grade 1 and 2 braille.

Residential: Short-term only.

Montreal Association for the Blind

7000 Sherbrooke Street West
Montreal, PQ H4B 1R3
(514) 489-8201
FAX: (514) 489-3477
E-mail: mabinfo@axess.com
URL: http://www.canpub.com/mab
Paul Gareau, Executive Director
Bill Rudkin, Director of Rehabilitation

Type of Agency: Public; non-profit.

Mission: To offer timely quality rehabilitation adjustment and social services to blind and visually impaired persons as well as support services to their families.

Funded by: Government and private donations.

Budget: $6,841,837.

Hours of Operation: 8:30 AM-4:30 PM.

Staff: 136.

History/Date: Est. 1908.

Number of Clients Served: 5,000.

Eligibility: Visually impaired; Canadian landed immigrant or citizen or by special permit.

Area Served: Province of Quebec.

Counseling/Social Work/Self-Help: Counseling available.

Educational: Specialized school and itinerant services.

Reading: Braille, large-print, recordings, high-tech aids; talking book library.

Residential: Seniors residence and school residential services.

Rehabilitation: Comprehensive program.

Recreational: Variety of programs.

Employment: Employment services.

Computer Training: Training for equipment provided.

Low Vision: Low vision clinic (multidisciplinary team, 3 optometrists).

Low Vision Aids: Full range of aids available; mandated centre for government aids program.

Low Vision Follow-up: Therapists and social workers maintain contact.

DOG GUIDE SCHOOLS

Foundation Mira

1820 Rang North West
Sainte-Madeleine, PQ J0H 1S0
(514) 795-3725
FAX: (514) 795-3789
Eric St. Pierre, General Director

Type of Agency: Guide dog school.

Mission: To provide guide dogs for blind persons.

Funded by: Public and corporation donations and fund-raising events.

Hours of Operation: 8:30 AM-5:00 PM.

Staff: 50.

History/Date: Est. 1981.

Number of Clients Served: 500.

Area Served: Canada and France.

Age Requirements: 15 years and younger, depending on child's maturity.

SAS-KATCHEWAN

◆ Educational Services

PROVINCIAL SERVICES

Special Education Unit Saskatchewan Education
2220 College Avenue
Sixth Floor
Regina, SK S4P 3V7
(306) 787-6052
FAX: (306) 787-2223
E-mail: lcarlson@sasked.gov.sk.ca
Larry Carlson, Educational Consultant

Type of Agency: Provincial Department of Education.
Mission: To provide free and appropriate public education to students who are blind or visually impaired.
Funded by: Provincial government.
Hours of Operation: Mon.-Fri. 8:00 AM-5:00 PM.
Staff: 1 consultant. Students are served directly by professional and paraprofessional staff in public schools.
Number of Clients Served: 150.
Area Served: Saskatchewan - entire province.
Age Requirements: 3 to 21 years.

Reading: Special format library.

7 regional offices.

Monitors the provision of educational services to children and youths with disabilities.

◆ Information Services

LIBRARIES

Saskatchewan Provincial Library
1352 Winnipeg Street
Regina, SK S4P 3V7
(306) 787-2972
FAX: Administration (306) 787-2029 or interlibrary loans (306) 787-8866
E-mail: srp.ill@provlib.lib.sk.ca
Maureen Woods, Provincial Librarian

Type of Agency: Provincial government.
Mission: Provides centralized library programs and services and specialized library resources for municipal and regional library systems throughout the province.
Funded by: Provincial government.
Budget: $2.1 million.
Hours of Operation: Mon.-Fri. 8:00 AM-5:00 PM.
Staff: 37 full time.
History/Date: Est. 1953.
Eligibility: Do not serve public directly.

Professional Training: Provides workshops and seminars for library staff on issues pertaining to access to library services for people with disabilities.

Library services directly provided to the public at over 300 locations across the province. For names, addresses, and other information, contact the Provincial Library.

INFORMATION AND REFERRAL

Visually Impaired Persons' Action Council (VIPAC)
508 Main Street East
Suite 204
Saskatoon, SK S7N 0C1
(306) 242-1105
Brenda Cooke, Co-Director

Type of Agency: Non-profit membership organization for the blind and visually impaired persons.
Mission: To promote the full participation and integration of blind and visually impaired persons in society and to provide support, information, and advocacy efforts.

◆ Rehabilitation Services

PROVINCIAL SERVICES

Community Living Department of Social Services
1920 Broad Street, 11th floor
Regina, SK S4P 3V6
(306) 787-3844
Larry Moffat, Executive Director, Community Living Division
Donna Allen, Special Assistant, Deputy Minister's Office,
(306) 787-0916

Area Served: Western Canada.

Administers grants and contributions program to help fund services and integration efforts for blind and visually impaired and other disabled adults.

REHABILITATION

Canadian National Institute for the Blind
Saskatchewan Division
2550 Broad Street
Regina, SK S4P 3Z4
(306) 525-2571
FAX: (306) 565-3300
Dennis Tottenham, Executive Director

District Offices:

Saskatoon: 1705 McKercher Drive, Saskatoon, SK S7H 5N6, (306) 374-4545, FAX (306) 955-6224.

See Canadian National Institute for the Blind, National Office, in Canadian national listings.

YUKON TERRITORY

♦ Educational Services

PROVINCIAL SERVICES

Government of the Yukon
Special Programs
Department of Education
P.O. Box 2703
Whitehorse, YT Y1A 2C6
(403) 667-8000
FAX: (403) 363-6339

County/District Where Located:
Yukon Territory.

Monitors the provision of educational services to children and youths with disabilities.

♦ Information Services

LIBRARIES

Government of the Yukon
Libraries and Archives Branch
Department of Education
P.O. Box 2703
Whitehorse, YT Y1A 2C6
(403) 602-5309
FAX: (403) 667-4253
Linda Johnson, Director

Type of Agency: Public library and archives.
Funded by: Government funding.
Hours of Operation: Mon.-Fri. 10:00 AM-9:00 PM; Sat. 10:00 AM-6:00 PM; Sun. 1:00 PM-9:00 PM.
Number of Clients Served: 28,000.
Area Served: Yukon Territory.

♦ Rehabilitation Services

PROVINCIAL SERVICES

Department of Health and Social Services
Government of the Yukon
2071 Second Avenue
Yukon Government
Administration Building
P.O. Box 2703
Whitehorse, YT Y1A 2C6
(403) 667-3632 or (403) 667-5045
Anne Sheffield, Director of Family and Children's Services

Administers grants and contributions program to help fund services and integration efforts for blind and visually impaired and other disabled persons.

REHABILITATION

Canadian National Institute for the Blind
British Columbia-Yukon Division
100-5055 Joyce Street
Vancouver, BC V5R 6B2
(604) 431-2121
FAX: (604) 431-2099
Mary Ann Roscoe, Executive Director

See Canadian National Institute for the Blind, British Columbia-Yukon Division, in British Columbia provincial listings.

UNITED STATES
<u>FEDERAL AGENCIES</u>
NATIONAL <u>ORGANIZATIONS</u>
NATIONAL CONSUMER AND PROFESSIONAL MEMBERSHIP <u>ORGANIZATIONS</u>

FEDERAL AGENCIES

♦ *Americans with Disabilities Act Agencies*

Architectural and Transportation Barriers Compliance Board

1331 F Street, N.W.
Washington, DC 20004
ADA Information Line (800) 872-2253 (800) USA-ABLE

See Architectural and Transportation Barriers Compliance Board under Other Agencies listings.

Equal Employment Opportunity Commission

1801 L Street, N.W.
Washington, DC 20507
(202) 663-4900 or TDD (202) 663-4494 or (800) 669-4000
Discrimination Claims

See Equal Employment Opportunity Commission under Other Agencies listings.

Federal Transit Administration

Office of the Chief Counsel
400 Seventh Street, S.W.
Washington, DC 20590
(202) 366-4063 or TDD (202) 366-2979

See Federal Transit Administration under U.S. Department of Transportation.

National Institute on Disability and Rehabilitation Research

330 C Street, S. W.
Washington, DC 20202
(202) 205-8134

The National Institute on Disability and Rehabilitation Research funds grants to maintain Disability and Business Technical Assistance Centers, whose purpose is to ensure that information and expertise are available on how to make reasonable accommodation for disabled employees in the work setting.

See National Institute on Disability and Rehabilitation Research under U.S. Department of Education.

♦ *U.S. Department of Education*

U.S. Department of Education Office of the Secretary

600 Independence Avenue, S.W.
Washington, DC 20202
(202) 401-3000
Richard W. Riley, Secretary

The U.S. Department of Education maintains regional offices throughout the country. The following is a list of these offices and the states covered within each federal region:

Region I: Post Office Square, 540 McCormack Courthouse, Boston, MA 02109-4557, (617) 223-9317.

Connecticut, Maine, Massachusetts, New Hampshire, Rhode Island, and Vermont.

Region II: 75 Park Place, 12th Floor, New York, NY 10007, (212) 264-7005.

New Jersey, New York, Puerto Rico, and Virgin Islands.

Region III: 3535 Market Street, Room 16350, Philadelphia, PA 19104, (215) 596-1001.

Delaware, District of Columbia, Maryland, Pennsylvania, Virginia, and West Virginia.

Region IV: 61 Forsyth Street, SW, Atlanta, GA 30303, (404) 562-6006.

Alabama, Florida, Georgia, Kentucky, Mississippi, North Carolina, South Carolina, and Tennessee.

Region V: 401 South State Street, Chicago, IL 60605-1225, (312) 886-8215.

Illinois, Indiana, Michigan, Minnesota, Ohio, and Wisconsin.

Region VI: 1200 Main Tower Building, Dallas, TX 75202, (214) 767-3626.

Arkansas, Louisiana, New Mexico, Oklahoma, and Texas.

Region VII: 10220 North Executive Hills Boulevard, Kansas City, MO 64153-1367, (816) 880-4000.

Iowa, Kansas, Missouri, and Nebraska.

Region VIII: 1244 Speer Boulevard, Denver, CO 80204-3582, (303) 844-3544.

Colorado, Montana, North Dakota, South Dakota, Utah, and Wyoming.

Region IX: 50 United Nations Plaza, San Francisco, CA 94102-4987, (415) 437-7520.

Arizona, California, Hawaii, Nevada, American Samoa, Guam, and Trust Territories of the Pacific Islands.

Region X: 915 Second Avenue, Seattle, WA 98174-1099, (206) 220-7800.

Alaska, Idaho, Oregon, and Washington.

Assistant Secretary for Special Education and Rehabilitative Services

330 C Street, S.W., Room 3006
Washington, DC 20202
(202) 205-5465
Judith E. Heumann, Assistant Secretary

Mission: Has administrative supervision of Office of Special Education Programs, Rehabilitation Services Administration, and National Institute on Disability and Rehabilitation Research.

Division of Blind and Visually Impaired

330 C Street, S.W.
Room 3227
Washington, DC 20202
(202) 205-9316

Mission: Develops methods, standards, and procedures to assist state agencies in the rehabilitation of blind persons. Administers the Randolph-Sheppard Act, which assures priority for blind persons in the operation of vending facilities on federal property.

Assists the states in developing programs that provide vocational rehabilitation services to blind persons to enable them to become self-supporting and gainfully employed; assists the states in analyzing occupations to ascertain their suitability for performance without the use of sight, and demonstrates to employers the suitability for employment of blind persons who are properly selected and adequately prepared for work; promotes and supports institutes

and training programs; conducts studies and prepares descriptions of occupations in which blind persons are or may be successfully engaged; prepares technical guides and other materials for use of staff members of state agencies; develops, in cooperation with state agencies, new training facilities for blind persons, and assists in the expansion of existing facilities; maintains continuous relationships with other public and private agencies for the blind; administers the grant for the Helen Keller National Center established to provide a national center and network for the rehabilitation of deaf-blind youth and adults; cooperates in the development of the Independent Living Services program for older blind individuals.

National Council on Disability

1331 F Street, N.W.
Washington, DC 20004
(202) 272-2004
Marla Bristo, Chairperson

Mission: Develops policy for the National Institute on Disability and Rehabilitation Research; advises the Commissioner of the Rehabilitation Services Administration on policy.

National Institute on Disability and Rehabilitation Research

330 C Street, S. W.
Washington, DC 20202
(202) 205-8134
Katherine D. Seelman, Director

Mission: Administers grants and contracts for research and demonstration projects related to disabled persons; also administers research and training centers.

Office of Special Education Programs

330 C Street, S.W., Room 3086
Washington, DC 20202
(202) 205-5507
Thomas Hehir, Director

Mission: Administers the Individuals with Disabilities Education Act and related programs for the education of disabled children, including grants to institutions of higher learning and fellowships to train educational personnel; grants to states for the education of disabled children; research and demonstration projects; and special programs, such as centers and services for children who are deaf-blind.

Rehabilitation Services Administration (RSA)

330 C Street, S.W.
Washington, DC 20202
(202) 205-5482
Frederick K. Schroeder, Commissioner

Mission: Provides national leadership and technical guidance for the federal-state vocational rehabilitation program. Administers grants to the states for vocational rehabilitation of the disabled. Provides demonstrations, professional training, and independent living grants for disabled persons, including visually impaired persons.

◆ U.S. Department of Health and Human Services

U.S. Department of Health and Human Services
Office of the Secretary
200 Independence Avenue, S.W.
Room 615F
Washington, DC 20201
(202) 690-7000
Donna E. Shalala, Secretary

The U.S. Department of Health and Human Services maintains regional offices throughout the country. The following is a list of these offices:

Region I - Boston: J.F. Kennedy Federal Office Building, Room 2100 Government Center, Boston, MA 02203, (617) 565-1500.

Region II - New York: Jacob K. Javits Federal Building, 26 Federal Plaza, New York, NY 10278, (212) 264-2662.

Region III - Philadelphia: Gateway Building, 3535 Market Street, P.O. Box 13716, Philadelphia, PA 19104, (215) 596-6492.

Region IV - Atlanta: 101 Marietta Tower, Atlanta, GA 30323, (404) 331-2442.

Region V - Chicago: 105 West Adams Street, Chicago, IL 60603, (312) 353-5160.

Region VI - Dallas: 1200 Main Tower Building, Dallas, TX 75202, (214) 767-3301.

Region VII - Kansas City: 601 East 12th Street, Federal Building, Kansas City, MO 64106, (816) 426-2821.

Region VIII - Denver: 1961 Stout Street, Denver, CO 80294, (303) 844-3372.

Region IX - San Francisco: Federal Office Building, Room 431, 50 United Nations Plaza, San Francisco, CA 94102, (415) 437-8500.

Region X - Seattle: 2201 Sixth Avenue, Seattle, WA 98121, (206) 615-2010.

Administration for Children and Families
901 D Street, S.W.
Washington, DC 20447
(202) 401-9200
JoAnn B. Barnhurt, Assistant Secretary

Mission: Has administrative supervision of the President's Committee on Mental Retardation; the Administration on Aging; Administration on Developmental Disabilities; Administration for Children, Youth and Families; Administration for Native Americans; and the program under Title XX (social services) of the Social Security Act.

Administration for Children, Youth, and Families
2026 MES
330 C Street, S.W.
Washington, DC 20201
(202) 205-8347
Wade F. Horn, Commissioner

Mission: Advises the Secretary of Health and Human Services on department plans and programs related to early childhood development; operates the Head Start day care and other related child service programs; provides leadership, advice, and services that affect the general well-being of children and youths.

Administration on Aging
200 Independence Avenue, S.W.
Washington, DC 20201
(202) 401-4634
Robyn Stone, Acting Assistant Secretary

Mission: Administers the Older Americans Act of 1965 to assist states and local communities to develop programs for older persons.

Health Care Financing Administration
200 Independence Avenue, S.W.
Washington, DC 20201
(202) 690-6726
Bruce Vladek, Acting Administrator

Mission: Administers the Medicare program under Title XVIII of the Social Security Act. Administers grants to the states for Medicaid under Title XIX of the Social Security Act for individuals who are medically indigent.

Health Resources and Services Administration
Bureau of Health Professions
5600 Fishers Lane
Rockville, MD 20857
(301) 443-5794
Fitzhugh S.M. Mullen, Director

Mission: Through appropriated funds, supports education programs, credentialing, analysis, and development of human resources needed to staff the U.S. health care system.

Health Services Administration
Bureau for Maternal and Child Health
Health Care Resources Department
5600 Fishers Lane
Room 14-95 Parklawn
Rockville, MD 20857
(301) 443-2170
Audrey H. Nora, Director

Mission: Administers block grants to the states for maternal and child health, and crippled children's services under Title V of the Social Security Act.

National Center for Health Statistics
6525 Belcrest Road
Hyattsville, MD 20782
(301) 436-7016
Edward J. Sondik, Director

Mission: Collects, compiles, and disseminates data related to health and vital statistics, including information on prevalence of vision defects, based on household interview surveys.

National Institutes of Health National Eye Institute Information Center
9000 Rockville Pike
Building 31, Room 6A03
Bethesda, MD 20892
(301) 496-2234
Carl Kupfer, M.D., Director,
(301) 496-2234

Mission: Finances and conducts research on the eye and vision disorders; supports training of eye researchers; and publishes materials on visual impairment.

National Institutes of Health National Institute on Aging
9000 Rockville Pike
Building 31, Room 5C35
Bethesda, MD 20892
(301) 496-0216
Richard Hodes, Director

Mission: Finances intramural and extramural research on aging; supports training of researchers in aging.

Social Security Administration
6401 Security Boulevard
Baltimore, MD 21235
(410) 965-3120
Shirley S. Chater, Commissioner

Mission: Administers old age, survivors, and disability insurance programs under Title II of the Social Security Act. Also administers the federal income maintenance program (Supplemental Security Income for the aged, blind, and disabled) under Title XVI of the Social Security Act. Maintains network of local/regional offices nationwide.

◆ U.S. Department of Labor

U.S. Department of Labor Office of the Secretary
200 Constitution Avenue, N.W.
Washington, DC 20210
(202) 219-8271
Alexis S. Herman, Secretary

Employment Standards Administration National Office Program Administration
200 Constitution Avenue, N.W.
Washington, DC 20210
(202) 219-4907
Daniel Sweeney, Team Leader

Mission: Monitors compliance with sub-minimum wage requirements for disabled workers in sheltered workshops, competitive industry, and hospitals and institutions under Section 14(e) of the Fair Labor Standards Act of 1938.

Office of Federal Contract Compliance Programs
200 Constitution Avenue, N.W.
Washington, DC 20210
(202) 219-9475
Shirley Wilcher, Deputy Assistant Secretary

Mission: Monitors compliance with Section 503 of the Rehabilitation Act of 1973 providing for affirmative action in the employment of qualified disabled workers by contractors with the federal government, as well as similar provisions of law regarding disabled veterans (38 U.S.C. 2012); also investigates complaints.

U.S. Employment Service
Patrick Henry Building
601 D Street, N. W.
Washington, DC 20213
(202) 219-6643
John R. Beverly, Director

Mission: Administers the federal-state employment service program. Has selective placement personnel in state employment service offices to serve disabled individuals.

◆ U.S. Department of Transportation

U.S. Department of Transportation Office of the Secretary
400 Seventh Street, S.W. #10424
Washington, DC 20590
(202) 366-1111
Rodney E. Slater, Secretary

Federal Transit Administration
400 Seventh Street, S.W.
Washington, DC 20590
(202) 366-4040
Gordon J. Linton, Administrator

Mission: Administers federally assisted mass transit programs.

The Federal Transit Administration maintains regional offices throughout the country. The following is a list of these offices:

Region I: 55 Broadway, Kendall Square, Cambridge, MA 02142, (617) 494-2055.

Region II: 26 Federal Plaza, New York, NY 10278, (212) 264-8162.

Region III: 1760 Market Street, Philadelphia, PA 19103, (215) 656-6900.

Region IV: 100 Alabama Street, S.W., Atlanta, GA 30303, (404) 562-3500.

Region V: 55 E Monroe Street, Chicago, IL 60603, (312) 353-2789.

Region VI: 524 East Lamar Boulevard, Arlington, TX 76011, (817) 860-9663.

Region VII: 6301 Rockhill Road, Kansas City, MO 64131, (816) 523-0204.

Region VIII: Columbine Place, Suite 650, 216 16th Street, Denver, CO 80202, (303) 844-3242.

Region IX: 201 Mission Street, San Francisco, CA 94105, (415) 744-3133.

Region X: 915 Second Avenue, Jackson Federal Building, Seattle, WA 98174, (206) 220-7954.

♦ U.S. Department of Veterans Affairs

U.S. Department of Veterans Affairs
Office of the Secretary
810 Vermont Avenue, N.W.
Washington, DC 20420
(202) 223-3775
Jesse Brown, Secretary

Blind Rehabilitation Service
810 Vermont Avenue, N.W.
Room 1071
Washington, DC 20420
(202) 535-7637
Don E. Garner, Director

Mission: Oversees programs for blinded veterans within the Veterans Health Administration. Services offered include Visual Impairment Services Teams (VIST) assistance and Blind Rehabilitation Center and Clinic Programs. Visual Impairment Services Teams are diagnostic and treatment agents who provide periodic evaluations of physical, visual, hearing, and adjustment status and ongoing individualized treatment according to needs, goals, and eligibility. Their resources include health services, financial benefits, adaptive equipment, referral for comprehensive blind rehabilitation, low vision services, vocational training, and support and adjustment counseling. Blind Rehabilitation Center and Clinic Programs offer comprehensive rehabilitation services that encompass orientation/mobility skills; visual skills including ophthalmology, and optometry; manual skills; communication and personal management skills; physical education and recreation; avocational skills and leisure time activities; psychological counseling and social work; general medical care; audiology; education in personal health care and dietary management; family programs; community resources; and review of benefits.

Blind Rehabilitation Centers offer instruction in the use of specialized electronic travel aids and reading machines, computer access training as well as the latest technological devices. Clinic programs are designed for blinded veterans who have special problems and/or needs in addition to blindness. Blind Rehabilitation Centers and Clinics are authorized to provide prosthetic and sensory aids to blinded veterans to assist them in overcoming blindness.

There is at least one VIST designated for each state. Blind Rehabilitation Centers are located at VA Medical Centers in: Birmingham, Alabama; Palo Alto, California; West Haven, Connecticut; Hines, Illinois; and San Juan, Puerto Rico. A center is being planned in Tucson, Arizona. Blind Rehabilitation Clinics are located at West Haven, Connecticut; Waco, Texas; and Tacoma, Washington.

See individual state listings for facilities' addresses and phone numbers.

Veterans Benefits Administration (VBA)
810 Vermont Avenue, N.W.
Room 520
Washington, DC 20420
(202) 273-6763

Mission: Furnishes compensation and pensions for disability and death to veterans and their dependents. Provides vocational rehabilitation services, including counseling, training, and assistance toward employment, to blinded veterans disabled as a result of service in the armed forces during World War II, the Korean conflict, and the Vietnam era; also provides rehabilitation services to certain peace-time veterans. Offers and guarantees loans for the purchase or construction of homes, farms, and businesses.

Veterans Health Administration (VHA)
810 Vermont Avenue, N.W.

Washington, DC 20420
(202) 273-5781
Kenneth W. Kizer, Under Secretary

Mission: Provides hospital and outpatient treatment as well as nursing home care for eligible veterans in Veterans Administration facilities. Services elsewhere provided on a contract basis in the United States and its territories. Provides non-vocational inpatient residential rehabilitation services to eligible legally blinded veterans of the armed forces of the United States.

◆ Other Agencies

Architectural and Transportation Barriers Compliance Board

1331 F Street, N.W.
Washington, DC 20004
(202) 272-5434
Lawrence W. Roffee, Executive Director

Mission: Administers Section 502 of the Rehabilitation Act of 1973 and enforces the Architectural Barriers Act of 1968, which prohibits architectural and transportation barriers to disabled persons in federally funded buildings.

Committee for Purchase from the Blind and Other Severely Handicapped

Crystal Square 5, Suite 1107
1755 Jefferson Davis Highway
Arlington, VA 22202-3509
(703) 557-1145
Beverly L. Milkman, Executive Director

Mission: Administers the Javits-Wagner-O'Day Act (P.L. 92-28), under which the federal government purchases products and services from non-profit workshops for the blind and other

handicapped outside the competitive bidding system.

Equal Employment Opportunity Commission

1801 L Street, N.W.
Washington, DC 20507
(202) 663-4001
Gilbert Casellas, Chairman

Mission: Enforces section 501 of the Rehabilitation Act of 1973, which prohibits discrimination on the basis of disability in federal employment, and the employment provisions of the American with Disabilities Act.

Library of Congress National Library Service for the Blind and Physically Handicapped

1291 Taylor Street, N.W.
Washington, DC 20542
(202) 707-5100 or (800) 424-8567
Frank Kurt Cylke, Director

Mission: Conducts national program to distribute free reading materials of a general nature— classics, current fiction, and nonfiction—to the nation's blind and physically disabled citizens who cannot utilize ordinary printed materials because of physical impairments. Provides reference information service on all aspects of blindness and other physical disabilities that affect reading. Conducts national correspondence courses to train sighted persons as braille transcribers and blind persons as braille proofreaders. With volunteer help, transcribes books into hand-copied braille, records books on magnetic tape, and repairs machines. Conducts a continuous program of testing, development, and evaluation of reading materials and related equipment.
Eligibility: Must be determined by competent authority.

Reading: Reading materials provided consist of talking books recorded on cassette tape or 33, 16, and 8 RPM disks, books in braille, and recorded and braille music. Reading materials also include approximately 70 magazines on flexible disks or in braille. Provides talking book machines and cassette machines for disk records and cassette tapes. Selects, orders, and distributes materials through a network of 160 libraries nationwide that function as circulating centers, using the mails to serve readers. Materials mailed postage free.

See individual state listings for regional libraries and distributors of talking book machines.

President's Committee on Employment of People with Disabilities

1331 F. Street, N.W.
Washington, DC 20004-1107
(202) 376-6200 or TDD (202) 376-6205
FAX: (202) 376-6200
Tony Coelho, Chairman
John Lancaster, Executive Director

Mission: Promotes the development of maximum employment opportunities for disabled persons. Consists of volunteer members throughout the country under a volunteer chairman and a paid secretariat.

Small Business Administration

409 Third Street, N.W.
Washington, DC 20416
(202) 205-6605
Aida Alvarez, Administrator

Mission: Administers the Small Business Act, including small business loans to disabled individuals; maintains local offices throughout the country.

U.S. Department of Justice
Civil Rights Division
Coordination and Review
Section
10th Street and Constitution
Avenue, N.W.
Washington, DC 20530
(202) 514-2151

Mission: Coordinates the
implementation by federal
agencies of Section 504 of the
Rehabilitation Act of 1973, as
amended, which prohibits
discrimination on the basis of
disability in federally assisted
programs and in programs and
activities conducted by federal
executive agencies. Also enforces
pattern or practice cases or cases of
general importance for Title III of
the Americans With Disabilities
Act on public accommodations
operated by private entities.

U.S. Office of Personnel
Management
Office of Human Resources and
Equal Employment
1900 E Street, N.W., Room 5431
Washington, DC 20415
(202) 606-2440
Alicia McPhie, Equal Opportunity
Division Chief

Mission: Establishes policy for
employment of disabled persons
within the federal service.
Administers a merit system for
federal employment that includes
recruiting, examining, training,
and promoting people on the basis
of knowledge and skills, regardless
of sex, race, religion, or other
factors.

NATIONAL ORGANI-ZATIONS

4-Sights Network
Upshaw Institute for the Blind

16625 Grand River Avenue
Detroit, MI 48227
(313) 272-3900
FAX: (313) 272-6893
E-mail: upshaw@wwnet.com
URL: http://www.wwnet.com/
~upshaw
Mary Beth Kullen, Information
Systems Supervisor

Mission: Acts as a national computer information service designed to collect and disseminate information of interest to people who are blind or visually impaired or who provide services to people with visual impairments.
Hours of Operation: 24 hours a day/7 days a week.
Age Requirements: None.

Information about technology, education, rehabilitation, the Americans with Disabilities Act, low vision, and other topics is available via computer-modem connection. The computer modem phone number is (313) 272-7111.

American Diabetes Association National Center

1660 Duke Street
P.O. Box 25757
Alexandria, VA 22314
(800) 342-2383
FAX: (703) 836-7439
John H. Graham, IV, Chief Executive Officer

Type of Agency: Not-for-profit professional health organization.
County/District Where Located: Fairfax County.

Mission: Promotes knowledge of diabetes through public and professional education. Seeks to prevent and cure diabetes and to improve the lives of all people affected by diabetes. All services provided at the local level by over 800 chapters throughout the United States and 54 affiliates in all 50 states.
Funded by: Voluntary contributions; membership fees.
Budget: $110 million.
Staff: 800.
History/Date: Est. 1940.
Area Served: Affiliates in all states; over 800 chapters.

Publications: *Diabetes Forecast; Diabetes; Clinical Diabetes; Diabetes Spectrum; Diabetes Care;* and *Diabetes Reviews.*

American Foundation for the Blind

11 Penn Plaza
Suite 300
New York, NY 10001
(212) 502-7600 or (800) 232-5463 or TDD (212) 502-7662
FAX: (212) 502-7777
E-mail: afbinfo@afb.org
URL: http://www.afb.org
Carl R. Augusto, President

Type of Agency: Non-profit.
Mission: To enable people who are blind or visually impaired to achieve equality of access and opportunity that will ensure freedom of choice in their lives. AFB accomplishes this mission through agency-wide program initiatives and through the delivery of a wide variety of services and publications. Current program initiatives include efforts on behalf of literacy for children and adults who are blind or visually impaired; implementation of the Americans with Disabilities Act; access to information; education of children who are blind or visually impaired and may have additional disabilities; specialized and general services; and employment and aging. Services and publications include governmental relations efforts; books, periodicals, other materials and videos for professional and consumer education; manufacture of talking books; technology evaluations; information and referral; a World Wide Web site and toll-free telephone information line; professional and consumer mentor networks; public education; social research; a professional library and archives; and consultation and training activities within and outside the blindness services field. AFB provides these services through headquarters in New York City; other offices in Atlanta, Chicago, Dallas, and San Francisco; and a governmental relations office in Washington, DC.
Funded by: Voluntary contributions and endowment.
History/Date: Est. and Inc. 1921.

Professional Training: Conducts the Josephine L. Taylor Leadership Institute annually and produces a wide variety of professional training materials through AFB Press.

Publications: *Journal of Visual Impairment & Blindness; AFB News;* regional newsletters, publications and other catalogs; *Current Projects & Activities;* and the *Directory of Services for Blind and Visually Impaired Persons in the United States and Canada.*

See individual state listings for other offices. The AFB Governmental Relations Group may be contacted at 820 First Street, NE, Suite 400, Washington, DC 20002, (202) 408-0200.

American Society for Contemporary Ophthalmology

4711 Golf Road
Suite 408
Skokie, IL 60076
(847) 568-1500
FAX: (847) 568-1527
Randall Bellows, M.D., Ph.D.,
Director

Mission: Promotes continuing education for ophthalmologists. Maintains computerized service, EYENET, for on-line communication of eye problems and access to selected journal articles.

Publications: *Annals of Ophthalmology; Glaucoma; Journal of Ocular Therapy and Surgery.*

AWARE (Associates for World Action in Rehabilitation and Education)

P.O. Box 96
Mohegan Lake, NY 10547
(914) 528-0567
FAX: (914) 528-0567
E-mail: aware usa@aol.com
Anne Yeadon, President

Type of Agency: Non-profit.
Mission: Collaborates with other human service agencies to develop and coordinate cost-effective outreach strategies to identify and serve hard-to-reach individuals with severe visual impairments in the United States and in the developing world. In partnership with local organizations, develops consumer and trainer materials for serving underserved populations. Conducts evaluations and organizational analyses; develops custom rehabilitation service strategies relevant to specific populations and human service organizations.
Funded by: Voluntary contributions, endowments, and special project grants.

Staff: Multidisciplinary national and international team of professionals.
History/Date: Est. 1991.
Area Served: United States and overseas.

Professional Training: Conducts workshops and long-term programs for human service professionals, paraprofessionals, and volunteers.
Publications: *New Independence! for Older Persons with Vision Loss in Long-Term Care Facilities* (a 3-volume in-service training kit). Booklets for consumers, family, and friends.

Better Vision Institute Vision Council of America

1800 North Kent Street
Suite 904
Rosslyn, VA 22209
(703) 243-1508
FAX: (703) 243-1537
Susan Burton, Executive Director

Type of Agency: Non-profit.
County/District Where Located: Arlington County.
Mission: Makes public aware of need for eye care. Publishes informational material and maintains library.
Funded by: International Vision Expo.
Budget: $2 million.
Hours of Operation: 9:00 AM-5:00 PM Eastern Standard Time.
Staff: 8.
Area Served: United States; international.

Publications: *BVI News.*

Blind Children's Fund

2875 Northwind Drive
Suite 211

East Lansing, MI 48823
(517) 333-1725
FAX: (517) 333-1730
Sherry Raynor, President

County/District Where Located: Ingham County.
Mission: Promotes the education and welfare of preschool blind and visually impaired infants and children by developing programs and disseminating information.

Publications: *VIP Newsletter.*

Blind Outdoor Leisure Development

533 East Main Street
Aspen, CO 81611
(970) 925-9511
Bill Dunaway, President
Francesca Campione, Program Director

Type of Agency: Private non-profit.
Mission: Provides guides for blind vistors engaging in outdoor sports. Trains guides, provides insurance for participants, and encourages reduced rates for local sports activities.
Funded by: Donations.
History/Date: Founded in 1968.
Number of Clients Served: 90 to 150 annually.
Eligibility: Participants must be legally blind.
Area Served: Aspen.
Transportation: Y.

Braille Authority of North America (BANA)

c/o Associated Service for the Blind
919 Walnut Street
Philadelphia, PA 19107
(215) 627-0600
FAX: (215) 922-0692
Dolores Ferrara-Godzieba, Chairperson

Type of Agency: U.S.-Canadian standard-setting organization whose member agencies strive to promulgate codes regarding the usage of braille and to encourage its use.
Mission: Promotes and facilitates the use, teaching, and production of braille.

Publications: *Annual Directory*.

DB-LINK: The National Information Clearinghouse on Children Who Are Deaf-Blind

c/o Teaching Research
Western Oregon State College
345 North Monmouth Avenue
Monmouth, OR 97361
(800) 854-7013 or TDD (800) 438-9376
FAX: (503) 838-8150
E-mail: dblink@tr.wosc.osshe.edu
URL: http://www.tr.wosc.osshe.edu/dblink/
John Rieman, Director

Type of Agency: A collaborative effort of the Helen Keller National Center for Deaf-Blind Youths and Adults, Perkins School for the Blind, and Teaching Research.
Mission: To identify, coordinate and disseminate information related to children and youth who are deaf-blind.
Funded by: Office of Special Education Programs.
Hours of Operation: 9:00 A.M.-5:00 P.M.

Delta Gamma Foundation

3250 Riverside Drive
P.O. Box 21397
Columbus, OH 43221-0397
(614) 481-8169
FAX: (614) 481-0133
Margaret Hess Watkins, Executive Director and Director of Development

Type of Agency: Non-profit.
Mission: Provides a means for its members to act in concert to further exclusively charitable, scientific, literary, and educational objectives. Conducts Delta Gamma Project on Sight Conservation and Aid to the Blind. Promotes local community service by members. Local services carried out through direct sponsorship or cooperation with agencies for blind and visually impaired persons.
Funded by: Voluntary donations from individuals and organized collegiate and alumnae groups of Delta Gamma.
Hours of Operation: Mon.-Fri. 8:30 AM-5:00 PM.
History/Date: Est. 1951.

Publications: *Anchora of Delta Gamma; Shield*.

Eye Bank Association of America

1001 Connecticut Avenue N.W.
Suite 601
Washington, DC 20036-5504
(202) 775-4999
FAX: (202) 429-6036
Patricia Aiken-O'Neill, President and Chief Executive Officer

County/District Where Located: District of Columbia.
Mission: Establishes medical standards for evaluating and distributing corneal transplants. Certifies eye banks and technicians entrusted with caring for donated tissue. Awards annual research grants to promote and encourage transplantation.

Publications: *Insight*.

Eye Bank for Sight Restoration

210 East 64th Street

New York, NY 10021
(212) 980-6700
FAX: (212) 319-6211
Mary Jane O'Neill, Executive Director

Mission: Collects and distributes healthy donated corneas for transplant, research and medical education. Maintains public education, professional education, research programs.
Funded by: Processing fees and general public contributions.
Budget: $2 million.
Hours of Operation: Office: Mon.-Fri. 9:00 AM-5:00 PM. Laboratory coverage: 24 hours.
Staff: 20 full and part-time.
History/Date: Est. 1944.
Number of Clients Served: 1,300 annually.
Eligibility: Referral by surgeon.
Area Served: New York City and six adjacent counties.

Educational: Videos and speakers bureau.
Professional Training: In-service training provided to hospital staffs.
Publications: *Eye-to-Eye Newsletter*.

Fight for Sight

160 East 56th Street
Eighth Floor
New York, NY 10022
(212) 751-1118
FAX: (212) 688-9641
Mildred Weisenfeld, Executive Director

Mission: Funds eye research awards to accredited institutions, fellowships to students of medicine or of the basic sciences, postdoctoral research fellowships and grants-in-aid to qualified investigators.
Funded by: Contributions, special events, and Fight for Sight Leagues.

Budget: $850,000.
Hours of Operation: 9:30 AM - 6:30 PM.
Staff: 5 full time; 2 part time.
History/Date: Est. and Inc. 1946; under National Council to Combat Blindness, Fight for Sight Inc. 1959.
Area Served: United States primarily, but accepts applications for research supported from accredited medical colleges, hospitals, and eye centers throughout the world.

The Foundation Fighting Blindness (National Retinitis Pigmentosa Foundation Inc.)
Executive Plaza 1
Suite 800
11350 McCormick Road
Hunt Valley, MD 21031-1014
(410) 785-1414 or TDD (410) 785-9687 or (888) 394-3937 or TDD (800) 683-5551
FAX: (410) 771-7470
URL: http://www.blindness.org
Jessica Beach, Outreach Program Coordinator
Stephanie Horney, Information and Referral Coordinator

Type of Agency: Non-profit research organization.
Mission: To find treatments and cures for blinding retinal degenerative diseases such as retinitis pigmentosa, macular degeneration and Usher syndrome, and to serve as an information source for affected individuals, their families, and eye care professionals.
Funded by: Contributions.
Budget: $9.5 million.
Hours of Operation: Mon.-Fri. 8:30 AM-5:00 PM.
Program Accessibility: All materials are in an accessible format.
History/Date: Est. and Inc. 1971.
Area Served: United States.

Publications: *Fighting Blindness News, Macular Update.*

See state listings for local affiliates.

The Glaucoma Foundation
33 Maiden Lane 7th Floor
New York, NY 10038
(212) 504-1901 or (800) 452-8266
FAX: (212) 504-1933
E-mail: glaucomafdn@mindspring.com
URL: http://www.glaucoma-foundation.org/info
John W. Corwin, Executive Director

Type of Agency: Private; non-profit.
Mission: Provides free literature and referrals to the public, available through toll-free worldwide hotline: 1-800-GLAUCOMA. Promotes and funds research into the causes of glaucoma and potential cures for the disease, and funds public education projects to provide information about glaucoma and the importance of early detection and treatment. The Foundation also hosts an annual Scientific Think Tank which brings together leading scientists to pool their insights regarding the protection and regeneration of the optic nerve.
Funded by: Donations.
Budget: $1.1 million.
Hours of Operation: 9:00 AM-5:00 PM.
Staff: 6.
History/Date: Est. 1985.
Number of Clients Served: Approximately 4,000 calls annually on hot line.
Area Served: United States.
Age Requirements: None.

Counseling/Social Work/Self-Help: Information and referral.

Educational: Public service announcements, brochures, information about glaucoma.

Glaucoma Research Foundation
490 Post Street
Suite 830
San Francisco, CA 94102
(415) 986-3162 or (800) 826-6693
FAX: (415) 986-3763
E-mail: info@glaucoma.org
URL: http://www.glaucoma.org
Tara L. Steele, Executive Director
Brad Curnow, Information Coordinator

Type of Agency: Non-profit.
Mission: To protect the sight of individuals with glaucoma through research and education.
Funded by: Private donations, grants.
Budget: $3,000,000.
Staff: 13.
History/Date: Est. 1978.
Area Served: United States.

Counseling/Social Work/Self-Help: Nationwide telephone glaucoma peer support network.
Publications: *Gleams Newsletter*; patient guide *Understanding & Living with Glaucoma*; fact sheets on variety of glaucoma-related issues.

See state listings for local affiliates.

Governmental Relations Group American Foundation for the Blind
820 First Street, N.E.
Suite 400
Washington, DC 20002
(202) 480-0200
FAX: (202) 289-7880
E-mail: afbgov@afb.org
URL: http://www.afb.org

See American Foundation for the Blind in U.S. national listings.

Hadley School for the Blind
700 Elm Street

Winnetka, IL 60093
(847) 446-8111 or (800) 323-4238
FAX: (847) 446-9916
Dr. Robert J. Winn, President

Type of Agency: International distance education school.
Mission: To enable blind persons at every stage of life to acquire specialized skills in order to participate successfully in the mainstream of society through home study.
Funded by: Contributions, endowment, and nonfederal grants.
Hours of Operation: Switchboard open Mon.-Fri. 8:00 AM-4:30 PM.
History/Date: Est. 1920; inc. 1922.
Number of Clients Served: Over 11,000 annually.

Educational: Provides academic, personal enrichment, and compensatory/rehabilitation education and technical education through free home study courses, including braille reading and writing. Also offers courses for parents of blind children and family members of blind adults. Accredited by Accrediting Commission of the Distance Education and Training Council and North Central Association of Colleges and Schools.

Helen Keller International

90 Washington Street, 15th Floor
New York, NY 10006
(212) 807-5800
John M. Palmer III, Executive Director

Type of Agency: Non-profit.
Mission: Promotes programs in the prevention of eye disease and blindness. Assists governments and voluntary agencies in developing countries to establish and integrate services to prevent or cure eye diseases and blindness into their national health and welfare systems and to rehabilitate and educate blind and visually impaired persons. Initiates programs for the integration of blind children and adults into community life. Trains field workers for rural areas.
Funded by: Voluntary contributions; bequests; grants from corporations; foundations; governmental agencies (both national and international).
History/Date: Est. 1915.
Area Served: More than 22 developing countries.

Publications: *Helen Keller International Newsletter.*

Helen Keller National Center for Deaf-Blind Youths and Adults

111 Middle Neck Road
Sands Point, NY 11050
(516) 944-8900 (voice/TDD)
FAX: (516) 944-7302
Joseph J. McNulty, Director, Helen Keller National Center
Fred W. McPhilliamy, President, Helen Keller Services for the Blind

Type of Agency: Non-profit. Operated by Helen Keller Services for the Blind under an agreement with the U.S. Department of Education.
Mission: To facilitate a national, cordinated effort to meet the social, rehabilitative, and independent living needs of America's deaf-blind population through demonstration of appropriate rehabilitative training techniques, methods, and technologies.
Funded by: Federal, state, private.
Budget: $5 million.
Hours of Operation: Mon.-Fri. 8:45-4:30 PM–Training Building; 24 hours a day, 7 days a week–Residence Building.
Staff: Approximately 120 nationwide.
History/Date: Est. 1969.

Number of Clients Served: Approximately 1,700 nationwide annually.
Eligibility: Legal blindness and deafness (a chronic hearing impairment so severe that speech cannot be understood with optimum amplification) which causes extreme difficulty in attaining independence in daily life activities. Must be 18 years of age and older.
Area Served: United States and territories.
Age Requirements: 18 years of age and up.

Counseling/Social Work/Self-Help: Available.
Professional Training: Offers training seminars at headquarters and nationwide through a national training team.
Residential: At headquarters in Sands Point, NY, during training only.
Rehabilitation: Provides diagnostic evaluation, short-term comprehensive vocational rehabilitation, and job preparation and placement for all Americans who are deaf-blind. Local services and training are offered nationwide to these individuals, their parents and professionals in the field through HKNC's 10 regional offices, some 30 affiliated agencies, a National Training Team, Services for Older Adults, and National Technical Assistance Consortium.
Recreational: Available for students.
Employment: Job and residential placement in local community.
Computer Training: Available for students.
Low Vision: Services available for students.
Low Vision Aids: Services available for students.

Publications: *National Center News,* 3 times per year in large print and braille, free to deaf-blind readers and libraries; brochures.

Local Offices:

Atlanta: Helen Keller National Center for Deaf-Blind Youths and Adults, Southeastern Region Office, 1005 Virginia Avenue, Suite 104, Atlanta, GA 30354, (404) 766-9625 (voice) or (TDD) (404) 766-2820.

Boston: Helen Keller National Center for Deaf-Blind Youths and Adults, New England Region Office, 313 Washington Street, Boston, MA 02158, (617) 630-1580 (voice/TDD).

Chicago: Helen Keller National Center for Deaf-Blind Youths and Adults, North Central Region Office, 205 West Wacker Drive, Chicago, IL 60606, (312) 726-2090 (voice/TDD).

Dallas: Helen Keller National Center for Deaf-Blind Youths and Adults, South Central Region Office, 4455 LBJ Freeway, LB#3, Dallas, TX 75244-5998, (214) 490-9677 (voice/TDD).

Lakewood: Helen Keller National Center for Deaf-Blind Youths and Adults, Rocky Mountain Region Office, 1880 South Pierce Street, Lakewood, CO 80232, (303) 934-8637 (voice/TDD).

Mission: Helen Keller National Center for Deaf-Blind Youths and Adults, Great Plains Region Office, 4330 Shawnee Mission Parkway, Mission, KS 66205, (913) 677-4562 (voice/TDD).

Riverdale: Helen Keller National Center for Deaf-Blind Youths and Adults, East Central Region Office, 6801 Kenilworth Avneue, Riverdale, MD 20737, (301) 699-2255 (voice) or (TDD) (301) 699-8490.

Sands Point: Helen Keller National Center for Deaf-Blind Youths and Adults, Mid-Atlantic Region Office, 111 Middle Neck Road, Sands Point, NY 11050, (516) 944-8900 (voice/TDD).

Seattle: Helen Keller National Center for Deaf-Blind Youths and Adults, Northwestern Region Office, 2366 East Lake Avenue East, Suite 209, Seattle, WA 98102-3366, (206) 324-9120 (voice/TDD).

Van Nuys: Helen Keller National Center for Deaf-Blind Youths and Adults, Southwest Region Office, 6851 Lennox Avenue, Van Nuys, CA 91405-4097, (818) 782-9935 or TDD (818) 782-9936.

Hilton/Perkins Program Perkins School for the Blind

175 North Beacon Street
Watertown, MA 02172
(617) 972-7220
FAX: (617) 923-8076
Michael T. Collins, Director

Mission: Improves the quality of life for underserved, multiply disabled blind and deaf-blind children and their families through collaborative efforts with local, regional and national organizations. Determines program needs and provides direct and support services to children, their families, and professionals in the U.S. and developing countries around the world. Encourages persons with visual impairments and their families to participate more actively in program planning and development. Provides leadership and advocacy for programs for multiply disabled blind and deaf-blind children.
Funded by: Conrad N. Hilton Foundation of Reno, Nevada.
Staff: 14.
History/Date: Est. 1989.
Area Served: Worldwide.

Educational: Works with direct-service providing organizations worldwide to establish new or improved services to multiply disabled children and their families.
Preschools: Works with agencies worldwide to create new services for multiply disabled blind or deaf-blind infants and toddlers and their families.
Professional Training: Provides preservice and in-service training for teachers of multiply disabled blind and deaf-blind children and for administrators of school and agency programs. Collaborates with colleges, universities, and agencies worldwide to create new training programs for teachers of children who are multiply disabled, blind or deaf-blind.
Publications: Develops and disseminates training materials and curricula for professionals and families.

International Society on Metabolic Eye Disease

1125 Park Avenue
New York, NY 10128
(212) 427-1246
FAX: (212) 360-7009
Heskel M. Haddad, M.D.,
Executive Director

Type of Agency: Organization of ophthalmologists, pediatricians, endocrinologists, internists, and paramedical personnel.
Mission: Promotes the study of metabolic eye problems and related biochemical and genetic aspects.
History/Date: Est. 1973.
Number of Clients Served: 600.
Eligibility: All ophthalmologists.
Area Served: Unlimited.
Age Requirements: None.

Publications: *Metabolic Pediatric & Systemic Ophthamology.*

IN TOUCH Networks
15 West 65th Street
New York, NY 10023
(212) 769-6270
FAX: (212) 769-6266
E-mail: bemass@aol.com
Bruce Massis, General Manager

Type of Agency: Non-profit.
Mission: Maintains volunteer service that allows blind or physically impaired people to listen to readings of articles from more than 100 newspapers and magazines via closed circuit and cable radio. Broadcasts are nationally accessible via satellite.
Funded by: Contributions from foundations, corporations, individuals.
Budget: $450,000.
Hours of Operation: 24 hours/day.
Program Accessibility: Special receiver of FM cable radio required.
Staff: 9.
History/Date: Est. 1974.
Number of Clients Served: Accessible to 11 million households in the United States and Canada and Virgin Islands.
Eligibility: Inability to read standard print.
Area Served: Mainland United States, Alaska and Hawaii.

Publications: *Annual Program Guide to In Touch Networks* (in large-print or audio cassette).

Joint Commission on Allied Health Personnel in Ophthalmology
2025 Woodlane Drive
St. Paul, MN 55125-2995
(612) 731-2944 or (800) 284-3937
FAX: (612) 731-0410
E-mail: jcahpo@jcahpo.org
URL: http://www.jcahpo.org
M. Edward Wilson Jr. M.D., Chairman

Mission: Serves to enhance the quality and availability of ophthalmic patient care by providing continuing education and certification.
Hours of Operation: Mon. - Fri. 8:00 AM - 5:00 PM.

Publications: *Outlook*; newsletter. Criteria booklets also available, including subspecialty certification in Assisting in Low Vision.

Joslin Diabetes Center
One Joslin Place
Boston, MA 02215
(617) 732-2400
Kenneth Quickel, M.D., President

County/District Where Located: Suffolk County.
Mission: Investigates new clinical treatment methods for diabetes. Supports camps for diabetic children. Conducts professional education courses.

Publications: *Joslin Magazine*.

Knights Templar Eye Foundation
5097 North Elston Avenue
Chicago, IL 60630
(773) 205-3838
Blair Mayford, President

County/District Where Located: Cook County.
Mission: Provides funding for eye treatment, surgery, and hospitilization for needy persons.
Funded by: Support from Knights Templar members.

The Lighthouse Inc.
111 East 59th Street
New York, NY 10022
(212) 821-9200 or (800) 334-5497 or TDD (212) 821-9713
FAX: (212) 821-9705
Barbara Silverstone, DSW, President and CEO

Type of Agency: Private; non-profit.
Mission: To overcome vision impairment for people of all ages through worldwide leadership in rehabilitation services, education, research, and advocacy. Undertakes regional, national, and international programs to enable people who are blind or have partial sight to lead independent lives. Maintains The Lighthouse Center for Education, which is composed of The Lighthouse Continuing Education Program, The Lighthouse National Center for Vision and Child Development, The Lighthouse National Center for Vision and Aging, and The Lighthouse International Center on Low Vision. The Arlene R. Gordon Research Institute conducts vision, research. Also conducts scientific inquiry into the physical, functional, and psychosocial consequences of vision impairment and maintains a toll-free information and resource service.
Funded by: Fees, government and private grants, product sales, investment income, contributions.

Professional Training: Offers continuing education courses and seminars on low vision care and vision rehabilitation course work for rehabilitation professionals, social workers, architects, interior designers, nursing home administrators and staff, career, and employment specialists. Also offers educational programs for consumers.
Publications: *Lighthouse News*; *Aging and Vision News*; *Envision* and *Sharing Solutions* newsletters.

Lions Clubs International
300 22nd Street

Oak Brook, IL 60521
(630) 571-5466
FAX: (630) 571-8890
Mark C. Lukas, Executive
Administrator

Type of Agency: Administrative
headquarters serving over 43,000
Lions Clubs throughout the world.
County/District Where Located:
DuPage County.
Mission: Provides community
service and promotes better
international relations. Has major
service interests relating to
visually impaired persons. In 1990,
announced Sightfirst Program to
eliminate preventable and
reversible blindness worldwide.
Service projects include Lions eye
bank programs in which Lions
enlist eye donor pledges and serve
as a clearinghouse to provide
ophthalmologists with corneal
tissue for transplant and research.
Programs to foster detection,
education, and awareness of
diabetes are also conducted. Clubs
provide glaucoma and other vision
testing screenings; sponsor
rehabilitation programs for newly
blind persons; provide aids and
devices for visually impaired
persons; make computer training
available through individual
Lions-supported and vocational
facilities; and finance subscriptions
to *Juvenile Braille Monthly
Magazine*.
Hours of Operation: Mon.-Fri.
8:00 AM-4:30 PM.

Publications: *Lion Magazine.*

March of Dimes Birth Defects Foundation

1275 Mamaroneck Avenue

White Plains, NY 10605
(914) 428-7100
FAX: (914) 997-4763
E-mail: resourcecenter@modimes.
org
URL: http://www.modimes.org
Dr. Jennifer Howse, President

County/District Where Located:
Westchester County.
Mission: To improve the health of
babies by preventing birth defects
and infant mortalities through
research, community services,
education and advocacy.

Publications: Wide variety of
materials relating to maternal and
infant health. Also publishes
professional educational material
for nurses.
For information on local offices,
call toll-free 888-MODIMES.

Myasthenia Gravis Foundation

222 South Riverside Plaza
Suite 1540
Chicago, IL 60606
(800) 541-5454 or (312) 258-0522
URL: http://www.med.unc.edu/
mgfa/
Anna El-Qudsi, Executive Director

Type of Agency: Non-profit.
Mission: Promotes detection,
treatment, and cure of myasthenia
gravis. Conducts professional and
public education, scientific
symposia. Has 40 chapters
nationwide.
Budget: $300,000.
Hours of Operation: Mon. - Fri.
9:00 AM - 4:30 PM.
Staff: 20.
History/Date: Est. 1952.
Number of Clients Served:
30,000.
Area Served: United States.

Publications: *MG Newsletter.*

Myopia International Research Foundation

1265 Broadway, Room 608
New York, NY 10001
(212) 684-2777
Sylvia N. Rachlin, President

Mission: Promotes research into
the causes, treatment, and
prevention of progressive myopia.
Launched the Myopia
International Research Network to
promote worldwide coordinated
scientific research on myopia by
doctors.

National Accreditation Council for Agencies Serving the Blind and Visually Handicapped

15 East 40th Street, Suite 1004
New York, NY 10016
(212) 683-5068
FAX: (212) 683-4475
E-mail: 104257.60@compuserve.
com
Ruth Westman, Executive Director

Mission: Administers program of
standards development and
accreditation for programs,
agencies and schools serving
children and adults who are blind
or visually impaired. Publishes
standards available in print,
braille, cassette tape, and disk.
Funded by: Individual
contributions, grants from
corporations and foundations, and
dues from accredited members,
sponsors, and supporters.
History/Date: Est. 1967.

National Association for Visually Handicapped

22 West 21st Street
New York, NY 10010
(212) 889-3141
FAX: (212) 727-2951
Lorraine H. Marchi, Founder/
Executive Director

Type of Agency: Health.

Mission: To provide services, solely for the benefit of the partially seeing, which include counseling in the testing and use of visual aids; supplying kits of information to low vision persons, their families, friends and professionals who serve them; providing large-print publications and a large-print loan library, by mail; furnishing large-print standards to publishers, corporations, and public agencies; offering one to one emotional and peer support sessions; participating in and sponsoring educational outreach programs for laypersons and professionals in the field of low vision.

Funded by: Contributions and membership dues.

Hours of Operation: Mon.-Fri. 9:00 AM-5:00 PM.

Program Accessibility: Fully accessible.

History/Date: Est. 1954 and Inc. 1959.

Number of Clients Served: 111,000.

Area Served: United States and Canada primarily, with information, literature, large-print books, and visual aids supplied internationally as well. Maintains office in San Francisco serving 13 western states.

Transportation: Y.

Counseling/Social Work/Self-Help: Counseling and guidance to partially seeing adults, including parents of low vision children, their families, friends, and professionals who serve them.

Educational: Conducts adult discussion groups, and seminars for professionals in the low vision field.

Preschools: Serves parents and teaching professionals.

Professional Training: Educates the professional and paraprofessional working with the partially seeing about the nature of partial vision and the special needs of the partially seeing.

Reading: Y.

Rehabilitation: Conducts rehabilitation, recreational, social, and educational programs for partially seeing adults.

Recreational: Y.

Low Vision: Y.

Low Vision Aids: Y.

Low Vision Follow-up: Y.

Publications: *In Focus* (children); *Seeing Clearly* (adults).

Local Offices:

San Francisco: National Association for Visually Handicapped, 3201 Balboa Street, San Francisco, CA 94121, (415) 221-3201.

National Association of Area Agencies on Aging

1112 16th Street, N.W.
Suite 100
Washington, DC 20036
(202) 296-8130
FAX: (202) 296-8134
E-mail: jjfn4a@erols.com
Janice Fiegener, Executive Director

County/District Where Located: District of Columbia.

Mission: Advocates at the national level for the needs of older persons. Disseminates information to the federal government, other national organizations, and the public.

Hours of Operation: Mon.-Fri. 9:00 AM-5:00 PM.

Staff: 6.

Area Served: Nationwide.

Publications: *Directory of State and Area Agencies on Aging* (annual).

National Association of Radio Reading Services

1430 Confederate Avenue
Columbia, SC 29201
(800) 280-5325
FAX: (803) 734-7885
Beth Jones, President

Type of Agency: Professional organization.

Mission: Promotes radio reading services. Has closed circuit radio broadcasts of daily newspapers plus other materials.

Funded by: Membership.

History/Date: Est. 1977.

Professional Training: Holds an annual conference with workshops to train staff and volunteers of new and established radio reading services.

Publications: *Hearsay Newsletter; Directory of Radio Reading Services.*

National Association of State Units on Aging

1225 I Street, N.W.
Suite 725
Washington, DC 20005
(202) 898-2578
FAX: (202) 898-2583
E-mail: staff@nasua.org
Daniel A. Quirk, Executive Director

Mission: Provides information on state services to older persons and advocates for legislation and funding for such services.

Staff: 14.

History/Date: Est. 1966.

National Birth Defects Center

40 Second Avenue,
Suite 460
Waltham, MA 02154
(617) 466-9555
FAX: (617) 487-2361
Caroline Hobbs, Administrative Director

Type of Agency: Nonprofit clinic. Evaluates, treats, and provides follow-up to children with birth defects and mental retardation.

County/District Where Located: Suffolk County.
Funded by: Genesis Fund.
Hours of Operation: Mon.-Fri. 8:30 AM-5:00 PM; on call off hours.
Staff: Pediatric-geneticists, physicians assistant, genetic fellow, genetic counselor. Pregnancy environmental hot line staff and administrative staff.
History/Date: Est. 1984.
Number of Clients Served: 2,000 patient visits per year.
Eligibility: Children with birth defects and their parents.
Area Served: Primarily New England but patients are seen from all over the United States.
Age Requirements: Most patients are under 18.

Counseling/Social Work/Self-Help: Genetic counseling; access to other counseling services.

Satellite clinics in Massachusetts, New Hampshire, and Maine.

National Camps for Blind Children

4444 South 52nd Street
Lincoln, NE 68506
(402) 488-0981
FAX: (402) 488-7582
Tom Lowe, Director
Art Grayman, Director
Peggy Hansen, Secretary

Type of Agency: Non-profit.
Mission: Operates summer camps for blind and visually impaired children and adults.
Funded by: Donations; contributions.
Staff: Full-time counselors, nurse, food service personnel.
History/Date: Est. 1967.
Eligibility: Legally or totally blind.
Area Served: United States and Canada.
Age Requirements: 9 years-adult.

Counseling/Social Work/Self-Help: CRS (Christian Record Services) representatives available for assistance and counseling.
Recreational: Biking, water skiing, hiking, crafts, horseback riding, beeper baseball, archery, swimming, tandem bicycling.
Publications: *Campfire Light*.

National Council of Private Agencies for the Blind

Carroll Center for the Blind
770 Centre Street
Newton, MA 02158-2597
(617) 969-6200 or (800) 852-3131
FAX: (617) 969-6204
E-mail: carrollb@tiac.net
URL: http://www.tiac.net/users/carrollb
Rachel Rosenbaum, President

County/District Where Located: Middlesex County.
Mission: Serves as an advocate concerning issues that relate to programs, operations, and funding affecting voluntary agencies serving blind and visually impaired persons. Acts as a unified voice in negotiating with federal and state agencies about fees and other matters concerning private agencies.

National Early Childhood Technical Assistance System (NEC*TAS)

Frank Porter Graham Child Development Center
University of North Carolina at Chapel Hill
Nations Bank Plaza
137 East Franklin Street, Suite 500
Chapel Hill, NC 27514
(919) 962-2001
FAX: (919) 966-7463
URL: http://www.nectas.unc.edu
Pascal Trohanis, Director

County/District Where Located: Orange County.

Mission: Provides technical assistance to four primary target populations–Part H staff, Interagency Coordinating Council members, Part B– Section 619 staff, and Early Education Program for Children with Disabilities project staff–as well as to various secondary populations to assist them in developing and providing multidisciplinary, comprehensive, culturally sensitive, and coordinated services for young children with special needs (birth through 8 years of age) and their families. Also strives to link the target populations to facilitate the exchange of information about models of service delivery and best practices.
Funded by: Federal funds.
History/Date: Est. 1987.

Publications: Publications list available.

National Easter Seals Society

230 W. Monroe
Suite 1800
Chicago, IL 60606-4802
(312) 726-6200
FAX: (312) 726-1494
E-mail: nessinfo@seals.com
James E. Williams, Jr., President

Type of Agency: Non-profit.
Hours of Operation: Mon.-Fri. 8:30 AM-5:00 PM.
Number of Clients Served: Over 1 million annually.
Eligibility: Varies site to site, program to program.

Publications: *Rehabilitation Literature*.

National Eye Care Project (NECP)

P.O. Box 429098
San Francisco, CA 94102-9098
(800) 222-3937
FAX: (415) 561-8567
Tom Juring, Manager

Mission: To provide eye care to the elderly poor.
Funded by: Grants, donations.
History/Date: Est. 1986.

Health: Medical and surgical eye care.
Educational: Can provide literature on eye diseases and procedures.
Low Vision: Literature and resource list available.

National Eye Research Foundation (Optometry)
910 Skokie Boulevard
Suite 207A
Northbrook, IL 60062
(847) 564-4652
FAX: (847) 564-0807
E-mail: nerf1955@aol.com
URL: http://www.eyemac.com/nerf
Andrew K. Kim, Co-President.

Type of Agency: Non-profit.
County/District Where Located: Cook County.
Mission: Promotes educational and informational services for doctors and the public.
Funded by: Memberships, donations.
Budget: $300,000.
Hours of Operation: Mon. - Fri. 8:30 AM - 5:00 PM.
Staff: 5.
History/Date: Est. 1955.
Number of Clients Served: 400.

Health: Refers for social evaluation/psychological testing and evaluation, school/training placement, nursing homes, community services.
Counseling/Social Work/Self-Help: Refers for counseling.
Educational: Referral for appropriate level.
Professional Training: In-service programs, open enrollment from other agencies (doctors of optometry, optometric and ophthalmic assistants).
Rehabilitation: Refers for daily living skills; offers a full-service clinic.
Recreational: Refers for continuing education, arts/crafts, hobby groups, camps.
Employment: Refers for prevocational evaluation, career/skill counseling, occupational development, vocational training, placement.
Publications: *Global Contacto, Pinnacle.*

Research: Support of clinical research projects.

National Glaucoma Research Program of the American Health Assistance Foundation
15825 Shady Grove Road
Suite 140
Rockville, MD 20850
(301) 948-3244
Eugene H. Michaels, President

County/District Where Located: Montgomery County.
Mission: Supports glaucoma research. Maintains programs within the foundation: National Heart Foundation, National Glaucoma Research, Alzheimer's Disease Research and Alzheimer's Family Relief Program.

National Industries for the Blind
1901 North Beauregard Street
Suite 200
Alexandria, VA 22311-1727
(703) 998-0770
FAX: (703) 820-7816
E-mail: nibva@aol.com
URL: http://www.nib.org
Judith Moore, President

Mission: To enhance opportunities for economic and personal independence for persons who are blind through creating, sustaining and improving employment. Allocates among qualified industries for blind persons purchase orders of the federal government for approved goods and services as designed by the President's Committee for Purchase from the Blind and Other Severely Handicapped. Coordinates the production of 106 industries in 36 states. Researches and recommends new products, prices, and price revisions to the President's Committee. Devises quality control systems, provides management and engineering services to increase plant efficiency and broaden production opportunities for people who are blind.
Funded by: Commission fees paid by the associated industries for the blind.
Hours of Operation: Mon.-Fri. 8:30AM-5:00PM.
Staff: 105.
History/Date: Est. and Inc. 1938.
Area Served: United States.

Professional Training: Conducts management and technical training programs for personnel from NIB - associated industries.
Publications: *Opportunity; Annual Report.*

National Information Center for Children and Youth with Disabilities
P.O. Box 1492
Washington, DC 20013-1492
(202) 884-8200 or TDD (800) 695-0285
FAX: (202) 884-8441
Susan Ripley, Director

Type of Agency: Non-profit.
County/District Where Located: District of Columbia.
Mission: Acts as a national information clearinghouse on subjects relating to children and youths with disabilities.

Funded by: Contracts with the U.S. Department of Education.
Hours of Operation: Mon.-Fri. 9:00 AM-6:00 PM.
Area Served: United States.

National Multiple Sclerosis Society

733 Third Avenue
New York, NY 10017
(212) 986-3240 or (800) 344-4867
FAX: (212) 986-7981
E-mail: nat@nmss.org
URL: http://www.nmss.org
Michael J. Dugan, President and Chief Executive Officer

County/District Where Located: Manhattan County.
Mission: Sponsors research; provides information and education, recreational counseling, and therapeutic services.
Funded by: Donations.
Budget: $89 million.
Hours of Operation: 9:00 AM - 5:00 PM.
History/Date: Est. 1946.
Number of Clients Served: Information Resource Center serves 2,300,000 people annually.
Area Served: United States.

Counseling/Social Work/Self-Help: Referrals to services at local chapters.
Educational: Informational materials about multiple sclerosis and related issues.
Rehabilitation: Referral to local chapters.
Recreational: Referral to local chapters.
Employment: Referral to local chapters.
Computer Training: Referral to local chapters.
Low Vision: Information and referral to low vision agencies.

Publications: *Inside MS* (members only); Additional list of publications available on request.

144 chapters and branches throughout the United States.

National Self-Help Clearinghouse

25 West 43rd Street, Room 620
New York, NY 10036
(212) 354-8525
FAX: (212) 642-1956
URL: http://www.selfhelpweb.org
Audrey Gartner, Director

Type of Agency: Information and referral.
County/District Where Located: Manhattan County.
Mission: Trains leaders of self-help groups; publishes and distributes pamphlets on how to start self-help groups; conducts research on the effectiveness of self-help groups; sponsors conferences; provides information and referral.
Hours of Operation: Mon.-Fri. 9:00 AM-5:00 PM.
History/Date: Est. 1978.
Area Served: Nationwide.

Publications: Publishes newsletter, *Self-Help Reporter*, four times a year.

New Eyes for the Needy

549 Millburn Avenue
P.O. Box 332
Short Hills, NJ 07078
(201) 376-4903
Joyce Wiggin, Office Manager

Type of Agency: Non-profit.
Mission: Provides eyeglasses for those who cannot afford to buy them.
Funded by: Donations.
Budget: $231,000.

Hours of Operation: Mon.-Thurs. 9:00 AM-4:00 PM; Fri. 9:00 AM-12:00 noon.
Staff: 3 part time; 200 volunteers.
History/Date: Est. 1932.
Number of Clients Served: Approximately 3,500.
Eligibility: Medically indigent. Letter to referral from social service agency, with copy of presciption.
Area Served: United States.

Publications: Newsletter.

NTAC (National Technical Assistance Consortium for Children and Young Adults who are Deaf-Blind)
Teaching Research Division

Western Oregon State College
345 North Monmouth Avenue
Monmouth, OR 97361
(503) 838-8391 or TDD (503) 838-9623
FAX: (503) 838-8150
E-mail: ntac@fstr.wosc.osshe.edu
URL: http://www.tr.wosc.osshe.edu/ntac
Bruce A. Dalke, Director, (503) 838-8807
Kathy McNulty, Area Director, (516) 944-8900
Janet Stevely, Area Director, (516) 944-8900

Mission: Provides technical assistance to families and agencies serving children and young adults who are deaf-blind. Primary mission is to (a) assist states in improving the quality of services for the deaf-blind; and (b) to increase the numbers of people who will benefit from these services.

Orbis International

330 West 42nd Street, Suite 1900

New York, NY 10036
(212) 244-2525
FAX: (212) 244-2744
Pina Taormira, President and
Executive Director

Mission: Combats eye disease by
sending opthalmologists to foreign
countries to train and educate eye
personnel via Orbis Flying
Hospital, a specially equipped
airplane.

Publications: *Orbis Observer
Newsletter.*

Overbrook International
Overbrook School for the Blind

6333 Malvern Avenue
Philadelphia, PA 19151
(215) 878-8700
FAX: (215) 878-8886
E-mail: larry@obs.org
Lawrence F. Campbell,
Administrator, International
Program

Type of Agency: Private; non-
profit.
Mission: The International
Program provides training in
computer technology and ESL to
blind youth (16-21 years of age)
with leadership potential and to
educators of the visually impaired
to promote the more widespread
use of access technologies in
education and employment. The
Program also provides outreach
services in selected regions of the
world and works in collaboration
with other international
organizations to accomplish this
objective.
Funded by: Endowments,
contributions, tuition.
History/Date: Est. 1985.
Number of Clients Served: 20
foreign students and teachers
annually (approximate).
Area Served: All countries are
eligible for participation.

Prevent Blindness America

500 East Remington Road
Schaumburg, IL 60173
(847) 843-2020 or (800) 221-3004 or
(800) 331-2020 PBA Center for
Sight
FAX: (847) 843-8458
E-mail: preventblindness
@compuserve.com
URL: http://www.prevent-
blindness.org
Richard Hellner, President and
CEO

Type of Agency: Non-profit.
Mission: Through state affiliates,
conducts a program of public and
professional education, research,
and industrial and community
services to prevent blindness.
Services include promotion and
support of local glaucoma and
preschool vision screening
programs, industrial eye safety,
collection of statistical and other
data on nature and extent of causes
of blindness and defective vision,
support groups, and improvement
of environmental conditions
affecting eye health in schools and
colleges. Supports research on eye
diseases in laboratories and
medical schools. Conducts public
and professional education
programs including publications,
films, exhibits, and conferences.
Maintains the PBA Fight for Sight
research division, and the PBA
Center for Sight toll-free
information line, and information
center.
Funded by: Contributions, Federal
Service Campaign, and
endowment.
Budget: $20 million.
Hours of Operation: Mon.-Fri.
8:30AM - 5:00PM.
Staff: 30.
History/Date: Est. 1908 and Inc.
1918.
Area Served: United States.

Publications: *Prevent Blindness
News; Sightsaving.*

See state listing for local affiliates.

Research to Prevent Blindness

645 Madison Avenue
New York, NY 10022-1010
(212) 752-4333 or (800) 621-0026
Toll-free
FAX: (212) 688-6231
David F. Weeks, President

Type of Agency: Voluntary health
agency.
Mission: Supports clinical and
basic eye research into causes,
treatment, and prevention of all
eye diseases through annual
financial grants to more than 55 U.
S. medical institutions and through
awards, professorships, and
fellowships to selected vision
scientists. Stimulates growth of
modern eye research facilities by
underwriting major laboratory
construction programs. Assists
departments of ophthalmology in
the development and
improvement of advances in
technological equipment for eye
research, diagnosis, and therapy.
Provides incentives to attract
scientists to eye research and
serves as a medium for the
exchange of scientific information.
Provides a voice for eye research
among the nation's health
interests. The Board of Trustees
plans programs with the advice of
a permanent scientific advisory
panel drawn from many scientific
disciplines and an ad hoc
committee of ophthalmic
investigators. Provides
information on eye research to the
public, press, and other
institutions.
Funded by: Contributions from
individuals, foundations,
corporations.
Hours of Operation: Mon.-Fri.
9:00AM-5:00PM.

Staff: 11 full time. Uses volunteers.
History/Date: Est. and Inc. 1960.
Area Served: United States.

Publications: *Progress Report Newsletter; Biennial Eye Research Seminar Papers; Eye Research News Briefs.*

Schepens Eye Research Institute

20 Stanford Street
Boston, MA 02114
(617) 742-3140
Christie Whitcomb, Assistant for Trustee Affairs

County/District Where Located: Suffolk County.
Mission: Pursues research activities and fields relating to the retina, vitreous, and cornea, with strong collaboration between clinic and laboratory studies in the fields of retinal and corneal diseases. Dedicated to research that improves the understanding, management and prevention of eye diseases and visual deficiencies.
Funded by: U.S. government, foundations, private agencies, and individuals.
History/Date: Est. 1950. Formerly called the Retina Foundation.

Publications: *Sundial Newsletter.*

Smith-Kettlewell Eye Research Institute Rehabilitation Engineering Center

2232 Webster Street
San Francisco, CA 94115
(415) 561-1619 (as of 8/1/97 area code 415 becomes 650) or
(415) 561-1620
FAX: (415) 581-1610
E-mail: rerc@skivs.ski.org
URL: http://www.ski.org/rerc
John Brabyn, Director
Deborah Gilden, Associate Director
William Gerrey, Vocational Devices Manager

Mission: Conducts rehabilitation engineering research and development in orientation/mobility, low vision, vocational educational, recreational, and deaf-blind aids. Can provide expert consultation on specialized jobsite adaptations.
Funded by: Federal and private grants.
Hours of Operation: Mon.-Fri. 9:00 AM-5:00 PM.
History/Date: Est. 1975.
Eligibility: Blind, visually impaired, deaf-blind.
Area Served: National.

Publications: Publishes a variety of materials on technical issues, including the *Smith-Kettlewell Technical File*, a technical journal for the blind and visually impaired.

Taping for the Blind

3935 Essex Lane
Houston, TX 77027
(713) 622-2767
FAX: (713) 622-2772
E-mail: 102677.2656@compuserve.com
Beth O'Callaghen, Executive Director

Type of Agency: Non-profit.
Mission: To provide audio versions of written materials for all persons whose reading ability is impaired, in order to expand their access to printed information.
Funded by: Private donations.
Budget: $200,000.
Hours of Operation: 24 hours a day.
Staff: 4 full time and more than 200 volunteers.
History/Date: Est. 1967.
Eligibility: Print handicapped.
Area Served: Radio reading service. 33 neighboring counties. Special request service. National.

Educational: Request, will record textbooks on audio cassette.
Reading: On request, will record any printed material not available on tape elsewhere. A 24 hour/day radio reading service of local and national publications, books, newspapers, and other materials.
Low Vision: Audio description of local theater productions, museum exhibits, rodeos, IMAX, and large theater films, etc.
Publications: *Open Mike* news letter.

United Cerebral Palsy

1660 L Street, NW
Washington, DC 20036
(800) 872-5827
FAX: (202) 776-0414
Michael Morris, Executive Director

Mission: To advocate for individuals with cerebral palsy and their families; and to provide these individuals with lifelong opportunities and choices that promote their independence, inclusion and quality of life.

United States Braille Chess Foundation

428 West Lima Street
Findlay, OH 45840
(419) 422-2833
Richard McShaw, President

Mission: Popularizes chess for blind persons. Sponsors tournaments.

Publications: *Newsletter* (on cassette).

MEMBERSHIP ORGANI- ZATIONS

Affiliated Leadership League of and for the Blind of America

2915 34th Street, N.W.
Washington, DC 20008
(202) 298-8151
FAX: (202) 298-8151
Robert Humphreys, Executive
Director

Type of Agency: Coalition of public and private organizations of and for the blind to advance services and the rights of blind and visually impaired people.
Mission: Advocates for improvement of the social and economic conditions of the blind and visually impaired.

American Academy of Ophthalmology

655 Beach Street
P.O. Box 7424
San Francisco, CA 94120-7424
(415) 561-8500
Davis J. Noonan, Deputy
Executive Vice President

Mission: Promotes continuing education for ophthalmologists and quality care in ophthalmology. Publishes informational material for professionals and the public. Sponsors the National Eye Care Project to give free eye care to the elderly.

Publications: *Argus Newsletter; Ophthalmology; Biographical Directory of AAO.*

American Association for Pediatric Ophthalmology and Strabismus

P.O. Box 193832

San Francisco, CA 94119-3832
(415) 561-8505
FAX: (415) 561-8575
Denise DeLosada, Services
Coordinator

Mission: Advances quality eye care for children through educational training programs for pediatric ophthalmologists. Sets ethical standards of practice and informs professionals of latest developments in the field. Conducts research programs.

Publications: *Journal of Pediatric Ophthalmology and Strabismus.*

American Association for the Deaf-Blind

814 Thayer Avenue
Silver Spring, MD 20910
(301) 588-6545
FAX: (301) 588-8705
E-mail: aadb@erols.com
Joy Larson

Type of Agency: Membership association.
Mission: Provides information and technical assistance to deaf-blind persons, families, educators, and service providers; holds an annual convention; has network of chapters around the country.
Staff: 2.
History/Date: Est. 1937.
Number of Clients Served: 600 members.
Area Served: National.

Publications: Quarterly magazine, *Deaf-Blind American.*

American Association of Certified Orthoptists

Eye Clinic
Shands Hospital
Gainesville, FL 32610
(352) 392-3111
Diana Shamisin, Director

County/District Where Located: Alachua County.

Mission: Promotes education, training, and placement of orthoptists. Maintains library in Georgia relating to treatment of defects in binocular function and low visual acuity.

Publications: *Prism; American Orthoptic Journal.*

American Association of Retired Persons Disability Initiative

601 E Street, N.W.
Washington, DC 20049
(202) 434-2477 or TDD (202) 434-6554
FAX: (202) 434-6499
Carmel Cang, Disability Initiative
Director

Type of Agency: Consumer.
County/District Where Located: District of Columbia.
Mission: Serves its membership of midlife and older Americans by offering a range of community services and educational programs, including technical assistance on legal issues, insurance, and a wide variety of consumer products and services and information dissemination on consumer issues, health and disability issues, and advocacy.
Hours of Operation: Mon.-Fri. 9:00 AM-5:00 PM EST.
Staff: Approximately 2,000.
Number of Clients Served: 33 million members.

Publications: Publishes a wide range of public education and consumer materials as well as *Modern Maturity* and *the Bulletin.*

American Blind Bowling Association

315 North Main
Houston, PA 15342
(412) 745-5986
Ron Marcase, Secretary/Treasurer

County/District Where Located:
Washington County.
Mission: Promotes bowling for blind people. Sanctions leagues and sponsors tournaments.

Publications: *The Blind Bowler.* 3 times yearly (Oct., Jan., April).

American Blind Lawyers Association

P.O. Box 1590
Indianola, MS 38751
(601) 887-5398
Gary Austin, President

County/District Where Located:
Sunflower County.
Mission: Addresses special problems of blind people in the legal profession. Promotes production of braille or recorded law materials and maintains an index of these materials.

American Blind Skiing Foundation

610 South William Street
Mt. Prospect, IL 60056
(847) 255-1739
Sam Skobel, Executive Director

Mission: Volunteers teach skiing and hold races.
Area Served: Chicago and its suburbs; nationwide for information.

Educational: Skiing instruction.
Recreational: Skiing and other activities.

American Council of the Blind

1155 15th Street, N.W.
Suite 720
Washington, DC 20005
(202) 467-5081 or (800) 424-8666
FAX: (202) 467-5085
E-mail: ncrabb@access.digex.net
URL: http://www.acb.org
Oral O. Miller, Executive Director

Type of Agency: Affiliation of individual members and occupational, special interest, and state groups.
Mission: Promotes effective participation of blind people in all aspects of society. Acts as national information clearinghouse. Provides information and referral; legal assistance and representation; scholarships; leadership and legislative training; consumer advocate support; assistance in technological research; speaker referral service; consultative and advisory services to individuals, organizations, and agencies; and program development assistance. Maintains offices across the United States.
Funded by: Contributions and membership fees.
Hours of Operation: Mon.-Fri. 9:00 AM-5:30 PM.
Program Accessibility: Accommadation for physically disabled individuals.
Staff: 15 in national office.
History/Date: Est. and Inc. 1961.
Number of Clients Served: 40,000 annually.
Area Served: United States and its territories.

Publications: *The Braille Forum* (braille, large print, cassette, and computer disk).

American Council on Rural Special Education (ACRES)

Department of Special Education
University of Utah
221 Milton Bennion Hall
Salt Lake City, UT 84112
(801) 585-5659
FAX: (801) 585-7291
E-mail: acres@gse.utah.edu
Joan Sebastian, Coordinator
M. Winston Egan, Coordinator

Mission: Improves direct services to rural agencies and individuals that serve disabled persons and increases educational opportunities for rural handicapped and gifted students. Serves as advocate for rural special education at federal, state, regional, and local levels; distributes information on rural special education needs; conducts task forces on rural problems and professional training; maintains resource linkage system.
Hours of Operation: 8:00AM-5:00PM.

Publications: *Rural Special Education Quarterly; Ruralink* (newsletter).

American Optometric Association

243 North Lindbergh Boulevard
St. Louis, MO 63141
(314) 991-4100
FAX: (314) 991-4101
Jeff Mays, Executive Director

Type of Agency: Joint United States-Canadian membership organization.
Mission: Improves the quality of vision care through promoting high standards, continuing education, information dissemination, and professional involvement. Conducts conferences; operates placement service; maintains optometric museum and library; also maintains Virginia office.
Hours of Operation: 8:00 AM-5:00 PM.

Publications: *AOA News; Journal of the American Optometric Association.*

Maintains low vision section, consisting of optometric practitioners in low vision field provides continuing education for low vision optometricsts. Referral source for low vision professionals in optometry.

American Society of Cataract and Refractive Surgery

4000 Legato Road
Suite 850
Fairfax, VA 22033
(703) 591-2220
FAX: (703) 591-0614
David A. Karcher, Executive Director

Type of Agency: Non-profit medical association.
Mission: Promotes continuing education for ophthalmologists doing cataract and refraction surgery. Informs public about intraocular implantation. Conducts research.
Hours of Operation: Mon. - Fri. 8:00 AM - 5:00 PM.
Staff: 23.

Publications: *Journal of Cataract and Refractive Surgery; Administrative Eye Care;* monthly Washington newsletter.

American Society of Ophthalmic Registered Nurses

P.O. Box 193030
San Francisco, CA 94119
(415) 561-8513
FAX: (415) 561-8575
Carol Ruehl, President
Sue Brown, Administrator.

Mission: Advances quality eye nursing care through continuing education, certification, research, and administration.
Hours of Operation: 8:30 AM-5:00 PM.
Eligibility: Must be a registered nurse.
Area Served: International.

Publications: *Insight, The Journal of the American Society of Ophthalmic Registered Nurses.*

Association for Education and Rehabilitation of the Blind and Visually Impaired

4600 Duke Street, Suite 430
Alexandria, VA 22304
(703) 823-9690
FAX: (703) 823-9695
E-mail: aernet@laser.net
Kathleen Megivern, Executive Director

Type of Agency: Joint United States-Canadian membership organization.
Mission: To render all possible support and assistance to professionals who work with blind and visually impaired persons of all ages. Offers conferences, workshops, publications and other professional development opportunities; certifies teachers; advocates for public policies which benefit blind and visually impaired persons and the professionals who work with them.

Publications: *AER Report; Job Exchange Monthly; RE: View.*

Association for Macular Diseases

210 East 64th Street
New York, NY 10021
(212) 605-3719
Nikolai Stevenson, President

Type of Agency: Non-profit.
Mission: Provides information and education. Maintains support group for persons with macular degeneration. Funds eye bank devoted to research on macular degeneration.
Funded by: Membership dues; contributions.
Staff: Volunteer.
History/Date: Est. 1978.
Number of Clients Served: Over 6,000 members.
Eligibility: Services restricted to current members.

Area Served: International.

Counseling/Social Work/Self-Help: Individual counseling by phone and mail.
Publications: *Eyes Only.*

The Association for Persons with Severe Handicaps (TASH)

29 West Susquehanna Avenue
Suite 210
Baltimore, MD 21204
(410) 828-8274
FAX: (410) 828-6706
E-mail: nweiss@tash.org
Nancy Weiss, Executive Director

Type of Agency: Non-profit membership organization.
Mission: To actively promote the full inclusion and participation of persons with disabilities in all aspects of life.
Funded by: Membership dues.
Hours of Operation: 9:00 AM - 12 noon and 1:00 PM - 4:00 PM.
History/Date: Inc. 1975.
Area Served: Unlimited.

Publications: Monthly newsletter, quarterly journal, and special publications of interest disseminated through *Tash Publication List.*

Contact central office for listing of chapters in local areas.

Association of Junior Leagues

660 First Avenue
New York, NY 10016
(212) 683-1515
FAX: (212) 481-7196
Holly Sloan, Executive Director

County/District Where Located: New York County.
Mission: Serves in an advisory and coordinating capacity to 293 Junior Leagues throughout the United States, Canada, London, and Mexico City. Through many Junior Leagues, volunteers are provided to organizations for the

blind; to educational and informational community projects focused on the prevention of blindness; and to community rehabilitation programs for blind persons.

Association of Visual Science Librarians

c/o Indiana School of Optometry
Bloomington, IN 47405
(812) 855-8629
FAX: (812) 855-6616
Douglas Freeman, President

Mission: Promotes information services in ophthalmology and optometry. Conducts institutes, workshops, and training courses for professional personnel. Provides legislative consultation.

Association on Higher Education and Disability (AHEAD)

P.O. Box 21192
Columbus, OH 43221
(614) 488-4972 (voice/TDD)
FAX: (614) 488-1174
E-mail: ahead@postbox.acs.
ohio.state.edu
URL: http://www.ahead.org
Ed Suddath, Executive President
Stephan Smith, Operations

County/District Where Located: Franklin County.
Mission: Provides leadership, focus, and expertise for professionals. Committed to promoting full participation of individuals with disabilities in postsecondary education and to upgrading quality of services available. Provides workshops, training programs, publications, conferences. Has special interest group for blindness; visual impairment.

Publications: *Journal of Postsecondary Education and Disability; ALERT Newsletter, BVI*

News (Blindness and Visual Impairment News).

Blinded Veterans Association

477 H. Street, N.W.
Washington, DC 20001-2694
(202) 371-8880 or (800) 669-7079
FAX: (202) 371-8258
Tom Miller, Executive Director

Type of Agency: Veterans service organization.
Mission: Encourages and assists all blinded veterans to take advantage of rehabilitation and vocational training benefits, job placement assistance, and other aid from federal, state, and local resources by means of a field service program. Promotes extension of sound legislation and rehabilitation through liaison with other agencies. Through 48 regional groups and field service offices, operates volunteer service program for blinded veterans in their communities and provides information and referral services.
Funded by: Contributions, membership dues.
Budget: $1.7 million.
Hours of Operation: Mon.-Fri. 8:00 AM-4:30 PM.
Staff: 15.
History/Date: Est. 1945.
Number of Clients Served: 2,000 yearly.
Eligibility: Any blind or legally blind veteran.
Area Served: United States and its territories.
Age Requirements: 17 years and over.

Educational: Public education and publications program.
Publications: *BVA Bulletin* (published six times per year and sent free in large print to all blinded veterans known in U.S.).

Local Offices:

Region I: VA Regional Office, 1200 Main Street, JFK Federal Building, Boston, MA 02203, (617) 565-2565, (800) 669-7079, Stephen Mathews.
Region II: Blinded Veterans Association, VA Regional Office, 1120 Vermont Avenue N.W., Washington, DC 20421, (202) 418-4267, (800) 669-7079.
Region III: VA Regional Office, Room 645, 730 Peachtree Street, N.E., Atlanta, GA 30308, (404) 347-3760, (800) 669-7079, Norman Jones.
Region IV: 536 South Clark Street, Room 478, P.O. Box 8136, M/P 80, Chicago, IL 60680, (312) 353-1740, (800) 669-7079, Robert Del Malak.
Region V: VA Regional Office, P.O. Box 25126, 155 Van Gordon, Denver, CO 80225, (303) 914-5831, (800) 669-7079, Peter Link.
Region VI: VA Outpatient Clinic, 4600 Broadway, Room 188, Sacramento, CA 95820, (916) 731-7329, (800) 669-7079, Lazaro Martinez, Jr.

Contact Lens Association of Ophthalmologists

523 Decatur Street, Suite#1
New Orleans, LA 70130-1027
(504) 581-4000
FAX: (504) 581-5884
John S. Massare, MSC, Executive Director

County/District Where Located: Orleans Parish.
Mission: Disseminates information on ophthalmology. Addresses problems related to contact lenses.

Publications: *CLAO: Journal of the Contact Lens Association*; also: "CONTACT LENSES: The CLAO To Basic Science and Clinical Practice"(book) and "*CLAO Pocket Guide*""(book).

Council for Exceptional Children

1920 Association Drive
Reston, VA 20191-1589
(703) 620-3660 or (800) 328-0272
FAX: (703) 264-9494
Dr. Nancy Safer, Executive
Director

Type of Agency: Joint United
States-Canadian membership
organization.
County/District Where Located:
Fairfax County.
Mission: Strives to improve
educational outcomes for
individuals with exceptionalities.
Accomplishes its worldwide
mission on behalf of special
educators and others working with
children with exceptionalities by
advocating for appropriate
government policies; setting
professional standards; providing
continuing professional
development; and assisting
professionals to obtain conditions
and resources necessary for
effective professional practice.
Budget: $6 million.
History/Date: Est. 1922.

Council of Citizens with Low Vision International

c/o American Council of the Blind
1155 15th Street N.W., Suite 720
Washington, DC 20005
(800) 733-2258
FAX: (317) 251-6588

Mission: Promotes rights of
partially sighted individuals to
maximize use of their residual
vision. Educates the public to the
needs of the visually impaired.
Informs persons with low vision of
available services. Support groups
and chapters throughout the
United States.
Funded by: Membership dues and
donations; publication
subscriptions.
Budget: $50,000.

Hours of Operation: Messages
can be left 24 hours a day.
Staff: All volunteers.
History/Date: Est. 1978.
Area Served: Unlimited.

**Counseling/Social Work/Self-
Help:** Peer support and adovacy.
Educational: Scholarship
programs.
Rehabilitation: Refferral to
appropritate sources.
Publications: *The New Vision
Access.*

Council of Families with Visual Impairment

c/o American Council of the Blind
1155 15th Street, N.W., Suite 720
Washington, DC 20005
(202) 393-3666 or (202) 467-5081
FAX: (202) 467-5085
URL: http://www.acb.org
Roy Ward, Director

Type of Agency: Support group of
parents of blind and visually
impaired children.

Publications: *Reflections
Newsletter.*

Council of Schools for the Blind

c/o St. Joseph's School for the
Blind
253 Baldwin Avenue
Jersey City, NJ 07306
(201) 653-0578
FAX: (201) 653-4087
Herbert Miller, Administrator

Type of Agency: Organization of
chief executive officers of
residential schools for the blind
and visually impaired in the
United States and Canada.
Mission: Serves as an information
clearinghouse and advocate for
areas of interest relating to
residential schools for blind and
visually impaired persons.

Guide Dog Users

14311 Astrodome Drive
Silver Spring, MD 20906
(310) 598-2131
E-mail: jcsheehan@smart.net
Jenine Stanley, President

Type of Agency: Support group.
Mission: Education and advocacy
for guide dog users.
Funded by: Dues, donations and
product sales.
Area Served: Nationwide.

Independent Visually Impaired Enterprises

c/o American Council of the Blind
1155 15th Street N.W.
Suite 720
Washington, DC 20005
(202) 467-5081 or (800) 424-8666
Carla Hayes, President

Mission: Promotes small business
opportunities for blind and
visually impaired persons.
Affiliated with American Council
of the Blind.

Laurence-Moon Bardet-Biedl Syndrome Self-Help Support Network

c/o The Foundation Fighting
Blindness
Executive Plaza, Suite 800, 11350
McCormick Road
Hunt Valley, MD 21031-1014
(410) 785-1414 or (800) 683-5555
FAX: (410) 771-9470
Jessica Beach, Outreach
Coordinator

Mission: To discover the causes,
treatments, preventions and cures
for retinal degenerative diseases.
Funded by: Private donations.
Hours of Operation: Mon.-Fri.
8:30AM-5:00PM.
Staff: 40.
History/Date: Est. 1971.
Area Served: Nationwide.

Counseling/Social Work/Self-Help: Provides support to individuals and families affected by LMBB Syndrome.
Publications: *LMBBS Newsletter.*

National Association for Parents of the Visually Impaired

P.O. Box 317
Watertown, MA 02272-0317
(800) 562-6265
FAX: (617) 972-7444
Susan E. Laventure, Executive Director
Kevin O'Connor, President

Type of Agency: Organization for parents and agencies.
Mission: Provides support to parents and families of visually impaired children and youths. Operates national clearinghouse for information, education, and referral. Fosters communication among federal, state, and local agencies that provide services or funding for services to visually impaired children and youths. Promotes public understanding of the needs and rights of visually impaired children and youths; supports state and local parents groups and workshops that educate and train parents in service potential and their children's rights.
Funded by: Private grants.
Hours of Operation: Mon.-Fri. 9:00 AM - 5:00 PM.

Publications: *Awareness* (newsletter).

National Association of Blind Teachers

c/o American Council of the Blind
1155 15th Street, N.W., Suite 720
Washington, DC 20005
(202) 467-5081
FAX: (202) 467-5085
URL: http://www.acb.org
Patty Slaby, President

Mission: Supports blind teachers in addressing problems involved in the performance of their professional duties. Promotes employment. Disseminates information.

Publications: *Work Center Memo; Newsletter; Work Center Directory.*

National Association of State Directors of Special Education

1800 Diagonal Road
Suite 320
Alexandria, VA 22314
(703) 519-3800
FAX: (703) 519-3808
Martha Fields, Executive Director

Type of Agency: Professional society to improve educational opportunities of exceptional children.
County/District Where Located: Fairfax County.
Budget: $2 million.
Hours of Operation: Mon.-Fri. 8:00 AM-5:00 PM.
Staff: 20.
History/Date: Est. 1938.
Area Served: Nationwide.

Publications: *SpecialNet* electronic communications network and numerous bulletin boards.

National Association of Vision Professionals

1775 Church Street, N.W.
Washington, DC 20036
(202) 234-1010
FAX: (202) 234-1020
Arnold Simonse, Executive Secretary

Type of Agency: Association of persons working in vision screening and eye health education.
Mission: Promotes intercommunication among vision professionals conducting programs in organizations.

Promotes professional standards. Certifies vision screening personnel.
Funded by: Dues.
Budget: $25,000.
Hours of Operation: Mon. - Fri. 9:00 AM - 4:00 PM.
Staff: 1.
History/Date: Est. 1976.

National Coalition on Deaf-Blindness

175 North Beacon Street
Watertown, MA 02172
(617) 972-7347
FAX: (617) 923-8076
Steven Davies, Executive Secretary
Michael Collins, Chairperson
Joseph McNulty, Co-Chairperson

Type of Agency: Private; non-profit.
Mission: Advocates on behalf of the interests of deaf-blind children and adults via maintaining contact with legislators and policymaking agencies. The coalition is comprised of national organizations that have an interest in services to deaf-blind people, and individual members including professionals, parents, and consumers interested in influencing such services.
Funded by: Membership dues.
Hours of Operation: Mon.-Fri. 9:00 AM-5:00 PM.
History/Date: Est. 1987.
Area Served: National.

Publications: Legislative updates sent to membership as necessary.

National Council of State Agencies for the Blind

1213 29th Street, N.W.
Washington, DC 20007
(202) 298-8468
FAX: (202) 333-5881
Charles Crawford, President

County/District Where Located: District of Columbia.
Mission: Promotes communication among agencies involved in preventing blindness and offering services to severely visually impaired individuals.

National Federation of the Blind

1800 Johnson Street
Baltimore, MD 21230
(410) 659-9314
FAX: (410) 685-5653
URL: http://www.hfb.org
Marc Maurer, President

Mission: Works to improve social and economic conditions of blind persons. Provides evaluations of present programs and assistance in establishing new ones. Grants scholarships to blind persons. Has a public education program including speakers' bureau. Has several special interest divisions, including those for diabetics, educators, lawyers, parents of blind children, students, and public employees. Has affiliates in all states, the District of Columbia, and Puerto Rico.
Funded by: Contributions.
History/Date: Est. 1940 and Inc. 1949.
Area Served: United States.

Publications: *The Braille Monitor; Future Reflections* (for parents of blind children); *Voice of the Diabetic.*

National Marfan Foundation

382 Main Street
Port Washington, NY 11050
(516) 883-8712 or (800) 862-7326
Carolyn Levering, Executive Director

County/District Where Located: Nassau County.
Mission: Disseminates information about Marfan syndrome and related connective tissue disorders to patients, family members, and physicians; provides means for patients and relatives to share experiences and support; fosters research and public education.
Funded by: Members.
Budget: $300,000.
Hours of Operation: 8:00 AM-3:30 PM.
Staff: 3 full time, 2 part time.
History/Date: Est. 1981.
Number of Clients Served: 13,000 on mailing list.
Area Served: Wordwide.

Counseling/Social Work/Self-Help: Self-help.
Educational: Current informational materials on Marfan syndrome available on request; annual conference sponsored.
Low Vision Follow-up: A variety of publications and educational materials, including *A Bibliography of the Marfan Syndrome and Associated Disorders, The Marfan Syndrome,* and *NMF Fact Sheet.*

National Organization for Albinism and Hypopigmentation (NOAH)

1530 Locust Street, #29
Philadelphia, PA 19102-4415
(215) 545-2322 or (800) 473-2310
E-mail: noah@albinism.org
URL: http://www.albinism.org
Charla McMillan, President

Type of Agency: Non-profit consumer organization; self-help group.
Mission: Provides information on albinism and hypopigmentation; provides peer support; sponsors conferences on the subject; publishes a newsletter regularly. Has network of state chapters. Founding-member of Albinism World Alliance.
Funded by: Membership dues, contributions, and grants.

Budget: 1996: $21,000.
Hours of Operation: 24-hour voice mail.
Program Accessibility: All print materials provided in 14-point type.
Staff: No paid staff. Operated by members on a volunteer basis.
History/Date: Est. 1982.
Number of Clients Served: 850 members. Local chapters in 28 states and 1 province in Canada.
Eligibility: Persons with albinism, their families, friends, and the professionals working with them.
Area Served: Primarily United States, but no restrictions.

Counseling/Social Work/Self-Help: Self-help groups.
Low Vision: Informational bulletin on low vision.
Low Vision Aids: Information is available.
Publications: Informational bulletins and newsletters.

Opticians Association of America

10341 Democracy Lane
Fairfax, VA 22030
(703) 691-8355
FAX: (703) 691-3929
Paul Houghland, Jr., C.A.E., Executive Director

Type of Agency: Private, nonprofit.
County/District Where Located: Fairfax County.
Mission: Strives to advance the science of prescribing and grinding corrective lenses and optical instruments; disseminates information about the field.
Staff: 20.

Publications: *Dispensing Optician.*

Randolph-Sheppard Vendors of America

1901 Commercial Drive
Suite 7
Harvey, LA 70058-2300
(504) 347-5299
FAX: (504) 347-5152
Ray Washburn, President
Kim Tromatroe, Office Manager

County/District Where Located:
Jefferson Parrish.
Mission: Promotes education and legislation to improve vending facility programs for blind persons.
Funded by: Membership.
Staff: Board of Directors.
Number of Clients Served:
Approximately 3,000 nationwide.
Area Served: United States.

Publications: *Vendorscope.*

RESNA

1700 North Moore Street
Suite 1540
Arlington, VA 22209-1903
(703) 524-6686 or TDD (703) 524-6639
FAX: (703) 524-6630
URL: http://www.resna.org/resna/reshome.htm
Nashiydah Anderson, Executive Director

Type of Agency: Non-profit.
Mission: Serves as an information center to address research, and the development, dissemination, integration, and utilization of knowledge in rehabilitation and assistive technology.
Hours of Operation: 9:00 AM-5:00 PM.
Program Accessibility: Fully accessible.
Area Served: United States/International.

Publications: List available on request.

United States Association for Blind Athletes

33 North Institute Street
Colorado Springs, CO 80903
(719) 630-0422
FAX: (719) 630-0616
E-mail: usaba@usa.net
Charlie Huebner, Executive Director
Mark Lucas, Assistant Executive Director

Type of Agency: Non-profit.
Mission: Promotes sports involvement for people who are blind or visually impaired.
Funded by: Membership, foundation grants, corporate gifts, contributions.
Budget: $750,000.
Hours of Operation: Mon.-Fri. 8:00 AM-5:00 PM.
Staff: 3-full time. Uses volunteers.
History/Date: Est. 1976.
Number of Clients Served: 3,000.
Eligibility: Legally blind.
Area Served: National. Has representatives in each state.
Transportation: Y.
Age Requirements: None.

Professional Training: Regular in-service training; short-term or summer training; open to enrollment from other agencies.
Recreational: Training camps and competitions in the following sports: swimming; track & field; wrestling; gymnastics; goal ball; skiing; skating; power lifting; judo, tandem cycling.
Publications: Quarterly newletters; *Visions.*

United States Blind Golfers Association

3094 Shamrock Street N.
Tallahassee, FL 32308
(904) 893-4511
URL: http://www.midnightgolf/delphi.com
Bob Andrews, President

Mission: To help blind persons return to or learn to play golf.
Hours of Operation: Mon.-Sat. 9:00 AM-6:00 PM.
History/Date: Est. 1953.
Eligibility: Must be totally blind to play in national championship, but membership open to all visually impaired persons.
Area Served: Nationwide.

CANADA
FEDERAL AGENCIES
NATIONAL ORGANIZATIONS
NATIONAL CONSUMER AND PROFESSIONAL MEMBERSHIP ORGANIZATIONS

FEDERAL AGENCIES

The Adaptive Computer Technology Centre (The ACT Centre)

10 Wellington Street
Second Floor
Hull, PQ K1A 0H3
(819) 953-2491
FAX: (819) 953-5995

Mission: Provides federal government employees who have disabilities with a wide range of adaptive computer technology support and service. Conducts workplace assessments and offers training, technical support, and information on adaptive tools for persons with visual, mobility, hearing, speaking, or learning disabilities.

Canadian Human Rights Commission

320 Queen Street
Place de Ville, Tower A
Ottawa, ON K1A 1E1
(613) 995-1151 or TTY (613) 996-5211
FAX: (613) 996-9661

Mission: Acts as a watchdog against discrimination in federally regulated organizations and administers the Canadian Human Rights Act.

Canadian Transportation Agency
Accessible Transportation Directorate

15 Eddy Street
Hull, PQ K1A 0N9
(819) 953-2749
FAX: (819) 953-6019

Mission: Attends to the removal of undue obstacles to the mobility of travelers with disabilities in Canada's national transportation system through the resolution of complaints by travelers and through the formulation and implementation of regulations to improve accessibility.

Human Resources Development Canada
Office for Disability Issues

25 Eddy Street
Terrasses de la Chandiere, Suite 100
Hull, PQ K1A 0M5
(819) 997-2412
FAX: (819) 953-4797
Cathy Chapman, Director

Mission: Assists in the development of policies and programs that promote equality and independence for persons with disabilities. Advocates regarding issues of concern to disabled persons and promotes research and the development of resources and information.

Human Resources Development Canada
Vocational Rehabilitation of Disabled Persons Program

Place du Portage
Phase IV, Federal Provincial Programs, Fifth Floor
Hull, PQ K1A 0J9
(819) 997-1471 or TTY (819) 997-2858
FAX: (819) 997-2056

Mission: Helps persons with disabilities obtain and sustain employment.

National Library of Canada

395 Wellington Street
Ottawa, ON K1A 0N4
(613) 995-3904
FAX: (613) 947-2916

Mission: Maintains comprehensive information on Canadian libraries and agencies serving people with disabilities, as well as on special format materials available to disabled persons.

The Public Works and Government Services Canada (PWGSC)
Accessibility Office

Place du Portage
Phase IV
Hull, PQ K1A 0M2
(819) 775-4660
FAX: (819) 775-4914

Mission: Ensures that government buildings are accessible to persons with disabilities, both employees and members of the general public who use government services. Provides support and consultation in the area of barrier-free design of federal buildings and develops design standards and guidelines.

Transport Canada
Accessible Transportation Policy and Programs

Place de Ville
Tower C, 26th Floor
Ottawa, ON K1A 0N5
(613) 991-6407
FAX: (613) 993-7930
Jean Corbiel, Minister of Transport

Mission: Enhances progress toward an accessible national transportation system by developing transportation policy and by providing advice and financial support.

Treasury Board of Canada

300 Laurier Avenue West
West Tower, Seventh Floor

Ottawa, ON K1A 0R5
(613) 952-2870
FAX: (613) 952-3231
Gilles Loiselle, President, Treasury
Board
Claudette Barré, Director,
Legislation and Policy,
Employment Equity Division,
Human Resources Branch

Mission: Develops and
administers a broad range of
policies and guidelines for all
government departments with
respect to the provision of services
to persons with disabilities.

Veterans Affairs Canada
Health Care Division, Veteran
Services Branch
P.O. Box 7700
Charlottetown, PE C1A 8M9
(902) 566-8611
FAX: (902) 566-8039
Gerald Merrithew, Minister of
Veterans Affairs

Mission: Operates programs
through which blind veterans are
equally eligible with other veterans
for a wide range of benefits and
services and receive special
equipment and supplementary
benefits specifically related to their
blindness.

NATIONAL ORGANI- ZATIONS

Alternate Media Canada
The National Broadcast Reading Service

150 Laird Drive Annex
Toronto, ON M4G 3V7
(416) 422-4222
FAX: (416) 422-1633
E-mail: nbrs@idirect.com
John Stubbs, Director

Mission: Researches and develops communication products for the blind.

Braille Authority of North America

1155 15th Street, N.W.
Suite 720
Washington, DC 20005
(202) 467-5081
FAX: (202) 467-5085
Delores Ferrara-Godzieba, Director

See Braille Authority of North America in U.S. national listings.

Canadian Blind Sports Association

1600 James Naismith Drive
Gloucester, ON K1B 5N4
(613) 748-5609
FAX: (613) 748-5899
Ross Bales, Executive Director

Type of Agency: Non-profit national sport organization.
Mission: To facilitate the provision of national and international sport opportunities for Canadians who are legally blind.
Funded by: Government, membership, internal fund raising, corporate donations.

Budget: $325,000.
Hours of Operation: Mon.-Fri. 8:30 AM-4:30 PM.
Staff: 2 full time.
Number of Clients Served: 10 provincial associations; 1,400 athletes, coaches, and volunteers.
Area Served: Canada.
Age Requirements: All ages.

Recreational: Offers a wide range of programs to promote integration of blind athletes into sports and recreation programs.
Publications: *Moving to Inclusion,* formerly titled *Activity Integration Program: Integrating the Visually Impaired Student into Physical Education, A Teacher's Resource Manual.*

Provincial affiliates in Alberta, British Columbia, New Brunswick, Newfoundland and Labrador, Manitoba, Nova Scotia, Ontario, Quebec, and Saskatchewan.

Canadian National Institute for the Blind
Department of Government Relations and International Services

320 McLeod Street
Ottawa, ON K2P 1A3
(613) 563-4021
FAX: (613) 232-9070
James W. Sanders, National Director, Government Relations and International Services

Canadian National Institute for the Blind
National Office

1929 Bayview Avenue
Toronto, ON M4G 3E8
(416) 480-7580
FAX: (416) 480-7677
E-mail: nat-government@east.cnib.ca
URL: http://www.cnib.ca
Euclid J. Herie, President

Type of Agency: Service and rehabilitation.
Mission: To ameliorate the lives of blind persons in Canada; to prevent blindness, and to promote sight-enhancement services.
Funded by: Government funds, United Way, private donations.
Budget: $52 million.
Hours of Operation: Mon.-Fri., business hours.
Staff: Approximately 1,500 nationally.
History/Date: Est. 1918.
Number of Clients Served: 90,000 clients on record; 10,000 new clients added annually.
Area Served: All of Canada, through a network of divisional offices.
Transportation: Y.
Age Requirements: None.

Counseling/Social Work/Self-Help: Available.
Reading: Y.
Rehabilitation: Seven core services of CNIB are counseling and referral; rehabilitation teaching; orientation/mobility instruction; sight enhancement; technical aids; career development and employment; and library services.
Employment: Employment counseling.
Computer Training: Y.
Low Vision: Assessments.
Low Vision Aids: Y.
Low Vision Follow-up: Y.
Publications: A wide variety.

Provides a wide variety of rehabilitation and other services, including the operation of a career development center, eye bank, CNIB Library for the Blind, Information Resource Centre.

Guide Dogs for the Blind
P.O. Box 151200

San Rafael, CA 94915
(415) 499-4000
FAX: (415) 499-4035
Sue Sullivan, Admissions

See Guide Dogs for the Blind in U.S. state listings.

John Milton Society for the Blind in Canada

40 St. Clair Avenue, East, Suite 202
Toronto, ON M4T 1M9
(416) 960-3953

Mission: Provides ecumenical Christian materials in large print and braille or on audiotape to Canada's blind and visually impaired population. Publishes quarterly magazines and maintains an audio cassette library.

Leader Dogs for the Blind

1039 South Rochester Road
Rochester, MI 48307
(810) 651-9011 or (810) 650-7115
FAX: (810) 651-5812
William Hansen, Executive Director

County/District Where Located: Oakland County.

See Leader Dogs for the Blind in U.S. state listings.

National Camps for Blind Children

4444 South 52nd Street
Lincoln, NE 68506
(402) 488-0981
FAX: (402) 488-7582
Art Grayman, Director

See National Camps for Blind Children in U.S. national listings.

Operation Eyesight Universal (OEU)

#4 Parkdale Crescent N.W.

Calgary, AB T2N 3T8
(403) 283-6323
FAX: (403) 270-1899
E-mail: oeuca@cadvision.com

Mission: To encourage, develop, and fund sight restoration and blindness prevention programs in the developing world.

Local Offices:

Central Canada Region: 2100 Ellesmere Road, Scarborough, ON M1L 3B7, (416) 759-8011.

Pilot Dogs, Inc.

625 West Town Street
Columbus, OH 43215-4496
(614) 221-6367
J. Jay Gray, Executive Director

See Pilot Dogs, Inc. in U.S. state listings.

Retinitis Pigmentosa Eye Research Foundation

36 Toronto Street
Suite 910
Toronto, ON M5C 2C5
(416) 360-4200
FAX: (416) 360-0060
Donna Raffa, Administrator
Sharon Colle, National Executive Director

Mission: Promotes and supports research on the cause, treatment, and cure of retinitis pigmentosa and other retinal degenerative diseases. Has a network of local chapters through which it strives to create public awareness and provide support for persons with retinitis pigmentosa and their families.
Funded by: Individual donations.
Budget: $1.25 million.
Hours of Operation: Mon.-Fri. 9:00 AM-5:00 PM.
Staff: 6.
History/Date: Founded 1974. Registered non-profit in province

of Ontario and Canadian registered charity.
Area Served: Canada.

The Seeing Eye, Inc.

Washington Valley Road
Morristown, NJ 07960
(201) 539-4425
Kenneth Rosenthal, President

See The Seeing Eye, Inc. in U.S. state listings.

Ski for Light (Canada) Inc.

2520 Glenview Avenue
Kamloops, BC V2B 4L4
(250) 376-6504
Leonard Thoen, Treasurer

Mission: Promotes programs of cross-country skiing, or ski touring, for visually impaired and physically disabled persons.
Funded by: Donations.

MEMBERSHIP ORGANI- ZATIONS

Alberta Sports and Recreation Association for the Blind

Box 85056 Alberta Park Postal Outlet
Calgary, AB T2A 7R7
(403) 262-5332
Shelley Allen, Executive Director

Mission: To promote sports and recreational activities for blind and visually impaired persons.

American Optometric Association

243 North Lindbergh Boulevard
St. Louis, MO 63141
(314) 991-4100
FAX: (314) 991-4101
Jeff Mays, Executive Director

See American Optometric Association in U.S. national listings.

Atlantic Provinces Special Education Authority

5940 South Street
Halifax, NS B3H 1S6
(902) 424-8500
FAX: (902) 424-0543
Deborah Pottie, Superintendent
Dr. P. Ann MacCuspie, Director

Mission: To promote the use of braille in Canada, encourage research in the development of braille technology, and establish, adopt, and monitor standards for the production and teaching of English and French braille.
Area Served: Eastern Canada.

Publications: Membership newsletter published in English print and braille and French print and braille.

Canadian Association of Optometrists

234 Argyle Avenue
Ottawa, ON K2P 1B9
(613) 235-7924
FAX: (613) 235-2025
E-mail: eyedocs@opto.ca
URL: http://www.opto.ca
Michale J. DiCola, President

Type of Agency: Professional association of optometrists in Canada.
Mission: To advance the quality, availability and accessibility of eye, vision and related healthcare.
Funded by: Members' dues.
Staff: 6.
History/Date: Est. 1948.

Canadian Council for Exceptional Children Division for the Visually Handicapped

1010 Polytek Court
Unit 36
Gloucestor, ON K1J 9J2
(613) 747-9226
FAX: (613) 745-9282
Bill Gowling, Director

Type of Agency: Non-profit.
Staff: 2.
Area Served: Canada.

See Council for Exceptional Children in U.S. national listings.

Canadian Council of the Blind

Suite 200
396 Cooper Street
Ottawa, ON K2P 2H7
(613) 567-0311
FAX: (613) 567-2728
Mary Lee Moran, Executive Director

Type of Agency: National consumer advocacy.
Mission: To provide social, recreational, and blindness prevention programs. To advocate on behalf of blind and visually impaired persons.
Funded by: Government, donations, membership dues.
Hours of Operation: Mon.-Fri. 8:30 AM-4:30 PM.
Staff: 2.
History/Date: Est. 1945.
Number of Clients Served: Membership over 4,000.
Area Served: Canada.

Canadian National Society of the Deaf-Blind

422 Willowdale Avenue
Suite 405
Toronto, ON M2N 5B1
(416) 480-7417 (voice/TDD)
Dan Udell, President

Mission: To represent the interests of and improve services to deaf-blind persons in Canada.

Canadian Ophthalmological Society

1525 Carling Avenue
Suite 610
Ottawa, ON K1Z 8R9
(613) 729-6779
FAX: (613) 729-7209
Hubert Drouin, Executive Director

County/District Where Located: Regional Municipality of Ottawa-Careleton.
Mission: Membership organization of opthalmologists. Provide information about eye conditions and related issues.
Funded by: Membership.
Budget: $1,000,000.
Hours of Operation: 8:30 AM - 4:30 PM.
Staff: 3 permanent.
History/Date: Founded in 1937.
Number of Clients Served: 800 members.
Area Served: Canada.

Employment: Job referral program for opthamologists.

Publications: *Canadian Journal of Ophthalmology*, published seven times per year; newsletter, published quarterly; patient information pamphlets (English and French).

CDBRA (Canadian Deaf Blind Research Association) National Office

c/o W. Ross Macdonald School
350 Brant Avenue
Brantford, ON N3T 3J9
(905) 527-2110
FAX: (905) 527-6384
Linda Mamer, President

Type of Agency: Social services.
Mission: To assist all persons who are deaf-blind and their families in achieving the best possible quality of life.
Funded by: Self-funded with assistance from the federal and provincial governments.
Budget: $1.7 million.
History/Date: Est. 1975; federal charter in 1976.
Eligibility: Congenital deaf-blindness and early-acquired deaf-blindness.
Area Served: Canada.

Counseling/Social Work/Self-Help: Counseling and self-help.
Educational: Assistance with special schools and individual programs.
Preschools: Consultation.
Professional Training: Available.
Residential: Assistance in education and programs.
Recreational: Use of community facilities.
Computer Training: Some training available.
Publications: *Intervention* published biannually.

Chapters in New Brunswick, Manitoba, Ontario, British Columbia, Nova Scotia and Saskatchewan.

Council for Exceptional Children

1920 Association Drive
Reston, VA 20191-1589
(703) 620-3660
FAX: (703) 264-9494
Dr. Nancy Safer, Executive Director

County/District Where Located: Fairfax County.

See Council for Exceptional Children in U.S. national listings.

Council of Schools for the Blind

c/o St Joseph's School for the Blind
253 Baldwin Avenue
Jersey City, NJ 07306
(201) 653-0578
FAX: (201) 653-4087
Herbert Miller, Administrator

Type of Agency: Organization of chief executive officers of specialized residential schools for the blind and visually impaired in the United States and Canada.
Mission: Serves as an information clearinghouse and advocate for areas of interest relating to specialized residential schools for the blind and visually impaired persons.

See Council of Schools for the Blind in U.S. national listings.

Low Vision Association of Ontario

263 Russell Hill Road, Suite 101
Toronto, ON M4V 2T4
(416) 921-6609

Mission: Offers self-help/peer support programs and counseling on vision aids and training in their use.

Regroupement des Aveugles et Amblyopes du Quebec

3740 Berri Street
Second Floor, Bureau 240
Montreal, PQ H2L 4G9
(514) 849-2018
FAX: (514) 849-2754
Yves Fleury, General Director

Type of Agency: Consumer advocacy organization fully administered and directed by blind and visually impaired persons.
Mission: Works for the social integration of blind and visually impaired people by representing the interests of people with visual impairments in all fields of life.
Funded by: Quebec government (Ministry of Health and Social Services and of Education); private and corporate funding.
Hours of Operation: Mon.-Fri. 9:00 AM-5:00 PM.
Staff: 2 full-time, 3 part time.
History/Date: Est. 1975.
Number of Clients Served: 1,400 blind and visually impaired members; 47 corporate subscribers to *INFO-RAAQ*.
Area Served: Province of Quebec; maintains 11 regional affiliate associations.
Age Requirements: Voting blind and visually impaired members, age 16 and over; parents of blind and visually impaired children.

Publications: *INFO-RAAQ* newsletter, edited in French, produced in braille and large print and on cassette and disk.

VIEWS for the Visually Impaired
95 Wareside Road
Etobicoke, ON M9C 3B5
(416) 620-1410
FAX: (416) 620-1472
Judy Chudoba, Administrative
Assistant

Mission: Membership
organization that strives to ensure
that children who are visually
impaired have the opportunity to
reach their full potential and that
the families of these children

receive the information, resources,
and support that they need.

UNITED STATES
PRODUCERS AND PUBLISHERS OF BRAILLE AND OTHER ALTERNATE MEDIA SOURCES OF ADAPTED PRODUCTS AND DEVICES

PRODUCERS OF ALTERNATE MEDIA

♦ Media Producers and Publishers

American Action Fund for Blind Children and Adults

18440 Oxnard Street
Tarzana, CA 91356
(818) 343-2022
Jean Dyon Norris, Program
Director

Publications: Books made available in print/braille Twin Vision format to children pre-K through high school. Free braille newspaper for deaf blind individuals and organizations that serve the deaf blind. Free braille calendars.

American Bible Society

1865 Broadway
New York, NY 10023
(212) 408-1200
FAX: (212) 408-1512

Mission: Translates, publishes, and distributes the Scriptures in braille, large print, and recorded forms.
Funded by: Personal and church donations and endowments.
History/Date: Est. 1816 and Inc. 1841.
Area Served: Worldwide services.

American Foundation for the Blind

11 Penn Plaza
Suite 300
New York, NY 10001
(212) 502-7600 or (800) 232-5463 or
TDD (212) 502-7662
FAX: (212) 502-7777
E-mail: afbinfo@afb.org
URL: http://www.afb.org

Mission: Publishes a wide variety of professional, reference, and consumer titles in various media, including print, braille, large print, disk, audio cassette, and CD-ROM. Publishes the *Journal of Visual Impairment & Blindness* in print and braille and on audiocassette. Issues selected videos with audiodescription. Records and manufactures talking books on audiocassette for the National Library Service for the Blind and Physically Handicapped and for commercial and nonprofit organizations.

American Printing House for the Blind, Inc.

1839 Frankfort Avenue
P.O. Box 6085
Louisville, KY 40206-0085
(502) 895-2405 or (800) 223-1839
FAX: (502) 899-2274
E-mail: info@aph.org
URL: http://www.aph.org
Dr. Tuck Tinsley III, President

Type of Agency: National organization for the production of literature and the manufacture of educational aids for visually impaired persons.
Mission: Publishes braille books, music, and magazines; large-type textbooks; talking books and magazines; microcomputer software; tactile graphics; and electronic books. Provides on-line reference-catalog service for volunteer-produced textbooks in all media for visually impaired

students, plus information about other sources of materials for those interested in the education of visually impaired. Manufactures special educational aids for blind and visually impaired persons. Maintains an educational research and development program concerned with educational procedures and methods and the development of educational aids.
Funded by: Contracts, public funds, and contributions; since 1879, through the federal "Act To Promote the Education of the Blind," receives an annual appropriation from Congress to provide textbooks and educational aids for all students attending schools or special educational institutions of less than college grade.
History/Date: Est. and Inc. 1858.
Area Served: United States primarily; worldwide services on a contract basis.

Publications: Through funds donated by the public, publishes braille and talking book editions of the *Reader's Digest*, braille and large type editions of *My Weekly Reader*, and a weekly talking book edition of *Newsweek Magazine*, and *The Century Braille Book Club*. Free newsletters include *APH Slate* and *Micro Materials Update*.

Associated Services for the Blind

919 Walnut Street
Philadelphia, PA 19107
(215) 627-0600
FAX: (215) 922-0692
E-mail: asbinfo@libertynet.org
Patricia C. Johnson, CEO
Dolores Ferrara-Godzieba,
Director: Braille, Radio/Recording

Mission: Produces braille and large-print books, under contract to the Library of Congress, for distribution throughout the United

States or for schools, businesses, and non-profit organizations.

Audio Studio for the Reading Impaired
P.O. Box 23043
Anchorage, KY 40223
(502) 245-5422
Robert J. Knoll, Chairman
Sandra Koukola, Director

County/District Where Located:
Jefferson County.
Area Served: Entire United States and Canada.
Groups Served: K-12, college students, other adults.

Types/Content: Textbooks, recreational, career/vocational, religious.
Media Formats: Talking books/cassettes.
Title Listings: No title listings available.

Austin Junior Women's Federation
1406 Wilshire Boulevard
Austin, TX 78722
(512) 385-6935 or (512) 451-4802
Margarine G. Beaman, Project Director

County/District Where Located:
Travis County.
Area Served: United States.
Groups Served: K-12, college students, other adults.

Types/Content: Career/vocational, miscellaneous.
Media Formats: Braille, large print, and raised characters for brochures, metal trails, elevator numbers, menus, bank automatic teller machines, bank statements, directories and malls.
Title Listings: None specified.

Bantam-Doubleday-Dell
1540 Broadway

New York, NY 10036
(212) 765-6500
FAX: (212) 782-9600

Mission: Publishes large-print and audio books, including fiction, nonfiction, and reference books.

Beach Cities Braille Guild
P.O. Box 712
Huntington Beach, CA 92648
(714) 969-7992
FAX: (714) 960-1815
Linda Mc Govern, President

Area Served: Most of the English speaking world.
Groups Served: K-12, college students, other adults, touch-impaired blind persons.

Types/Content: Textbooks, recreational, career/vocational, religious.
Media Formats: Braille/large-print books. Jumbo braille. Also computer-assisted transcription.
Title Listings: Title listings in preparation.

Provides resource counseling for blind and visually impaired individuals.

Bible Alliance
P.O. Box 621
Bradenton, FL 34206
(941) 748-3031
FAX: (941) 748-2625
Joseph Aleppo, Executive Director

County/District Where Located:
Manatee County.
Mission: Distributes the Bible on cassette in many languages at no charge. Also produces talking book tapes; translations to other languages.

Reading: The Bible is available in more than 50 languages free of charge to individuals who cannot read standard print because of visual impairment. A verification of the impairment is necessary.

Blindskills, Inc.
P.O. Box 5181
Salem, OR 97304
(800) 860-1224 or (503) 581-4224
FAX: (503) 581-0178
E-mail: blindskl@teleport.com
URL: http://www.teleport.com/~blindskl
Carol M. McCarl, Editor
Richard L. Belgard, Assistant Editor

County/District Where Located:
Marion County.
Mission: To provide blind and visually impaired people with a magazine by and for them as well as resources, support and information.
Funded by: Group and individual subscriptions, donations and organization grants.
History/Date: Est. 1983.
Number of Clients Served: 1,200.
Area Served: Worldwide.

Publications: *DIALOGUE* magazine in braille, large print, on 4-track cassette and IBM-compatible diskette. A quarterly publication written by blind and visually impaired authors, *DIALOGUE* contains articles on resources and new products for the newly blind and those experiencing sight loss as well as support for coping and daily living skills.

Books Aloud
180 West San Carlos
San Jose, CA 95113-2096
(408) 277-4878
FAX: (408) 277-4818
URL: http://www.booksaloud.org/
Barbara Niemann, Contact Person

Area Served: United States and Canada.
Groups Served: Blind and physically handicapped, all ages.

Types/Content: All subjects but no textbooks.
Media Formats: Cassette books.
Title Listings: Catalogs available for adults and children.

Braille Communication Services

P.O. Box 16126
Lansing, MI 48901
(517) 627-9849
Duane Rolison, Manager

Area Served: Worldwide.
Groups Served: All groups.

Types/Content: Text materials in English other than mathematics or music, including computer-related materials.
Media Formats: Braille and large print.

Braille Inc.

184 Seapit Road
P.O. Box 457
East Falmouth, MA 02536-0457
(508) 540-0800
FAX: (508) 548-6116
E-mail: braillinc@c2pecod.net
Joan B. Rose

County/District Where Located: Barnstable County.
Area Served: Unlimited.
Groups Served: Departments of Education, schools, colleges, Departments of Human Services, public and private corporations.
Types/Content: Library braille, mathematics, computer and technical materials and diagrams, music.
Media Formats: Braille.
Title Listings: Individual listings are too numerous for inclusion here.

Braille International

3290 S.E. Slater Street

Stuart, FL 34997
(407) 286-8366 or (800) 336-3142
FAX: (407) 286-8909
Jeffrey Bull, President

County/District Where Located: Martin County.
Area Served: Continental United States, Canada, and abroad.
Groups Served: All groups.

Types/Content: Literary braille; reference books, menus, greeting cards, brochures, catalogs, technical manuals, children's books.
Media Formats: Braille and children's listening cassettes.
Title Listings: Catalog available.

Chivers North America

1 Lafayette Road
P.O. Box 1450
Hampton, NH 03842-0015
(603) 926-8744 or (800) 621-0182
FAX: (603) 929-3890

County/District Where Located: Rockingham County.
Mission: Publishes large-print and audio books, including fiction and nonfiction.

Choice Magazine Listening

Dept 12
P.O. Box 10
Port Washington, NY 11050
(516) 883-8280
FAX: (516) 944-6849
Doris Fields, Editor

Mission: Provides quality recorded reading for blind and visually impaired persons.
Funded by: Sponsor contributions and investment income.
History/Date: Est. 1961 and Inc. 1965.
Area Served: United States.

Records on 4-track tape free bimonthly anthology of unabridged articles, fiction, and poetry selected from current

periodicals; distributed throughout the U.S. free of charge through regional libraries and individual subscription.

Christian Education for the Blind

P.O. Box 6399
Fort Worth, TX 76115
(817) 923-0603
James Wiles, Program Director

Mission: Tape-records and distributes the *Evangel Voice Magazine,* Sunday school lessons, the Christian Education Library for the Blind, and sacred music. Publishes the *Evangel Hymn Book* (words only), and *Evangel Hymn Book* (words and music) in braille. Distributes Scriptures in braille and on recordings. Reading services are offered to blind persons without cost through a library loan system.
Funded by: Contributions; church groups; foundations.

Christian Mission for the Blind

5354 Boy Scout Road
Indianapolis, IN 46226
(317) 549-2386
William B. Schalk, Executive Director

County/District Where Located: Marion County.
Mission: Distributes religious material in braille, large type, and on cassette tapes.
Funded by: Churches and private contributions.
History/Date: Est. 1958.
Area Served: North America and nine foreign countries.

Publications: *Spiritual Light* (large-print newsletter and cassette tapes). *Christian Talking Magazine* (cassette tape only). Lending library (free catalog of large-print and cassette tape materials on request).

Christian Record Services

4444 South 52nd Street
P.O. Box 6097
Lincoln, NE 68506
(402) 488-0981 or (402) 488-1902
TDD
FAX: (402) 488-7582
Larry J. Pitcher, President

County/District Where Located:
Lancaster County.
Mission: Produces braille books,
talking books/cassettes, and
large-print books. Has lending
library.

Publications: *Christian Record;*
Children's Friend (braille); *Student;*
Encounter; Young and Alive;
Christian Record Talking Magazine;
Lifeflow; Review and Herald;
Campfire Light.

Christian Science Publishing Society

1 Norway Street
Boston, MA 02115
(617) 450-2000 or (800) 288-7090,
ext. 2694
FAX: (617) 450-2500
Stephanie Gaylord, Account
Manager

County/District Where Located:
Suffolk County.
Mission: Sells talking book
editions of Bible lessons and
articles from *Christian Science*
Journal and *Sentinel.*
Funded by: Income from
publications.
History/Date: Est. 1898.
Area Served: Worldwide.

Publications: *The Herald of*
Christian Science and *Christian*
Science Bible Lessons (braille).

Church of Jesus Christ of Latter-Day Saints Special Curriculum

50 East North Temple
Floor 24
Salt Lake City, UT 84150
(801) 240-2509
FAX: (801) 240-5732
E-mail: hinddl@chq.byu.edu
Douglas L. Hind, Manager

Mission: Prepares spiritual books,
lessons and auxiliary handbooks in
braille, disk, and cassette formats.
Funded by: Church funds.
Area Served: Worldwide services.

Publications: *The Ensign*
(monthly talking book magazine);
Friend (monthly, braille magazine);
New Era (monthly braille
magazine).

Cleveland Sight Center of the Cleveland Society for the Blind

1909 East 101st Street
Cleveland, OH 44106
(216) 791-8118
FAX: (216) 791-1101
Alice Miller, Coordinator, Taping
Services
Marlene Smith, Coordinator,
Braille and Large-Print
Transcription Services

County/District Where Located:
Cuyahoga County.
Area Served: Unlimited.
Groups Served: All ages.

Types/Content: General, all
academic subjects.
Media Formats: Braille books;
cassettes; large-print books.
Title Listings: Provided on
request.

The Clovernook Center Opportunities for the Blind

7000 Hamilton Avenue
Cincinnati, OH 45231
(513) 522-3860
FAX: (513) 728-3946
Marvin Kramer, Ed.D., Executive
Director

Mission: Provides visually
impaired persons, particularly
those with multiple disabilities,
with services and training
necessary for the attainment and
maintenance of each individual's
optimal level of independence.
Funded by: Income from printing
operations and contributions.
History/Date: Est. 1915.
Area Served: United States.

Publications: Embosses braille
books, magazines, catalogs, and
other publications for individuals
and national organizations,
including the Library of Congress,
American Foundation for the
Blind, Lions Clubs International,
United States Internal Revenue
Service, United States Department
of Education, and the Social
Security Administration.
Publishes *Tactic Magazine*, a
consumer oriented quarterly on
adaptive technology.

Contra Costa Braille Transcribers

514 Freya Way
Pleasant Hill, CA 94523
(510) 682-4734
FAX: (510) 682-0101
E-mail: akelt@juno.com
Ann Kelt, Chairperson

Area Served: Nationwide, with
emphasis on California.
Groups Served: K-12, college
students, and other adults.

Types/Content: Textbooks;
recreational; career/vocational.
Media Formats: Braille books.
Title Listings: No title listings
available.

Deaf-Blind Program The National Academy, Gallaudet University

Peet Hall, Third Floor
800 Florida Avenue, N.E.
Washington, DC 20002
(202) 651-5256
FAX: (202) 651-5887
Arthur Roehrig, Coordinator

Area Served: United States.
Groups Served: Deaf-blind persons, their families, and the professionals who work with them.

Types/Content: Continuing education.
Media Formats: Braille/large-print books.
Title Listings: No title listings available.

Vocational training for computer-related careers.

ELCA (Evangelical Lutheran Church in America) Braille and Tape Service

426 South Fifth Street
P.O. Box 1209
Minneapolis, MN 55440
(612) 330-3502
Karen Hoppe, Coordinator

County/District Where Located: Hennepin County.
Groups Served: Blind and visually impaired members of the Evangelical Lutheran Church in America.

Media Formats: Braille and audiotape.

G.K. Hall and Company Simon and Schuster

200 Old Tappan Road
Old Tappan, NJ 07675
(800) 223-2348

County/District Where Located: Bergen County.
Mission: Publishes large-print books.

Gospel Association for the Blind

P.O. Box 62
Delray Beach, FL 33447
(407) 274-9700
Rev. Ralph Montanus, Jr., President

County/District Where Located: Palm Beach County.
Funded by: Contributions and affiliated churches.
History/Date: Est. 1945 and Inc. 1947.
Area Served: United States, Canada, and islands of the Caribbean.

Reading: Has a large free circulating library of braille, books, and cassettes.
Publications: Monthly cassette magazine, *The Gospel Messenger*, for adults.

Grey House Publishing Company

8 Holly Street
P.O. Box 1958
Lakeville, CT 06039
(860) 435-0868 or (800) 562-2139
FAX: (860) 435-0867
Amy Lignor, Contact Person

Mission: Publishes large-print books, including fiction and nonfiction.

HarperCollins Publishers

10 East 53rd Street
New York, NY 10022
(212) 207-7000

Mission: Publishes large-print and audio books, including fiction, nonfiction, and reference.

Helen Keller Services for the Blind/Braille Library

One Helen Keller Way
Hempstead, NY 11550
(516) 485-1234
FAX: (516) 538-6785
Edith Magee, Assistant Director

County/District Where Located: Nassau County.
Area Served: United States.
Groups Served: K-12.

Types/Content: Textbooks; novels.
Media Formats: Braille/large-print books.
Title Listings: No title listings available.

Braille and large print text book masters created and copies provided to students within New York State. Copies of masters available for sale outside of New York State.

Herald House

Drawer 1770
Independence, MO 64055
(816) 252-5010

Mission: Publishes large-print and audio books, including fiction, nonfiction, and reference books.

Howe Press of Perkins School for the Blind

175 North Beacon Street
Watertown, MA 02172
(617) 924-3490
FAX: (617) 926-2027
Sarah A. McPhillips, Office Manager

County/District Where Located: Middlesex County.
Mission: Manufactures and sells the Perkins Brailler, manual or electric; standard, large cell, jumbo dot braille; slates; styli; mathematical aids; braille games; heavy and light-grade braille paper.
Funded by: Sale of products.
Area Served: Worldwide services.

Isis Large Print Books Transaction Publishers

Rutgers—The State University of New Jersey
New Brunswick, NJ 08903
(732) 445-2280
FAX: (732) 445-3138
Scott Bramson, President

County/District Where Located:
Middlesex County.

Offers wide variety of fiction and non-fiction books in large print.

Jewish Braille Institute of America

110 East 30th Street
New York, NY 10016
(212) 889-2525 or (800) 433-1531
FAX: (212) 689-3692
Gerald M. Kass, Executive Vice President

Mission: Serves the Jewish religious, cultural, educational, and communal needs of blind, visually impaired, and reading disabled persons by providing information on Judaism. Publishes braille books in Hebrew and English; talking books in Hebrew, Yiddish, English, French, Hungarian, Russian, German, and Romanian and large-print books in English and Hebrew. Transcribes and records other special material. Maintains free circulating braille, talking book, and large-print library meeting the needs of children as well as adult readers. Serves as a counseling and referral resource.
Funded by: Contributions, endowment, synagogues, and foundations.
History/Date: Est. and Inc. 1931.
Area Served: Worldwide services.

Professional Training: Training institutes for librarians and professionals working with the elderly persons.
Publications: *Jewish Braille Review*; *JBI Voice*; *Likkotin* (in Hebrew); and *JBI Cultural Series*.

Jewish Guild for the Blind (The Guild)

15 West 65th Street

New York, NY 10023
(212) 769-6331
FAX: (212) 769-6266
E-mail: bemass@aol.com
Bruce Massis, Director of Library Services

Area Served: Worldwide.
Groups Served: Adults.

Types/Content: Recreational.
Media Formats: Talking books/cassettes.
Title Listings: $25 charge (in large-print or on cassette) or Medicaid exemption.

John Milton Society for the Blind

475 Riverside Drive
Room 455
New York, NY 10115
(212) 870-3335
FAX: (212) 870-3229
Darcy Quigley, Managing Director and Editor-in-Chief

Type of Agency: Non-profit. Worldwide interdenominational ministry in Christian literature and education.
Mission: Publishes in Braille and large print and on cassette quarterly magazines for adults and teens free of charge.

Publications: *Discovery* (Braille, for youth); *John Milton Magazine* (large type); *Adult Lessons Quarterly* (Braille and cassette); *Directory of Resources*; *Annual Bible Commentary* (Braille); *Motto Calendar*(Braille). Publishes in Braille, large-print, and on cassette quarterly magazines for adults and teens free of charge. Accepts unsolicited manuscripts and poetry.

Library Reproduction Service

14214 South Figueroa Street

Los Angeles, CA 90011-1096
(800) 255-5002
FAX: (213) 749-8943
E-mail: lrsprint@aol.com
Joan Hudson-Miller, President

County/District Where Located:
Los Angeles County.
Mission: Provides large print reproductions of any and all educational and reading materials for purchase. Reproductions are produced from either titles already available or from originals sent to service. Catalog available on request at no charge.

Lutheran Braille Evangelism Association

1740 Eugene Street
White Bear Lake, MN 55110
(612) 426-0469
Rev. Dennis A. Hawkinson, Executive Director

Mission: Publishes and distributes Christian literature for blind and visually impaired persons. Strives to serve the spiritual needs of blind persons via publications in large-print and braille and on audio cassette and computer disk.

Publications: *Christian Magnifier*; *Tract Messenger*; *Lutheran Braille Evangelism Bulletin*.
Revised standard Braille bible available; King James 4 track cassette album available.

Lutheran Braille Workers

Box 5000
Yucaipa, CA 92399-1450
(909) 795-8977
FAX: (909) 795-8970
LeRoy Delafosse, Executive Director

Mission: Provides religious and educational materials in braille and large print. Maintains 200 work centers worldwide staffed by volunteers to help make the Bible accessible to the blind and visually impaired. All material provided free upon certification of being blind or visually impaired.

Publications: *Work Center Memo; Lutheran Braille Workers Newsletter; Work Center Directory.*

Types/Content: Provides braille copies of limited reference and textbook materials for blind students and of bible studies materials.

Lutheran Library for the Blind

1333 South Kirkwood Road
St. Louis, MO 63122
(314) 965-9000, ext. 1322 or
(800) 433-3954
FAX: (314) 965-0959
Lynne Borchelt, Assistant

Mission: Provides braille, large-print, cassette periodicals, and books.
Funded by: Lutheran Church, Missouri Synod.
History/Date: Est. 1951.
Area Served: Worldwide.

Publications: *The Lutheran Messenger, The Lutheran Witness, The Lutheran Digest, The Lutheran Women Missionary League Quarterly, The Lutheran Layman, My Devotions, My Delight, Christian Life, Happy Times, My Pleasure, Teacher's Interaction, Portals of Prayer, Strength for the Day, Teen Time, Our Life in Christ Sunday School Lessons, Catechisms.*

Matilda Ziegler Magazine for the Blind

80 Eighth Avenue, Room 1304
New York, NY 10011
(212) 242-0263
FAX: (212) 633-1601
E-mail: zieglermag@ibm.net
URL: http://www.zieglermag.org
Michael Mellor, Editor

County/District Where Located: Manhattan.

Mission: Publishes in braille and on four-track, half-speed cassette the *Matilda Ziegler Magazine for the Blind*, a free, general-interest, monthly covering a wide range of subjects, which includes news of special interest to blind and visually impaired people, pen pals, and a letter column where readers can seek or give advice or express their opinions sent to any visually impaired person requesting it.
Funded by: Endowment.
History/Date: Est. and Inc. 1907.
Area Served: Worldwide services.

Metrolina Association for the Blind

704 Louise Avenue
Charlotte, NC 28204
(704) 372-3870 or (800) 926-5466
FAX: (704) 373-3872
Robert Scheffel, Director

County/District Where Located: Mecklenburg County.
Mission: Produces braille and large-print documents, textbooks, bank statements, utility statements.

Michigan Braille Transcribing Service

4000 Cooper Street
Jackson, MI 49241
(517) 788-7560, ext. 494
Francelia Wonders, Director

Area Served: United States and Canada.
Groups Served: K-12, adults, businesses.

Types/Content: Textbooks, math and computer-related materials.
Media Formats: Braille books.
Title Listings: Print lists available at no charge.

Monterey County Braille Transcribers

P.O. Box DF

Pacific Grove, CA 93950
(408) 372-2944
Margaret Parenti, Work Coordinator

County/District Where Located: Monterey County.
Area Served: United States and Canada.
Groups Served: K-12; college students and other adults.

Types/Content: None specified.
Media Formats: Textbook braille.
Title Listings: None specified.

MSMT Braille Center

11 West Barham Avenue
Santa Rosa, CA 95407
(707) 579-1115
FAX: (707) 579-1246
Carolyn Colclough, Contact Person

County/District Where Located: Sonoma County.
Area Served: United States.

Types/Content: Text materials (other than music and math), including computer-related materials, graphs, maps, charts, and diagrams.
Media Formats: Braille; large-print.

National Association for Visually Handicapped

22 West 21st Street
New York, NY 10010
(212) 889-3141
FAX: (212) 727-2931
E-mail: staff@navh.org
URL: http://www.navh.org
Eva Cohen, Director's Assistant

Mission: Provides large-print and audio books, including fiction, nonfiction, newsletters for adults and children.

National Association to Promote the Use of Braille

3618 Dayton Avenue
Louisville, KY 40207
(502) 897-2632
FAX: (502) 899-1610
Betty Nicely, President

County/District Where Located: Jefferson County.

Mission: Makes the *Random House Concise Dictionary* available in a VersaBraille II Plus disk version.

National Braille Association

3 Townline Circle
Rochester, NY 14623
(716) 427-8260
FAX: (716) 427-0263
Angela Coffaro, Executive Director

County/District Where Located: Monroe County.

Mission: Assists all involved in the development and improvement of skills and techniques required for the production of reading materials for individuals who are print handicapped.

Funded by: Membership fees; contributions; grants.

History/Date: Est. 1945.

Area Served: Unlimited.

Educational: Provides continuing education to groups and individuals who prepare reading materials for print handicapped persons through seminars, workshops, consultations, and the publication of instruction manuals.

Publications: *Tape Recording Manual; Tape Recording Lessons; Guidelines for Administration of Groups Producing Reading Materials for the Visually Handicapped; Manual for Large-type Transcribing; NBA Bulletin* (quarterly to membership, available in print, braille, and on disk and cassette tape; available to agencies by subscription); reprints and workshops pertaining to all

advanced braille codes, tactile graphics, and computer-assisted transcription.

Types/Content: Provides braille textbooks, music, career, and technical materials at below cost to blind students and professionals and helps meet other braille needs of a more general nature.

National Braille Press

88 St. Stephen Street
Boston, MA 02115
(617) 266-6160 or (800) 548-7323
FAX: (617) 437-0456
E-mail: orders@nbp.org
William M. Raeder, Executive Director

Mission: Provides braille printing services for organizations, including the Library of Congress. Sponsors children's Braille Book-of-the-Month Club.

Publications: *Syndicated Columnists Weekly; Our Special; National Braille Press Release.*

Types/Content: Sells braille books, including computer manuals, tutorials and reference guides, cookbooks, baby and child care information, Christmas cards, an employment guide, AIDS information, and books on writing skills and etiquette.

Northern Nevada Braille Transcribers

1015 Oxford Avenue
Sparks, NV 89431-3037
(702) 358-2456 (voice/TDD)
Lois Baskerville, Advocate

Area Served: United States and some foreign English-speaking areas.

Groups Served: Teens and adults; original transcription requests taken from deaf-blind persons, with additional copies available for loan to others. A list of young

children and elementary level books is available.

Types/Content: Recreational, any requests, with priority to deaf-blind persons' requests.

Media Formats: Braille books.

Title Listings: Braille lists available on request; some print lists available.

Print Access Center The Lighthouse Inc.

111 East 59th Street
New York, NY 10022
(212) 821-9681
FAX: (212) 821-9707
E-mail: braille@lighthouse.org or astevenson@lighthouse.
org
URL: http://www.lighthouse.org.
Andrew Stevenson, Director, Information Resources

Area Served: Worldwide.

Groups Served: Individuals, businesses, libraries, schools, training centers.

Media Formats: Braille, large print and cassette. Provides braille and large print for business organizations.

Provides consultation on braille and large print needs.

Prose & Cons Braille Unit

P.O. Box 2500
Lincoln, NE 68542-2500
(402) 471-3161, ext. 3373
FAX: (402) 471-3472
Dominic Inzodda, Shop Operator

County/District Where Located: Lancaster County.

Area Served: United States and Canada.

Groups Served: K-12, college students, other adults.

Types/Content: Textbooks, menus, tests (mathematics, science, computer, etc.).

Media Formats: Braille/large print books.
Title Listings: Printed at no charge.
Braille writer repair, tactiles, and grading literary lessons.

Random House Large Print

201 East 50th Street
New York, NY 10022
(212) 572-2600 or (800) 726-0600
FAX: (212) 872-8026

County/District Where Located: Manhattan County.
Mission: Publishes large-print and audio books, including fiction, nonfiction, and reference books.

Recording for the Blind and Dyslexic

20 Roszel Road
Princeton, NJ 08540
(609) 452-0606 or (800) 221-4792
FAX: (609) 987-8116
E-mail: info@rfbd.org
URL: http://www.rfbd.org
Ritchie L. Geisel, President and CEO

Type of Agency: Non-profit.
Mission: Provides recorded and computerized textbooks, library services, and other educational resources to people who cannot read standard print because of a visual, physical, or perceptual disability. Maintains a lending library of recorded books and acts as a recording service for additional titles.
Funded by: Individual corporations and foundations.
Hours of Operation: Customer services: Mon.-Fri. 8:30 AM-5:00 PM, EST; administration: Mon.-Fri. 8:30 AM-4:45 PM.
Staff: 4,800 trained volunteers.
History/Date: Est. 1948; inc. 1951.
Number of Clients Served: 30,000.

Eligibility: Documented print disability--blindness, low vision, learning disability, or other physical impairment that impedes reading.
Area Served: United States, Canada, and other countries.

Publications: *RFB&D Impact* (newsletter); *RFB&D Annual Report.*

Resources for Rehabilitation

33 Bedford Street
Suite 19A
Lexington, MA 02173
(617) 862-6455
Susan Greenblatt, Contact Person

Mission: Publishes large-print computer disk, and audio books, including nonfiction, and reference books that enable consumers and service providers to locate resources that contribute to independence.

Conducts custom-designed training programs for consumers and service providers related to vision loss, rehabilitation, and assistive technology. Conducts program evaluations.

St. Martin's Press

175 Fifth Avenue
New York, NY 10010
(800) 221-7945
FAX: (212) 420-9314

County/District Where Located: Manhattan County.
Mission: Publishes audio books, including fiction, nonfiction, and reference books.

Seedlings: Braille Books for Children

P.O. Box 51924

Livonia, MI 48151-5924
(313) 427-8552 or (800) 777-8552
FAX: (313) 427-8552
E-mail: seedlink@aol.com
URL: http://www.22cent.com/seedlings/

Type of Agency: Non-profit.
Mission: Publishes braille books for children.

Seedlings publishes low-cost braille books for children ages 1-14 (some are available in print-and-braille format). Free catalog on request.

Services to the Blind Reorganized Church of Jesus Christ of Latter-Day Saints

1001 West Walnut
P.O. Box 1059
Independence, MO 64051
(816) 833-1000, ext. 1460
FAX: (816) 521-3043
Carol White, Supervisor

Area Served: United States; Canada; requests world wide considered.
Groups Served: K-12; college students; other adults; agencies who need braille adapted.

Types/Content: Textbooks; recreational; career/vocational; religious; any requests considered.
Media Formats: Braille books; talking books/cassettes.
Title Listings: Print and braille lists available at no charge from Free Lending Library.

Braille adaptations done for clients on request. Free Lending Library-both braille and cassette. Free calendars on request.

Sight Line Productions

505 Paradise Road
Suite 200

Swampscott, MA 01907
(617) 595-9800
FAX: (617) 595-9800
E-mail: psudore@datablast.net
Pamela S. Sudore, President

Mission: Publishes materials in braille and large type.
Area Served: National.
Groups Served: Businesses, organizations, and agencies.

Types/Content: Maps, brochures, forms, menus, charts, diagrams, business cards, floor plans, and greeting cards.

Simon & Schuster Publishing

200 Old Tappan Road
Old Tappan, NJ 07675
(800) 223-2348
FAX: (800) 445-6991

County/District Where Located: Bergen County.
Mission: Publishes large-print and audio books, including fiction, nonfiction, and reference books.

Theosophical Book Association for the Blind

54 Krotona Hill
Ojai, CA 93023
(805) 646-2121
E-mail: 75457.633@compuserve.com

Mission: Supplies individuals and libraries with braille books. Operates free lending library of materials in braille and tape.
Funded by: Members of the Theosophical Societies, foundation grants, and endowments.
History/Date: Est. 1910; inc. 1943.
Eligibility: Worldwide.

Publications: Publishes theosophical material, esoteric philosophy, and metaphysical material in braille and on tapes and cassettes, including *The Braille Star Theosophist*, an occasional

magazine distributed internationally without charge.

Thorndike Press

P.O. Box 159
Thorndike, MI 04986-0159
(207) 948-2962
FAX: (207) 948-2863

County/District Where Located: Waldo County.
Mission: Publishes large-print and audio books, including fiction and nonfiction books.

Ulverscroft Large Print Books Limited

1881 Ridge Road
West Seneca, NY 14224
(716) 674-4270 or (800) 955-9659
FAX: (716) 694-4195

County/District Where Located: Erie County.
Mission: Publishes large-print and audio books, including fiction and nonfiction.

Visual Aid Volunteers, Inc.

617 State Street
Garland, TX 75040
(972) 272-1615
FAX: (972) 494-5002
Elizabeth Gross, Director

Area Served: Unlimited.
Groups Served: K-college level.

Types/Content: Textbooks, commercial materials, menus. LOC certified.
Media Formats: Braille books, computer disks.
Title Listings: None specified.

Volunteer Braille Services

3730 Toledo Avenue, North
Robbinsdale, MN 55422
(612) 521-0372
FAX: (612) 588-4912
Jean Zolik, Coordinator/Format Advisor

County/District Where Located: Hennepin County.
Area Served: United States.
Groups Served: Braille and large print readers.

Types/Content: Textbooks and text materials other than computer-related materials.
Media Formats: Braille and large print.

Also maintains children's print/braille library for residents of the United States, serving kindergarten through grade 12.

Volunteer Braillists and Tapists

517 North Segoe Road
Suite 200
Madison, WI 53705
(608) 233-0222
Bonnie Crossman, President
Gail Yu, Office Coordinator

Area Served: All of United States and Canada, but primarily Wisconsin.
Groups Served: Preschool; K-12; college students; other adults.

Types/Content: Textbooks; career/vocational; religious; children's literature; adult fiction; cookbooks; handiwork.
Media Formats: Braille books; talking books/cassettes; braille-print children's books.
Title Listings: Print and braille lists available at no charge.

Volunteers of Vacaville

P.O. Box 670
Vacaville, CA 95696
(707) 448-6841
Dave Boult, Coordinator

Area Served: United States; worldwide.
Groups Served: K-12; college students; other adults.

Types/Content: Textbooks; recreational; career/vocational; religious.
Media Formats: Talking books/cassettes.

Repair services for braillers.

Volunteer Transcribing Services

205 East Third Avenue, Suite 200
San Mateo, CA 94401
(415) 344-8664 (as of 8/1/97 area code 415 becomes 650)
FAX: (415) 344-8676
Alanah Hoffman, Director

Area Served: United States and Canada.
Groups Served: K-14.

Types/Content: Textbooks.
Media Formats: Large-print books.
Title Listings: Fee for service.

Wheeler Publishing, Inc.

P.O. Box 531
Accord, MA 02018-0531
(617) 871-9170
FAX: (617) 871-9173

County/District Where Located: Plymouth County.

Reading: Large print books for the visually handicapped. Primary focus is bestsellers.

Xavier Society for the Blind

154 East 23rd Street
New York, NY 10010
(212) 473-7800 or (800) 945-5565
FAX: (212) 888-4183
Rev. Alfred Caruana, S.J., Director

County/District Where Located: Manhattan County.
Mission: Makes available various weekly and monthly Catholic periodicals; maintains free lending library of Braille, large-type, and tape books of exclusively religious nature; provides a variety of devotional materials in accessible

forms. Catalogs available in all three media.
History/Date: Inc. 1904.
Area Served: United States and Canada; certain services extended to blind persons overseas.

Publications: Spiritual and inspirational literature in the Catholic tradition (in braille, large print, and on tape).

Zondervan Publishing House

5300 Patterson Avenue, S.E.
Grand Rapids, MI 49530
(616) 698-6900
FAX: (616) 698-3421

County/District Where Located: Kent County.
Mission: Publishes large-print and audio books, including fiction, nonfiction, and reference.

◆ Audiodescription Services

Audio Description
Metropolitan Washington Ear

35 University Boulevard East
Silver Spring, MD 20901
(301) 681-6636
Dr. Margaret Rockwell Pfanstiehl, President and Founder
Cody Pfanstiehl, Audiodescription Services

County/District Where Located: Montgomery County.

Trains describers, guides, and docents in audiodescription; publishes a newsletter for individuals interested in audiodescription; and helps other organizations launch audiodescription services.

Audio Optics, Inc.

24 Hutton Avenue, #26

West Orange, NJ 07052
(201) 736-1704
Albert D. Hecht, Director

Audiodescribes movies for home video release as well as select television programs.

Audio Vision

416 Holladay Avenue
San Francisco, CA 94110
(415) 641-4589
FAX: (415) 641-4461
Ida C. Johnson, Executive Director

County/District Where Located: San Francisco County.

Offers training for audiodescribers and production services for audiodescribed films, plays, and exhibits.

Descriptive Video Service
WGBH-TV

125 Western Avenue
Boston, MA 02134
(617) 492-2777
FAX: (617) 783-8668
E-mail: laurie_everett@wgbh.org
URL: http://www.boston.com/wgbh/dvs
Laurie Everett

Produces audiodescription for national series on PBS (Public Broadcasting Service) and TCM (Turner Classic Movies), as well as non-broadcast films and videos. Provides description in IMAX and OMNI MAX theatres. Operates DVS Home Video, a mail order catalog of described Hollywood movies and public television documentaries. Publishes a quarterly newsletter (The DVS Guide) and new releases for *DVS* Home Video (2 times per year).

Narrative Television Network

5840 South Memorial Drive
Suite 312

Tulsa, OK 74145
(918) 627-1000
FAX: (918) 627-4101
E-mail: narrative@aol.com

County/District Where Located:
Tulsa County.

Produces audiodescription for
movies for cable television
systems.

**National Academy of Audio
Description
RP International**
P.O. Box 900
Woodland Hills, CA 91365
(818) 992-0500
Helen Harris, Director

Mission: Provides
audiodescriptions of motion
pictures in theaters, on home video
and on television.

SOURCES OF PRODUCTS

♦ *Mail Order, Catalogs, and Distributors*

Includes organizations and companies that carry a wide variety of products, including independent living, health care, and recreation products; low vision devices; and communication aids. Products can usually be ordered by catalog, which can be obtained from the individual companies listed.

American Printing House for the Blind
P.O. Box 6085, Department 0086
Louisville, KY 40206-0085
(502) 895-2405

Ann Morris Enterprises Inc.
890 Fams Court
East Meadow, NY 11554
(516) 292-9232 or (800) 454-3175
FAX: (516) 292-2522
E-mail: annmor@netcom.com
URL: http://tribeca.ios.com/tildaannm2

Automagic Corporation
195 South Beverly Drive
Suite 406
Beverly Hills, CA 90212
(310) 552-2101 or (310) 552-1412
FAX: (310) 275-1550

Carolyn's
1415 57th Avenue

West Bradenton, FL 34207
(800) 648-2266
FAX: (941) 739-5503
E-mail: magnify@bhip.infi.net

Enabling Technologies Company
3102 S.E. Jay Street
Stuart, FL 34997
(407) 283-4817
FAX: (407) 220-2920

Enhanced Vision Systems, Inc.
2915 Redhill Avenue, Suite B201
Costa Mesa, CA 92626
(800) 440-9476 or (714) 957-0155
FAX: (714) 957-0722

Environmental Lighting, Inc
3923 Coconut Palm Drive
Tampa, FL 33619

Independent Living Aids, Inc.
27 East Mall
Plainview, NY 11803
(800) 537-2118 or (516) 752-8080
FAX: (516) 752-3135

The Lighthouse Inc.
36-20 Northern Boulevard
Long Island City, NY 11101
(718) 786-5620

LS&S Group, Inc.
P.O. Box 673
Northbrook, IL 60065
(800) 468-4789 or (847) 498-9777
FAX: (847) 498-1482
E-mail: lsgrp@aol.com
URL: http://www.lssgroup.com

Maddak, Inc.
Bel-Art Products Subsidiary
6 Industrial Road

Pequannock, NJ 07440-1993
(201) 628-7600, ext. 9
FAX: (201) 305-0841
E-mail: custservice@maddak.com
URL: http://www.maddak.com
or http://www.ableware.com

Massachusetts Association for the Blind
The Store
200 Ivy Street
Brookline, MA 02146
(800) 682-9200 or (617) 738-5110

Maxi-Aids
42 Executive Boulevard
P.O. Box 3209
Farmingdale, NY 11735
(800) 522-6294 or (516) 752-0521
FAX: (516) 752-0689
E-mail: sales@maxiaids.com
URL: http://www.lighthouse.org

Mid-Michigan Center for the Blind
3200 South Pennsylvania Avenue
Lansing, MI 48910
(517) 887-6646

National Federation of the Blind
1800 Johnson Street
Baltimore, MD 21230
(410) 659-9314
FAX: (410) 685-5653

Rose Resnick Lighthouse for the Blind and Visually Impaired
214 Van Ness Avenue
San Francisco, CA 94102
(415) 431-1481

Science Products
P.O. Box 888
Southeastern, PA 19399
(800) 888-7400 or (800) 888-7401
FAX: (610) 296-0488

Visionics Corporation Inc.
1000 Boone Avenue North
Suite 600
Minneapolis, MN 55427
(800) 507-4448 or (612) 544-4950
FAX: (612) 544-4784
E-mail: insight@visionics.com
URL: http://www.visionics.com

◆ Household, Personal, and Independent Living Products

Includes such products as kitchen utensils and measuring devices; canes; talking clocks, scales, and calculators; games and toys; and braille watches.

Adaptive Living Institute
P.O. Box 57640
Tucson, AZ 85732
(520) 884-4229
FAX: (602) 745-9749

Ann Morris Enterprises Inc.
890 Fams Court
East Meadow, NY 11554
(516) 292-9232 or (800) 454-3175
FAX: (516) 292-2522
E-mail: annmor@netcom.com

Autofold, Inc.
208 Coleman Street Extension
Gardner, MA 01440-1063
(508) 632-0667

Braille Greeting Cards
246 Dale Avenue
Mansfield, OH 44902
(419) 522-5708

Fotofonics
315 Larkspur Turn

Peachtree City, GA 30269
(770) 487-5854

Gladys Loeb Foundation
2002 Forest Hill Drive
Silver Spring, MD 20903-1532
(301) 434-7748

Howe Press of Perkins School for the Blind
175 North Beacon Street
Watertown, MA 02172
(617) 924-3490
FAX: (617) 926-2027

Innovative Rehabilitation Technology
1411 West El Camino Real
Mt. View, CA 94040
(415) 961-3161 (as of 8/1/97 area code 415 becomes 650)

Kentucky Industries for the Blind
1900 Brownsboro Road
Louisville, KY 40206-2199
(502) 893-0211

The Lighthouse Inc.
Lighthouse Enterprises
36-20 Northern Boulevard
Long Island City, NY 11101
(800) 829-0500
FAX: (718) 786-5620

LS&S Group, Inc.
P.O. Box 673
Northbrook, IL 60065
(800) 468-4789 or (847) 498-9777
FAX: (847) 498-1482
E-mail: lsgrp@aol.com
URL: http://www.lssgroup.com

Lucent/ACPC
14250 Clayton Road
Town and Country, MO 63017
(800) 233-1222
FAX: (314) 891-7896

Maddak, Inc.
Bel-Art Products Subsidiary
6 Industrial Road
Pequannock, NJ 07440-1993
(201) 628-7600, ext. 9
FAX: (201) 305-0841
E-mail: cservice@maddak.com
URL: http://www.maddak.com
or http://www.ableware.com

Massachusetts Association for the Blind
The Store
200 Ivy Street
Brookline, MA 02146
(800) 682-9200 or (617) 738-5110
FAX: (617) 738-1247

Mattel Consumer Affairs
Mattel Toys
333 Continental Boulevard
El Segundo, CA 90245
(310) 252-2000

Maxi-Aids
42 Executive Boulevard
P.O. Box 3209
Farmingdale, NY 11735
(800) 522-6294 or (516) 752-0521
FAX: (516) 752-0689
E-mail: sales@maxiaids.com
URL: http://www.lighthouse.org

Mid-Michigan Center for the Blind
3200 South Pennsylvania Avenue
Lansing, MI 48910
(517) 887-6646

National Association for Visually Handicapped
22 West 21st Street
New York, NY 10010
(212) 889-3141 or (415) 221-3201

National Federation of the Blind
1800 Johnson Street

Baltimore, MD 21230
(410) 659-9314
FAX: (410) 685-5653

Nurion Industries
Station Square
Building 2
Paoli, PA 19301
(610) 640-2345

Phillip Barton Vision Systems
3911 York Lane
Bowie, MD 20715
(301) 262-3665

Precision Grinding & Manufacturing
8019 Flood Road
Baltimore, MD 21222
(410) 285-1135

Prophecy Designs
P.O. Box 84
Round Pond, MA 04564
(207) 529-5318
FAX: (207) 529-6418

Rainshine Company
2017 1/2 Corscot Court
Madison, WI 53704
(608) 249-8231

Rose Resnick Lighthouse for the Blind and Visually Impaired
214 Van Ness Avenue
San Francisco, CA 94102
(415) 431-1481

Rubbermaid Health Care Products
3124 Valley Avenue
Winchester, VA 22601
(800) 526-8051
FAX: (800) 775-6303

Sears, Roebuck and Company New Account Center
3000-A North Mall Road

Knoxville, TN 37924
(800) 323-3274 or (423) 521-3700

Spectrum, The Lighthouse Store
111 East 59th Street
New York, NY 10022
(212) 821-9384
FAX: (212) 821-9707

Technology for Independence
529 Main Street
Boston, MA 02129
(617) 242-7007
FAX: (617) 242-2007

Whirlpool Corporation Appliance Information Services
2303 Pipestone Road
Benton Harbor, MI 49022
(800) 253-1301 or (800) 632-2243

White Cane Institute for the Blind
Route 3, Box 89A
Jenkins, MO 65605
(417) 574-6368

Wildlife Materials, Inc.
1031 Autumn Ridge Road
Carbondale, IL 62901
(618) 549-6330

◆ Low Vision

Ir.cludes such products as magnifiers, loupes, lamps, and closed-circuit televisions; encompasses optical and nonoptical devices, both electronic and nonelectronic.

4X Products, Inc
P.O. Box 555
Millwood, NY 10546
(914) 762-3555
FAX: (914) 944-0605

Audio Visual Marts
P.O. Box 23020
Harahan, LA 70183
(800) 737-6278 or (504) 733-1500

Automagic Corporation
195 South Beverly Drive
Suite 406
Beverly Hills, CA 90212
(310) 552-2101 or (310) 552-1412
FAX: (310) 275-1550

Bausch & Lomb Company
1 Bausch & Lomb Place
Rochester, NY 14604
(800) 344-8815 or (716) 338-6000

Bernell Corporation
750 Lincolnway East
P.O. Box 4637
South Bend, IN 46634-4637
(219) 234-3200 or (800) 348-2225
FAX: (219) 233-8422

Big Eye Lamps, Inc.
133 Yellowbrook Road
Farmingdale, NJ 07727
(908) 938-2490 or (800) 242-8311
FAX: (908) 938-5921 or Toll-free
(888) 424-4393

Bossert Specialties, Inc. Magnification Center
3620 East Thomas Road, D-124
Phoenix, AZ 85018
(602) 956-6637 or (800) 776-5885
FAX: (602) 965-1008

Celexx Trading Company, Inc.
2535 Seminole
Detroit, MI 48214
(800) 886-3259
FAX: (309) 827-5450

Charles Nusinov and Sons, Inc.
8720 Satyr Hill Road
Baltimore, MD 21234
(410) 661-5050
FAX: (410) 882-8883

Coburn Optical Industries, Inc.
4606 South Garnett Road
Suite 200
Tulsa, OK 74146
(800) 262-8761 or (918) 665-1815
FAX: (918) 665-1821

Contact East, Inc.
335 Willow Street, South
North Andover, MA 01845
(508) 682-2000
FAX: (508) 688-7829
URL: http://
www.contacteast.com

Dazor Manufacturing Corporation
4483 Duncan Avenue
St. Louis, MO 63110
(800) 345-9103 or (314) 652-2400
FAX: (314) 652-2069
URL: http://www.dazor.com

Deluxe Check Printers, Inc.
1020 West County Road F
Shoreview, MN 55126
(800) 328-9546 or (612) 483-7200
FAX: (612) 787-1614

Designs for Vision, Inc.
760 Koehler Avenue
Ronkonkoma, NY 11779
(800) 345-4009 or (516) 585-3300
FAX: (516) 585-3404

Electronic Visual Aid Specialists
P.O. Box 371
Westerly, RI 02891
(800) 872-3827 or (401) 596-3155
FAX: (401) 596-3979
URL: http://www.evas.com

Eschenbach Optik of America
904 Ethan Allen Highway
Ridgefield, CT 06877
(203) 438-7471
FAX: (203) 438-1670
URL: http://
www.eschenbach.com

Exceptional Teaching Aids
20102 Woodbine Avenue
Castro Valley, CA 94546
(510) 582-4859 or (800) 549-6999
FAX: (510) 582-5911

Fishburne Enterprises
140 East Stetson Avenue
#319
Hemet, CA 92543
(909) 765-9276
FAX: (909) 766-0843

Florida New Concepts Marketing
P.O. Box 261
Port Richey, FL 34673-0261
(800) 456-7097 or (813) 842-3231
FAX: (813) 845-7544
URL: http://gulfaide.com/
compulenz

Fred Sammons, Inc.
P.O. Box 5071
Bolingbrook, IL 60440
(800) 323-5547
FAX: (800) 547-4333
URL: http://
www.samonspreston.com

General Electric
G.E. Appliance Park
Building 6
Room 106
Louisville, KY 40225
(502) 452-4311 or (502) 452-5691
FAX: (502) 452-0213

Gladys Loeb Foundation
2002 Forest Hill Drive
Silver Spring, MD 20903-1532
(301) 434-7748

Hexagon Products
P.O. Box 1295

Park Ridge, IL 60068-7295
(847) 692-3355
E-mail: 76064.1776@compuserve.
com
URL: http://
ourworld.compuserve.com/
homepages/hexagon

Honeywell Residential Controls
1985 Douglas Drive, North
Golden Valley, MN 55422-3992
(612) 951-1000

HumanWare, Inc.
6245 King Road
Loomis, CA 95650
(800) 722-3393 or (916) 652-7253
FAX: (916) 652-7296
E-mail: info@humanware.com
URL: http://
www.humanware.com

Innoventions, Inc.
5921 S. Middlefield Road, Suite 102
Littleton, CO 80123-2877
(800) 854-6554 or (303) 797-6554
FAX: (303) 727-4940
E-mail:
magnicam@magnicam.com
URL: http://
www.magnicam.com/magnicam

Jesana Ltd.
979 Saw Mill River Road
Yonkers, NY 10710
(800) 443-4728
FAX: (914) 376-0021

J P Trading, Inc.
300 Industrial Way
Brisbane, CA 94005
(415) 468-0775
FAX: (415) 469-8038
E-mail: jptusa@a.crl.com

Keeler Instruments, Inc.
456 Parkway

Broomall, PA 19008
(800) 523-5620 or (610) 353-4350
FAX: (610) 353-7814

The Lighthouse Inc.
Lighthouse Enterprises
36-20 Northern Boulevard
Long Island City, NY 11101
(800) 829-0500
FAX: (718) 786-0437

LS&S Group, Inc.
P.O. Box 673
Northbrook, IL 60065
(800) 468-4789 or (847) 498-9777
FAX: (847) 498-1482
E-mail: lsgrp@aol.com
URL: http://www.lssgroup.com

Luxo Corporation
36 Midland Avenue
P.O. Box 951
Port Chester, NY 10573
(914) 937-4433 or (800) 222-5896

Magnisight
P.O. Box 2653
Colorado Springs, CO 80901
(800) 753-4767
FAX: (719) 578-9887

Maitland Vision Center
600 South Orlando Avenue
Suite 300
Maitland, FL 32751
(407) 628-3133
FAX: (407) 628-1216

Massachusetts Association for the Blind
The Store
200 Ivy Street
Brookline, MA 02146
(800) 682-9200 or (617) 738-5110

Mattingly International, Inc.
938-K Andreason Drive

Escondido, CA 92029
(800) 826-4200
FAX: (800) 368-4111

Maxi-Aids
42 Executive Boulevard
P.O. Box 3209
Farmingdale, NY 11735
(800) 522-6294 or (516) 752-0521
FAX: (516) 752-0689
E-mail: sales@maxiaids.com
URL: http://www.lighthouse.org

McLeod Optical, Inc.
100 Jefferson Park Road
Warwick, RI 02888
(401) 467-3000

Mons International
6595 Roswell Road
#224
Atlanta, GA 30328
(800) 541-7903 or (770) 551-8455
FAX: (770) 551-8460
URL: http://www.negia.net

M-Tech Optics Corporation
P.O. Box 12110
Birmingham, MI 48012
(313) 531-3577

National Association for Visually Handicapped
22 West 21st Street
New York, NY 10010
(212) 889-3141 or (415) 221-3201

National Federation of the Blind
1800 Johnson Street
Baltimore, MD 21230
(410) 659-9314
FAX: (410) 685-5653

National Pen Corporation
342 Shelbyville Mills Road
Shelbyville, TN 37160
(800) 854-1000 or (800) 347-7367

New Concepts Marketing, Inc.
P.O. Box 261
Port Richey, FL 34673-0261
(813) 842-3231

Ocutech, Inc.
P.O. Box 625
Chapel Hill, NC 27515
(800) 326-6460 or (919) 967-6460
FAX: (919) 968-4601

Okay Vision-Aide Corporation
14811 Myford
Tustin, CA 92680
(800) 325-4488
FAX: (714) 669-1081

Overseer Electronic Visual Aids
6826 Logan Avenue, South
Richfield, MN 55423
(612) 866-7606

Pencar Associates
137-75 Geranium Avenue
Flushing, NY 11355
(718) 939-7031
FAX: (718) 359-5782

Phillip Barton Vision Systems
3911 York Lane
Bowie, MD 20715
(301) 262-3665

Prodigy Products Company
1823 Oakmount Road
South Euclid, OH 44121
(216) 381-0500

PulseData International, Inc.
4994 Austell Road
Austell, GA 30001
(888) 734-8439
FAX: (770) 732-8580
E-mail: pulse_data@compuserve.com

Reed EZ-Reader, Inc.
9780 Hope Acres Road
P.O. Box 433
White Plains, MD 20695
(301) 932-6565
FAX: (301) 934-4365

Reflection Technology
230 Second Avenue
Waltham, MA 02154
(617) 890-5905, ext. 235
FAX: (617) 890-5918

Replogle Globes, Inc.
2801 South 25th Avenue
Broadview, IL 60153
(708) 343-0900 or (708) 343-0923

Science Products
P.O. Box 888
Southeastern, PA 19399
(800) 888-7400 or (800) 888-7401
FAX: (610) 296-0488

Sears, Roebuck and Company New Account Center
3000-A North Mall Road
Knoxville, TN 37924
(800) 323-3274 or (423) 521-3700

Seemore Vision Products
42 Executive Boulevard
Farmingdale, NY 11735
(800) 462-3738
FAX: (516) 752-0687

Sped Publications
2010 Eagle View
Colorado Springs, CO 80909
(719) 473-6991

Stocker and Yale, Inc.
32 Hampshire Road
Salem, NH 03079
(603) 893-8778
FAX: (603) 893-5604
URL: http://www.stakr.com

Strieter Laboratories, Inc.
222 Vandalia Street
Collinsville, IL 62234
(800) 851-4557 or (618) 345-5814

S. Walters, Inc.
30423 Canwood Street
Suite 115
Agoura Hills, CA 91301
(800) 992-5837 or (818) 706-2202
FAX: (818) 706-2206

Tagarno of America, Inc.
615 Otis Drive
Dover, DE 19901
(800) 441-8439 or (302) 734-9630
FAX: (302) 734-9654

Talking and Visual Aids
8136 Appoline
Detroit, MI 48228
(313) 935-1266
E-mail: leeghume@aol.com

Tekvision Products
5383 Orchard Drive
Paradise, CA 95969
(800) 554-4544

TeleSensory Corporation
455 North Bernardo
P.O. Box 7455
Mountain View, CA 94039-7455
(800) 286-8484
FAX: (415) 969-9064 (as of 8/1/97 area code 415 becomes 650)
URL: http://www.telesensory.com

Typewriting Institute for the Handicapped
3102 West Augusta Avenue
Phoenix, AZ 85051
(602) 939-5344

Universal Low Vision Aids
1550 College Hill Drive

Columbus, OH 43221
(614) 486-0098
FAX: (614) 486-1043
E-mail: ulval@aol.com

Vision Technology, Inc.
40 Worthington Drive
Maryland Heights, MO 63043
(800) 560-7226 or (314) 879-0933
FAX: (314) 878-6562

Visual Methods, Inc.
35 Charles Street
Westwood, NJ 07675
(201) 666-3950 or (201) 666-7931

Winco Optical Inc.
555 Mulberry Street
P.O. Box 1675
Reading, PA 19603
(800) 345-1567 or (610) 372-6612

Xerox Adaptive Products
9 Centennial Drive
Peabody, MA 01960
(800) 248-6550
FAX: (508) 977-2148
E-mail: doihon@xis.xerox.com
URL: http://www.outlookcctv.com

◆ Computer Hardware

Includes adaptive equipment such as laptop computers, braille displays, key caps, braille embossers, and optical character recognition systems.

Acrontech International, Inc.
5500 Main Street
Williamsville, NY 14221
(716) 854-3814 or (800) 245-2020
FAX: (716) 854-4014
E-mail: acrontec@idirect.com

Adaptec Systems
6909 Rufus Drive
Austin, TX 78752-3123
(512) 451-1717
E-mail: tecraig@bga.com

AICOM Corporation
2381 Zanker Road
Suite 160
San Jose, CA 95131
(408) 577-0370
FAX: (408) 577-0373

A.I. Kurzweil, Inc.
411 Waverley Oaks Road
Waltham, MA 02154
(617) 893-5151 or (800) 634-8723
FAX: (617) 893-6525
URL: http://www.kurzweil.com

American Thermoform Corporation
2311 Travers Avenue
City of Commerce, CA 90040
(213) 723-9021
FAX: (213) 728-8877

Ann Morris Enterprises Inc.
890 Fams Court
East Meadow, NY 11554
(516) 292-9232 or (800) 454-3175
FAX: (516) 292-2522
E-mail: annmor@netcom.com

Apple Computer, Inc.
20525 Marianni Avenue
Cupertino, CA 95014
(800) 767-2775 or (408) 996-1010

Arkenstone, Inc.
555 Oakmead Parkway
Sunnyvale, CA 94086
(408) 245-5900 or (800) 444-4443
FAX: (408) 745-6739
URL: http://www.arkenstone.org

Artic Technologies
55 Park Street
Suite 2

Troy, MI 48083-2753
(810) 588-7370 or (810) 588-1425
FAX: (810) 588-2650

Automated Functions, Inc.
7700 Leesburg Pike
Suite 420
Falls Church, VA 22043
(703) 883-9797
FAX: (703) 883-9798
E-mail: autofunc@tmn.com

Blazie Engineering
105 East Jerretsville Road
Forest Hill, MD 21050
(410) 893-9333
FAX: (410) 836-5040
URL: http://www.blazie.com/

Braille Sterling Christiansen Studios
P.O. Box 583
Hanover, NH 03755
(603) 448-6166

Centigram Communications Corporation
91 East Tasman Drive
San Jose, CA 95134
(408) 944-0250 or (408) 428-3732

ComputAbility Corporation
7271 51st Boulevard
Milwaukee, WI 53223
(800) 896-1334 or (414) 357-8182
FAX: (414) 357-7814
URL: http://
www.computability.com

Cotrax Consumer Products Group
24027 Research Drive
Farmington Hills, MI 48335
(800) 521-1350 or (810) 442-0900
FAX: (810) 442-0922

C TECH
2 North Williams Street
P.O. Box 30

Pearl River, NY 10965-9998
(914) 735-7907 or (800) 228-7798
FAX: (914) 735-0513

Don Johnston Developmental Equipment
1000 North Rand Road, Building 115
P.O. Box 639
Wauconda, IL 60084
(847) 526-2682 or (800) 999-4660
FAX: (847) 526-4177
E-mail: djde@aol.com

Dragon Systems, Inc.
320 Nevada Street
Newton, MA 02160
(617) 965-5200
FAX: (617) 527-0372
URL: http://www.dragons.com

Echo
6460 Via Real
Carpinteria, CA 93013
(805) 684-4593

Edmark
P.O. Box 97021
Redmund, WA 98052
(800) 426-0856

Electronic Learning Systems
5200 N.W. 43rd Street
Gainesville, FL 32606
(800) 443-7971
FAX: (352) 375-5679
E-mail: elstech@elsin.com

Electronic Visual Aid Specialists
P.O. Box 371
Westerly, RI 02891
(800) 872-3827 or (401) 596-3155
FAX: (401) 596-3979
URL: http://www.evas.com

Enabling Technologies Company
3102 S.E. Jay Street

Stuart, FL 34997
(407) 283-4817
FAX: (407) 220-2920

First Byte Inc.
19840 Pioneer Avenue
Torrance, CA 90503-1660
(310) 793-0610
FAX: (310) 793-0606
URL: http://www.davd.com

Health Science
418 Wall Street
Princeton, NJ 08540
(800) 841-8923 or (609) 924-7616

Henter-Joyce, Inc.
2100 62nd Avenue North
St. Petersburg, FL 33702
(800) 336-5658 or (813) 528-8900
FAX: (813) 528-8901
E-mail: info@hj.com
URL: http://www.hj.com

Hooleon Corporation
411 South 6th Street
Building B
Cottonwood, AZ 86326
(520) 634-7515
FAX: (520) 634-4620
E-mail: sales@hooleon.com

HumanWare, Inc.
6245 King Road
Loomis, CA 95650
(800) 722-3393 or (916) 652-7253
FAX: (916) 652-7296
E-mail: info@humanware.com
URL: http://
www.humanware.com

Hy-Tek Manufacturing CO.
1998 Bucktail Lane
Sugar Grove, IL 60554
(630) 466-7664
FAX: (630) 466-7678

IBM Special Needs Systems
11400 Burnet Road
Building 904/6 internal zip 9448
Austin, TX 78758
(800) 426-4832 or (512) 838-4598

**Innovative Rehabilitation
Technology**
1605 West El Camino Real
Mt. View, CA 94040
(415) 961-3161 (as of 8/1/97 area
code 415 becomes 650)

**Institute on Applied Technology
Children's Hospital of Boston**
300 Longwood Avenue
Boston, MA 02115
(617) 735-8391

IntelliTools
55 Leverom Court
Novato, CA 94949
(415) 382-5959
FAX: (415) 382-5950
E-mail: info@intellitools.com
URL: http://
www.intellitools.com

**Intex Micro Systems
Corporation**
P.O. Box 12310
Birmingham, MI 48012
(313) 540-7601

Kinetic Designs, Inc.
14231 Anatezka Lane S.E.
Olalla, WA 98359
(206) 857-7943

Kurzweil Educational Systems
411 Waverly Oaks Road
Waltham, MA 02154
(800) 894-5374 or (617) 893-8200
FAX: (617) 893-4157
E-mail: info@kurzweiledu.com
URL: http://http:/
www.kurzweiledu.com

Maxi-Aids
42 Executive Boulevard
P.O. Box 3209
Farmingdale, NY 11735
(800) 522-6294 or (516) 752-0521
FAX: (516) 752-0689
E-mail: sales@maxiaids.com
URL: http://www.lighthouse.org

OMS Development
1921 Highland Avenue
Wilmette, IL 60091
(708) 251-5787

Optelec
4 Lyberty Way
Westford, MA 01886
(508) 392-0707 or (800) 828-1056
FAX: (508) 692-6073
E-mail: optelec@optelec.com
URL: http://www.optelec.com

Personal Data Systems, Inc.
P.O. Box 1008
Campbell, CA 95009-1008
(408) 866-1126
FAX: (408) 866-1128

Personal Interface
3333 South Wadsworth
Lakewood, CO 80227
(303) 987-0557

Phillip Barton Vision Systems
3911 York Lane
Bowie, MD 20715
(301) 262-3665

Prodigy Products Company
1823 Oakmount Road
South Euclid, OH 44121
(216) 381-0500

R.C. Systems, Inc.
1609 England Avenue
Everett, WA 98203
(206) 355-3800

Reflection Technology
230 Second Avenue
Waltham, MA 02154
(617) 890-5905, ext. 235
FAX: (617) 890-5918

Royal Data Systems
Speech and Learning Center
Systems
413 Highridge Drive
Morganton, NC 28655
(704) 433-5909

Schamex Research
19201 Parthenia Street, Suite H
Northridge, CA 91324
(818) 772-6644
FAX: (818) 993-2946

Science Products
P.O. Box 888
Southeastern, PA 19399
(800) 888-7400 or (800) 888-7401
FAX: (610) 296-0488

Scientific Capital Corporation
3235 Vishaal Drive
Orlando, FL 32817
(407) 275-8395
FAX: (407) 275-0142

Talking Computer Systems
12 Riverside Street
1-3
Watertown, MA 02172
(617) 926-1919

Talktronics, Inc.
27341 Eastridge Drive
El Toro, CA 92630
(716) 768-4220

Technologies for the Visually
Impaired, Inc.
9 Nolan Court
Hauppauge, NY 11788
(516) 724-4479
E-mail: tvii@concentric.com
URL: http://villagenet/~tvinc

TeleSensory Corporation
455 North Bernardo
P.O. Box 7455
Mountain View, CA 94039-7455
(800) 286-8484 or (415) 960-0920 (as
of 8/1/97 area code 415 becomes
650)
FAX: (415) 969-9064
URL: http://
www.telesensory.com

T.S. Microtech, Inc.
12565 Crenshaw Boulevard
Hawthorne, CA 90250
(800) 356-5906 or (213) 644-0859

Western Center for
Microcomputers
1259 El Camino Real
Suite 275
Menlo Park, CA 94025
(415) 326-6997 (as of 8/1/97 area
code 415 becomes 650)

Words Plus, Inc.
40015 Sierra Highway
Building B-145
Palmdale, CA 93550
(805) 266-8500

Xerox Imaging Systems
9 Centennial Drive
Peabody, MA 01960
(800) 248-6550
FAX: (508) 977-2148
E-mail: doiron@xis.xerox.com
URL: http://www.xerox. com

Zygo Industries, Inc.
P.O. Box 1008
Portland, OR 97207
(800) 234-6006 or (503) 684-6006
FAX: (503) 684-6011

◆ *Computer*
Software

Includes adaptive software such
as large-print and synthetic-
speech programs, braille
translation software, and
educational software and
computer tutorial programs.

Access-Ability Systems
P.O. Box 97
Wilmette, IL 60091
(708) 251-5787

Adaptec Systems
6909 Rufus Drive
Austin, TX 78752-3123
(512) 451-1717
E-mail: tecraig@bga.com

Ai Squared
P.O. Box 669
Manchester Center, VT 05225-0669
(802) 362-3612
FAX: (802) 362-1670
E-mail: zoomtext@aisquared.com

Alva Access
5801 Christie Avenue
Suite 475
Emeryville, CA 94608
(510) 923-6280
FAX: (510) 923-6270
E-mail: info@aagi.com

American Printing House for the
Blind
P.O. Box 6085, Department 0086
Louisville, KY 40206-0085
(502) 895-2405 or (800) 223-1839

Andromina, Inc.
326 East Mason Avenue
Alexandria, VA 22301
(703) 549-3214

Apple Computer, Inc.
20525 Marianni Avenue
Cupertino, CA 95014
(800) 776-2333 or (408) 996-1010

Apple Talk
3015 South Tyler Street
Little Rock, AR 72204
(813) 595-7890

Aquarius Instructional
P.O. Box 128
Indiana Rocks Beach, FL 34635
(813) 595-7890
FAX: (813) 595-2685

Aristo Computer, Inc.
6700 S.W. 105th Avenue
Suite 307
Beaverton, OR 97005
(800) 327-4786 or (503) 626-6333

Arkenstone, Inc.
555 Oakmead Parkway
Sunnyvale, CA 94086
(408) 245-5900 or (800) 444-4443
FAX: (408) 745-6739
URL: http://www.arkenstone.org

Artic Technologies
55 Park Street
Suite 2
Troy, MI 48083-2753
(810) 588-7370 or (800) 588-1425
FAX: (810) 588-2650

Arts Computer Products, Inc.
145 Tremont Street
Suite 407
Boston, MA 02111
(617) 482-8248

Automagic Corporation
195 South Beverly Drive
Suite 406
Beverly Hills, CA 90212
(213) 552-2101

Automated Functions, Inc.
7700 Leesburg Pike
Suite 420

Falls Church, VA 22043
(703) 883-9797
FAX: (703) 883-9798
E-mail: autofunc@tmn.com

Blazie Engineering
105 East Jerrettsville Road
Forest Hill, MD 21050
(410) 893-9333
FAX: (410) 836-5040
URL: http://www.blazie.com

Bobcat Computer Applications
5200 West 68
Shawnee Mission, KS 66208
(913) 262-7440

Borland International
1700 Green Hills Road
Scotts Valley, CA 95066-0001
(408) 438-8400

Boston Educational Computing, Inc.
78 Dartmouth Street
Department R
Boston, MA 02116
(617) 536-5116

Braille Sterling Christiansen Studios
P.O. Box 583
Hanover, NH 03755
(603) 448-6166

Castle Special Computer Services
9801 San Gabriel, N.E.
Albuquerque, NM 87111
(505) 293-8379

Comp Tech Systems Design
P.O. Box 107
Waconia, MN 55387
(612) 442-9776

ComputAbility Corporation
7271 N. 51st Boulevard

Milwaukee, WI 53223
(800) 896-1334 or (414) 357-8182

Cornucopia Software, Inc.
P.O. Box 6111
Albany, CA 94706
(415) 528-7000 (as of 8/1/97 area
code 415 becomes 650)

Cross Educational Software
504 East Kentucky
Ruston, LA 71270
(318) 255-8921

Data Transforms
616 Washington Street
Denver, CO 80203
(303) 832-1501

Digital Equipment Corporation
P.O. Box 9501
Merrimac, NH 03054
(800) 344-4825
FAX: (800) 234-2298

Don Johnston Developmental Equipment
1000 North Rand Road, Building 115
P.O. Box 639
Wauconda, IL 60084
(847) 526-2682 or (800) 999-4660
FAX: (847) 526-4177
E-mail: djde@aol.com

Dunamis, Inc.
3620 Highway 317
Suwanee, GA 30174
(800) 828-2443

Duxbury Systems, Inc.
435 King Street
P.O. Box 1504
Littleton, MA 01460
(508) 486-9766
FAX: (508) 486-9712

Electronic Learning Systems
5200 N.W. 43rd Street
Suite 102-323
Gainesville, FL 32606
(800) 443-7971
FAX: (352) 375-5679
E-mail: elstech@elsin.com

Enabling Technologies Company
3102 S.E. Jay Street
Stuart, FL 34997
(407) 283-4817
FAX: (407) 220-2920

E.V.A.S.
16 David Avenue
P.O. Box 371
Westerly, RI 02891
(800) 872-3827 or (401) 596-3155
FAX: (401) 596-3979
URL: http://www.evas.com

Exceptional Teaching Aids
20102 Woodbine Avenue
Castro Valley, CA 94546
(510) 582-4859 or (800) 549-6999
FAX: (510) 582-5911

FDLRS
5555 S.W. 93rd Avenue
Miami, FL 33165
(305) 274-3501

First Byte Inc.
19840 Pioneer Avenue
Torrance, CA 90503-1660
(310) 793-0610
FAX: (310) 793-0606
URL: http://www.davd.com

Flexible Software
Laird Communications
P.O. Box 334
Manchester, MA 01944
(508) 526-7490

GW Micro
725 Airport North Office Park

Ft. Wayne, IN 46825
(219) 489-3671
FAX: (219) 482-2492
URL: http://www.gwmicro.com

Harbor Computing Services
P.O. Box 2181
Gig Harbor, WA 98355
(206) 858-9459

Hartley Courseware, Inc.
9920 Pacific Heights Boulevard
Suite 500
San Diego, CA 92121
(800) 247-1380
FAX: (619) 622-7873
URL: http://www.jlc.com

Henter-Joyce, Inc.
2100 62nd Avenue North
St. Petersburg, FL 33702
(800) 336-5658 or (813) 528-8900
FAX: (813) 528-8901
E-mail: info@hj.com
URL: http://www.hj.com

Hexagon Products
P.O. Box 1295
Park Ridge, IL 60068-7295
(847) 692-3355
E-mail: 76064.1776@compuserve.com
URL: http://ourworld.compuserve.com/homepages/hexaxon

HFK Software, Inc.
68 Wells Road
Lincoln, MA 01773
(617) 259-0059

HumanWare, Inc.
6245 King Road
Loomis, CA 95650
(800) 722-3393 or (916) 652-7253
FAX: (916) 652-7296
E-mail: info@humanware.com
URL: http://www.humanware.com

IBM Special Needs Systems
11400 Burnett Road
Building 904/6 Internal Zip 9448
Austin, TX 78758
(800) 426-2133 or (512) 838-4598

Innovative Rehabilitation Technology
1605 West El Camino Real
Mt. View, CA 94040
(415) 961-3161 (as of 8/1/97 area cod 415 becomes 650)

Intelligent Info Technologies Corporation
P.O. Box 5002, Station A
Champaign, IL 61801
(217) 359-7933

Interface Systems International
P.O. Box 20415
Portland, OR 97220
(503) 665-0965

Kidsview Software, Inc.
P.O. Box 98
Warner, NH 03278
(603) 927-4428

Kinetic Designs, Inc.
14231 Anatezka Lane S.E.
Olalla, WA 98359
(206) 857-7943

Laureate Learning Systems, Inc.
110 East Spring Street
Winooski, VT 05404-1837
(800) 562-6801 or (802) 655-4755

Life Science Associates
One Fennimore Road
Bayport, NY 11705
(516) 472-2111

Lorin Software
1106 Summit Pointe Way
Atlanta, GA 30329
(407) 872-3245

Marblesoft
21805 Zumbrota, N.E.
Cedar, MN 55011
(612) 434-3704

Microsystems Software, Inc.
600 Worcester Road
Suite 5A
Framingham, MA 01701-5342
(508) 879-9000
FAX: (508) 879-1069
URL: http://www.microsys.com

MicroTalk Software
721 Olive Street
Texarkana, TX 75501
(903) 792-2570
FAX: (903) 792-5140
URL: http://
www.screenaccess.com

Mirage Multimedia Systems, Inc.
4286 Lincoln Boulevard
Marina del Rey, CA 90292
(800) 228-3349 or (310) 649-9199
FAX: (310) 649-9177

Myna Corporation
239 Western Avenue
Essex, MA 01929
(800) 370-6962 or (508) 768-9000
FAX: (508) 768-9911
E-mail: mynacorporation@aol.com

**National Institute for
Rehabilitation Engineering**
Drawer T
Hewitt, NJ 07421
(201) 853-6585

Omnichron
1438 Oxford Avenue
Berkeley, CA 94709
(510) 540-6455

OMS Development
1921 Highland Avenue
Wilmette, IL 60091
(708) 251-5787

One on One Computer Training
2055 Army Trail Road
Suite 100
Addison, IL 60101
(800) 222-3547 or (708) 790-1117

Optelec
4 Lyberty Way
Westford, MA 01886
(508) 392-0707 or (800) 828-1056
FAX: (508) 692-6073
E-mail: optelec@optelec.com
URL: http://www.optelec.com

PC-SIG
1030D East Duane Avenue
Sunnyvale, CA 94086
(408) 730-9291

Peal Software, Inc.
5000 North Parkway Calabasas
Suite 105
Calabasas, CA 91302
(818) 883-7849

Peripheral Technologies, Inc.
1109 Hilcrest Road
Narberth, PA 19072
(215) 667-2190

Personal Interface
3333 South Wadsworth
Lakewood, CO 80227
(303) 987-0557

Phillip Barton Vision Systems
3911 York Lane
Bowie, MD 20715
(301) 262-3665

**Productivity Software
International**
211 East 43rd Street
Suite 2202
New York, NY 10017-4707
(212) 818-1144

The Productivity Works
7 Belmont Circle
Trenton, NJ 08618
(609) 984-8044
FAX: (609) 984-8048
E-mail: info@prodworks.com
URL: http://
www.prodworks.com

Raised Dot Computing, Inc.
408 South Baldwin Street
Madison, WI 53703
(608) 257-9595 or (608) 241-2498
FAX: (608) 257-4143
URL: http://www.well.com/
www/dnavy

R.C. Systems, Inc.
1609 England Avenue
Everett, WA 98203
(206) 355-3800

Replogle Globes, Inc.
2801 South 25th Avenue
Broadview, IL 60153
(708) 343-0900 or (708) 343-0923

Roundley Associates
P.O. Box 608
Owings Mills, MD 21117
(800) 333-7049

**Royal Data Systems
Speech and Learning Center
Systems**
413 Highridge Drive
Morganton, NC 28655
(704) 433-5909

Scholastic, Inc.
2931 East McCarty Street
P.O. Box 7501
Jefferson City, MO 65102
(800) 325-6149 or (800) 392-2179

Seemore Vision Products
42 Executive Boulevard

Farmingdale, NY 11735
(800) 462-3738
FAX: (516) 752-0687

SkiSoft, Inc.
1644 Massachusetts Avenue
Suite 79
Lexingotn, MA 02173
(617) 863-1876
E-mail: info@skisoft.com
URL: http://www.skisoft.com

Soft Key International
6160 Summit Drive
Minneapolis, MN 55430
(612) 569-1500

Spies Laboratories
4040 Spencer Street
Suite Q
Torrance, CA 90503
(213) 538-8166

Stat Talk Computer Products
285 Hardenburgh Avenue
Demerest, NJ 07267
(201) 581-8291

Syn-Talk Systems and Services
70 Estero Avenue
San Francisco, CA 94127
(415) 334-0586

Talking and Visual Aids
8136 Appoline
Detroit, MI 48228
(313) 935-1266
E-mail: leeghume@aol.com

Talking Computer Products
P.O. Box 142
Wallace, KS 67761
(913) 891-3532

Talking Computers, Inc.
140 Little Falls Street
Suite 208

Falls Church, VA 22046
(800) 485-6338 or (703) 241-8224

Talking Computer Systems
12 Riverside Street
1-3
Watertown, MA 02172
(617) 926-1919

Tandy/Radio Shack
1800 One Tandy Center
Fort Worth, TX 76102
(817) 390-3011

Technologies for the Visually Impaired, Inc.
9 Nolan Court
Hauppauge, NY 11788
(516) 724-4479

TeleSensory Corporation
455 North Bernardo
P.O. Box 7455
Mountain View, CA 94039-7455
(800) 286-8484
FAX: (415) 969-9064 (as of 8/1/97 area code 415 becomes 650)
URL: http://www.telesensory.com

Texas Instruments
P.O. Box 53
Lubbock, TX 79408
(800) 842-2737

T.F.I. Engineering, Inc.
529 Main Street
Boston, MA 02129
(617) 242-7007

Traxler Enterprises
6504 West Girard Avenue
Milwaukee, WI 53210
(414) 445-5925

Turbo Power
P.O. Box 49009

Colorado Springs, CO 80949-9009
(719) 260-6641

The Voice Connection
17835 Skypark Circle
Suite C
Irvine, CA 92714
(714) 261-2366

Worthington Data Solutions
3004 Mission Street
Santa Cruz, CA 95060
(408) 458-9938

◆ Braille and Other Literacy Materials

Includes such products as slates and styli, braille computer paper and other braille accessories, braille typewriters, and tactile materials and kits.

Advanced Access Devices
2066-C Walsh Avenue
Santa Clara, CA 95050
(408) 970-9760
FAX: (408) 727-9351
E-mail: aadbrl@aol.com

American Printing House for the Blind
P.O. Box 6085, Department 0086
Louisville, KY 40206-0085
(502) 895-2405 or (800) 223-1839
FAX: (502) 895-1509

American Thermoform Corporation
2311 Travers Avenue
City of Commerce, CA 90040
(213) 723-9021
FAX: (213) 728-8877

Esselte Pendaflex Corporation
71 Clinton Road
Garden City, NY 11530
(516) 741-3200

Fishburne Enterprises
140 E. Stetson Avenue
#319
Hemet, CA 92543
(909) 765-9276
FAX: (909) 766-0843

General Electric
G.E. Appliance Park
Building 6
Room 106
Louisville, KY 40225
(502) 452-4311 or (502) 452-5691
FAX: (502) 452-0213

Howe Press of Perkins School for the Blind
175 North Beacon Street
Watertown, MA 02172
(617) 924-3490

HumanWare, Inc.
6245 King Road
Loomis, CA 95650
(800) 722-3393 or (916) 652-7253
FAX: (916) 652-7296
E-mail: info@humanware.com
URL: http://
www.humanware.com

Learning Express
8029 Danwood
Little Rock, AR 72204
(501) 565-8208

Mattel Consumer Affairs Mattel Toys
333 Continental Boulevard
El Segundo, CA 90245
(310) 252-2000

Mid-Michigan Center for the Blind
3200 South Pennsylvania Avenue

Lansing, MI 48910
(517) 887-6646

National Federation of the Blind
1800 Johnson Street
Baltimore, MD 21230
(410) 659-9314
FAX: (410) 685-5653

Rose Resnick Lighthouse for the Blind and Visually Impaired
214 Van Ness Avenue
San Francisco, CA 94102
(415) 431-1481

Sighted Electronics
464 Tappan Raod
Northvale, NJ 07647
(201) 767-3977
FAX: (201) 767-0612
E-mail: sighted@village.ios.com

◆ *Medical Products*

Includes such products as talking blood glucose monitors and blood pressure meters, syringes, and medical alert systems.

American Medical Alert Corporation
3265 Lawson Boulevard
Oceanside, NY 11572
(800) 645-3244 or (516) 536-5850

Andros Analyzers, Inc.
2332 Fourth Street
Berkeley, CA 94710
(415) 849-5700

Becton-Dickinson
1 Beckton Drive
Franklin Lakes, NJ 07417
(201) 847-6800

Bentham International
4291 N.W. 18th Street
Suite P-104
Lauderhill, FL 33313
(305) 485-6629

Boehringer Mannheim Diagnostics
9115 Hague Road
Indianapolis, IN 46250-0100
(800) 858-8072

Conney Safety Products
P.O. Box 44190
Madison, WI 53744-0190
(800) 356-9100 or (800) 362-9150

Home Diagnostics, Inc.
2300 North West 55th Court
Fort Lauderdale, FL 33309
(800) 342-7226

Independent Living Aids, Inc.
27 East Mall
Plainview, NY 11803
(800) 537-2118 or (516) 752-8080

LS&S Group, Inc.
P.O. Box 673
Northbrook, IL 60065
(800) 468-4789 or (847) 498-9777
FAX: (847) 498-1482
E-mail: lsgrp@aol.com
URL: http://lssgroup.com

Medical Monitoring System, Inc.
2070 Helena Street
Madison, WI 53704
(608) 241-2341

National Federation of the Blind
1800 Johnson Street
Baltimore, MD 21230
(410) 659-9314
FAX: (410) 685-5653

Palco Labs
830 Soquel Avenue

Santa Cruz, CA 95062
(408) 476-3151

**Sears, Roebuck and Company
New Account Center**
3000-A North Mall Road
Knoxville, TN 37924
(800) 323-3274 or (423) 521-3700

Tandy/Radio Shack
1800 One Tandy Center
Fort Worth, TX 76102
(817) 390-3011

◆ Products for Deaf-Blind/ Multiply Disabled Persons

Includes such products as vibratory alert systems and amplification and communication systems.

Beltone Hearing Aid Service
71 Park Avenue
West Springfield, MA 01089
(413) 733-3196

Canon, U.S.A., Inc.
One Canon Plaza
Lake Success, NY 11042-9979
(516) 488-6700

Comp Tech Systems Design
P.O. Box 107
Waconia, MN 55387
(612) 442-9776

Digital Equipment Corporation
MK01-2/89
P.O. Box 9501
Merrimac, NH 03054
(800) 344-4825
FAX: (800) 234-2298

Don Johnston Developmental Equipment
1000 North Rand Road
Building 115
P.O. Box 639
Wauconda, IL 60084
(847) 526-2682 or (800) 999-4660
FAX: (847) 526-4177
E-mail: djde@aol.com

Dunamis, Inc.
3620 Highway 317
Suwanee, GA 30174
(800) 828-2443

**Enable
Schneier Communication Unit**
1603 Court Street
Syracuse, NY 13208
(315) 455-7591

Fotofonics
315 Larkspur Turn
Peachtree City, GA 30269
(404) 487-5854

Fred Sammons, Inc.
P.O. Box 5071
Bolingbrook, IL 60440
(800) 323-5547
FAX: (800) 547-4333
URL: http://
www.samonspreston.com

Haskill Hearing Aid Center
255 Main Street
Hackensack, NJ 07601
(201) 342-7947

Health Science
418 Wall Street
Princeton, NJ 08540
(609) 924-7616 or (800) 841-8923

Helen Keller National Center for Deaf-Blind Youths and Adults
111 Middle Neck Road
Sands Point, NY 11050
(516) 944-8900

Hitec Special Needs Center
8160 Madison
Burr Ridge, IL 60521
(630) 654-9200
URL: http://www.hitec.com

Hy-Tek Manufacturing Company, Inc.
1998 Bucktail Lane
Sugar Grove, IL 60554
(630) 466-7664
FAX: (630) 466-7678

Independent Living Aids, Inc.
27 East Mall
Plainview, NY 11803
(800) 537-2118 or (516) 752-8080
FAX: (516) 752-3135

IntelliTools
55 Leverom Court 9
Novato, CA 94949
(415) 382-5959
FAX: (415) 382-5950
E-mail: info@intellitools.com
URL: http://
www.intellitools.com

Lucent/ACPC
14250 Clayton Road
Town and Country, MO 63017
(800) 233-1222
FAX: (314) 891-7896

Luminaud, Inc.
8688 Tyler Boulevard
Mentor, OH 44060
(216) 255-9082

Maddak, Inc.
Bel-Art Products Subsidiary
6 Industrial Road
Pequannock, NJ 07440-1993
(201) 628-7600, ext. 9
FAX: (201) 305-0841
E-mail: cservice@maddak.com
URL: http://www.maddak.com

National Catalog House of the Deaf
4300 North Kilpatrick Avenue
Chicago, IL 60641
(312) 283-2907

Royal Data Systems
Speech and Learning Center Systems
413 Highridge Drive
Morganton, NC 28655
(704) 433-5909

Science Applications International Corporation
200 Harry S. Truman Parkway
Suite 400
Annapolis, MD 21401
(301) 266-0994 or (301) 261-8424

Sonic Alert
1750 West Hamlin Road
Rochester Hills, MI 48309
(313) 656-3110

Texas Instruments
P.O. Box 53
Lubbock, TX 79408
(800) 842-2737

Words Plus, Inc.
40015 Sierra Highway
Building B-145
Palmdale, CA 93550
(805) 266-8500

Zygo Industries, Inc.
P.O. Box 1008
Portland, OR 97207
(800) 234-6006 or (503) 684-6006
FAX: (503) 684-6011

◆ Audible and Tactile Signs and Detectable Warning Surfaces

Includes such products as braille and raised-letter signs and detectable warning tiles, intended to provide access to information about the environment.

Accessories Plus
7717 North Kenton
Skokie, IL 60076
(708) 674-7717

AccuBraille
30 Cleveland Street
San Francisco, CA 94103
(415) 863-8450
FAX: (415) 863-9659

Advance Corporation
327 East York Avenue
St. Paul, MN 55101
(612) 771-9297

Advantage Metal Systems, Inc.
685 Oak Street, #13-1
Brockton, MA 02401
(617) 297-7117
FAX: (617) 344-0912

American Olean Tile Company
1000 Cannon Avenue
P.O. Box 271
Lansdale, PA 19446-0271
(215) 855-1111
FAX: (215) 362-6050

Balcon, Inc.
2630 Conway Road
P.O. Box 3388
Crofton, MD 21114
(410) 721-1900 or (410) 793-0657

Best Manufacturing Company
1202 North Park Avenue
Montrose, CO 81401-3170
(800) 235-2378 or (800) 432-2378

Bomanite Corporation
232 South Schnoor Avenue
Madera, CA 93636
(800) 854-2094
FAX: (209) 673-2411

Carsonite International
1301 Hot Springs Road
Carson City, NV 89701
(800) 648-7974
FAX: (701) 883-0525

Castek, Inc.
Transpo Industries, Inc.
20 Jones Street
New Rochelle, NY 10801-6024
(800) 321-7870 or (914) 636-1000
FAX: (914) 636-1282

Crossville Ceramics
Cumberland County Industrial Park
Crossville, TN 38555
(615) 484-2110
FAX: (615) 484-8418

CT Concrete Company
394 Whitehall Street
Allentown, PA 18104
(215) 433-2757

Diversified Enterprises International
5584 Willow Highway
Grand Ledge, MI 48837
(517) 627-3137

Emed Company, Inc.
330 Greene Street
P.O. Box 369
Buffalo, NY 13208
(716) 891-4434

Engineered Plastics, Inc.
300 Pearl Street
Suite 200
Buffalo, NY 14202
(717) 642-6049
FAX: (717) 842-6039

**G.A.L. Manufacturing
Corporation**
50 East 153rd Street
Bronx, NY 10451
(212) 292-9000

SCS
547 West County Road
Shoreview, MN 55126
(612) 483-4600

**Stampcrete Decorative
Concrete, Inc.**
17 Blackwood Drive
Liverpool, NY 13090
(315) 451-2837
FAX: (315) 451-2290

Summitville Tiles, Inc.
P.O. Box 644
Summitville, OH 43962
(216) 223-1511
FAX: (216) 223-1414

Suprarock Block Company
3301 27th Avenue North
P.O. Box 5326
Birmingham, AL 35207
(205) 324-8624
FAX: (205) 324-8671

Traconex, Inc.
3510 Basset Stret
Santa Clara, CA 95054
(408) 727-0260

**Truxes Company
Signage Division**
16 Stone Hill
Oswego, IL 60543
(708) 554-8448

Universal Engraving, Inc.
9090 Neiman Road
Overland Park, KS 66214
(913) 599-0600

CANADA
PRODUCERS AND PUBLISHERS OF BRAILLE AND OTHER ALTERNATE MEDIA SOURCES OF ADAPTED PRODUCTS AND DEVICES

PRODUCERS OF ALTERNATE MEDIA

♦ *Media Producers and Publishers*

Audio Studio for the Reading Impaired
P.O. Box 23043
Anchorage, KY 40223
(502) 245-5422
Robert J. Knoll, Chairman
Sandra Koukola, Director

County/District Where Located:
Jefferson County.

See Audio Studio for the Reading Impaired in U.S. national listings.

Blindskills
P.O. Box 5181
Salem, OR 97304
(503) 581-4224
FAX: (503) 581-0178
E-mail: blindskl@teleport.com
Carol M. McCarl, Editor

County/District Where Located:
Marion County.

See Blindskills in U.S. national listings.

Books Aloud
180 West San Carlos
San Jose, CA 95113-2096
(408) 277-4878

County/District Where Located:
Santa Clara County.

See Books Aloud in U.S. national listings.

Braille International
3142 S.E. Jay Street
Stuart, FL 34997
(407) 286-8366 or (800) 336-3142
FAX: (407) 286-8909
Jeri Brubaker

See Braille International in U.S. national listings.

Christian Blind Mission International
P.O. Box 800
Stouffville, ON L4A 7Z9
(905) 640-6464, ext. 230
FAX: (905) 640-4332
E-mail: 10200.3725@compusgrve. com

County/District Where Located:
Ontario.
Mission: Provides Christian tapes to people in Canada.

Talking Book Library.

Christian Mission for the Blind
5354 Boy Scout Road
Indianapolis, IN 46226
(317) 549-2386
FAX: (317) 549-2386
William B. Schalk, Executive Director

County/District Where Located:
Marion County.

See Christian Mission for the Blind in U.S. national listings.

Christian Record Services
1300 King Street
Suite 119
Oshawa, ON L1H 8N9
(905) 436-6938
FAX: (905) 436-7102
Pat Page, Executive Director

Mission: Provides braille, large-print, and audiotape materials for legally blind and hearing impaired persons. Operates an extensive free lending library and a national camp program.

Church of Jesus Christ of Latter-Day Saints Special Curriculum
50 East North Temple
Floor 24
Salt Lake City, UT 84150
(801) 240-2477
FAX: (801) 240-5732
E-mail: hinddl@chq.byu.edu
Douglas L. Hind, Special Curriculum Manager

See Church of Jesus Christ of Latter-Day Saints in U.S. national listings.

Cleveland Sight Center of the Cleveland Society for the Blind
1909 East 101st Street
Cleveland, OH 44106
(216) 791-8118
FAX: (216) 791-1101
Alice Miller, Coordinator, Taping Services
Marlene Smith, Coordinator, Braille and Large-Print Transcription Services

See Cleveland Sight Center of the Cleveland Society for the Blind in U.S. national listings.

Crane Resource Centre University of British Columbia
1874 East Mall
Vancouver, BC V6T 1Z1
(604) 822-6111
FAX: (604) 822-6113
E-mail: crane@unixg.ubc.ca
URL: http://www.library. ubc.ca
Paul E. Thiele, Director

Area Served: Local, national and international.
Groups Served: Blind, visually impaired, physically disabled, and print disabled persons requiring alternatives to print.

Types/Content: University texts; support, reference, and materials; general literature; Canadiana; support materials for teachers of blind students.

Media Formats: Braille, talking books, large-type, computer disks, regular print.
Title Listings: Approximately 60,000 titles.
Contract braille and audio book production; inter-library/agency resource sharing; technology training; academic support services; coping techniques for vision and print impaired students; liason with instructors, employers; reference collection in braille, audiobook and large print;

Eyes of Faith Ministries
P.O. Box 743336
Dallas, TX 75374-3336
(214) 669-1103
Gayle Gould, Administrator and Braille Coordinator

See Eyes of Faith Ministries in U.S. national listings.

Gospel Association for the Blind
P.O. Box 62
Delray Beach, FL 33447
(407) 274-9700
Rev. Ralph Montanus, Jr., President

County/District Where Located: Palm Beach County.

See Gospel Association for the Blind in U.S. national listings.

I Can See Books
88 Captain Morgan Boulevard
Nanaimo, BC V9R 6R1
(250) 753-3096

Mission: Publishes tactile reading-readiness books and children's books with clear plastic braille pages inserted in the text and includes detailed picture descriptions.

Institut Nazareth et Louis-Braille
1111 St. Charles West

Longueuil, PQ J4K 5G4
(514) 463-1710
FAX: (514) 463-0243
E-mail: phbuteau@login.net
Paul-Henri Buteau, Coordinateur

Area Served: Canada and USA.
Groups Served: All ages, French speaking.

Types/Content: Textbooks, cultural materials, general information documents, adapted materials.
Media Formats: Hard copy (braille), thermoform, tactile material.
Title Listings: More than 400 titles.
Braille production of textbooks and literary material; production of graphics and other adopted material.

Library for the Blind
Canadian National Institute for the Blind
1929 Bayview Avenue
Toronto, ON M4G 3E8
(416) 480-7520
FAX: (416) 480-7700
Rosemary Kavanagh, Executive Director
Victora Owen, Director, Library Services
Ellen Stroud, Manager

Type of Agency: Non-profit.
Mission: To ensure that blind and print disabled Canadians have equitable access to information, culture, education, and life-long learning.
Funded by: Donations; reader assessment fee charged to geographic divisions of CNIB; sales; and fees for service.
Budget: $5 million.
Hours of Operation: Mon.-Fri. 8:00 AM-5:00 PM.
Staff: 82 and 500 volunteers.
History/Date: Founded in 1906.

Number of Clients Served: More than 17,000 registered users; more than 400 agencies.
Eligibility: Blind and visually impaired Canadians registered with CNIB. Blind persons whose visual acuity, as determined by competent authority, is 20/200 or less in the better eye with corrective lenses, or whose widest diameter of visual field subtends an anular distance no greater than 20 degrees.
Area Served: National.

Educational: Transcribes textbooks.
Reading: Transcribes books of various kinds into alternative formats. Operates an audiotape and braille lending library and reference service. Collects braille, audio, descriptive video and electronic texts.
Publications: Catalog; *Off the Shelf* newsletter; *Wordsworthy*, client newsletter.

Lutheran Library for the Blind
1333 South Kirkwood Road
St. Louis, MO 63122
(314) 965-9000, ext. 1322 or
(800) 433-3954
FAX: (314) 965-0959
Lynne Borchelt, Assistant

See Lutheran Library for the Blind in U.S. national listings.

Monterey County Braille Transcribers
P.O. Box DF
Pacific Grove, CA 93950
(408) 372-2944
Margaret Parenti, Coordinator

County/District Where Located: Monterey County.

See Monterey County Braille Transcribers in U.S. national listings.

Multi-Lingual Braille and Large Print Association

146 Colborne Street
Brantford, ON N3T 2G6
(519) 758-8509
FAX: (519) 753-8397
URL: http://gwdgraphics.com/braille
Janice Buckley, CEO

County/District Where Located: Brant County.
Area Served: Unlimited.
Groups Served: Adults and children.

Types/Content: All types.
Media Formats: Braille and large print.

National Braille Association

Three Townline Circle
Rochester, NY 14623-2513
(716) 427-8260
FAX: (716) 427-0263
Angela Coffaro, Executive Director

County/District Where Located: Monroe County.

See National Braille Association in U.S. national listings.

National Braille Press

88 St. Stephen Street
Boston, MA 02115
(617) 266-6160 or (800) 548-7323
E-mail: orders@nbp.org

See National Braille Press in U.S. national listings.

PAL Reading Services

252 Bloor Street West
Suite 5-105
Toronto, ON M5S 1V5
(416) 960-1177
E-mail: pal.radio@utoronto.ca
Valerie Veinotte, Coordinator

Area Served: Canada.
Groups Served: Persons who are print handicapped: blind, low vision, learning disabled.

Media Formats: 2-track and 4-track audio cassette; computer disk from scanned material.

People Helping People

151 Colborne Street
Brantford, ON N3T 2G7
(519) 753-1362
Claire Jesney, General Manager

Area Served: Unlimited.
Groups Served: Adults and children.

Types/Content: All types.
Media Formats: Talking books.

Prose & Cons Braille Unit

P.O. Box 2500
Lincoln, NE 68542-2500
(402) 471-3161, ext. 3373
FAX: (402) 471-3472
Dominic Inzodda, Shop Operator

County/District Where Located: Lancaster County.

See Prose & Cons Braille Unit in U.S. national listings.

Recording for the Blind and Dyslexic

20 Roszel Road
Princeton, NJ 08540
(609) 452-0606 or (800) 221-4792
FAX: (609) 987-8116
E-mail: info@rfbd.org
URL: http://http//www.rfbd.org
Ritchie L. Geisel, President and CEO

See Recording for the Blind and Dyslexic in U.S. national listings.

VoicePrint
The National Broadcast Reading Service, Inc.

150 Laird Drive Annex
Toronto, ON M4G 3V7
(416) 422-4222
FAX: (416) 422-5430
E-mail: nbrs@idirect.com
Heather Lusignan, Director

Hours of Operation: 24 hours per day.
History/Date: Est. 1990.
Area Served: Broadcast via cable-TV to 5 million homes across Canada.

Broadcasts published news in audio format.

Volunteers of Vacaville

P.O. Box 670
Vacaville, CA 95696
(707) 448-6841
Steve Norris, Coordinator

See Volunteers of Vacaville in U.S. national listings.

Volunteer Transcribing Services

205 East Third Avenue
Suite 200
San Mateo, CA 94401
(415) 344-8664
Alanah Hoffman, Director

See Volunteer Transcribing Services in U.S. national listings.

Xavier Society for the Blind

154 East 23rd Street
New York, NY 10010
(212) 473-7800 or (800) 945-5565
FAX: (212) 888-4183
Rev. Alfred Caruana, S. J., Director

See Xavier Society for the Blind in U.S. national listings.

♦ *Audiodescription Services*

Audio Vision Canada
The National Broadcast Reading Service, Inc.
150 Laird Drive Annex

Toronto, ON M4G 3V7
(416) 422-4222
FAX: (416) 422-1633
E-mail: nbrs@idirect.com
Marc Rosen, Director

Type of Agency: Audio
description center.
Hours of Operation: Mon.-Fri.
9:00AM-5:00PM.
History/Date: Est. 1995.

SOURCES OF PRODUCTS

◆ Mail Order, Catalogs, and Distributors

Includes organizations and companies that carry a wide variety of products, including independent living, health care, and recreation products; low vision devices; and communication aids. Products can usually be ordered by catalog, which can be obtained from the individual companies listed.

Microcomputer Science Centre, Inc.
88 General Road
Unit 6
Mississauga, ON L4W 1Z8
(905) 629-1654
FAX: (905) 629-2321
E-mail: microsci@ican.net
URL: http://home.ican.net/~microsci

◆ Household, Personal, and Independent Living Products

Includes such products as kitchen utensils and measuring devices; canes; talking clocks, scales, and calculators; games and toys; and braille watches.

AmbuTech

Melet Plastics, Inc.
34 DeBaets Street
Winnipeg, ON R2J 3S9
(204) 663-3340
FAX: (204) 663-9345

Canadian National Institute for the Blind
1929 Bayview Avenue
Toronto, ON M4G 3E8
(416) 480-7594

◆ Low Vision

Includes such products as magnifiers, loupes, lamps, and closed-circuit televisions; encompasses optical and nonoptical devices, both electronic and nonelectronic.

Acrontech
2 Thorncliffe Park Drive
Unit 32
Toronto, ON M4H 1H2
(416) 467-6800
FAX: (416) 467-1994
E-mail: info@acrontech.com
URL: http://www.acrontech.com

Microcomputer Science Centre, Inc.
88 General Road
Unit 6
Mississauga, ON L4W 1Z8
(905) 629-1654
FAX: (905) 629-2321
E-mail: microsci@ican.net
URL: http://home.ican.net/~microsci

Octopus Audio Visual
P.O. Box 1120
Berry's Bay, ON K0J 1B0
(613) 756-3938
FAX: (613) 756-2560

◆ Computer Hardware

Includes adaptive equipment such as laptop computers, braille displays, key caps, braille embossers, and optical character recognition systems.

Acrontech
2 Thorncliffe Park Drive
Unit 32
Toronto, ON M4H 1H2
(416) 467-6800 or (800) 245-2020
FAX: (416) 467-1994
E-mail: info@acrontech.com
URL: http://www.acrontech.com

**Betacom Group
Montreal Betacom**
2670 Sabourin
St. Laurent, PQ H4S 1M2
(514) 332-7000
FAX: (514) 332-7500

**Betacom Group
Toronto Betacom**
2999 King Street West
Inglewood, ON L0N 1K0
(905) 838-1411
FAX: (905) 838-1487
E-mail: peter@betacom.com
URL: http://www.betacom.com

Canadian National Institute for the Blind
1929 Bayview Avenue
Toronto, ON M4G 3E8
(416) 480-7594

Frontier Computing
250 Davisville Avenue
Suite 205
Toronto, ON M4S 1H2
(416) 489-6690
FAX: (416) 489-6693

IBM
Special Needs Department
105 Moatfield
North York, ON M3B 3R1
(800) 426-4968 or (416) 383-5003
URL: http://www.can.ibm.com/specialneeds

Microcomputer Science Centre, Inc.
88 General Road
Unit 6
Mississauga, ON L4W 1Z8
(905) 629-1654
FAX: (905) 629-2321
E-mail: microsci@ican.net
URL: http://home.ican.net/~microsci

Octopus Audio Visual
P.O. Box 1120
Barry's Bay, ON K0J 1B0
(613) 756-3938
FAX: (613) 756-2560

Syntha-Voice Computers, Inc.
800 Queenstone Road
Suite 304
Stony Creek, ON L8G 1A7
(800) 263-4540 or (905) 662-0565 or
BBS (905) 662-0569
FAX: (905) 662-0568

Visualaide, Inc.
841 Jean-Paul-Vincent Boulevard
Longueuil, PQ J4G 1R3
(514) 463-1717
FAX: (514) 463-0243

♦ Computer Software

Includes adaptive software such as large-print and synthetic-speech programs, braille translation software, and educational software and computer tutorial programs.

Betacom Group
Montreal Betacom
2670 Sabourin
St. Laurent, PQ H4S 1M2
(514) 332-7000
FAX: (514) 332-7500

Betacom Group
Toronto Betacom
2999 King Street West
Inglewood, ON L0N 1K0
(905) 838-1411
FAX: (905) 838-1487
E-mail: peter@betacom.com
URL: http://www.betacom.com

Frontier Computing
250 Davisville Avenue
Suite 205
Toronto, ON M4S 1H2
(416) 489-6690
FAX: (416) 489-6693

Microcomputer Science Centre, Inc.
88 General Road
Unit 6
Mississauga, ON L4W 1Z8
(905) 629-1654
FAX: (905) 629-2321
E-mail: microsci@ican.net
URL: http://home.ican.net/~microsci

Syntha-Voice Computers, Inc.
800 Queenstone Road
Suite 304
Stony Creek, ON L8G 1A7
(800) 263-4540 or (905) 662-0565 or
BBS (905) 662-0569
FAX: (905) 662-0568

♦ Braille and Other Literacy Materials

Includes such products as slates and styli, braille computer paper and other braille accessories, braille typewriters, and tactile materials and kits.

Inegra Products
10728 18th Street
Dawson Creek, BC V1G 4E2
(604) 782-3380

Microcomputer Science Centre, Inc.
88 General Road
Unit 6
Mississauga, ON L4W 1Z8
(905) 629-1654
FAX: (905) 629-2321
E-mail: microsci@ican.net
URL: http://home.ican.net/~microsci

♦ Products for Deaf-Blind/ Multiply Disabled Persons

Includes such products as vibratory alert systems and amplification and communication systems.

Canadian National Institute for the Blind
1929 Bayview Avenue
Toronto, ON M4G 3E8
(416) 480-7594

SuData Consulting
50 Overlee Drive
Toronto, ON M4H 1B9
(416) 696-9590
FAX: (416) 425-4858

ORGANIZATION INDEX

UNITED STATES

A

Access-Ability Systems 527
Accessories Plus 534
AccuBraille 534
Acrontech International, Inc. 524
Adaptec Systems 525, 527
Adaptive Living Institute 520
Addie McBryde Rehabilitation Center for the Blind .. 216, 217
ADEC Resources for Independence 142
Administration for Children and Families 467
Administration for Children, Youth, and Families 467
Administration on Aging 467
Advance Corporation 534
Advanced Access Devices 531
Advantage Metal Systems, Inc. 534
Affiliated Blind of Louisiana, Inc. 165
Affiliated Leadership League of and for the Blind of
    America 487
Aging and Adult Administration / Arizona Department
    of Economic Security 24
Aging and Adult Services Administration / Washington
    State Department of Social and Health Services 415
Aging Services Division / North Dakota Department of
    Human Services 296
Aging Services Division / Oklahoma Department of
    Human Services 317
AICOM Corporation 525
Aid to Visually Handicapped 301
A.I. Kurzweil, Inc. 525
A.I.R.R.E.S. Radio Reading Service 14
Ai Squared 527
Akron Blind Center and Workshop 304
Alabama Academy of Ophthalmology 10
Alabama Department of Rehabilitation / Volunteer
    Information Resource Center 6
Alabama Division of Rehabilitation Services 6
Alabama Industries for the Blind / Alabama Institute
    for Deaf and Blind 7
Alabama Institute for Deaf and Blind 4
Alabama Instructional Resource Center 4
Alabama Optometric Association, Inc. 10
Alabama Radio Reading Service Network 6
Alabama Regional Library for the Blind and Physically
    Handicapped 4, 5
Alabama School for the Blind / Alabama Institute for
    Deaf and Blind 3
Alabama's Early Intervention System / Alabama
    Department of Rehabilitation Services 3
Alabama State Department of Education 3
Alaska Department of Education 13

Alaska Division of Vocational Rehabilitation 14
Alaska Optometric Association 15
Alaska State Library / Talking Book Center 14
Alaska State Ophthalmological Society 15
Albany Library for the Blind and Handicapped 99
Allegheny Intermediate Unit / Project Dart 327
Allegheny Intermediate Unit Vision Program 329
Alliance for the Blind and Visually Impaired 371
Alpena-Montmorency-Alcona Intermediate Schools 192
Alphapointe Association for the Blind 223
Alva Access 527
American Academy of Ophthalmology 487
American Action Fund for Blind Children and Adults 507
American Association for Pediatric Ophthalmology
    and Strabismus 487
American Association for the Deaf-Blind 487
American Association of Certified Orthoptists 487
American Association of Retired Persons / Disability
    Initiative 487
American Bible Society 507
American Blind Bowling Association 487
American Blind Lawyers Association 488
American Blind Skiing Foundation 488
American Council of the Blind 488
American Council on Rural Special Education (ACRES) .. 488
American Diabetes Association / National Center 472
American Foundation for the Blind 264, 472, 507
American Foundation for the Blind Midwest 125
American Foundation for the Blind Southeast 101
American Foundation for the Blind Southwest 380
American Foundation for the Blind West 39
American Lake Blind Rehabilitation Clinic / U.S.
    Department of Veterans Affairs 412
American Medical Alert Corporation 532
American Olean Tile Company 534
American Optometric Association 403, 488
American Printing House for the Blind 519, 527, 531
American Printing House for the Blind, Inc. 507
American Red Cross / Braille Division 37
American Red Cross / Midway-Kansas Chapter 150
American Society for Contemporary Ophthalmology 473
American Society of Cataract and Refractive Surgery 489
American Society of Ophthalmic Registered Nurses 489
American Thermoform Corporation 525, 531
Anchor Center for Blind Children 59
Andrew Heiskell Library for the Blind and Physically
    Handicapped / New York Public Library 260
Andromina, Inc. 527
Andros Analyzers, Inc. 532
Ann Morris Enterprises Inc. 519, 520, 525
Apple Computer, Inc. 525, 527
Apple Talk 528

APRIS 124

Aquarius Instructional 528

Architectural and Transportation Barriers Compliance
Board 465, 470

Aristo Computer, Inc. 528

Arizona Center for the Blind and Visually Impaired 21

Arizona Industries for the Blind 22

Arizona Instructional Resource Center 18

Arizona Ophthalmological Society 23

Arizona Optometric Association 23

Arizona State Braille and Talking Book Library 19

Arizona State Schools for the Deaf
and the Blind 16, 18, 19, 23

Arizona State Schools for the Deaf and the Blind/
Visually Impaired Preschoolers Program 17

Arkansas Department of Correction 27

Arkansas Department of Education/Special Education
Department 25

Arkansas Division of Services for the Blind 28, 29

Arkansas Lighthouse for the Blind 28

Arkansas Ophthalmological Society 29

Arkansas Optometric Association 29

Arkansas Radio Reading Service 27

Arkansas School for the Blind 25, 26

Arkansas Technology Resource Center 29

Arkenstone, Inc. 525, 528

Artic Technologies 525, 528

Arts Computer Products, Inc. 528

Asheville Lions Club Eye Clinic 292

Assistance League of Santa Clara County 42

Assistant Secretary for Special Education and
Rehabilitative Services 466

Assistive Technology Center 355

Assistive Technology Clinics/The Childrens' Hospital 63

Assistive Technology Services/Kentucky Department
for the Blind 159

Associated Blind 266

Associated Services for the Blind 332, 347, 507

Association for Education and Rehabilitation of the
Blind and Visually Impaired 489

Association for Macular Diseases 489

The Association for Persons with Severe Handicaps
(TASH) 489

Association for the Advancement of Blind and
Retarded, Inc. 266

Association for the Blind 360

Association for the Blind and Visually Impaired
(formerly Vision Enrichment Services) 201, 202

Association for the Blind and Visually Impaired/
(formerly Vision Enrichment Services) 197

Association for the Blind and Visually Impaired of
Greater Rochester, Inc. 266

Association for the Blind and Visually Impaired of
Greater Rochester, Inc./Low Vision Clinic 280

Association for the Blind and Visually Impaired of
Lehigh County/Pennsylvania Association for the
Blind 332

Association for the Visually Impaired 267

Association of Junior Leagues 489

Association of Pleasant Hills Community Church 329

Association of Visual Science Librarians 490

Association on Higher Education and Disability
(AHEAD) 490

ATLA Adaptive Materials Center 14

Atlanta Braille Volunteers 100

Audio Description/Metropolitan Washington Ear 517

Audio Journal 182

Audio Optics, Inc. 517

Audio Reader of Cloud County 151

Audio Studio for the Reading Impaired 508

Audio Vision 517

Audiovision/New Jersey Library for the Blind and
Handicapped 246

Audio Vision Radio Reading Service 39

Audio Visual Marts 521

Augusta Blind Rehabilitation Center/U. S. Department
of Veterans Affairs 103

Aurora of Central New York 267, 278

Austin Junior Women's Federation 508

Autofold, Inc. 520

Automagic Corporation 519, 521, 528

Automated Functions, Inc. 525, 528

AWARE (Associates for World Action in Rehabilitation
and Education) 473

B

Baby Net/South Carolina Department of Health and
Environmental Control 357

Badger Association for the Blind 429

Bainbridge Subregional Library for the Blind and
Physically Handicapped 99

Balcon, Inc. 534

Baltimore Infants and Toddlers Program 170

Bantam-Doubleday-Dell 508

Barnes Eye Clinic 225

Barrett School 5

Bartholomew County Public Library 137

Baruch College/Computer Center for Visually
Impaired People 278

Bascom Palmer Eye Institute/Anne Bates Leach Eye
Hospital 93

Bausch & Lomb Company 521

Beach Cities Braille Guild 508

Beacon Lighthouse for the Blind 382

Beaver County/Association for the Blind 333

Becton-Dickinson.. 532

Bedford Branch/Pennsylvania Association for the
    Blind... 333

BEGIN/(Babies Early Growth Intervention Network)/
    Center for the Visually Impaired........................ 98

Beltone Hearing Aid Service................................. 533

Bentham International.. 532

Berks County Association for the Blind/Pennsylvania
    Association for the Blind................................... 333

Bernell Corporation.. 521

BESB Industries... 68

Best Manufacturing Company............................. 534

Bestwork Industries for the Blind....................... 247

Beth Shalom Braille Committee.......................... 221

Better Vision Institute/Vision Council of America..... 473

Bible Alliance... 508

Big Eye Lamps, Inc. 521

Birth to Three Early Intervention/Division of
    Supportive Living/Wisconsin Department of Health
    and Family Services.. 424

Birth to Three Early Intervention Program/
    Washington Department of Social and Health
    Services... 409

Blair County Association for the Blind and Visually
    Handicapped 334

Blazie Engineering.. 525, 528

Blind and Low Vision Services of North Georgia....... 103, 106

Blind and Physically Handicapped Services......... 137

Blind and Visually Impaired Center of Monterey
    County... 42

Blind and Visually Impaired Services/Indiana Family
    and Social Services Administration.................. 138

Blind Association of Western New York........ 268, 280

Blind Babies Foundation... 33

Blind Children's Center... 33

Blind Children's Fund... 473

Blind Children's Learning Center.......................... 34

Blinded Veterans Association.............................. 490

Blind Enterprises of Oregon................................ 322

Blind, Inc. 209

Blind Industries and Services of Maryland.......... 174

Blind Industries and Services of Maryland/Eastern
    Shore Division... 174

Blind Industries and Services of Maryland/Western
    Maryland Division 174

Blind Outdoor Leisure Development.................... 473

Blind Rehabilitation Center/U.S. Department of
    Veterans Affairs.. 382

Blind Rehabilitation Service................................ 469

Blind Relief Fund of Philadelphia....................... 334

Blind San Franciscans.. 40

Blind Service Association..................................... 127

Blindskills, Inc.. 508

Blind Work Association.. 268

Blue Ridge Braillers... 287

Blue Springs Special Services Center.................. 219

Blue Water Library Foundation/Blind and Physically
    Handicapped Library 194

Board on Aging... 212

Bobcat Computer Applications............................ 528

Boehringer Mannheim Diagnostics.................... 532

Boise Public Schools... 114

Bomanite Corporation.. 534

Books Aloud... 508

Borland International.. 528

Bosma Industries for the Blind........................... 139

Bossert Specialties, Inc./Magnification Center...... 521

Boston Aid to the Blind.. 183

Boston Center for Blind Children................. 178, 184

Boston College/Graduate School of Education...... 180

Boston Educational Computing, Inc. 528

Boston Medical Center... 188

Bower Hill Braille Foundation............................. 329

Braille Association of Kansas............................... 150

Braille Authority of North America (BANA)....... 473

Braille Communication Services.......................... 509

Braille Computer Center/Boulder Public Library...... 60

Braille Greeting Cards.. 520

Braille Inc. 509

Braille Institute Library Services........................... 36

Braille Institute of America, Inc. 37, 40, 42

Braille Institute of America, Inc./Youth Center...... 34

Braille International... 509

Braille Sterling/Christiansen Studios.......... 525, 528

Braille Transcribers... 37

Braille Transcribers Club of Illinois.................... 121

Braille Transcribers of Central New York, Inc. 261

Braille Transcribers of Humboldt.......................... 37

Braille Transcription Project of Santa Clara County,
    Inc. 37

Brevard County Library System Talking Books Library...... 80

Brooklyn Bureau of Community Service............. 268

Broward County Talking Book Library.................. 80

Bucks County Association for the Blind/Pennsylvania
    Association for the Blind................................... 334

Buffalo General Hospital/Wettlaufer Eye Clinic...... 280

Bureau for Sensory Disabilities/Wisconsin Division of
    Supportive Living... 429

Bureau of Aging/In-Home Services.................... 143

Bureau of Aging/Wisconsin Division of Community
    Services... 432

Bureau of Blindness and Visual Services/Pennsylvania
    Department of Public Welfare........................... 331

Bureau of Braille and Talking Book Services........ 81

Bureau of Developmental Disabilities/Idaho Department of Health and Welfare 113

Bureau of Early Childhood Education and Social Services/Connecticut Department of Education 65

Bureau of Elder and Adult Services/Maine Department of Human Services 169

Bureau of Instructional Support and Community Services/Florida Department of Education 78

Bureau of Special Education/Iowa State Department of Education 144

Bureau of Vocational Rehabilitation/New Hampshire Department of Education 243

Burns Clinic Medical Center/Low Vision Clinic 202

Butler County Association for the Blind/Pennsylvania Association for the Blind 335

C

Cabell-Wayne Services for the Blind and Visually Impaired 420

California Association of Ophthalmology 52

California Department of Aging 57

California Department of Education/Special Education Division 31

California Early Intervention Technical Assistance Network 31

California Optometric Association 52

California Pacific Medical Center/Department of Ophthalmology/Low Vision Service 52

California School for the Blind 31, 35, 50

California State Library/Braille and Talking Book Services 36

California State University at Sacramento 35

California State University, Los Angeles 36

Cambria County Association for the Blind and Visually Handicapped/Pennsylvania Association for the Blind 335

Camden Optometric Center 249

Camp Allen, Inc. 241

Canon, U.S.A., Inc. 533

Canton Program for the Visually Handicapped/Canton City Schools 301

Capital Area Intermediate Unit 325, 329

Carnegie Library of Pittsburgh/Library for the Blind and Physically Handicapped 328

Carolyn's 519

Carroll Center for the Blind 184

Carsonite International 534

Castek, Inc./Transpo Industries, Inc. 534

Castle Special Computer Services 528

Castro Valley School District 37

Catholic Charities/Office for Disabled Persons 269

Catholic Charities Services for Visually Impaired Persons 269

Catholic Community Services 247

Catholic Guild for the Blind 269, 270

Cattaraugus County Association for the Blind and Visually Handicapped, Inc. 264

Celexx Trading Company, Inc. 521

Center and Homebound Preschool Intervention Program 391

Center for Blind Adults 15

Center for Blind and Visually Impaired Children 424, 427

Center for Blindness and Low Vision/Rehabilitation Institute 223

Center for Computer Assistance to the Disabled 387

Center for Independence 62, 63

Center for Living Independence for Multi-Handicapped Blind (CLIMB) 43

Center for Sight and Hearing Impaired 127

Center for the Blind and Visually Impaired 51

Center for the Partially Sighted 43, 53

Center for the Visually Impaired 103

Center for the Visually Impaired, Inc. 84

Center for Vision Rehabilitation 348

Center for Visual Independence/Eye Foundation Hospital 10

Centigram Communications Corporation 525

Central Alabama Easter Seal Rehabilitation Center 8

Central Association for the Blind and Visually Impaired 270

Central Blind Rehabilitation Center 122, 131

Central Blind Rehabilitation Center/U.S. Department of Veterans Affairs 128

Central Illinois Sight Center/TCRC Sight Center 128

Central Indiana Radio Reading, Inc. 138

Central Instructional Support Center 328

Central Instruction Support Center 329

Central Kentucky Radio Eye 157

Central Ohio Radio Reading Service 302

Central Piedmont Community College Radio Reading Service 287

Central Savannah River Area Radio Reading Service, Inc. 101

Central Susquehanna Sight Services, Inc. 336

Charles Nusinov and Sons, Inc. 521

Charleston County School District/Pupil Personnel Services 359

Chautauqua Blind Association, Inc. 271

Cherry Creek School District 59

Chester County Association for the Blind/Pennsylvania Association for the Blind 336

Chicagoland Radio Information Service, Inc. 124

Chicago Lighthouse for People Who Are Blind or Visually Impaired 128, 131, 132

Chicago Lighthouse for People Who Are Blind or Visually Impaired/Development Center 119

Chicago Public Library / Illinois Regional Library for the Blind and Physically Handicapped........................ 121, 122
Chicago Public Library / Talking Book Center 121
Child Development Center / The Lighthouse Inc. 256
Children's Center for the Visually Impaired (CCVI)............ 220
Children's Medical Services 78
Children's Rehabilitation Center / University of Virginia Hospital 400
Children's Vision Center / Department of Ophthalmology / University of California, Davis Medical Center 32
Children's Vision Rehabilitation Project / West Virginia University, Department of Ophthalmology 422
Chivers North America.. 509
Choice Magazine Listening 509
Christian Education for the Blind 509
Christian Mission for the Blind 509
Christian Record Services 510
Christian Science Publishing Society 510
Church of Jesus Christ of Latter-Day Saints / Special Curriculum 510
Cincinnati Association for the Blind............... 298, 304, 309, 310
CITE (Center for Independence, Technology and Education)... 85, 92
CITE (Center for Independence, Technology and Education) / Low Vision Screening and Education Clinic 94
Clark County School District 237
Clearinghouse for Specialized Media and Technology / California Department of Education............. 35
Cleveland Public Library / Library for the Blind and Physically Handicapped... 300
Cleveland Radio Reading Service 302
Cleveland Sight Center of the Cleveland Society for the Blind 299, 305, 310, 510
Cleveland Skilled Industries.. 305
Clover Bottom Developmental Center................................ 369
The Clovernook Center / Opportunities for the Blind 306, 510
Coburn Optical Industries, Inc... 522
College of Optometry / Ferris State University 203
College of Optometry / Northeastern State University 317
College of the Redwoods / High Tech Center..................... 51
Colorado Department of Education / Special Education Services Unit 58
Colorado Easter Seal Society... 63
Colorado Instructional Materials Center for the Visually Handicapped 59
Colorado Ophthalmological Society................................... 63
Colorado Optometric Association....................................... 63
Colorado Optometric Center / Low Vision Clinic.............. 63
Colorado Rehabilitation Center / Colorado Division of Vocational Rehabilitation 62

Colorado Rehabilitation Center / Communications for the Visually Impaired.. 63
Colorado School for the Deaf and the Blind 58, 59, 63
Colorado Talking Book Library 60
Columbia Lighthouse for the Blind................................ 74, 75
Columbia Lighthouse for the Blind / Ferd Nauheim Low Vision Clinic 76
Commission for the Blind / Family Independence Agency.. 196, 205
Commission on Aging 12, 115, 375
Committee for Purchase from the Blind and Other Severely Handicapped... 470
Community Blind Center... 44
Community Services for the Blind and Partially Sighted 412, 414
Comp Tech Systems Design... 528, 533
CompuBraille.. 37
ComputAbility Corporation 525, 528
Computer Access Laboratory / California State University, Students with Disabilities Resources............... 51
Computer Center for Citizens with Disabilities.................... 394
Computers to Help People 431
Conklin Center for Multihandicapped Blind....................... 86
Connecticut Association of Optometrists............................. 69
Connecticut Board of Education and Services for the Blind 69
Connecticut Braille Association 66, 67
Connecticut Department of Social Services / Elderly Services Division 69
Connecticut Radio Information System (CRIS) 67
Connecticut Society of Eye Physicians 69
Connecticut State Board of Education and Services for the Blind... 65, 66, 67, 68
Connecticut State Library / Library for the Blind and Physically Handicapped 66
Conney Safety Products 532
Consolidated Industries of Greater Syracuse, Inc............... 271
Contact East, Inc.. 522
Contact Lens Association of Ophthalmologists.................... 490
Contra Costa Braille Transcribers 510
Cooperative Preschool for Visually Handicapped 18
Cornucopia Software, Inc.. 528
Cotrax Consumer Products Group 525
Council for Exceptional Children... 491
Council of Citizens with Low Vision International 491
Council of Families with Visual Impairment....................... 491
Council of Schools for the Blind.. 491
Council on Aging / Division of Aging and Adult Services 218
Cross Educational Software 528
Crossroads Rehabilitation Center 142
Crossville Ceramics... 534

CT Concrete Company 534
C TECH 525

D

Dade County Talking Book Library 81
Dallas Lighthouse for the Blind, Inc. 382
Dallas Services for the Visually Impaired 379
Dallas Services for the Visually Impaired/Low Vision
    Clinic 388
Dallas Services for Visually Impaired Children 376, 383
Darien Community Association Program for the Blind 67
Data Transforms 528
Dayton Public Schools 301
Dazor Manufacturing Corporation 522
DB-LINK: The National Information Clearinghouse on
    Children Who Are Deaf-Blind 474
Deaf-Blind Program/The National Academy,
    Gallaudet University 510
Dean A. McGee Eye Institute 317
Debbie School/Mailman Center for Child
    Development 79
Deicke Center for Visual Rehabilitation 132
DeKalb County School System 100
Delaware Academy of Ophthalmology/Delaware Eye
    Associates 72
Delaware Association for the Blind 71
Delaware Department of Public Instruction 70
Delaware Division for the Visually Impaired 70
Delaware Industries for the Blind 71
Delaware Optometric Association, Inc. 72
Delco Blind/Sight Center 336
Delta Gamma Center for Children with Visual
    Impairments 220
Delta Gamma Foundation 474
Deluxe Check Printers, Inc. 522
Department for the Blind and Physically Handicapped 5
Department of Human Resources/Division of Services
    for the Blind 293
Department of Public Health and Human Services/
    Blind and Low Vision Services 231
Department of Public Health and Human Services
    Office on Aging 231
Department of Rehabilitation Services 12
Department of Social Services/New York State
    Commission for the Blind and Visually Handicapped .. 285
Descriptive Video Service/WGBH-TV 517
Desert Blind Association 44
Designs for Vision, Inc. 522
Detroit Institute of Ophthalmology/Low Vision
    Program/Friends of Vision 203
Detroit Radio Information Service 196
Developmental Disabilities Division/New Mexico
    Department of Health 251

Developmental Disabilities Division/North Dakota
    Department of Human Services 294
Developmental Disabilities Program/Department of
    Public Health and Human Services 228
Developmental Disabilities Section/Division of Mental
    Health, Mental Retardation and Substance Abuse
    Services/North Carolina Department of Human
    Services 286
Developmental Disabilities Services/Arkansas
    Department of Human Services 25
Developmental Education Birth through Two (DEBT
    Project) 377
Devers Eye Institute 323
Dialing-In/Metropolitan Washington Ear 172
Digital Equipment Corporation 528, 533
District of Columbia Department of Human Services 77
District of Columbia Library for the Blind and
    Physically Handicapped 73, 74
District of Columbia Rehabilitation Services
    Administration/Visual Impairment Section 75
District of Columbia Special Education Branch 73
Diversified Enterprises International 534
Division for Aging Services/Nevada Department of
    Human Resources 239
Division for the Blind and Visually Impaired/Bureau
    of Rehabilitation Services/Department of Labor 169
Division for the Blind and Visually Impaired/Maine
    Department of Human Services 167
Division for the Blind and Visually Impaired/Maine
    Department of Labor 168
Division for the Blind and Visually Impaired/Vermont
    Agency of Human Services 397, 398
Division for the Visually Impaired/Delaware
    Department of Health and Social Services 71, 72
Division for the Visually Impaired/Delaware Health
    and Social Services 72
Division of Aging 293
Division of Aging/Missouri Department of Social
    Services 227
Division of Aging and Adult Services/Arkansas
    Department of Human Services 30
Division of Aging and Adult Services/Colorado
    Department of Human Services 64
Division of Aging and Adult Services/Utah
    Department of Social Services 395
Division of Aging Services/Cabinet for Human
    Resources 160
Division of Blind and Visually Impaired 466
Division of Blind Services/Florida Department of
    Labor 79, 83
Division of Blind Services/Florida Department of
    Labor and Employment Security 92
Division of Community Program Development/Office
    of Mental Retardation/Pennsylvania Department of
    Public Welfare 325

Division of Developmental Disabilities/Wyoming Department of Health 433

Division of Disabilities and Rehabilitation Services/ Virgin Islands Department of Human Services 407

Division of Elderly and Adult Services/New Hampshire Department of Health and Human Services 243

Division of Family Health/Rhode Island Department of Health 354

Division of Health/Wisconsin Department of Health and Family Services 424

Division of Management Services/Delaware Health and Social Services Birth to Three 70

Division of Maternal and Child Health Care and Crippled Children Services/Virgin Islands Department of Health/Knud Hansen Complex 407

Division of Rehabilitation Services/West Virginia Division of Rehabilitation Services 421

Division of Rehabilitation Services/West Virginia State Board of Rehabilitation 419

Division of Senior Citizens/Guam Department of Public Health and Social Services 108

Division of Senior Services/Alaska Department of Administration 15

Division of Services for Aging and Adults with Physical Disabilities/Delaware Department of Health and Social Services 72

Division of Services for the Blind/Arkansas Department of Human Services 30

Division of Service to the Blind and Visually Impaired/South Dakota Department of Human Services 364, 366

Division of Special Education/Minnesota Department of Children, Families and Learning 206

Division of Supportive Living/Wisconsin Department of Health and Family Services 432

Division of Vocational Rehabilitation 15

Division of Vocational Rehabilitation/Hawaii Department of Human Services 112

Division of Vocational Rehabilitation/Wyoming Department of Employment 433, 434

Division on Aging 434

Division on Aging/New Jersey Department of Community Affairs 250

Dominican College 259

Don Johnston Developmental Equipment 525, 528, 533

Doran Resource Center for the Blind 44

Downtown Detroit Subregional Library for the Blind and Physically Handicapped 194

Dragon Systems, Inc. 525

Duke University Eye Center/Duke University Medical Center 292

Dunamis, Inc. 528, 533

DuPage/West Cook Regional Special Education Association 119

Duxbury Systems, Inc. 528

D'Youville College/Division of Education 259

E

Early Childhood Division/Illinois State Board of Education 117

Early Childhood Education/Michigan Department of Education 192

Early Childhood Initiatives Unit/Colorado Department of Education 58

Early Childhood Program/Texas Department of Health 376

Early Childhood Services/Division of Child and Family Services/Nevada Department of Human Resources 237

Early Childhood Special Education Services/Omaha Public Schools 232

Early Education Center/Training and Evaluation Center of Hutchinson 148

Early Intervention and Early Childhood Special Education Programs/Oregon Department of Education 318

Early Intervention Program/Alaska Department of Health and Social Services 13

Early Intervention Program/California Department of Developmental Services 31

Early Intervention Program/District of Columbia Department of Human Services 73

Early Intervention Program/Division of Family Services/Utah Department of Health 391

Early Intervention Program/New York Department of Health 255

Early Intervention Programs/Division of Public Health/Georgia Department of Human Resources 97

Early Intervention Services/Massachusetts Department of Public Health 178

East Bay Center for the Blind, Inc. 44

Eastern Blind Rehabilitation Center/U.S. Department of Veterans Affairs 68

Eastern Blind Rehabilition Center Eye Clinic 69

Eastern Michigan University 193

Eastern Shore Radio Reading Service/WESM-FM 172

Easter Seals Occupational Rehabilitation Center 8

East Texas Lighthouse for the Blind 383

Echo 525

Edith R. Rudolphy Residence for the Blind 337

Ed Lindsey Industries for the Blind 372

Edmark 525

Educational Services for Visually Impaired/Arkansas School for the Blind 26

Educational Vision Services/New York City Public Schools, District 75 261

Education and Reading Service (EARS) 428
E.H. Gentry Technical Facility 10
E.H. Gentry Technical Facility / Alabama Institute for
    Deaf and Blind 9
ELCA (Evangelical Lutheran Church in America)/
    Braille and Tape Service 511
Eleanor E. Faye Low Vision Service / The Lighthouse
    Inc. 281
Electronic Information and Education Service 246
Electronic Learning Systems 525, 529
Electronic Visual Aid Specialists 522, 525
El Paso Lighthouse for the Blind 384
El Paso Lighthouse for the Blind / Low Vision Center 388
El Paso Radio Reading Service 379
Emed Company, Inc. 534
Emil Fries Piano Hospital and Training Center 412
Employment Standards Administration / National
    Office Program Administration 468
ENABLE 278
Enable / Schneier Communication Unit 533
Enabling Technologies Company 519, 525, 529
Engineered Plastics, Inc. 535
Enhanced Vision Systems, Inc. 519
Environmental Lighting, Inc. 519
Equal Employment Opportunity Commission 465, 470
Erie Center for the Blind and Visually Handicapped /
    Pennsylvania Association for the Blind 337
Erie County Medical Center 281
Erlanger Medical Center / Lions Low Vision Service 374
Escambia County School District 81
Eschenbach Optik of America 522
Esselte Pendaflex Corporation 532
Evansville Association for the Blind, Inc. 139
E.V.A.S. 529
Evergreen Radio Reading Service 411
Exceptional Student Education 82
Exceptional Student Services / Arizona Department of
    Education 16
Exceptional Teaching Aids 522, 529
Executive Office of Elder Affairs 190
Executive Office on Aging / Office of the Governor 112
Eye and Ear Clinic 415
Eye Bank Association of America 474
Eye Bank for Sight Restoration 474
Eye Clinic / Grady Memorial Hospital 106
Eye Clinic, Children's Memorial Hospital 132
Eye Dog Foundation for the Blind 51
The Eye Institute / Pennsylvania College of
    Optometry / William Feinbloom Vision
    Rehabilitation Center 348
Eye Institute / St. Louis University 226
Eye Institute of New Jersey / University of Medicine
    and Dentistry 249
Eye of the Pacific Guide Dogs and Mobility Services,
    Inc. 111

F
FACES Access Services 211
Fairfield Regional Vision Rehabilitation Center 306
Family and Social Service Federation 248
Family and Social Services Administration / Disability,
    Aging and Rehabilitation Services 143
Father Palmer Memorial Braille Service / Lilac Blind
    Foundation 411
Fayette County Association for the Blind /
    Pennsylvania Association for the Blind 338
La Fayette Subregional Library for the Blind and
    Physically Handicapped 99
FDLRS 529
Federal Transit Administration 465, 468
Ferguson Industries for the Blind 185
The Fernald Center 178
Fidelco Guide Dog Foundation 68
Fight for Sight 474
Finger Lakes Independent Center 278
First Byte Inc. 526, 529
First Steps / Family and Social Services Administration 135
Fishburne Enterprises 522, 532
Flexible Software / Laird Communications 529
Florida Association of Workers for the Blind 92
Florida Association of Workers for the Blind (Miami
    Lighthouse) 86
Florida Center for the Blind Incorporated 87
Florida Department of Elder Affairs 95
Florida Division of Blind Services 96
Florida Instructional Materials Center for the Visually
    Handicapped 80
Florida New Concepts Marketing 522
Florida Optometric Association 93
Florida School for the Deaf and Blind 78
Florida Society of Ophthalmology 93
Florida State University / Visual Impairments 80
Focus for Newly Blind and Family 429
Fort Smith Public Library for the Blind and
    Handicapped 27
Fotofonics 520, 533
The Foundation Fighting Blindness / Alaska Affiliate 14
The Foundation Fighting Blindness / Arizona Affiliate 20
The Foundation Fighting Blindness / Arkansas Affiliate 27
The Foundation Fighting Blindness / Atlanta Affiliate 101
The Foundation Fighting Blindness / Bronx-
    Westchester-Rockland Affiliate 264
The Foundation Fighting Blindness / Brooklyn Affiliate 264
The Foundation Fighting Blindness / Central Florida
    Affiliate 83

The Foundation Fighting Blindness/Central Virginia Affiliate 403

The Foundation Fighting Blindness/Chicago Affiliate 125

The Foundation Fighting Blindness/Connecticut Affiliate 67

The Foundation Fighting Blindness/Dallas Affiliate 380

The Foundation Fighting Blindness/Delaware Affiliate 71

The Foundation Fighting Blindness/Eastern Kentucky Affiliate 157

The Foundation Fighting Blindness/Eastern Ohio Affiliate 303

The Foundation Fighting Blindness/Fresno Affiliate........... 40

The Foundation Fighting Blindness/Greater Kansas City Affiliate 222

The Foundation Fighting Blindness/Greater St. Louis Affiliate 222

The Foundation Fighting Blindness/Greater Washington, DC Chapter 74

The Foundation Fighting Blindness/Hawaii Affiliate 110

The Foundation Fighting Blindness/Iowa Affiliate 145

The Foundation Fighting Blindness/Long Island Affiliate 264

The Foundation Fighting Blindness/Maine Affiliate 167

The Foundation Fighting Blindness/Manhattan Affiliate 264

The Foundation Fighting Blindness/Maryland Affiliate ... 173

The Foundation Fighting Blindness/Massachusetts Affiliate 182

The Foundation Fighting Blindness/Michigan Affiliate..... 196

The Foundation Fighting Blindness/Minnesota Affiliate 208

The Foundation Fighting Blindness/Nebraska/Iowa Affiliate 234

The Foundation Fighting Blindness/New Jersey Affiliate 246

The Foundation Fighting Blindness/North Carolina Affiliate 288

The Foundation Fighting Blindness/Northern California Affiliate 40

The Foundation Fighting Blindness/Northern New Jersey Affiliate 246

The Foundation Fighting Blindness/North Florida Affiliate 83

The Foundation Fighting Blindness/Ormond Beach Affiliate 83

The Foundation Fighting Blindness/Philadelphia Affiliate 331

The Foundation Fighting Blindness/Piedmont Affiliate ... 288

The Foundation Fighting Blindness/Raleigh Affiliate 288

The Foundation Fighting Blindness/Rhode Island Affiliate 354

The Foundation Fighting Blindness/Rocky Mountain Affiliate 60

The Foundation Fighting Blindness/San Diego Affiliate 40

The Foundation Fighting Blindness/Seattle Affiliate 411

The Foundation Fighting Blindness/Southern California Affiliate 40

The Foundation Fighting Blindness/South Florida Affiliate 83

The Foundation Fighting Blindness/Syracuse Affiliate 264

The Foundation Fighting Blindness/Texas Panhandle Affiliate 380

The Foundation Fighting Blindness/Toledo Affiliate 303

The Foundation Fighting Blindness/Utah Chapter 393

The Foundation Fighting Blindness/Vermont Affiliate 397

The Foundation Fighting Blindness (National Retinitis Pigmentosa Foundation, Inc.) 173

The Foundation Fighting Blindness (National Retinitis Pigmentosa Foundation Inc.) 475

Foundation for Blind Children 17, 20

Foundation for the Junior Blind 32

4-Sights Network/Upshaw Institute for the Blind............. 472

4X Products, Inc 521

Fredericksburg Area Subregional Library 401

Fred Sammons, Inc. 522, 533

Free Library of Philadelphia/Library for the Blind and Physically Handicapped 329

Fresno County Free Library/Blind and Handicapped Services 36

Friendship Center for the Blind and Visually Impaired 45

G

G.A.L. Manufacturing Corporation 535

Gary Community Public Schools Corporation 136

Gary Public Schools, V.I.P. Resource Center 137

General Electric 522, 532

George Meyer Instructional Resource Center 245

Georgetown University Medical Center/Center for Sight 76

George Washington University Medical Center/ Department of Ophthalmology 76

Georgia Academy for the Blind 97, 98, 106

Georgia Department of Human Resources/Division of Rehabilitation Services 107

Georgia Division of Rehabilitation Services 100, 101

Georgia Industries for the Blind 104

Georgia Lions Lighthouse Foundation, Inc. 104

Georgia Optometric Association 106

Georgia Radio Reading Service, Inc. 101

Georgia Regional Library for the Blind and Physically Handicapped 99

Georgia Society of Ophthalmology 106

Georgia State Department of Education/Division of Exceptional Students 97

Georgia State University 98

The Gerald E. Fonda, M.D., Low Vision Center of Saint Barnabas 249

Gillette Children's Hospital 211
G.K. Hall and Company / Simon and Schuster 511
Gladys Loeb Foundation 520, 522
The Glaucoma Foundation 475
Glaucoma Research Foundation 475
Glens Falls Association for the Blind 272
Golden Gate Braille Transcribers, Inc. 37
Golden Hours, Inc. 321
Goodwill Industries of Dayton 306
Goodwill Industries of Greater Detroit 198
Goodwill Industries of Mid-Michigan, Inc. 198
Goodwill Industries of the Coastal Empire, Inc. 104
Gospel Association for the Blind 511
Governmental Relations Group / American Foundation
     for the Blind 475
Governor Morehead School 286
Governor's Interagency Coordinating Council on
     Infants and Toddlers / Arizona Department of
     Economic Security 16
Governor's Office for Elderly Affairs 353
Grand Traverse Area Library for the Blind and
     Physically Handicapped 194
Greater Akron Low Vision Clinic 311
Greater Pittsburgh Guild for the Blind 349
Greater Pittsburgh Guild for the Blind (now known as
     Pittsburgh Vision Services) 338, 348
Greater Wilkes-Barre Association for the Blind 339
Green Bay Public Schools 428
Grey House Publishing Company 511
Group Health Cooperative of Puget Sound 415
Guam Department of Education 108
Guam Department of Education / Division of Special
     Education 108
Guam Department of Vocational Rehabilitation 108
Guam Public Library for the Blind and Physically
     Handicapped 108
Guide Dog Foundation for the Blind, Inc. 279
Guide Dogs for the Blind 51, 323
Guide Dogs of America 52
Guide Dogs of the Desert 52
Guide Dog Users 491
Guiding Eyes for the Blind, Inc. 279
Guiding Light for the Blind 339
Guild for the Blind 122
GW Micro 529

H

Hadley School for the Blind 475
Halifax Hospital Medical Center Eye Clinic 94
Hampton Roads Voice of the Print Handicapped 402
Hampton Subregional Library for the Blind and
     Physically Handicapped 401

Harbor Computing Services 529
HarperCollins Publishers 511
Harrisburg Area Radio Reading Service 330
Hartley Courseware, Inc. 529
Haskill Hearing Aid Center 533
Hawaii Center for the Deaf and Blind 109
Hawaii Department of Education / Hawaii Center for
     the Deaf and the Blind 109
Hawaii Library for the Blind and Physically
     Handicapped 109, 110
Hawaii Ophthalmological Society 111
Hawaii Optometric Association 111
Hazleton Blind Association / Pennsylvania Association
     for the Blind 339
Health Care Financing Administration 467
Health Resources and Services Administration / Bureau
     of Health Professions 467
Health Science 526, 533
Health Services Administration / Bureau for Maternal
     and Child Health / Health Care Resources
     Department 467
Heart of Illinois Talking Book Center 121
Helen Keller International 476
Helen Keller National Center for Deaf-Blind Youths
     and Adults 278, 476, 533
Helen Keller National Center for Deaf-Blind Youths
     and Adults / East Central Region Office 174
Helen Keller National Center for Deaf-Blind Youths
     and Adults / Great Plains Region Office 152
Helen Keller National Center for Deaf-Blind Youths
     and Adults / Mid-Atlantic Region Office 272
Helen Keller National Center for Deaf-Blind Youths
     and Adults / New England Region Office 185
Helen Keller National Center for Deaf-Blind Youths
     and Adults / North Central Region Office 129
Helen Keller National Center for Deaf-Blind Youths
     and Adults / Northwest Region Office 413
Helen Keller National Center for Deaf-Blind Youths
     and Adults / Rocky Mountain Region Office 63
Helen Keller National Center for Deaf-Blind Youths
     and Adults / South Central Region Office 384
Helen Keller National Center for Deaf-Blind Youths
     and Adults / Southeast Region Office 105
Helen Keller National Center for Deaf-Blind Youths
     and Adults / Southwest Region Office 45
Helen Keller Services for the Blind 257, 272, 278
Helen Keller Services for the Blind / Braille Library 262, 511
Henter-Joyce, Inc. 526, 529
Herald House 511
Hexagon Products 522, 529
HFK Software, Inc. 529
Hillsborough County Talking Book Library 81
Hilton / Perkins Program / Perkins School for the Blind 477

Hitec Special Needs Center 533
Home Diagnostics, Inc. 532
Honeywell Residential Controls 522
Hooleon Corporation 526
Ho'opono Services for the Blind / Hawaii Department
   of Human Services / Vocational Rehabilitation and
   Services for the Blind Division 110
Ho'opono Workshop for the Blind 111
Hope Family Support Program 34
Hope Haven Children's Clinic / Low Vision Clinic 94
The Hope School 117
Horizons for the Blind 122
Houston Taping for the Blind Radio 380
Howe Press of Perkins School for the Blind 511, 520, 532
HumanWare, Inc. 522, 526, 529, 532
Hunter College, City University of New York /
   Department of Special Education 259
Huntsville Subregional Library for the Blind and
   Physically Handicapped 5
Hy-Tek Manufacturing CO. 526
Hy-Tek Manufacturing Company, Inc. 533

I

IBM Special Needs Systems 526, 529
Idaho Commission for the Blind and Visually Impaired
                                                                           115, 116
Idaho Optometric Association 115
Idaho Radio Reading Service 115
Idaho School for the Deaf and the Blind 113, 114
Idaho Society of Ophthalmology 115
Idaho State Department of Education 113
Idaho State Library / Services for Blind and Physically
   Handicapped 114, 115
Illinois Association of Ophthalmology 131
Illinois Center for Rehabilitation and Education 133
Illinois Department of Rehabilitation Services 126, 134
Illinois Department of Rehabilitation Services / Bureau
   of Blind Services 131
Illinois Department on Aging 134
Illinois Eye Institute / Illinois College of Optometry 133
Illinois Industrial Materials 120
Illinois Instructional Materials Center 122
Illinois Optometric Association 131
Illinois Radio Reader 124
Illinois School for the
   Visually Impaired 117, 119, 120, 122, 131
Illinois Society for the Prevention of Blindness 125
Illinois State Board of Education 117
Illinois State University 120
Independence for the Blind 88, 93
Independent Living Aids, Inc. 519, 532, 533
Independent Living for Adult Blind (ILAB) 88

Independent Living Resources 320, 322
Independent Visually Impaired Enterprises 491
Indiana Academy of Ophthalmology 142
Indiana County Blind Association 340
Indiana Department of Education / Division of Special
   Education 135
Indiana Educational Resource Center / Indiana School
   for the Blind 136
Indiana Optometric Association 142
Indianapolis Eye Care Center / Indiana University
   School of Optometry 142
Indiana School for the Blind 135, 136
Indiana State Library / Special Services Division 137
Industries for the Blind, Inc. 429
Industries for the Blind of New York State 273
Industries of the Blind 289
Infant and Child Development Program / Columbia
   Lighthouse for the Blind 73
Infant and Toddler Program / Mississippi Department
   of Health 213
Infant and Toddler Program / Virginia Department of
   Mental Health, Mental Retardation and Substance
   Abuse Services 399
Infant-Family Program of the Foundation for the Junior
   Blind 35
Infants and Toddlers with Handicaps / Puerto Rico
   Department of Health 351
Infant-Toddler Program / Kentucky Department of
   Mental Health and Mental Retardation Services 155
Innovative Rehabilitation Technology 520, 526, 529
Innoventions, Inc. 522
IN-SIGHT Radio—Division of IN-SIGHT 354
IN-SIGHT (Rhode Island Association for the Blind) . 355, 356
INSIGHT / WYMS 428
Institute for Families of Blind Children 40
Institute on Applied Technology / Children's Hospital
   of Boston 526
Instituto Loaíza Cordero para Niños Ciegos 351
Instructional Materials Center for the Blind 167
Intelligent Info Technologies Corporation 529
IntelliTools 526, 533
Interagency Coordinating Council for Early Childhood
   Intervention / Oklahoma Commission on Children
   and Youth 313
Interagency Early Intervention Planning Project /
   Minnesota Department of Children, Families and
   Learning 206
Intercommunity Blind Center 45
Interdepartmental Coordinating Council on Early
   Intervention / Child Development Services 167
Interface Systems International 529
International Society on Metabolic Eye Disease 477
Intex Micro Systems Corporation 526

IN TOUCH Networks 263, 478
Iowa Academy of Ophthalmology 146
Iowa Braille and Sight Saving School 144, 145
Iowa Department for the Blind 145, 146, 147
Iowa Department of Education 144
Iowa Department of Elder Affairs 147
Iowa Library for the Blind and Physically
    Handicapped/Iowa Department for the Blind 145
Iowa Optometric Association 146
Iowa Radio Reading Information Service (IRIS) 145
Isis Large Print Books/Transaction Publishers 511

J
Jackson State University/Department of Special
    Education and Rehabilitative Services 214
Jefferson County Association for the Blind 273
Jefferson County Public Schools 157
Jesana Ltd. 522
Jewish Braille Institute of America 512
Jewish Guild for the Blind/Home for Aged Blind/
    Kramer Vision Rehabilitation Center 281
Jewish Guild for the Blind (The Guild) 257, 273, 512
Jewish Heritage for the Blind 262
J.I.S.D. #287 206
Johanna Bureau for the Blind and Physically
    Handicapped, Inc. 123
John Milton Society for the Blind 512
Joint Commission on Allied Health Personnel in
    Ophthalmology 478
Joslin Diabetes Center 478
Joslin Diabetes Center/William P. Beetham Eye
    Research and Treatment Unit 188
J P Trading, Inc. 522
Jules Stein Eye Institute 53
Juniata Association for the Blind 340

K
Kagan Home for the Blind 129
Kansas Audio-Reader Network 151
Kansas City, Kansas Public Library/Kansas Braille
    Library 149
Kansas City Veterans Affairs Medical Center/
    VICTORS Program 226
Kansas Department of Health and Environment 148
Kansas Department on Aging 154
Kansas Division of Services for the Blind 151
Kansas Eye Center/University of Kansas Medical
    Center/Low Vision Rehabilitation Service 153
Kansas Industries for the Blind 152
Kansas Instructional Resource Center for the Blind and
    Visually Impaired 149
Kansas Optometric Association 153
Kansas Rehabilitation Center for the Blind 150, 153

Kansas Specialty Dog Service 153
Kansas State Department of Education/Student
    Support Services 148
Kansas State Ophthalmological Society 153
Kansas State School for the Blind 148, 149
Kansas Talking Book Service/Kansas State Library 150
KBPS Seeing Sound 321
KCHO-FM Radio Reading Service 39
Keeler Instruments, Inc. 522
Kent County Library for the Blind and Physically
    Handicapped 194
Kentucky Academy of Eye Physicians and Surgeons 159
Kentucky Clinic/University of Kentucky/Department
    of Ophthalmology 159
Kentucky Department for the Blind 158, 160
Kentucky Department of Education/Division of
    Exceptional Children Services 155
Kentucky Industries for the Blind 158, 520
Kentucky Instructional Materials Resource Center 156
Kentucky Library for the Blind and Physically
    Handicapped 157
Kentucky Lions Eye Center, Low Vision Clinic/
    University of Louisville Department of
    Ophthalmology 159
Kentucky Optometric Association 159
Kentucky School for the Blind 155, 156
Keystone Blind Association 341
Keystone Radio Information Service/Blair County
    Association for the Blind and Visually Handicapped 330
Kidsview Software, Inc. 529
Kinetic Designs, Inc. 526, 529
King-Drew Medical Center 53
Kings Tape Library for the Blind 38
Knights Templar Eye Foundation 478
KPBS-FM Radio Reading Service 39
Kresge Eye Institute Low Vision Service 203
Kurzweil Educational Systems 526
KUT 90.5FM 380
Kutztown University/Department of Special
    Education 328

L
Lackawanna Branch/Pennsylvania Association for the
    Blind 341
Laureate Learning Systems, Inc. 529
Laurence-Moon Bardet-Biedl Syndrome Self-Help
    Support Network 491
Lavelle School for the Blind 255, 258, 278
Lawrence County Branch/Pennsylvania Association
    for the Blind 342
Leader Dogs for the Blind 202
League for the Blind and Disabled 142
League for the Blind and Disabled, Inc. 140

LEA Resource Center.. 98
Learning Express.. 532
Lee County Subregional Library for the Blind and
    Physically Handicapped....................................... 81
Lehigh Valley Braille Guild..................................... 329
Library and Resource Center/Virginia Department for
    the Visually Handicapped................................... 401
Library and Resource Center for the Blind and
    Physically Handicapped... 5
Library for the Blind and Handicapped, Northwest....... 27
Library for the Blind and Handicapped, Southwest...... 27
Library for the Blind and Physically Handicapped 5, 27, 99
Library for the Blind and Physically Handicapped/
    Delaware Division of Libraries............................ 70
Library for the Blind and Physically Handicapped/
    Newport News Public Library System.................. 402
Library for the Blind and Print Handicapped............. 36
Library of Congress National Library Service for the
    Blind and Physically Handicapped..................... 470
Library of Michigan/Services for the Blind and
    Physically Handicapped............................... 194, 195
Library Reproduction Service................................. 512
LICA-NSSEO Infant Vision Program.................... 120
LICA-NSSEO Vision East....................................... 123
LICA-NSSEO Vision West...................................... 123
Life Science Associates.. 529
LIFT... 278
LIFTT Radio Reading Service................................ 229
Lighthouse for the Blind................................. 209, 224
The Lighthouse for the Blind, Inc.......................... 413
Lighthouse for the Blind in New Orleans............... 164
Lighthouse for the Blind of Fort Worth........... 384, 387
Lighthouse for the Blind of the Palm Beaches 89, 93, 94
Lighthouse for the Visually Impaired and Blind........ 89
The Lighthouse Inc.......................... 264, 274, 279, 478, 519
The Lighthouse Inc./Hudson Valley................. 258, 279
The Lighthouse Inc./Lighthouse Enterprises........ 520, 523
Lighthouse of Broward County.............................. 90
Lighthouse of Houston.............................. 379, 385, 387
Lighthouse of Houston/Low Vision Clinic............. 388
Lilac Blind Foundation.. 413
Lions Blind Center of Diablo Valley...................... 45
Lions Blind Center of the Santa Clara Valley.......... 46
Lions Center for the Blind............................... 46, 51
Lions Club Industries for the Blind, Inc............... 289
Lions Clubs International..................................... 478
Lions Industries for the Blind............................. 290
Lions Low Vision Clinic of the Inland Empire....... 415
Lions Services... 290
Lions Vision Research and Rehabilitation Center/
    Wilmer Ophthalmological Institute................... 175
Lions Volunteer Blind Industries......................... 372

Lions World Services for the Blind..................... 28, 29
Little Light House, Inc... 314
Living Skills Center for the Visually Impaired......... 46
Liz Moore Low Vision Center................................ 11
Long Island Jewish Medical Center/Eye Care Center....... 282
Lorin Software.. 529
Louisiana Association for the Blind...................... 164
Louisiana Center for the Blind............................ 164
Louisiana Council for the Blind........................... 162
Louisiana Learning Resources System/Louisiana State
    Department of Education............................ 161, 162
Louisiana Ophthalmological Association............... 165
Louisiana Rehabilitation Services........................ 163
Louisiana Rehabilitation Services/Department of
    Social Services... 166
Louisiana School for the Visually Impaired....... 161, 162
Louisiana State Association of Optometrists.......... 165
Louisiana State Library/Section for the Blind and
    Physically Handicapped................................. 162
Louisiana State University Eye Center/Low Vision
    Clinic.. 165
Lowell Association for the Blind/Center for the Blind
    and Visually Impaired.................................... 185
Low Vision Center/Tampa Lighthouse for the Blind.......... 95
Low Vision Clinic... 165
Low Vision Clinic/Department of Ophthalmology,
    University of Iowa Hospitals and Clinics.......... 146
Low Vision Clinic/Helen Keller Services for the Blind
    (HKSB)... 282
Low Vision Clinic/Ho'opono Rehabilitation Center for
    the Blind and Visually Impaired..................... 111
Low Vision Clinic/Nevada Bureau of Services to the
    Blind.. 239
Low Vision Clinic/University of California, San
    Francisco Eye Clinic....................................... 54
Low Vision Clinic/University of California School of
    Optometry... 54
Low Vision Clinic/West Virginia University/
    Department of Ophthalmology......................... 422
Low Vision Consultants....................................... 203
Low Vision/Contact Lens Service......................... 146
Low Vision Facility of Boswell Eye Institute........... 23
Low Vision Information Center............................. 173
Low Vision Library/Kansas City Association for the
    Blind... 221, 225
Low Vision Rehabilitation Center/Carroll Center for
    the Blind... 189
Low Vision Rehabilitation Program/University of
    Missouri - Kansas City/Department of
    Ophthalmology... 226
Low Vision Rehabilitation Service/University Station
    Clinics.. 431
Low Vision Service/The Lighthouse Inc................ 282

Low Vision Service/Perkins School for the Blind.............. 189

Low Vision Service/State University of New York/
  College of Optometry... 283

Low Vision Service of Jessamine Optometric
  Association.. 159

Low Vision Services/The Lighthouse Inc..................... 283

Low Vision Services/Utah Division of Services for the
  Blind and Visually Impaired................................... 394

Low Vision Services of Kentucky............................... 160

Low Vision Unit/Hermann Eye Center......................... 389

Loyola University Medical Center/Department of
  Ophthalmology.. 133

LS&S Group, Inc.............................. 519, 520, 523, 532

Lucent/ACPC.. 520, 533

Luminaud, Inc... 533

Lutheran Braille Evangelism Association.................... 512

Lutheran Braille Workers... 512

Lutheran Library for the Blind................................. 513

Luxo Corporation... 523

M

Macomb Library for the Blind and Physically
  Handicapped... 194

Macon Subregional Library for the Blind and
  Physically Handicapped... 99

Maddak, Inc.................................... 519, 520, 533

Madison-Chatham Braille Association........................ 245

Magnisight.. 523

Maine Center for the Blind and Visually Impaired..... 168, 169

Maine Division for the Blind and Visually Impaired...... 167

Maine Optometric Association, Inc........................... 169

Maine Society of Eye Physicians and Surgeons.......... 169

Maine State Library/Library Services for the Blind and
  Physically Handicapped... 167

Maitland Vision Center... 523

Mana-Sota Lighthouse for the Blind........................... 90

Manhattan Public Library.. 150

Mankato State University.. 207

Marblesoft.. 530

March of Dimes Birth Defects Foundation.................. 479

Marin Low Vision Clinic.. 54

Mary Bryant Home for the Blind................................ 130

The Mary Culver Home.. 224

Maryland Division of Vocational Rehabilitation
  Services.. 174, 175, 177

Maryland Optometric Association, Inc....................... 175

Maryland School for the Blind................... 170, 171, 175

Maryland Society For Sight..................................... 173

Maryland Society of Eye Physicians and Surgeons..... 175

Maryland State Department of Education................... 170

Maryland State Library for the Blind and Physically
  Handicapped... 171

Massachusetts Association for the Blind.............. 181, 185

Massachusetts Association for the Blind/
  The Store.................................... 519, 520, 523

Massachusetts Braille and Talking Book Library........ 181

Massachusetts Commission for the Blind................... 191

Massachusetts Department of Education/Educational
  Improvement Group... 178

Massachusetts Eye and Ear Infirmary/Vision
  Rehabilitation Services... 189

Massachusetts Society of Eye Physicians and Surgeons.... 188

Massachusetts Society of Optometrists, Inc............... 188

Massachusetts State Commission for the Blind......... 183, 188

Matheny School and Hospital.................................... 244

Matilda Ziegler Magazine for the Blind...................... 513

Mattel Consumer Affairs/Mattel Toys................ 520, 532

Mattingly International, Inc...................................... 523

Maxi-Aids.................................... 519, 520, 523, 526

Maxwell Low Vision Clinic/Center for the Visually
  Impaired.. 106

Mayo Clinic.. 211

McLeod Optical, Inc.. 523

M.C. Migel Memorial Library/Information Center/
  American Foundation for the Blind.......................... 260

Medical College of Georgia/Low Vision Clinic............. 107

Medical Monitoring System, Inc................................ 532

Memphis City Schools.. 367

Merrick Educational Center....................................... 80

Metrolina Association for the Blind...................... 290, 513

Metropolitan Nashville Public Schools/Visually
  Impaired/Multihandicapped Program....................... 368

Metropolitan Washington Ear, Inc....................... 74, 172

Michigan Association of Transcribers for the Visually
  Impaired.. 195

Michigan Braille Transcribing Service........................ 513

Michigan Commission for the Blind
  Training Center.. 198, 201

Michigan Department of Education/Special Education
  Services... 192

Michigan Ophthalmological Society........................... 202

Michigan Optometric Association.............................. 202

Michigan School for the Deaf and Blind............... 192, 193

Michigan State University.. 193

Microsystems Software, Inc..................................... 530

MicroTalk Software.. 530

Middle Tennessee Reception Center.......................... 369

Mideastern Michigan Library Co-op/Library for the
  Blind and Physically Handicapped........................... 195

Mid-Illinois Talking Book.. 121

Mid-Michigan Center for the Blind.............. 519, 520, 532

Midwest Enterprises for the Blind............................. 199

Midwestern Braille Volunteers.................................. 222

Milwaukee Area Technical College............................ 431

Minnesota Academy of Ophthalmology 211
Minnesota Library for the Blind and Physically
    Handicapped 207, 208
Minnesota Optometric Association 211
Minnesota Resource Center/Blind/Visually Impaired 207
Minnesota Services for the Blind/Career and
    Independent Living Services 212
Minnesota State Academy for the Blind 206, 207, 211
Minnesota State Services for the Blind 208
Minnesota State Services for the Blind/
    Communication Center 207
Minnesota State Services for the Blind and Visually
    Handicapped 209
Mirage Multimedia Systems, Inc. 530
Mississippi Department of Education 213
Mississippi Eye, Ear, Nose, and Throat Association 217
Mississippi Industries for the Blind 216
Mississippi Library Commission/Talking Book and
    Braille Services 214
Mississippi Optometric Association, Inc. 217
Mississippi School for the Blind 213, 214, 217
Mississippi State University/Rehabilitation Research
    and Training Center on Blindness and Low Vision 214
Missouri Department of Elementary and Secondary
    Education 219
Missouri Ophthalmological Society 225
Missouri Optometric Association, Inc. 225
Missouri Rehabilitation Services for the Blind 222
Missouri School for the Blind 219, 221, 225
Mobile Association for the Blind 9
Mobility Services, Inc. 105
Mons International 523
Montana Academy of Ophthalmology 230
Montana Department of Curriculum/Division of
    Special Education 228
Montana Low Vision Service, Inc. 230
Montana Optometric Association, Inc. 230
Montana School for the Deaf and the Blind 228, 229
Montana Talking Books Library 229
Montefiore Hospital/Medical Center/Low Vision
    Service 283
Monterey County Braille Transcribers 513
Montgomery County Association for the Blind 342
Montgomery County Public Schools Vision Services
    Center 172
Montgomery Home for the Blind/Wyoming Pioneer
    Home 434
Moore Eye Foundation 349
Morgan Memorial Goodwill Industries, Inc. 186
MSMT Braille Center 513
M-Tech Optics Corporation 523
Multi-Sensory Intervention Through Consultation and
    Education (MICE) 240

Muskegon County Library for the Blind and Physically
    Handicapped 195
Myasthenia Gravis Foundation 479
Myna Corporation 530
Myopia International Research Foundation 479

N

Naperville Area Transcribing for the Blind 123
Narrative Television Network 517
Nassau Community College Library 262
National Academy of Audio Description/RP
    International 518
National Accreditation Council for Agencies Serving
    the Blind and Visually Handicapped 479
National Association for Parents of the Visually
    Impaired 492
National Association for
    Visually Handicapped 40, 479, 513, 520, 523
National Association of Area Agencies on Aging 480
National Association of Blind Teachers 492
National Association of Radio Reading Services 480
National Association of State Directors of Special
    Education 492
National Association of State Units on Aging 480
National Association of Vision Professionals 492
National Association to Promote the Use of Braille 514
National Birth Defects Center 480
National Braille Association 514
National Braille Press 514
National Camps for Blind Children 481
National Catalog House of the Deaf 534
National Center for Health Statistics 468
National Coalition on Deaf-Blindness 492
National Council of Private Agencies for the Blind 481
National Council of State Agencies for the Blind 492
National Council on Disability 466
National Early Childhood Technical Assistance System
    (NEC*TAS) 481
National Easter Seals Society 481
National Eye Care Project (NECP) 481
National Eye Research Foundation (Optometry) 482
National Federation of the Blind 493, 519, 520, 523, 532
National Federation of the Blind of Utah 393
National Glaucoma Research Program of the American
    Health Assistance Foundation 482
National Industries for the Blind 482
National Information Center for Children and Youth
    with Disabilities 482
National Institute for Rehabilitation Engineering 248, 530
National Institute on Disability and Rehabilitation
    Research 465, 466
National Institutes of Health/National Eye Institute
    Information Center 468

National Institutes of Health/National Institute on Aging.. 468
National Marfan Foundation 493
National Multiple Sclerosis Society 483
National Naval Medical Center/Ophthalmology Service 176
National Organization for Albinism and Hypopigmentation (NOAH) 493
National Pen Corporation.. 523
National Self-Help Clearinghouse......................... 483
Nebraska Academy of Ophthalmology 235
Nebraska Department of Education................. 232, 233
Nebraska Department on Aging............................. 236
Nebraska Division of Rehabilitation Services for the Visually Impaired 234, 235
Nebraska Optometric Association, Inc................... 235
Nebraska School for the Visually Handicapped 232, 233, 235
NEGA RESA 100
Neighborhood News for the Blind 288
Nevada Bureau of Services to the Blind.......... 237, 238
Nevada Department of Education 237
Nevada Ophthalmological Society.......................... 239
Nevada Optometric Association, Inc....................... 239
Nevada Public Radio Corporation/KNPR 238
Nevada State Library/Regional Library for the Blind 238
Nevada State Library and Archives/Regional Library for the Blind/Talking Book Program 237
New Concepts Marketing, Inc.................................. 523
New England Eye Institute of the New England College of Optometry, Low Vision Clinic 190
New England Home for the Deaf (Aged, Blind or Infirm).. 186
New England Medical Center/New England Eye Center 190
New Eyes for the Needy 483
New Hampshire Association for the Blind 242
New Hampshire Association for the Blind/Low Vision Program 242
New Hampshire Department of Education............. 240
New Hampshire Educational Services for the Sensory Impaired 240, 241
New Hampshire Optometric Association, Inc........ 242
New Hampshire's Early Support and Services/ Division of Mental Health and Developmental Services/New Hampshire Department of Health and Human Services 240
New Hampshire Society of Eye Physicians and Surgeons 242
New Hampshire State Library/Library Services to the Handicapped Division... 241
New Jersey Academy of Ophthalmology 249
New Jersey College Resource Center for Adaptive Aids.. 246
New Jersey Commission for the Blind and Visually Impaired 247, 250

New Jersey Foundation for the Blind..................... 248
New Jersey Library for the Blind and Handicapped........... 245
New Jersey Optometric Association 249
New Mexico Commission for the Blind............ 253, 254
New Mexico Commission for the Blind/Low Vision Clinic 254
New Mexico Ophthalomological Society................ 254
New Mexico Optometric Association, Inc............... 254
New Mexico School for the Visually Handicapped 251, 252, 254
New Mexico School for the Visually Handicapped Preschool 252
New Mexico State Department of Education/Special Education Office.. 251
New Mexico State Library for the Blind and Physically Handicapped 252
Newsline for the Blind... 252
Newspapers for the Blind.. 196
New York City Industries for the Blind.................. 275
New York Eye and Ear Infirmary 284
New York Institute for Special Education 255, 279
New York Public Library Project ACCESS/Mid-Manhattan Library 260
New York State Commission for the Blind and Visually Handicapped 265
New York State Education Department/Office for Special Education Services 255
New York State Ophthalmological Society............. 280
New York State Optometric Association, Inc.......... 280
New York State School for the Blind 256
New York State Talking Book and Braille Library 260
New York University/School of Education/ Rehabilitation Counseling Program 259
Niagara Frontier Radio Reading Service 263
North Carolina Department of Human Resources/ Division of Services for the Blind 287, 288
North Carolina Department of Public Instruction/ Exceptional Children Division 286
North Carolina Library for the Blind and Physically Handicapped 287
North Carolina Lions Foundation........................... 290
North Carolina Memorial Hospital/Low Vision Clinic..... 292
North Carolina Rehabilitation Center for the Blind............. 291
North Carolina Society of Eye Physicians and Surgeons .. 291
North Carolina State Optometric Society, Inc........ 292
North Central Sight Services 330
North Central Sight Services/Pennsylvania Association for the Blind 342
Northcentral Technical College........................ 425, 431
North Country Association for the Visually Impaired 275
North Dakota Department of Human Services 296
North Dakota Department of Public Instruction.... 294

North Dakota Optometric Association, Inc. 296

North Dakota Society of Ophthalmology and
  Otolaryngology 296

North Dakota State Library Services for the Disabled 295

North Dakota Vision Services/
  School for the Blind 294, 295, 296

Northeastern Association of the Blind 276, 279, 284

North Eastern Indiana Radio Reading Service, Inc.
  (NEIRRS) 138

Northeastern University 180

Northeast Eye Institute 349

Northeast Radio Reading Service 263

Northeast Vision Consultants 178

Northern Illinois Radio Information Services/WNIJ 124

Northern Illinois Radio Information Services/WNIU-
  FM 124

Northern Illinois University 120

Northern Indiana Independent Living Service/ADEC
  Resources for Independence 140

Northern Kentucky Talking Book Library 157

Northern Nevada Braille Transcribers 514

Northern State College/Special Education Program 363

Northland Library Cooperative 195

Northland Public Library 330

Northport Veterans Affairs Medical Center/Low
  Vision Clinic and VICTORS Program 284

North Shore University Hospital Low Vision Services 284

North Texas Taping and Radio for the Blind 379, 380

Northwestern Medical Faculty Foundation 133

Northwest Indiana Subregional Library for the Blind
  and Physically Handicapped 137

Northwest Kansas Library System/Talking Books 150

NTAC (National Technical Assistance Consortium for
  Children and Young Adults who are Deaf-Blind)/
  Teaching Research Division 483

Nurion Industries 521

O

Oak Hill School/Connecticut Institute for the Blind 65, 66

Oakland County Library for the Blind and Physically
  Handicapped 195

Oakmont Visual Aids Workshop 38

The Occupational Rehabilitation Group, Inc. 187, 188

Ocutech, Inc. 523

Office for Special Education/Tennessee Department of
  Education 367

Office for the Aging 285

Office of Adult Services and Aging 365

Office of Aging 107, 422

Office of Early Intervention and School Readiness/
  Florida Division of Public Schools/Department of
  Education 78

Office of Elderly Affairs 166

Office of Federal Contract Compliance Programs 468

Office of Maternal and Child Health/Children with
  Special Health Care Needs Program/West Virginia
  Department of Health and Human Resources 417

Office of Programs for Exceptional Children/South
  Carolina Department of Education 357

Office of Services to the Aging 205

Office of Special Education/South Dakota Division of
  Education and Resources 362

Office of Special Education Programs 466

Office of Special Education Programs/New Jersey
  Department of Education 244

Office of Special Education Services 161

Office of Vocational Rehabilitation for the Blind/
  Mississippi Department of
  Rehabilitation Services 215, 218

Office on Aging 77, 177

Ohio Department of Aging 311

Ohio Department of Education/Division of Special
  Education 298

Ohio Department of Health/Bureau of Early
  Intervention Services 298

Ohio Educational Telecommunications Network
  Commission 302

Ohio Ophthalmological Society 310

Ohio Optometric Association, Inc. 310

Ohio Rehabilitation Services Commission/Bureau of
  Services for the Visually Impaired 303

Ohio State School for the Blind 298, 299, 309

Ohio State University/School of Teaching and
  Learning 300

Ohio State University College of Optometry/Low
  Vision Clinic 311

Ohio Valley Goodwill Industries/Rehabilitation Center .. 307

Okay Vision-Aide Corporation 523

Oklahoma League for the Blind 316

Oklahoma Library for the Blind and Physically
  Handicapped 315

Oklahoma Optometric Association 317

Oklahoma State Department of Education/Special
  Education Services 313

Oklahoma State Department of Education/Special
  Education Services/Sooner Start Program 313

Oklahoma State Society of Eye Physicians and
  Surgeons 317

Olympia Educational Service District 114 414

Omnichron 530

OMS Development 526, 530

One on One Computer Training 530

Onondaga Braillists 262

Ophthalmology Department/University of Nebraska
  Medical Center 235

Optelec 526, 530

Opticians Association of America 493
Optometric Center of Los Angeles 54
Optometric Center of St. Louis 226
Optometric Society of the District of Columbia 76
Orbis International 483
ORCLISH (Ohio Resource Center for Low Incidence and Severely Handicapped) 300
Oregon Academy of Ophthalmology 323
Oregon Commission for the Blind 321, 322, 324
Oregon Department of Education 318, 319
Oregon Health Sciences University / Department of Ophthalmology / Low Vision Aid Clinic 323
Oregon Office of Special Education / Services to Children and Youth with Deafblindness 318
Oregon Optometric Association 323
Oregon School for the Blind 318, 319, 320, 322
Oregon State Library / Talking Book and Braille Services 320, 321
Oregon Text and Media Center for the Visually Handicapped 320
Outreach Services / Perkins School for the Blind 180
Outreach Services to Elders / Perkins School for the Blind 187
Overbrook International / Overbrook School for the Blind 484
Overbrook School for the Blind 325, 327, 348
Overseer Electronic Visual Aids 523
Owensboro Recording Unit 157

P
Pacific University / College of Optometry 323
Palco Labs 532
Palm Beach County Schools 82
Palomar College 51
Parent Advocates for Visually Impaired Children (PAVIC) 61
Parents, Let's Unite for Kids (PLUK) 230
Parkview School (Oklahoma School for the Blind) 313, 314, 315, 316
PC-SIG 530
Peabody College of Vanderbilt University 369
Peal Software, Inc. 530
Pencar Associates 523
Peninsula Center for the Blind and Visually Impaired .. 47, 55
Pennsylvania Academy of Ophthalmology and Otolaryngology 348
Pennsylvania Association for the Blind 343
Pennsylvania Association for the Blind and Handicapped 330
Pennsylvania College of Optometry / Institute for the Visually Impaired 328
Pennsylvania Department of Aging 350
Pennsylvania Department of Education / Bureau of Special Education 325

Pennsylvania Department of Public Welfare 350
Pennsylvania Lions Beacon Lodge Camp 343
Pennsylvania Optometric Association, Inc. 348
Penrickton Center for Blind Children 199
Peoria Area Blind People's Center, Inc. 123, 130
Peripheral Technologies, Inc. 530
Perkins School for the Blind 179
Personal Data Systems, Inc. 526
Personal Interface 526, 530
Petaluma Braille Transcribers, Inc. 38
Philip J. Rock Center and School 118
Phillip Barton Vision Systems 521, 523, 526, 530
Philomatheon Society of the Blind, Inc. 307
PIA Media Center 193
Pilot Dogs, Inc. 310
Pinellas Center for the Visually Impaired, Inc. (PCVI) 91
Pinellas County Schools 82
Pittsburgh Blind Association / Pennsylvania Association for the Blind (now known as Pittsburgh Vision Services) 344
Pittsburgh Vision Services 344
Porter Memorial Hospital / Porter Low Vision Service 64
Portland Family Vision Center 323
Portland State University / Department of Special Education 320
Precision Grinding & Manufacturing 521
Prescott Talking Book Library 19
Preserve Sight Colorado 61
Preserve Sight Mississippi 215
President's Committee on Employment of People with Disabilities 470
Prevent Blindness America 125, 484
Prevent Blindness Connecticut 67
Prevent Blindness Florida 83
Prevent Blindness Georgia 101
Prevent Blindness Indiana 138
Prevent Blindness Iowa 145
Prevent Blindness Kentucky 157
Prevent Blindness Massachusetts 182
Prevent Blindness Nebraska 234
Prevent Blindness New Jersey 246
Prevent Blindness New York 264
Prevent Blindness North Carolina 288
Prevent Blindness Northern California 40
Prevent Blindness Ohio 303
Prevent Blindness Oklahoma 315
Prevent Blindness Southern California 40
Prevent Blindness Tennessee 370
Prevent Blindness Texas / Austin Branch 380
Prevent Blindness Texas / Dallas Branch 380
Prevent Blindness Texas / East Texas Branch 380
Prevent Blindness Texas / El Paso Branch 380

Prevent Blindness Texas/Fort Worth Branch............ 381
Prevent Blindness Texas/Galveston/Gulf Coast
   Branch.. 381
Prevent Blindness Texas/Lubbock Branch 381
Prevent Blindness Texas/Midland Branch 381
Prevent Blindness Texas/San Antonio Branch......... 381
Prevent Blindness Texas/State Office........................ 381
Prevent Blindness Utah... 393
Prevent Blindness Virginia 403
Prevent Blindness Wisconsin 428
Prevention of Blindness Society of Metropolitan
   Washington 74
Print Access Center/The Lighthouse Inc. 514
Prodigy Products Company 523, 526
Productivity Software International 530
The Productivity Works 530
Program for Visually Impaired/Milwaukee Area
   Technical College 425
Program for Visually Impaired Adults/Family Service
   Association 141
Programs for the Blind and Visually Impaired/
   Wisconsin Division of Vocational Rehabilitation Low
   Vision Services 431
Programs in Special Education 358
Project CABLE/Carroll Center for the Blind............ 188
Prophecy Designs 521
Prose & Cons Braille Unit 514
Public Library of Cincinnati and Hamilton County/
   Library for the Blind and Physically Handicapped 300
Puerto Rico Blind Rehabilitation Center/U.S.
   Department of Veterans Affairs 353
Puerto Rico Deaf-Blind Parents Association/Projecto
   Ninos Sordos-Ciegos 352
Puerto Rico Department of Education/Special
   Education Program 351, 352
Puerto Rico Ophthalmological Society 353
Puerto Rico Regional Library for the Blind and
   Physically Handicapped....................................... 352
PulseData International, Inc. 523

Q
Queens Borough Public Library/Special Services........ 261
Quik-Scrybe 38

R
Radio Information Center for the Blind (RICB)...................... 330
Radio Information Service 124
Radio Information Service for Blind and Print
   Handicapped 124
Radio Information Services 331
Radio Reading Network of Maryland 172
Radio Reading Service of Mississippi........................ 215
Radio Reading Service of the Rockies 60

Radio Reading Service of Western New England................. 182
Radio Reading Services, Inc. 288
Radio Reading Services of Greater Cincinnati, Inc. 302
Radio Talking Book Network 208
Radio Talking Book Service 234
Radio Vision-Ramapo Catskill Library System 263
Rainshine Company 521
Raised Dot Computing, Inc. 530
Raleigh Lions Clinic for the Blind 290
Raleigh Lions Clinic for the Blind/Evaluation Unit/
   North Carolina Division of Services for the Blind............ 292
Randolph-Sheppard Vendors of America................... 494
Random House Large Print.. 515
R.C. Systems, Inc. 526, 530
Readers' Services Department 137
Reading Radio Service 151
Recording for the Blind and Dyslexic................ 20, 38, 60, 100,
   123, 157, 181, 182, 195, 245, 246, 262, 330, 369, 379, 402, 515
Recording for the Blind and Dyslexic/Connecticut Unit..... 67
Recording for the Blind and Dyslexic/Florida Unit 82
Recording for the Blind and Dyslexic of Metropolitan
   Washington 74
Recording Library for the Blind and Physically
   Handicapped 379
Reed EZ-Reader, Inc. 524
Reflection Technology 524, 527
Regional Audio Information Service Enterprise
   (RAISE).. 288
Region IV Education Service Center........................... 379
Rehabilitation Center for the Blind/Kansas
   Department of Social Services 154
Rehabilitation Center Vision Rehabilitation Services............ 69
Rehabilitation Division/Nevada Department of
   Human Resources 239
Rehabilitation Services/Colorado Department of
   Human Services 61, 64
Rehabilitation Services Administration/Arizona
   Department of Economic Security 20, 24
Rehabilitation Services Administration (RSA)....................... 466
Rehabilitation Services Commission/Bureau of
   Services for the Visually Impaired 312
Rehabilitation Services for the Visually Impaired/
   Nebraska Department of Public Institutions..................... 236
Replogle Globes, Inc... 524, 530
Research to Prevent Blindness................................... 484
RESNA.. 494
Resource Center for the Visually Impaired/New York
   State School for the Blind 259
Resources for Rehabilitation...................................... 515
Rhode Island Department of Education..................... 354
Rhode Island Department of Elderly Affairs............. 356
Rhode Island Optometric Association 356

Rhode Island Regional Library for the Blind and
Physically Handicapped.. 354

Rhode Island Services for the Blind and Visually
Impaired.. 356

Rhode Island Services for the Blind and Visually
Impaired / Rhode Island Department of Human
Services.. 356

Rhode Island Society of Eye Physicians and Surgeons....... 356

Richard E. Hoover Services for Low Vision and
Blindness / Department of Ophthalmology / Greater
Baltimore Medical Center.. 176

Rio Salado Community College.. 17

RISE.. 263

Roanoke City Public Library / Outreach Services................ 402

Rocky Mountain Development Council................................ 230

Rodef Shalom Temple Sisterhood....................................... 330

Rome Subregional Library for the Blind and Physically
Handicapped.. 99

Roosevelt Warm Springs Institute for Rehabilitation.......... 101

Rose Resnick Lighthouse for the Blind and Visually
Impaired.................................. 47, 519, 521, 532

Roundley Associates 530

Royal Data Systems / Speech and Learning Center
Systems 527, 530, 534

Royer-Greaves School for Blind 326

RP International 48

RP International / Low Vision 55

Rubbermaid Health Care Products 521

Ruth M. Shellens Library / The Lighthouse Inc. 261

Ruth Parker Eason School 175

S

St. John's Episcopal Home for the Aged and Blind............. 276

St. Joseph's Home for the Blind.. 248

St. Joseph's Low Vision Services 24

St. Joseph's School for the Blind 244

St. Louis Society for the Blind
and Visually Impaired 224, 227

St. Lucy Day School for Children with Visual
Impairments 326

St. Martin's Press... 515

St. Mary Low Vision Center 55

St. Paul-Ramsey Medical Center Low Vision Clinic............ 211

Samuel W. Bell Home for Sightless, Inc. 307

San Antonio Lighthouse... 385

San Bernardino Valley Lighthouse for the Blind, Inc. 48

San Diego Center for the Blind and Vision Impaired 48

San Francisco State University... 36

San Gabriel Valley Braille Guild 38

Santa Barbara City Schools Program for Visually
Impaired / Special Education Services 33

Santa Barbara School District 38

Santa Rosa Low Vision Clinic... 389

Savannah Association for the Blind / Communications
Department, Inc 106

Savannah Association for the Blind, Inc. 105

Saving Sight Rhode Island 354

Schamex Research 527

Scheie Eye Institute Department of Ophthalmology /
University of Pennsylvania Health System / Low
Vision Research and Rehabilitation Center 349

Schepens Eye Research Institute 485

Schepens Retina Associates / Low Vision Rehabilitation
Center 190

Scholastic, Inc. 530

Science Applications International Corporation 534

Science Products 519, 524, 527

Scientific Capital Corporation 527

Scripps Memorial Hospital Mericos Eye Institute /
Partial Vision Center 55

SCS 535

Sears, Roebuck and Company /
New Account Center.......................... 521, 524, 533

Seattle Area Braillists, Inc. 411

Section of Special Education / Missouri Department of
Elementary and Secondary Education 219

Seedlings: Braille Books for Children.................................... 515

Seeing Eye, Inc. 249

Seeing Hand Association 421

Seemore Vision Products... 524, 530

Senior and Disabled Services Division................................ 324

Senior Citizen Affairs / Virgin Islands Department of
Human Services 408

Sensory Access Foundation 49

Sensory Program / Rehabilitation Research and
Development Center (151 R) / U.S. Department of
Veterans Affairs... 106

Sequoia Transcribers 39

Service Club for the Blind.. 225

Services for Blind and Physically Handicapped /
Kanawha County Public Library................................. 418

Services for Sensory Accommodations / University of
Illinois at Urbana-Champaign / Division of
Rehabilitation Education Services............................... 130

Services for the Blind / California Department of
Rehabilitation 41, 57

Services for the Blind / Tennessee Division of
Rehabilitation Services 368

Services for the Blind and Physically Handicapped /
Cabell County Public Library...................................... 418

Services for the Blind and Physically Handicapped /
Ohio County Public Library... 419

Services for the Blind and Physically Handicapped /
Parkersburg and Wood County Public Library 419

Services for the Blind and Visually Impaired 354

Services for the Blind and Visually Impaired / New
Hampshire Division of Vocational Rehabilitation.. 241, 242

Services for the Blind and Visually Impaired/
Tennessee Division of Rehabilitation Services 370
Services for the Visually Impaired/Wyoming
Department of Education 433
Services to the Blind/Reorganized Church of Jesus
Christ of Latter-Day Saints 515
Services to the Blind and Visually Impaired 363
Service to the Visually Impaired/Business and
Education Institute 365
Sight and Hearing Association/Minnesota Society for
the Prevention of Blindness and Preservation of
Hearing 208
Sight Center Audio Network 302
The Sight Center of the Toledo Society for the Blind. 301, 307
Sighted Electronics 532
Sight Line Productions 515
The Sight Seer 196
Sight Society of Ohio, Inc. 308
Signature Works, Inc. 216
Simon & Schuster Publishing 516
Sisterhood Braille Group of East Midwood Jewish
Center 262
Sisterhood of Temple Beth Hillel 39
Sisterhood of Temple Sinai 262
Sisterhood Temple Israel of Jamaica 262
Sister Kenny Institute 211
SkiSoft, Inc. 531
Small Business Administration 470
Smith-Kettlewell Eye Research Institute/Rehabilitation
Engineering Center 485
Social Security Administration 468
Society for the Blind 49
Society for the Blind/Visual Services Center/Low
Vision Clinic 56
Soft Key International 531
Sonic Alert 534
South Carolina Commission for the Blind... 358, 359, 360, 361
South Carolina Commission for the Blind/Columbia
Office 361
South Carolina Commission on Aging 361
South Carolina Educational Radio for the Blind 359
South Carolina Eye Institute/Department of
Ophthalmology/University of South Carolina School
of Medicine 361
South Carolina Optometric Association, Inc. 361
South Carolina School for the Deaf
and the Blind 357, 358, 359
South Carolina Society of Ophthalmology 360
South Carolina State Library/Department for the Blind
and Physically Handicapped 358, 359
South Central Kansas Library System/Talking Book
Division 150
South Dakota Academy of Ophthalmology 365

South Dakota Industries for the Blind 363, 364
South Dakota Low Vision Services/Service for the
Blind and Visually Impaired 365
South Dakota Optometric Society 365
South Dakota Rehabilitation Center for the Blind 365
South Dakota School for the Visually Handicapped . 362, 363
South Dakota State Library for the Handicapped 363
Southeastern Blind Rehabilitation Center 10
Southeastern Blind Rehabilitation Center/U.S.
Department of Veterans Affairs 10
Southeastern Guide Dogs, Inc. 93
Southeastern North Carolina Radio Reading Service 288
Southern California College of Optometry/Low Vision
Clinic 56
Southern College of Optometry 374
Southern Illinois Radio Information Service 125
Southern Illinois Talking Book Center 121
Southern Illinois University 121, 123
Southern Nevada Sightless 239
Southern Tier Association for the Visually Impaired 276
Southern Will County Cooperative 120
South Texas Lighthouse for the Blind 386
Southwest Alabama Regional School for the Deaf and
Blind 3, 6
Southwestern Blind Rehabilitation Center 22
Special Education Media Center 234
Special Education, Part H Program/Nebraska
Department of Education 232
Special Education Services Agency 13
Special Education Services Agency/Infant Learning
Program 13
Special Education Technology Center 153, 414
Special Education Unit/Vermont Department of
Education 396
Special Library and Transcription Services/Minnesota
State Services for the Blind Communication Center 208
Special Needs Center/Phoenix Public Library 19
Special Needs Library 172
Special Needs Vision Clinic 203
Special School District, Saint Louis County 222
Special Services/Fairfax County Public Library 402
Special Services/Tulsa City-County Library System 315
Special Services Division/Virginia Beach Public
Library 402
Spectrum, The Lighthouse Store 521
Sped Publications 524
Spencerport Braille Association 262
Spies Laboratories 531
Stampcrete Decorative Concrete, Inc. 535
Stanford/Department of Ophthalmology, Low Vision
Services 56
State Agency on Aging 254

State Department of Rehabilitation / Visual Services
   Division 317
Stat Talk Computer Products 531
Stephanie Joyce Kahn Foundation (SJK) 261
Stephen F. Austin State University 378
Stocker and Yale, Inc. 524
STORER Computer Access Center / Cleveland Sight
   Center of the Cleveland Society of the Blind 310
Strieter Laboratories, Inc. 524
Subregional Library for the Blind and Physically
   Handicapped 99
Subregional Library for the Blind and Physically
   Handicapped / Talking Book Center 100
Summitville Tiles, Inc. 535
Sunrise Care Center Inc. 430
Sun Sounds Radio Reading Service 20
Suprarock Block Company 535
Susquehanna Association for the Blind and Vision
   Impaired 344
S. Walters, Inc. 524
Syn-Talk Systems and Services 531

T
Tagarno of America, Inc. 524
Talking and Visual Aids 524, 531
Talking Book and Braille Service 233, 234
Talking Book Center 100, 101, 172
Talking Book Center / Staunton Public Library 402
Talking Book Center of Northwest Illinois 121
Talking Book Library 157, 181
Talking Book Library / Jacksonville Public Libraries 81
Talking Book Program / Las Vegas–Clark County
   Library 238
Talking Book Program / State Library of Ohio 300
Talking Book Program / Las Vegas-Clark County
   Library / Subregional Library for the Blind and
   Handicapped 237
Talking Books 150
Talking Books / Nassau Library System 261
Talking Books / Palm Beach County Library Annex 81
Talking Books Department 150
Talking Book Service 81
Talking Book Service / Alexandria Library 402
Talking Book Service / Arlington County Department
   of Libraries 402
Talking Book Service / Library for the Blind and
   Physically Handicapped 150
Talking Book Services 137
Talking Books Plus / Outreach Services 261
Talking Computer Products 531
Talking Computers, Inc. 531
Talking Computer Systems 527, 531

Talking Information Center 182
The Talking Library 370
Talking Tapes for the Blind 222
Talktronics, Inc. 527
Talladega College 4
Tampa Lighthouse for the Blind 91, 93
Tandy / Radio Shack 531, 533
Taping for the Blind 485
Teachers College, Columbia University / Department
   of Health and Behavioral Studies 260
Technical Aids Center / New Jersey Commission for the
   Blind and Visually Impaired 249
Technologies for the Visually Impaired, Inc. 527, 531
Technology Center / North Dakota School for the Blind 296
Technology for Independence 521
Techspress / RCIL 279
Tekvision Products 524
TeleSensory Corporation 524, 527, 531
Temple Israel Sisterhood 369
Temple Sinai Sisterhood 330
Temple Sisterhood Braille Group 82, 301
Temple University Hospital / Ophthalmology
   Department 350
Tennessee Academy of Ophthalmology 374
Tennessee Department of Education 367
Tennessee Department of Education / Resource Center
   for the Visually Impaired 369
Tennessee Department of Human Services / Division of
   Rehabilitation Services 375
Tennessee Library for the Blind and Physically
   Handicapped 369, 370
Tennessee Optometric Association, Inc. 374
Tennessee Rehabilitation Center 374
Tennessee Rehabilitation Center / Visually Impaired
   Services 372
Tennessee School for the Blind 367, 368, 369, 374
Texas Commission for the Blind 381, 387, 390
Texas Commission for the Blind / Criss Cole
   Rehabilitation Center 386
Texas Department on Aging 390
Texas Education Agency 376
Texas Instructional Materials Center for Students with
   Visual Handicaps / Texas Education Agency / Texas
   School for the Blind and Visually Impaired 378
Texas Instruments 531, 534
Texas Ophthalmological Association 388
Texas Optometric Association, Inc. 388
Texas School for the Blind
   and Visually Impaired 376, 377, 388
Texas State Library / Talking Book Program 378, 379
Texas Tech University / College of Education 378
Texas Tech University / School of Medicine / Health
   Sciences Center 389

TFB Publications 246

T.F.I. Engineering, Inc. 531

Theodore Lester Elementary School 359

Theosophical Book Association for the Blind 516

Therapeutic Living Centers for the Blind 50

Thorndike Press 516

Traconex, Inc. 535

Trade Winds Rehabilitation Center 141

Transcribers of Orange County 39

Travis Association for the Blind 386

Traxler Enterprises 531

Tri-County Branch/Pennsylvania Association for the
Blind 345

Tri-Valley Developmental Services 149

Tri-Visual Services 39, 50

Truxes Company/Signage Division 535

T.S. Microtech, Inc. 527

Tucson Association for the Blind and Visually
Impaired 22, 23

Tulane Medical Center Hospital and Clinic 165

Turbo Power 531

Tuscaloosa Subregional Library for the Blind and
Physically Handicapped 5

Typewriting Institute for the Handicapped 524

U

Ulverscroft Large Print Books Limited 516

United Cerebral Palsy 485

United States Association for Blind Athletes 494

United States Blind Golfers Association 494

United States Braille Chess Foundation 485

Universal Engraving, Inc. 535

Universal Low Vision Aids 524

University Eye Institute/SUNY Health Science Center
at Syracuse 285

University Medical Center/Department of
Ophthalmology/John A. Moran Eye Center 395

University Medical Center, Department of
Ophthalmology 217

University of Alabama at Birmingham 4

University of Alabama at Birmingham/The Medical
Center/School of Optometry/Low Vision
Rehabilitation Clinic 11

University of Arizona 19

University of Arkansas at Little Rock 27

University of Arkansas for Medical Sciences/
Department of Ophthalmology 30

University of California, Davis Department of
Ophthalmology Low Vision Services 56

University of Florida/Eye Center, Low Vision Service 95

University of Illinois at Urbana-Champaign/Division
of Rehabilitation Education Services 124

University of Kansas Audio Reader Network 151

University of Kentucky Deafblind Project 155

University of Louisville/School of Education 156

University of Maryland/Department of
Ophthalmology/Low Vision Program 176

University of Massachusetts at Boston 180

University of Minnesota/Department of Educational
Psychology 207

University of Minnesota/Department of
Ophthalmology 212

University of Nebraska 233

University of North Dakota 295

University of Northern Colorado 60

University of Pittsburgh/School of Education/
Department of Instruction and Learning 328

University of Puerto Rico 352

University of Texas/Health Science Center at Dallas/
Department of Ophthalmology Low Vision Clinic 389

University of Texas at Austin 378

University of Texas, Health Science Center 390

University of Toledo/Department of Special Education
Services 300

University of Washington 411

UPDATE 263

Upper Peninsula Library for the Blind and Physically
Handicapped 195

Upshaw Institute for the Blind 199

U.S. Department of Education/Office of the Secretary 465

U.S. Department of Health and Human Services/Office
of the Secretary 467

U.S. Department of Justice/Civil Rights Division/
Coordination and Review Section 471

U.S. Department of Labor/Office of the Secretary 468

U.S. Department of Transportation/Office of the
Secretary 468

U.S. Department of Veterans Affairs/Office of the
Secretary 469

U.S. Employment Service 468

U.S. Office of Personnel Management/Office of Human
Resources and Equal Employment 471

Utah Division of Services for the Blind and Visually
Impaired 393

Utah Educational Resource Center 392

Utah Industries for the Blind 394

Utah Ophthalmological Society 394

Utah Optometric Association 394

Utah Schools for the Deaf and the Blind 391, 392, 393

Utah Schools for the Deaf and the Blind/Parent-Infant
Program (PIP) 392

Utah State Library/Division for the Blind and
Physically Handicapped 392

Utah State Office of Education/Special Education
Section 391

Utah State Office of Rehabilitation 395

Utah State Radio Reading Service.................................. 393

V

Valley Voice Radio Reading Service............................... 402

Venango County Branch/Pennsylvania Association for
the Blind 345

Ventura County Braille Transcribers Association 39

Vermont Association for the Blind and Visually
Impaired 396, 397

Vermont Association of Business, Industry, and
Rehabilitation 398

Vermont Department of Aging and Disabilities.................. 398

Vermont Department of Libraries/Special Services
Unit... 396

Vermont Ophthalmological Society 398

Vermont Optometric Association 398

Veterans Administration/West Side Medical Center/
VICTORS Program 134

Veterans Administration Center 432

Veterans Administration Hospital/Low Vision Service,
Eye Clinic 95

Veterans Affairs Medical Center.. 56

Veterans Benefits Administration (VBA)............................ 469

Veterans Health Administration (VHA)............................... 469

Virginia Association of Workers for the Blind 405

Virginia Department for the Aging 406

Virginia Department for the
Visually Handicapped 400, 403, 406

Virginia Department for the Visually Handicapped/
Instructional Materials and Resource Center..................... 401

Virginia Department for the Visually Handicapped/
Program for Infants, Children, and Youth 399

Virginia Department for the Visually Handicapped/
Services Division 406

Virginia Industries for the Blind/Virginia Department
for the Visually Handicapped 405

Virginia Optometric Association.. 405

Virginia Optometric Center 406

Virginia Rehabilitation Center for the Blind............... 405, 406

Virginia School for the Deaf and Blind at Hampton .. 399, 401

Virginia School for the Deaf and the Blind 399

Virginia Society of Ophthalmology 405

Virginia Tech Radio Reading Service.................................. 403

Virginia Voice for the Print Handicapped 403

Virgin Islands Department of Education/State Office of
Special Education 407

Virgin Islands Department of Human Services..................... 408

Virgin Islands Regional Library for the Visually and
Physically Handicapped.. 407

Vision Center of Central Ohio 301, 308, 310

VISION Foundation 187

Visionics Corporation Inc. 520

Vision Loss Resources............................... 210, 211, 212

Vision Northwest.. 322

Vision Rehabilitation Center 154

Vision Rehabilitation Inc................................ 299, 309, 311

Vision Rehabilitation Institute/Genesis Medical Center .. 147

Vision Rehabilitation Institute, Sinai Hospital.................... 204

Vision Rehabilitation Service/Wisconsin Council of the
Blind.. 432

Vision Resources Library 180

Vision Resources Library/Massachusetts Department
of Education 181, 182

Vision Services/Early Childhood Learning Center/
Montgomery County Public Schools 171

VISIONS/Services for the Blind and Visually Impaired ... 277

Vision Technology, Inc... 524

Visual Aid Volunteers, Inc. 516

Visual Impairment and Blindness Services of
Northampton County, Inc. (VIABL) 346

Visually Handicapped Materials Center/Cincinnati
Public Schools.. 301

Visually Handicapped Services/Detroit Receiving
Hospital and University Health Center..................... 200, 201

Visually Impaired Center 200, 202

Visually Impaired Persons of Southwest Florida 92

Visually Impaired Preschool Services (VIPS) 156

Visually Impaired Program/Hillsborough County
Schools 79

Visual Methods, Inc... 524

Visual Rehabilitation and Research Center of Southeast
Michigan 204

Visual Services Division/Oklahoma Department of
Rehabilitation Services 315

VITAL (Visually Impaired Training and Learning)
Center 373

VITAL (Visually Impaired Training and Learning)
Center of Nashville 373

Vocational Guidance Services 309

Vocational Rehabilitation/North Dakota Department
of Human Services 295

Vocational Rehabilitation/Blind and Low Vision
Services/Montana Department of Public Health and
Human Services 229

Vocational Rehabilitation Program/Puerto Rico
Department of Social Services 352

The Voice Connection... 531

Voice of the Peninsula 403

Volunteer Blind Industries.. 373

Volunteer Braille Services... 516

Volunteer Braillists and Tapists 516

Volunteer Services for the Visually Handicapped 428

Volunteers for the Visually Handicapped 74, 76, 172, 174

Volunteers of Vacaville... 516

Volunteer Transcribing Services 517

W

Walter Reed Army Medical Center/Ophthalmology
   Service 76
Washington Academy of Eye Physicians and Surgeons.... 414
Washington Association of Optometric Physicians 414
Washington DC Ophthalmological Society 76
Washington Department of Services for the Blind 416
Washington-Greene Blind Association 346
Washington Instructional Resource Center/
   Washington State School for the Blind 410
Washington Library for the Blind and Physically
   Handicapped 410
Washington Office of Superintendent of Public
   Instruction/Special Education 409
Washington State Braille Access Center/Washington
   State School for the Blind 411
Washington State Department of Services for the Blind.... 411
Washington State School for the Blind 409, 410, 415
Washington State School for the Blind/Technical
   Center for Blind and Visually Handicapped Students ... 414
Washington University Eye Center/Department of
   Ophthalmology and Visual Sciences/Low Vision
   Service 227
Washtenaw County Library for the Blind and
   Physically Handicapped 195
Watts Health Foundation/United Health Plan 57
Wausau School District 426
Wayne County Regional/Library for the Blind and
   Physically Handicapped 195
Wayne State University 193
WCBU Radio Information Service 125
WCNY-READ-OUT Radio Reading Service 263
Welcome Home for the Blind 201
Westchester Independent Living Center, Inc. 277
Western Blind Rehabilitation Center/U.S. Department
   of Veterans Affairs 50, 57
Western Center for Microcomputers 527
Western Michigan University/Department of Special
   Education 193
Western Michigan University/Vision Rehabilitation
   Clinic 204
Western Montana Radio Reading Services 229
Western Pennsylvania School for Blind Children 327
West Florida Regional Library Subregional Talking
   Book Library 81
Westmoreland County Branch/Pennsylvania
   Association for the Blind 346
West Texas Lighthouse for the Blind 387
West Virginia Academy of Ophthalmology 421
West Virginia Department of Education 417
West Virginia Division of Rehabilitation Services............. 422

West Virginia Instructional Resource Center/West
   Virginia Schools for the Deaf and the Blind 418
West Virginia Library Commission of Services for the
   Blind and Physically Handicapped 419
West Virginia Optometric Association 422
West Virginia Radio Reading Service 419
West Virginia Rehabilitation Center/Low Vision Clinic .. 422
West Virginia Schools for the Deaf
   and the Blind 417, 418, 419, 421
West Virginia Society for the Blind and Severely
   Disabled 421
WGCU Radio Reading Service 82
Wheeler Publishing, Inc. 517
Whirlpool Corporation/Appliance Information
   Services 521
White Cane Institute for the Blind 521
White Station Lions Foundation 375
Wichita Industries and Services for the Blind 152
Wichita Radio Reading Service 151
Wildlife Materials, Inc. 521
William Judson Center/San Antonio Lighthouse 388
Wills Eye Hospital/Low Vision Service 350
Winco Optical Inc. 524
Winston-Salem Industries for the Blind 291
Winston-Salem Industries for the Blind/Ashville
   Division 291
Wisconsin Academy of Ophthalmology 431
Wisconsin Council for the Blind 430
Wisconsin Department of Public Instruction/
   Exceptional Education Team 424
Wisconsin Educational Services Center for the Visually
   Impaired 427, 428
Wisconsin Optometric Association, Inc. 431
Wisconsin Regional Library for the Blind and
   Physically Handicapped 428
Wisconsin School for the Visually Handicapped and
   Educational Services Center for the Visually
   Impaired 426, 427, 431
Wiscraft/Wisconsin Enterprises for the Blind 430
WIUM/WIUW Radio Information Service 125
WJGF Radio Station 419
WKAR Radio Talking Book 196
W.K. Kellogg Eye Center/Low Vision Services/
   University of Michigan Medical Center 204
WLRH Radio 6
WLRN Radio Reading Service 82
WMFE Radio Reading Service 82
WNIN Radio Reading Service 138
Wolfner Library for the Blind and Physically
   Handicapped 221
Wood County Office of Education 299
Words Plus, Inc. 527, 534

Workshops, Inc. 10
Worthington Data Solutions 531
WRBH-FM/Radio for the Blind 162
Written Communications Radio Service (WCRS) for
    the Print Handicapped 302
WRKC-Radio Home Visitor 331
WRRS/RADPRIN of Lehigh Valley 331
WTSU Radio Reading Service 6
WUAL Radio Reading Service 6
WUIS/WIPA Radio Information Service 125
WUSF Radio Reading Service 83
WXXI Reachout Radio 263
Wyoming Ophthalmological Society 434
Wyoming Optometric Association 434
WYPL-FM 370

X
Xavier Society for the Blind 517
Xerox Adaptive Products 524
Xerox Imaging Systems 527

Y
York County Blind Center 347
York County Blind Center Radio Reading Service 331
Youngstown Braille Service 302
Youngstown Radio Reading Service 302
Yuma Center for the Visually Impaired 23

Z
Zero to 3 Hawaii Project 109
Zondervan Publishing House 517
Zygo Industries, Inc. 527, 534

CANADA

A

Access 20/20.. 452
Acrontech... 543
The Adaptive Computer Technology Centre (The ACT
    Centre)... 497
Alberta Association of Optometrists.......................... 438
Alberta Sports and Recreation Association for the Blind.. 501
Alternate Media Canada/The National Broadcast
    Reading Service.. 499
AmbuTech/Melet Plastics, Inc................................... 543
American Optometric Association 501
Atlantic Provinces Special Education Authority 501
Atlantic Provinces Special Education Authority
    (APSEA)/Department of Education 444, 446, 448, 456
Audiobook Program/Province of British Columbia
    (BBLA) Library Services Branch............................ 440
Audio Studio for the Reading Impaired..................... 539
Audio Vision Canada/The National Broadcast
    Reading Service, Inc. 541

B

Balance... 453
Betacom Group/Montreal Betacom.................... 543, 544
Betacom Group/Toronto Betacom 543, 544
Blindskills 539
Books Aloud... 539
Braille Authority of North America 499
Braille International.. 539
British Columbia College and Institute Library Service
    for the Print Impaired.. 439
British Columbia Library Services to the Handicapped 439

C

Canadian Association of Optometrists....................... 501
Canadian Blind Sports Association............................ 499
Canadian Council for Exceptional Children/Division
    for the Visually Handicapped............................... 501
Canadian Council of the Blind 501
Canadian Guide Dogs for the Blind........................... 454
Canadian Human Rights Commission 497
Canadian National Institute for the Blind 543, 544
Canadian National Institute for the Blind/Alberta–
    Northwest Territories Division...................... 438, 447
Canadian National Institute for the Blind/British
    Columbia-Yukon Division.............................. 441, 462
Canadian National Institute for the Blind/Department
    of Government Relations and International Services 499
Canadian National Institute for the Blind/Manitoba
    Division... 442
Canadian National Institute for the Blind/National
    Office 499

Canadian National Institute for the Blind/New
    Brunswick Division... 444
Canadian National Institute for the Blind/
    Newfoundland and Labrador Division................. 446
Canadian National Institute for the Blind/Nova
    Scotia–Prince Edward Island Division 449, 456
Canadian National Institute for the Blind/Ontario
    Division 453
Canadian National Institute for the Blind/Quebec
    Division... 458
Canadian National Institute for the Blind/
    Saskatchewan Division 460
Canadian National Society of the Deaf-Blind 501
Canadian Ophthalmological Society.......................... 501
Canadian Transportation Agency/Accessible
    Transportation Directorate 497
Canine Vision Canada/Lions Foundation of Canada........ 455
CDBRA (Canadian Deaf Blind Research Association)
    National Office 502
Centre for Sight Enhancement.................................... 455
Centre Louis-Hébert... 458
Christian Blind Mission International 539
Christian Mission for the Blind................................... 539
Christian Record Services... 539
Church of Jesus Christ of Latter-Day Saints/Special
    Curriculum... 539
Cleveland Sight Center of the Cleveland Society for the
    Blind.. 539
Community Living/Department of Social Services........... 460
Community Support Services Division/Ministry of
    Social Services 440
Computer Braille Facility/University of Western
    Ontario.. 452
Council for Exceptional Children................................ 502
Council of Schools for the Blind 502
Crane Resource Centre/University of British Columbia
                                                           440, 539

D

Department of Education, Culture and Employment/
    Early Childhood and School Services 447
Department of Family Services/Community Living
    Division 442
Department of Health and Social Services/
    Government of the Yukon....................................... 462
Developmental Services Branch/Ministry of
    Community and Social Services 453
Direction de l'Adaption Scolaire et des Services
    Complémentaires.. 457
Direction des Bibliothèques Publiques/Ministère des
    Affaires Culturelles... 458

E

Eastern School District Unit.. 456

Eyes of Faith Ministries.. 540

F

Family and Community Social Services/New
   Brunswick Department of Health and Community
   Services.. 444
Family and Rehabilitative Services/Department of
   Social Services, Province of Newfoundland 446
Family and Social Services Department......................... 438
Ferguson Library for Print Handicapped Students............... 449
Foundation Mira.. 459
Frontier Computing.. 454, 543, 544

G

Gospel Association for the Blind...................................... 540
Government of the Yukon/Libraries and Archives
   Branch/Department of Education.................................. 462
Government of the Yukon/Special Programs/
   Department of Education... 462
Guide Dogs for the Blind.. 499

H

High Park Forest School/Ontario Foundation for
   Visually Impaired Children Inc. 451
Hollywood Public School.. 451
Human Resources Development Canada/Office for
   Disability Issues... 497
Human Resources Development Canada/Vocational
   Rehabilitation of Disabled Persons Program.................... 497

I

IBM/Special Needs Department....................................... 544
I Can See Books... 540
Inegra Products... 544
Institut Nazareth et Louis-Braille............................. 458, 540

J

John Milton Society for the Blind in Canada...................... 500

L

Leader Dogs for the Blind... 500
Library for the Blind/Canadian National Institute for
   the Blind... 540
Library Services/Alberta Community Development........... 437
Low Vision Association of Ontario................................... 502
Lutheran Library for the Blind.. 540

M

Manitoba Association of Optometrists............................. 443
Manitoba Blind Sport Association................................... 442
Materials Resource Centre for the Visually Impaired/
   Alberta Education (AEEM) 437
Metropolitan Toronto Reference Library/Centre for
   People with Disabilities.. 452
Metro Special Program (Vision) (Itinerant Program-
   Public and Special Schools) 451

Microcomputer Science Centre, Inc......................... 543, 544
Mohawk College of Applied Arts and Technology............. 452
Monterey County Braille Transcribers............................. 540
Montreal Association for the Blind........................... 457, 459
Multi-Lingual Braille and Large Print Association............. 541

N

National Braille Association.. 541
National Braille Press.. 541
National Camps for Blind Children................................. 500
National Library of Canada.. 497
New Brunswick Library Service/Department of
   Municipalities, Culture and Housing............................ 444
Newfoundland Provincial Public Libraries Board.............. 446
Northwest Territories Library Services/Department of
   Education, Culture and Employment............................ 447
Nova Scotia Provincial Library....................................... 449

O

Octopus Audio Visual.. 543, 544
Ontario Audio Library Service/Trent University............... 452
Operation Eyesight Universal (OEU)............................... 500
Organization for the Education of the Visually
   Handicapped (OEVH) 452

P

PAL Reading Services.. 541
PEI Health and Community Services................................ 456
People Helping People.. 541
Pilot Dogs, Inc.. 500
Policy and Planning/Family Services.............................. 442
Prose & Cons Braille Unit.. 541
Provincial Library... 456
Provincial Resource Centre for the Visually Impaired/
   Ministry of Education and Ministry Responsible for
   Multiculturalism and Human Rights............................ 439
Public Inquiries Unit/Communications Branch/
   Ministry of Education and Training............................... 451
Public Library InterLINK... 440
The Public Works and Government Services Canada
   (PWGSC)/Accessibility Office..................................... 497

R

Recording for the Blind and Dyslexic.............................. 541
Regroupement des Aveugles et Amblyopes du Quebec...... 502
Resource Services/Atlantic Provinces Special
   Education Authority.. 449
Retinitis Pigmentosa Eye Research Foundation................. 500

S

Saskatchewan Provincial Library.................................... 460
The Seeing Eye, Inc... 500
Service des Programmes aux Personnes Handicapées/
   Ministère de la Santé et des Services Sociaux,
   Gouvernement du Québec... 458

Sir Frederick Fraser School/Atlantic Provinces Special
  Education Authority 448
Ski for Light (Canada) Inc. 500
Special Education Branch/Alberta Department of
  Education 437
Special Education Unit/Saskatchewan Education 460
Special Materials Services/Manitoba Department of
  Education and Training (MWESM) 442
Special Programs Branch 439
Stanley A. Milner Public Library 437
Stanton Regional House Board 447
Strategic and Operational Planning and Policy
  Development/Department of Community Services,
  Province of Nova Scotia 449
Student Services Branch 444
Student Services Division/Department of Education 448
Student Support Services/Department of Education 446
SuData Consulting 544
Syntha-Voice Computers, Inc. 544

T
Transport Canada/Accessible Transportation Policy
  and Programs 497
Treasury Board of Canada 497

U
University of British Columbia/Educational
  Psychology and Special Education 439
University of Sherbrooke/Faculty of Education 457

V
Veterans Affairs Canada/Health Care Division,
  Veteran Services Branch 498
VIEWS for the Visually Impaired 502
Vision Institute 455
Visualaide, Inc. 544
Visually Impaired Persons' Action Council (VIPAC) 460
VoicePrint/The National Broadcast Reading Service,
  Inc. 541
Volunteers of Vacaville 541
Volunteer Transcribing Services 541

W
W. Ross Macdonald School 451
W. Ross Macdonald School/Resource Services Library 451

X
Xavier Society for the Blind 541

Y
York Regional Library/Talking Book Service 444